THE CHINESE HERBALIST'S HANDBOOK

There's a place on my shelf for *The Chinese Herbalist's Handbook,* but that spot is gathering dust. This reference is out on my table, is used with every patient, provides me with formulas and supports my thinking in a way that no other reference can. For every time I go back to other resources, I've used the *CHH* 50 times...

Kenneth Fielding Morehead,
BM, MM, MSOM, DOM, DAONB

The Chinese Herbalist's Handbook

A Practitioner's Reference Guide to Traditional Chinese Herbs and Formulas

DAGMAR EHLING
STEVE SWART

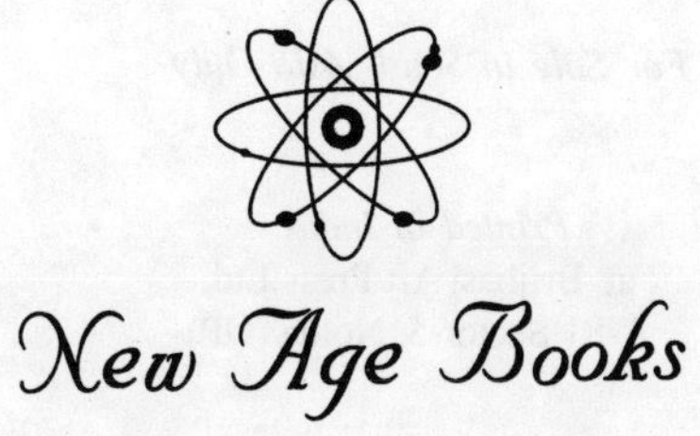

ISBN: 81-7822-196-9

First Indian Edition: Delhi, 2006
(Previously published 2002 by Lotus Press, USA)

First Edition 1994. Revised Edition 1996. 3rd Revised Edition 2002

Published by
NEW AGE BOOKS
A-44 Naraina Phase-I
New Delhi-110 028 (INDIA)
Email: nab@vsnl.in
Website: www.newagebooksindia.com

For Sale in South Asia Only

Printed in India
at Brijbasi Art Press Ltd.
A-81 Sector-5, Noida (UP)

Acknowledgements

I would like to express my sincere thanks to all my teachers, who have enabled me to write this book. I would like to thank especially Dr. Nancy Zeng, who broadened my perspective of TCM and imparted her vast knowledge of herbal medicine, and Dr. Jake Fratkin, who provided the foundation for my love of Chinese herbal medicine. I thank Steve Swart for his patience, and for contributing his knowledge and efforts to Parts Two and Three.

Dagmar Ehling

My deepest thanks and appreciation to my teachers of Chinese herbal medicine, Drs. Daoshing and Maoshing Ni, who taught me so much by their example and by their patience with my endless questions. And, to Dr. Nancy Zeng who has enlarged my whole understanding of the art of prescribing Chinese herbs. A very special thanks to Li Hua Chuang, who patiently taught me to read Chinese herbal characters. Finally, my respect and admiration to my colleague, Dagmar Ehling, for inviting me to participate in this project and for her unfailing excellence and friendship.

Steve Swart

We would like to thank Drs. Skya and Anthony Abbate, Ted Krueger, our reviewers Caylor Wadlington, Rory Kerr, Kelly Corbet, Astrid Brouwer, and Daniel Santos.

Chinese technical editors, Dr. Xiaorong Li and Dr. Chunyan Teng deserve our sincere thanks for their careful, meticulous work consulting many Chinese text relevant to Part 1 and 3. Thanks to Bruce Sturgeon for the thorough editing of Part 4.

Thanks to the InWord Press team who assisted in the first two editions of this book: Michelle Emmons, Barbara and Dan Raker, David Talbott, Carol Leyba, Lynne Egensteiner, Betsy Fogelman, Margaret Burns, Cary Cascio, Julie Mullen, Tierney Tully, and Dennis Jarrett.

Special appreciation goes to Dan Oldenburg, Helga und Dr. med. Jakob Ehling.

Warning and Disclaimer

This book is intended as a professional reference volume only, not as a medical manual or a guide to self-treatment. We caution lay persons not to attempt diagnosis or to embark upon self-treatment of a serious illness without competent professional assistance.

The information presented here is not intended to substitute for any treatment that may have been prescribed by your physician. The information contained in this book is given in good faith, but the authors and publisher cannot be held responsible for any error or omission, nor can they be held in any way responsible for treatment given on the basis of information contained herein. It you are in doubt concerning any aspect of this book, consult a qualified, licensed practitioner of Chinese medicine.

About the Illustrations

The illustrations throughout Part 1 of this book are traditional Chinese folk designs from paper cut-out motifs. They are combined with Chinese calligraphy representing the various disharmony names in Part 1. Thanks go to Robert Zeng for his contribution of the calligraphy.

Table of Contents

Part 2

Part 3

Part 4

Introduction

Historical Background

Within the context of Oriental medicine Chinese herbal medicine is one of the oldest treatment modalities. Though it is not as well known in the West, it is rapidly gaining popularity. About 5,000 years ago the emperor Shen Nong (3737 – 3697 BC) is said to have become fascinated with the use of various plants and their medicinal properties. The legends tell that he personally tried many of the various plants, minerals and animal substances, including many poisonous ones. His research culminated in the *Shen Nong Ben Cao Jing - Classic Materia Medica*, which included approximately 360 medicinals. Around 2700 BC the *Huang Di Nei Jing – Yellow Emperor's Inner Classic* conceptualized basic thoughts on Chinese philosophy. It included principles on Taoism, religion, and observations pertaining to the workings of nature and the universe, and their application to the functions within the body. This text set the foundation of Oriental medicine and, within that context, of Chinese herbal medicine.[1]

Over the next couple of centuries newly discovered functions of various medicinals were passed on from generation to generation. With the emergence of written documentation the *Nei Jing* appeared during the Warren States period 475 – 221 BC. Various scholars put forth the *Shen Nong Ben Cao Jing* into written form around that time. Concurrently, the famous Chinese physician Zhang Zhong Jing, who witnessed the death of many from infectious disease, wrote *Shan Han Lun - Treatise on Febrile Diseases Caused by Cold*.[1]

By approximately 200 AD, Hua Tuo was the first to use pain-relieving decoctions. Narcotic teas for minor surgical procedures were used around 1200 AD. By the Song dynasty (960-1279 AD) the pharmacopoeia embraced about 1,000 substances derived from the plant, animal and mineral worlds. The pharmacopoeia included herbal prescriptions, data on collecting and preparing medicinals, information regarding toxicity, instructions on herbal pastes, pills, wines and poultices and their uses for various ailments. From China, herbal medicine spread throughout the rest of Asia where it took on different flavors.

The Ben Cao Gang Mu – Grand Materia Medica, which was compiled by Li Shi Zhen around 1590 during the Ming dynasty, denoted a foundation of Chinese herbal medicine. His vast work was published in many other countries. During the Qing dynasty around 1700, Protestant missionaries introduced Western medicine into China, which led to a decline of its time-honored medicine. Establishment of the People's Republic of China in 1949, however, brought about a reappearance of Chinese medicine; since then it has become an integrated part of mainstream health care.

Jiangsu College of New Medicine published the *Zhong Yao Da Ci Dian – Encyclopedia of Traditional Chinese Medicinal Substances* in 1977. This monumental work includes over 5,000 medicinals and encompasses the entire pharmacopoeia to date. Each depicted medicinal is discussed with its respective actions and indications and includes descriptions regarding taste, temperature, dosage, preparation and contraindications.[2]

Chinese Herbal Medicine in Today's World

China has achieved full integration of traditional Chinese and Western medicine and practitioners are usually trained in both practices. Patients are cross-referred on a continuous basis; they view both types of medicines as complementary, consulting one form of medicine for certain ailments, the other for different ones, or using both styles concurrently. In many hospitals Chinese herbal and allopathic pharmacies are commonly right next to one another.

In today's China, an average of 80% of all traditional Chinese medical patients are treated with herbs, while the remaining 20% are treated with acupuncture, or other Oriental medical treatment modalities. Herbal medicine is particularly useful in the management of chronic disease.

In this country, acupuncture has established itself far more visibly. A cornerstone was James Reston's report of his personal experience of post-appendectomy pain while in China with President Nixon in 1972, which was published in the *New York Times*. Currently, there are still fewer Chinese herbal practitioners than acupuncturists in this country. However, with ever increasing standards for educational requirements, state licensure, and national certification their numbers are growing rapidly.

Why This Book Was Written

This book has grown out of my personal experience as a Western student and practitioner of Oriental medicine. I recall the early days of an herbal clinic class I attended. A patient would be brought in and a student would present the case. After thoroughly discussing the patient's case, arriving at patterns of disharmony and treatment principles, my instructor would ask: "What formula would you use?" This usually provoked a long silence. Even though we had studied single herb and prescriptionology most of us did not have the knowledge or clinical experience to prescribe formulas quickly, nor were we able to modify them.

As a clinical supervisor and instructor, I still work with many students who have difficulty integrating Chinese medicinals as a treatment modality. There is a gap between textbook knowledge and clinical application.

In China, students memorize formulas by rote using rhymes to remember the exact ingredients of each formula. The training in Western countries cannot implement this teaching tool, as these rhymes are not available in the English language.

The Chinese Herbalist's Handbook serves as a practical guide for the application of single herb prescribing in an Oriental medical practice. It aids the student or practitioner of Chinese herbal medicine in finding appropriate prescriptions once an Oriental medical differential diagnosis or pattern discrimination has been established. Its intention is to demystify Chinese herbal medicine, and to assist practitioners in making the transition from textbook knowledge to effective clinical application.

Cultural Context

In the Western world, alternative and complementary (CAM) treatment modalities have gained more popularity in the past twenty years and are growing steadily.[3] As herbal medicine is becoming more integrated into mainstream medicine and as more research is conducted its popularity is likely to continue.[4]

More and more patients are looking to herbs as a modality of treating their ailments. Chinese people have been taking herbs as far back as 3000 BC. Chinese children grow up with herbs and they are readily available in many stores. Taking herbs or even combining herbs with modern medical treatment is an integral part of Chinese culture.

In the West, we grow up with the quick-fix promise of pharmaceutical drugs. Many patients are tired of paying for expensive drugs with numerous undesirable side effects, and then taking other drugs to alleviate those side effects. As beneficial and life saving as drugs in many circumstances might be many patients are looking for alternatives, particularly for the management of chronic disorders. Oriental medicine has shown particular efficacy in the treatment of premorbid states; a patient feels sick and complains of certain symptoms but a Western medical workup fails to reveal any objective laboratory or diagnostic imaging data, hence sending the patient home without any constructive solution to their complaint.

Herbs vs. Pharmaceutical Drugs

It is crucial to understand the difference between the Chinese herbal (ingesting the whole plant/animal/mineral substance) versus the Western pharmacological approach (reducing a substance to its active ingredient). Western pharmacologists take a plant substance, find its active ingredient for treating a certain disease and extract it. The active ingredient(s) are then concentrated, patented and sold as pharmaceuticals.

In contrast, a medicinal effective in treating many ailments is considered superior in China. The more illnesses it treats, the more precious it becomes. Ren Shen / Radix Ginseng, for instance, is thought to be very precious because it is a tonic to many body systems. In Western medicine, the term 'tonic' does not exist. While Oriental medicine considers a certain drug to be superior, Western medicine may view it as inferior and vice versa. Chinese medicine is based on natural principles, and seeks treatment success on a broader, more gradual path.

Ephedrine was originally derived from the Chinese herb Ma Huang / Herba Ephedrae; it was then concentrated into a drug for the treatment of asthma in Western medicine. In its pharmaceutical form, ephedrine may overstimulate the heart, contribute to hypertension, rapid heartbeat and increased nervousness. In Chinese medicine, however, Ephedra is used in its natural form, where ephedrine has a concentration of about 0.7%. Although beneficial effects are more gradual, there are also fewer negative side effects. Ephedra in its natural form is gradually metabolized because the plant has natural moderators that offset side effects.[1] Nevertheless, even in Chinese medicine, Ephedra is one of the medicinals that needs to be used with caution. Transient hypertension has been observed even in healthy individuals if dosages exceeded 30 mg/day.[5] In the past few years overdosing with herbal 'energizers' to enhance athletic performance, create 'highs' or to lose weight with long-term use has caused serious side effects and in isolated cases even death.

Principles of Prescribing

In general, herbs work more gently and gradually, except in acute conditions where results can be dramatic. Many patients seeking herbal treatment have chronic ailments and usually herbs are slow and gradual in their effect since chronic problems and their respective energetic disharmonies have taken years to establish.

The Oriental diagnosis or pattern of disharmony dictates a certain treatment strategy and, subsequently, a formula is carefully tailored. It is important to note that no two patients are alike; this is reflected in the prescription of medicinals. Five patients with an identical Western diagnosis of headache will most likely all receive a different formula based on varying Oriental patterns of disharmony. Therefore, Chinese medicinals cannot be prescribed without careful analysis of the patient. Chinese medicinals are hardly ever given singly; a tailored prescription usually includes a variety of dried twigs, roots, barks, seeds, leaves, flowers and fruits numbering anywhere between six to twenty different herbs.

Quality Chinese herbs grow naturally in China and about 90% of Chinese medicinals are plant based. Cultivated herbs, which depend on artificial seed selection, fertilization and irrigation, grow well in various regions of China.[1] Over the past 30 – 40 years the cultivation of medicinal plants has become a major agricultural industry in China. The parts of the plant used for medicinal purposes differ for each herb. In some plants, only the roots are medically useful, while in others only the stems, flowers, seeds or leaves have medicinal value. Some plants are used whole. After the plants have been harvested they are dried. Various substances have to be specially prepared, i.e. cooked in ginger, boiled in vinegar, honey-fried or cut a certain way, so that they may reach their least toxic and greatest medicinal state.[6]

Animal substances are less commonly used within Chinese herbal prescribing although they are thought to be stronger medicinally. They are most commonly found in patent medicines — herbs in pill form — as one uses only a small amount of the animal substance.

The patterns of disharmony and their respective treatment plans dictate how to address the patient's individual disease process. A Chinese herbal prescription is the result of that process. Other treatment modalities such as acupuncture, moxibustion, cupping, diet therapy, tui na, or medical qi gong can be chosen simultaneously. All treatment modalities aim to return the patient to homeostasis or energetic balance thereby creating health within mind, body and spirit.

Patient Compliance

Practitioners in the West who utilize herbal medicine as a treatment modality use roughly 200 to 350 different herbs in a typical herbal pharmacy. Herbs are prescribed in their individual raw form and tailored exactly to the pattern diagnosis of each patient. After decocting the herbs into a medicinal tea the patient drinks it daily. Via this method of administration the ingredients are absorbed quickly after ingestion and take effect immediately. Taking herbs for a particular illness allows the patient to be treated daily, which may reduce the overall cost of care because patients require fewer acupuncture treatments. Herbal medicine can enhance the efficacy of the overall treatment, thereby increasing the speed of recovery, particularly if the pattern of disharmony includes body fluid imbalances such as yin deficiency, blood deficiency, or damp accumulation, which are more effectively treated with medicinals.

Patient education is one of the most effective tools for successful treatment outcome and is pivotal in Western countries because people are used to sugarcoated pills and sweet-tasting syrups, which are easy to ingest. When patients receive prescribed bulk herbs, they will find themselves with bags of strange ingredients, which they have to decoct. The resulting medicinal tea is unfamiliar and usually tastes and smells unpleasant. Contrary to Chinese patients where herbs are an integral part of their culture, Western patients may balk at this method of treatment. Thus, patient education is crucial.

It is helpful to provide written instructions to patients regarding preparation methods of the medicinals (see Appendix D). The Oriental medical practitioner should explain the decoction process, dosage and storage, as there is much room for confusion. If a patient is taking herbs for the first time, the practitioner may consider giving the patient only one bag on the first visit to test whether he/she is willing and able to follow through with the decoction process.

The prescription dosages in this text are based on daily amounts. However, most Chinese patients receive one package of herbs ranging from about 100 to 120 g per bag, which they cook fresh daily. As compliance in the West is already a challenging task it would be unreasonable to expect patients to cook herbs daily. Thus, many practitioners dispense two bags per week to patients, each weighing approximately 180 - 200 g. These are decocted twice with 1 cup of water (250 ml or 8 oz) per 30 g of herbs. For example, for a bag weighing 210 g, one uses 7 cups of water, which is decocted for a prescribed amount of time; the second cooking requires one cup less than the previous amount and is decocted for a separate specified amount of time. By mixing both decoctions the patient ends up with approximately 11 cups of medicinal tea since some liquid evaporates through steam. Thus, depending on the daily dose to be consumed, one bag may last anywhere from 3 to 5 days. Using this method patients prepare herbal teas only twice a week rather than daily, thus increasing compliance.

Patient brochures that provide details explaining the pros and cons of herbal therapy have proven to be helpful. It can serve as an introduction to general herbal therapy principles and their application.

By boiling their herbs, storing them properly, and self-administering them patients take an active role in their healing process. Like deciding to eat well, exercise, breathe properly, or curb an addiction, herbs can be viewed as part of a general process of conscious life-style choices leading to better health.

Patients should understand they are responsible for their healing process. Life-style changes and taking care of physical and psychological needs are key components in getting well. By completing the Oriental medical exam, the Ten Questions, patients gain a new awareness toward their bodies, which helps them listen to their bodily and emotional needs. This process fosters self-awareness and well being.

About Prepared Medicines

Many practitioners use prepackaged herbs in pill form, as patient compliance tends to be better. Prepared medicines include patent medicines, tinctures, capsules, and granules. Individual tailoring of a prescription for a specific patient, however, is impossible for most of these forms of administration. They are considerably weaker than herbal soups. Granules are preferred for infants, the elderly or patients that dislike herbal teas. They have the advantage of ease of use and may be dispensed into capsules. Some Chinese herbal suppliers are selling single herb granulates, which allows custom tailoring of prescriptions. A disadvantage is that the processing increases the price; the debate on whether they are as equally effective as decoctions continues.

Another alternative is to grind loose herbs and have patients ingest them in powder or capsule form or as drafts, in which the powder is boiled for a short period of time in a small amount of water. The resulting tea is strained and consumed. Some practitioners also make personalized alcohol tinctures using various extraction processes.

On occasion, it is useful to prescribe prepared medicines along with loose herbs, especially when using substances that are expensive, rare or derived from animals. For further reading please consult *Chinese Herbal Patent Medicines* by Jake Paul Fratkin and *Outline Guide to Chinese Herbal Patent Medicines* by Margaret Naeser.

Safety of Chinese Herbs

Several issues have emerged during the transition from an ancient culturally embedded folk medicine practiced for millennia in China to widespread utilization of herbs of international breadth. While for the most part Chinese herbs are extremely safe, particularly when compared to Western pharmaceutical incidences, a number of issues have been reported in the literature.[7] Problems have ranged from improper herb identification, lacing patent medicines with Western pharmaceuticals and heavy metal contamination to improper use of endangered species and herb/drug interactions.

Misidentification or mislabeling of herbs has lessened over the past decade as companies have increased quality and safety controls, although two cases of dispensing errors were reported in the United Kingdom in 1998.[11] Contamination of certain patent medicines made in China gave Chinese herbal medicine some negative press in the same year. Contaminants included various levels of heavy metals such as arsenic, lead and mercury whereas common drug contaminants included acetaminophen and caffeine.

The aristolochic acid debate of 2000 and the subsequent recall of certain herbs brought the importance of stringent testing to the forefront. This issue originated in 1992 with a questionably designed Belgian weight loss study where patients received a mixture of two Chinese herbal substances combined with the amphetamines fenfluramine and diethylproprion,[7] acetazolamide, belladonna, diuretics and theophylline. One of the two Chinese herbs appeared to be misidentified. Patients also were on a restricted diet. The result was that most of the women in this study went into renal failure.[8, 9] It remains largely unclear whether the Chinese herbs' aristolochic acid content, the mixture of Western pharmaceuticals or the combinations thereof were to blame.[10] Large amounts of the misidentified herb Guang Fang Ji - Radix Aristolochia were distributed elsewhere in Belgium but no adverse reactions were reported.[8] According to the FDA herbs can be sold in the United States if they are free of aristolochic acid.

Due to the increase of Chinese herb consumption certain animal substances such as Hai Mai/Hippocampus have become rare. Attempts are being made to make substitutions whenever possible. Sea horse breeding farms now supply a significant market share for the ever-increasing demand. The US Fish & Wildlife Endangered Species Act of 1973 contains a list of substances that can no longer be imported. These include Xi Jiao/Rhinoceros, Hu Gu/Tigris, Xiong Dan/Ursus and many others.

Structure of *The Chinese Herbalist's Handbook*

For clinical practicality, traditional prescriptions are arranged according to their diagnostic pattern of disharmony.

In Part One, "Herbal Prescriptions According to Syndrome Differentiation," the formulas are arranged according to those that pertain to all Zang Fu syndromes, Four Stages (Wen Bing), Six Divisions (Shang Han), and Body Fluid (Jin Ye) disharmonies. Selected internal medicine disorders and miscellaneous patterns are included as well.

Formulas are organized alphabetically by Pinyin name under each diagnostic syndrome. Primary formulas for each syndrome are indicated with special symbols. Each formula listing includes indications, ingredients with recommended dosages, tongue and pulse readings, contraindications, and preparation methods. All listings include English names. Contraindications and cautions for pregnancy noted in this section are rather conservative and do not necessarily appear in the traditional literature. This is done to warn the less experienced practitioner of dangers that could result from the use of a particular prescription during pregnancy.

Part Two is the "Clinical Quick Reference to Single Herbs." It is a selection of the most commonly used single herbs, broken down into traditional categories, and further divided into subcategories of specific herb functions. This is intended to help direct the practitioner in the right direction when making herb substitutions or modifications of a prescription.

Part Three is a "Table of Herbal Preparation Procedures" for single herbs. It is packed with information needed when mixing formulas, i.e., which herb needs to be powdered, cut in slices, cooked for longer or shorter periods of time, etc. Toxic herbs and those contraindicated during pregnancy are noted. The standard adult dosage range for each herb is included.

Part Four is a listing of herbs with names sorted alphabetically four different ways. It cross-references single herbs according to different naming conventions: Pinyin, botanical, pharmaceutical, and common names.

The appendices include information for new practitioners, a suggested start-up pharmacy herb list, and a supplier source list.

Naming System

Standard Pinyin formula names are used throughout this book. English formula names have been included here for those who prefer them. Most translations were adapted from Bensky/Barolet's *Formulas & Strategies* as standardization of English translations for Chinese formulas is crucial since they are also used in the NCCAOM (National Certification Commission of Acupuncture and Oriental Medicine) herbal examination.

Chinese herbal medicine is taught in a variety of ways in schools throughout this country. Some schools teach Pinyin and pharmaceutical names of single medicinals, some use the common English name. This book uses Pinyin and an abbreviated version of the botanical names. For animal and mineral substances without botanical names, either the zoological or the pharmaceutical name is used. If you are unsure about which medicinal or part of a specific substance is meant, please consult Part Four, the naming cross-reference, which details this information.

How To Use This Guide

After establishing a pattern discrimination and treatment principle for a specific patient, turn to that particular heading in Part One and scan the formula indications in that section. Several formulas might be possible for your patient.

Next, compare the ingredients in the formulas, then narrow down the possibilities until you arrive at the best formula for your patient. Depending on your experience, you may want to write a prescription, which is a combination of two or even three traditional formulas. Part Two will help you to further modify your individual formula.

As you are ready to mix your formula, check Part Three for special preparation methods for individual herbs.

For example, your patient has a pattern diagnosis of middle jiao damp and qi stagnation with Spleen and Stomach qi deficiency. The patient presents symptoms such as poor appetite, abdominal pain and fullness especially after eating, flatulence, belching, loose stools and low energy. His pulse is weak and slippery. His tongue is pale, swollen with teeth-marks, and has a thick white coat.

Your treatment principle is to dispel damp, rectify qi in the middle jiao, and supplement Spleen and Stomach qi.

Go to Part One and look under "Accumulation of Tan Yin (Damp and Phlegm)" and look at the varying indications. You will find several prescriptions, which might be possible for this patient:

1. Liu Jun Zi Tang – Six-Gentlemen Decoction treats Spleen qi deficiency with mild damp. Its ability to treat the damp accumulation is not very strong and it does not address the qi stagnation adequately.
2. Ping Wei San – Calm the Stomach Powder treats Spleen qi deficiency with damp and qi stagnation causing fullness and distention. When looking at the ingredients you will find that this formula is very strong for drying dampness but does not do enough for Spleen qi supplementation and rectification, which you desire. Continue your search.
3. Shen Ling Bai Zhu San – Ginseng, Poria, and Atractylodes Powder addresses Spleen qi deficiency with damp causing diarrhea but does not treat middle jiao qi stagnation sufficiently.
4. Xiang Sha Liu Jun Zi Tang – Six-Gentlemen Decoction with Aucklandia and Amomum treats Spleen qi deficiency, damp accumulation and middle jiao qi stagnation. You find that the ingredients in this formula address all three patterns of disharmony.

Your patient at times has severe abdominal pain hence you want to strengthen the qi rectifying effect. Go to Part Two and look under "Herbs that Regulate Qi." The first subtitle discusses middle jiao regulators. The three most appropriate herbs listed are: Zhi Shi / Citrus, Zhi Ke / Citrus, and Da Fu Pi / Areca. Depending on your single herb knowledge (you may want to consult a materia medica), one of these herbs is added to Xiang Sha Liu Jun Zi Tang – Six-Gentlemen Decoction with Aucklandia and Amomum.

Next, check each ingredient in Part Three to see whether any special preparation instructions exist. Ban Xia / Pinellia comes prepared as Fa Ban Xia from your supplier but is still slightly toxic. Therefore, caution during pregnancy is advised. Sha Ren / Amomum should be crushed into small pieces when mixing the formula. Mu Xiang / Saussurea and Sha Ren / Amomum should be added during the last five minutes of the first boiling to optimize their aromatic properties. Both of these herbs should be bagged separately when mixing the formula.

A thorough analysis of prescriptions, single herbs or discussion of the function of each herb in a given formula is beyond the scope of this book. Traditional modifications are not included. *The Chinese Herbalist's Handbook* is primarily a quick reference.

Knowing how to diagnose properly, form a treatment strategy, and utilize single herbs are all prerequisites for using this guide. An in-depth discussion of diagnostic skills is beyond the scope of this book.

For further research on a prescription, please consult the following comprehensive English language texts: *Chinese Herbal Medicine: Formulas & Strategies*, by Dan Bensky and Randall Barolet, and *Handbook of Chinese Herbs and Formulas – Vol 2*, by Him-che Yeung. For further information on single substances, please consult *Chinese Herbal Medicine: Materia Medica*, by Dan Bensky and Andrew Gamble, and *Handbook of Chinese Herbs and Formulas – Vol 1*, by Him-che Yeung.

General Implications of Prescribing Herbs

As discussed above, in order to prescribe herbs effectively a correct pattern diagnosis and treatment strategy are essential. There are many implications within the Oriental medical context and since the majority of patients are not textbook cases a delicate equilibrium needs to be achieved.

- Qi boosting formulas may cause heat, as most qi boosting medicinals are warm in nature. If this effect is not desired, cool qi tonics should be used instead. Boosting qi by itself may cause qi stagnation so one must add herbs to regulate qi as well.
- Most yin nourishing medicinals are sticky or cloying; therefore, they may aggravate a pre-existing damp condition. Likewise, herbs that dry dampness may injure yin.
- Blood nourishing medicinals, to a lesser degree than yin enriching herbs, may also contribute to dampness.
- Long-term yang supplementation may cause heat. Therefore, yang supplementation should be decreased and heat clearing or yin nourishing herbs added to a predominantly yang-supplementing formula, particularly once the patient begins to exhibit heat signs and symptoms.
- Quickening the blood in cases with severe blood stasis consumes qi. It takes qi to move qi and blood. To a lesser extent, strong qi regulation may also consume qi.
- The strategy of clearing heat damages Spleen qi as most of those medicinals are cold and/or bitter.
- Mostly warm and acrid herbs are used to resolve cold stagnation. This may damage the yin.
- Overuse of both wind heat and wind cold clearing medicinals consume qi and damage yin.
- Herbs that promote urination and resolve wind damp heat may dry up yin.
- Astringents may contribute to stagnation, as they promote holding fluids or stool inward.
- Heavy tranquilizing substances and downward bearing laxatives can damage the Spleen, as they tend to be cold in nature and hard to digest.
- In women, during the follicular phase — the phase between the onset of menstruation and ovulation — deficiencies may be exacerbated. Alternately, during the luteal phase — the phase between ovulation and the menstruation — problems of stagnation may be predominant.

These considerations are important when prescribing medicinals. During the course of treatment it is important that a patient's progress is continuously reevaluated. Close attention to the patient's symptom picture, pulse, tongue and any differences the patient may exhibit when reevaluating the treatment principle and formula is crucial to a positive outcome. A reevaluation should be done weekly on new patients, about every two to four weeks on an established patient. Additions or deletions to your prescription might be necessary as well as changing the formula altogether. This is a skill, which young practitioners develop with clinical practice.

Roughly 5% of the population will present with adverse reactions to herbs even after adjusting the formula. This is due to food allergies, odor sensitivities, or environmental illness. With those patients, a more intensive acupuncture program is needed, or perhaps another treatment modality.

Summary

The Chinese herbal pharmacopoeia is one of the most extensive in the world. Working within the Oriental tradition, the connection between natural substances and human health can be felt deeply. Touching and smelling Chinese medicinals is a soul-satisfying experience. I enjoy my herbal pharmacy immensely and feel that I have a relationship with the distinct personalities of each herb. There is a certain beauty involved in handling the herbs, which goes beyond intellectual knowledge.

Different practitioners have favorite herbs, which they use more frequently than others. This relates partly to subjectivity and is also partly a reflection of their training. The same preferences are true for substitutions in formulas. In working with Chinese herbs, there is space for varying interpretations and intuition.

The points discussed in this introduction are meant to clarify the implications of working within the Chinese herbal tradition and thereby empower the practitioner to move into this modality. Chinese herbal medicine can be a very enriching experience and is a never-ending learning process. When prescribing herbs we are using a part of our Mother Earth as a medium through which we touch other people's lives. Finding balance between East and West, heaven and earth, inner and outer, body and spirit, yin and yang – is experiencing the Tao. I wish you well in your herbal endeavors.

Dagmar Ehling
February 1993
Revised July 2001

[1] Reid D. *Chinese Herbal Medicine*. Boston, Mass. Shambhala Publications, INC. 1987.
[2] Bensky D, Gamble A. *Chinese Herbal Medicine: Materia Medica*. Seattle, WA 1993: Eastland Press.
[3] Eisenberg D, Davis R, Ettner S, et al. *Trends in alternative medicine use in the United States 1990-1997: results of follow-up survey*. JAMA, Nov 11, 1998 280: 1569-1577
[4] Bensoussan A, Talley N, Hing M, Menzies R, Guo A, Ngu M. *Treatment of irritable bowel syndrome with Chinese Herbal Medicine*. *JAMA*, Nov 11, 1998 280: 1585-1589
[5] Dharmananda S. *Safety Issues Affecting Chinese Herbs: The case of Ma Huang*. www.itmonline.org
[6] Sionneau P. Pao Zhi. *An Introduction to the Use of Processed Chinese Medicinals*. Boulder, CO: Blue Poppy Press; 1995.
[7] Blackwell R. *Cases of Toxicity*. J Chin Med.
[8] Maciocia G. *Safety of Chinese Herbal Medicine*. Buckinghamshire, UK 1999. Su Wen Press.
[9] Vanherweghem JL, Depierreux M, Tielemans C, et al. *Rapidly progressing interstitial renal fibrosis in young women. Association of slimming regimen indicating Chinese herbs*. Lancet:1993:341;387-391
[10] *The New England Journal of Medicine*, 2000,342(23)
[11] Lord GM, Tagore R, CookT, Gower P, Pusey CD. *Nephropathy caused by Chinese herbs in the UK*. Lancet, Aug 7, 1999; 354:481-482,494

the

Chinese Herbalist's Handbook

A Practitioner's Reference Guide to Traditional Chinese Herbs and Formulas

Part 1

Herbal Prescriptions According to Syndrome Differentiation

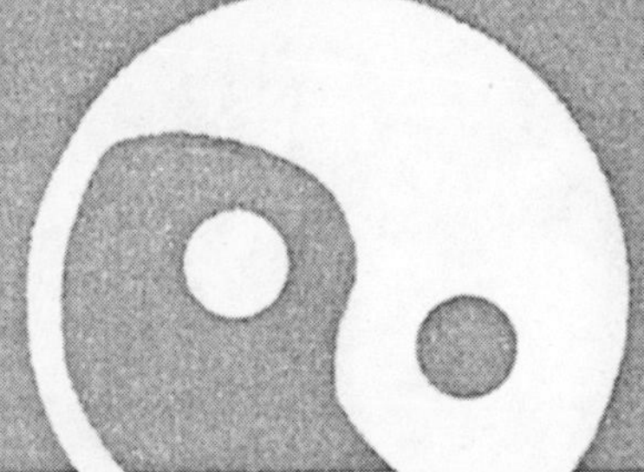

This chapter lists all prescriptions, with ingredients, dosages, tongue and pulse descriptions, preparation methods, and contraindications. The gray boxes above each syndrome listing depict the main signs and symptoms within each category.

Prescriptions are arranged in alphabetical order within each syndrome according to Chinese Pinyin names of each formula. Each prescription has a bold printed paragraph, which is a quick summary of indications with the most prevalent symptom picture. Within the box of each formula on the left the Pinyin names of herbs are listed whereas on the right the botanical names are noted. For animal and mineral substances the zoological or pharmaceutical names are used.

Herbs listed in brackets [...] are only sometimes included in the traditional formula.

Major formulas within each syndrome heading are indicated with a star ✪. Please note all formulas should be decocted unless otherwise noted except, of course, when one uses granules or single tincture extracts of medicinals.

In this chapter, there are several prescriptions for which the exact English translations were unavailable. (1) *Gui Xiong Si Wu Tang* is now translated as 'Altered Four-Substance Decoction', (2) *Qing Gan Zhi Lin Tang* is 'Clear Liver and Stop Leukorrhea Decoction', (3) *Wu Bi Shan Yao Wan* is 'Dioscorea Pill', (4) *He Che Da Zao Wan* is 'Pills of Human Placenta', (5) *Gui Shen Tang* is 'Comeback Kidney Decoction', and (6) *Qong Yu San* is 'Ginseng and Rehmannia Powder'.

Summary of Symbols

T Tongue

P Pulse

✘ Contraindications

✪ **Major Formula within Syndrome**

☞ Special instructions

LUNG DISHARMONIES

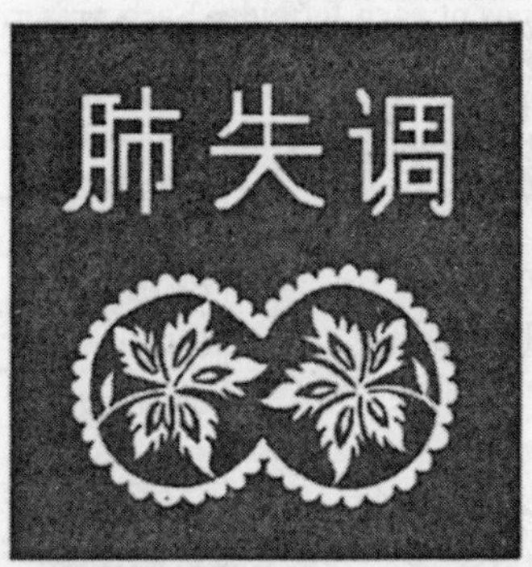

WIND COLD INVASION

- chills greater than fever
- sneezing with clear watery nasal discharge
- body aches
- itchy throat

T thin white coat

P superficial, tight

Wind Cold

External wind cold entering the Stomach causing severe damp accumulation, which then leads to fever and chills, diarrhea, vomiting, fullness, or abdominal bloating.

T sticky white coat

P slippery, superficial

BU HUAN JING ZHENG QI SAN

Rectify the Qi Powder Worth More Than Gold

Extract Formula Name: Pinellia, Atractylodes, and Agastache Formula

Hou Po	*Magnolia*	9 - 12 g
Cang Zhu	*Atractylodes*	3 - 9 g
Huo Xiang	*Agastache*	6 - 9 g
Ban Xia	*Pinellia*	6 - 9 g
Chen Pi	*Citrus*	3 - 6 g
Gan Cao	*Glycyrrhiza*	3 - 6 g
[Sheng Jiang	*Zingiber*	3 - 6 g]
[Da Zao	*Ziziphus*	3 - 5 pc]

Exterior wind cold or heat with more internal heat which starts to go from the wei to the qi level into the yangming channel. Only mild exterior symptoms are present. Thirst, constipation, full and painful eye orbits, severe bodyaches, or restlessness are the main symptoms.

T red, dry, thin yellow coat

P superficial, slightly flooding, rapid

CHAI GE JIE JI TANG

Bupleurum and Kudzu Decoction to Release the Muscle Layer

Extract Formula Name: Bupleurum and Pueraria Combination

Chai Hu	*Bupleurum*	3 - 9 g
Ge Gen	*Pueraria*	9 - 12 g
Bai Zhi	*Angelica*	3 - 9 g
Shi Gao	*Gypsum*	6 - 15 g
Bai Shao Yao	*Paeonia*	6 - 9 g
Qiang Huo	*Notopterygium*	3 - 6 g
Huang Qin	*Scutellaria*	6 - 9 g
Jie Geng	*Platycodon*	3 - 6 g
Da Zao	*Ziziphus*	3 - 4 pc
Sheng Jiang	*Zingiber*	3 - 6 g
Gan Cao	*Glycyrrhiza*	3 - 6 g

Wind cold in the superficial and channel layer causing headaches and a common cold.

T thin white coat

P superficial

CHUAN XIONG CHA TIAO SAN

Ligusticum Chuanxiong Powder to be Taken with Green Tea

Extract Formula Name: Cnidium and Tea Formula

Chuan Xiong	*Ligusticum*	3 - 9 g
Bo He	*Mentha*	9 - 12 g
Jing Jie	*Schizonepeta*	3 - 9 g
Xi Xin	*Asarum*	1 - 4 g
Qiang Huo	*Notopterygium*	3 - 6 g
Fang Feng	*Ledebouriella*	3 - 6 g
Bai Zhi	*Angelica*	3 - 6 g
Gan Cao	*Glycyrrhiza*	3 - 6 g

Wind cold or heat in the early stage leading to a common cold. Symptoms include mild fever and chills, a slight headache and a stuffy nose.

T thin white coat

P superficial

CONG CHI TANG

Scallion and Prepared Soybean Decoction

Dan Dou Chi	*Glycine*	9 - 25 g
Cong Bai	*Allium*	9 - 12 g

Exterior wind cold damp with internal heat. The fever is greater than the chills. Symptoms also include thirst, restlessness, or headache.

T thin yellow coat

P rapid

DA QIANG HUO TANG

Major Notopterygium Decoction

Qiang Huo	*Notopterygium*	9 - 12 g
Fang Feng	*Ledebouriella*	9 - 12 g
Xi Xin	*Asarum*	3 - 6 g
Du Huo	*Angelica*	9 - 12 g
Guang Fang Ji	*Aristolochia*	9 - 12 g
Huang Lian	*Coptis*	3 - 9 g
Huang Qin	*Scutellaria*	6 - 12 g
Bai Zhi	*Angelica*	6 - 12 g
Cang Zhu	*Atractylodes*	6 - 12 g
Zhi Mu	*Anemarrhena*	9 - 15 g
Sheng Di Huang	*Rehmannia*	9 - 15 g
Chuan Xiong	*Ligusticum*	9 - 15 g
Zhi Gan Cao	*Glycyrrhiza*	3 - 9 g

Wind cold with internal heat manifesting especially in the upper jiao. There is lack of sweating or slight sweating due to the internal heat. The fever is greater than the chills.

T red, dry, thin white or yellow coat

P superficial, tight, rapid

DA QING LONG TANG

Major Bluegreen Dragon Decoction

Extract Formula Name: Major Blue Dragon Combination

Ma Huang	*Ephedra*	6 - 9 g
Xing Ren	*Prunus*	6 - 9 g
Shi Gao	*Gypsum*	15 - 20 g
Gui Zhi	*Cinnamomum*	6 g
Sheng Jiang	*Zingiber*	6 - 9 g
Da Zao	*Ziziphus*	3 - 12 pc
Gan Cao	*Glycyrrhiza*	3 - 6 g

Wind cold in the exterior with phlegm heat in the interior causing cough and wheezing. The phlegm expectoration is thick and yellow.

T sticky yellow coat

P slippery, rapid

DING CHUAN TANG

Arrest Wheezing Decoction

Extract Formula Name: Ma-Huang and Ginkgo Combination

Bai Guo	*Gingko*	6 - 9 g
Ma Huang	*Ephedra*	6 - 9 g
Kuan Dong Hua	*Tussilago*	6 - 9 g
Zi Su Zi	*Perilla*	3 - 6 g
Xing Ren	*Prunus*	3 - 6 g
Ban Xia	*Pinellia*	6 - 9 g
Sang Bai Pi	*Morus*	6 - 9 g
Huang Qin	*Scutellaria*	6 - 9 g
Gan Cao	*Glycyrrhiza*	3 - 6 g

Wind cold (common cold) without sweating leading to muscle aches and a stiff neck primarily.

T thin white coat

P superficial, tight

GE GEN TANG

Kudzu Decoction

Extract Formula Name: Pueraria Combination

Ge Gen	*Pueraria*	9 - 12 g
Ma Huang	*Ephedra*	6 - 9 g
Gui Zhi	*Cinnamomum*	3 - 6 g
Bai Shao Yao	*Paeonia*	6 g
Sheng Jiang	*Zingiber*	3 - 6 g
Da Zao	*Ziziphus*	3 - 4 pc
Gan Cao	*Glycyrrhiza*	3 - 6 g

Wind cold is lodged in the taiyang channels which leads to severe upper body muscle pain and spasms.

T thin white coat

P superficial

GUI ZHI JIA GE GEN TANG

Cinnamon Twig Decoction plus Kudzu

Extract Formula Name: Cinnamon and Pueraria Combination

Gui Zhi	*Cinnamomum*	6 - 9 g
Bai Shao Yao	*Paeonia*	6 - 9 g
Ge Gen	*Pueraria*	9 - 12 g
Sheng Jiang	*Zingiber*	3 - 6 g
Da Zao	*Ziziphus*	3 - 4 pc
Gan Cao	*Glycyrrhiza*	3 - 6 g

Wind cold lasting for eight to ten days causes the patient to develop mild heat symptoms such as itching, flushed face, and thirst.

T red tip, thin white coat

P slightly slow

GUI ZHI MA HUANG GE BAN TANG

Combined Cinnamon Twig and Ephedra Decoction

Extract Formula Name: Cinnamon and Ma-Huang Combination

Gui Zhi	*Cinnamomum*	3 - 6 g
Bai Shao Yao	*Paeonia*	3 - 6 g
Xing Ren	*Prunus*	3 - 6 g
Ma Huang	*Ephedra*	3 - 6 g
Sheng Jiang	*Zingiber*	3 - 6 g
Da Zao	*Ziziphus*	3 - 4 pc
Gan Cao	*Glycyrrhiza*	3 - 6 g

Wind cold with sticky or clear phlegm expectoration, or patient with pre-existing phlegm accumulation gets a wind cold invasion.

T thick white coat
P superficial, slippery

HUA GAI SAN

Canopy Powder

Extract Formula Name: Ma-Huang and Morus Formula

Ma Huang	*Ephedra*	6 - 9 g
Sang Bai Pi	*Morus*	6 - 9 g
Fu Ling	*Poria*	6 - 9 g
Zi Su Zi	*Perilla*	6 - 9 g
Chen Pi	*Citrus*	3 - 6 g
Xing Ren	*Prunus*	3 - 6 g
Gan Cao	*Glycyrrhiza*	3 - 6 g

Wind cold and damp accumulation, with qi stagnation in the middle jiao causing diarrhea, nausea, vomiting, headache, or fever and chills.

T white sticky coat
P soggy or slippery
☞ All ingredients should be ground into a powder. Take 6 g two to three times a day.

HUO XIANG ZHENG QI SAN

Agastache Powder to Rectify the Qi

Extract Formula Name: Agastache Formula

Huo Xiang	*Agastache*	9 g
Hou Po	*Magnolia*	6 - 9 g
Bai Zhi	*Angelica*	3 - 6 g
Zi Su Ye	*Perilla*	3 - 6 g
Chen Pi	*Citrus*	6 g
Bai Zhu	*Atractylodes*	6 g
Fu Ling	*Poria*	3 - 6 g
Ban Xia	*Pinellia*	6 g
Da Fu Pi	*Areca*	3 - 6 g
Jie Geng	*Platycodon*	6 g
Gan Cao	*Glycyrrhiza*	6 - 9 g
[Da Zao	*Ziziphus*	1 - 3 g]
[Sheng Jiang	*Zingiber*	3 - 6 g]

Wind cold invasion without sweating; milder than Ma Huang Tang - Ephedra Decoction. Symptoms include fever and chills, headache, body aches, and a runny nose with clear mucus.

T white coat

P superficial

JIA WEI XIANG SU SAN

Augmented Cyperus and Perilla Leaf Powder

Xiang Fu	*Cyperus*	6 - 9 g
Zi Su Ye	*Perilla*	6 g
Jing Jie	*Schizonepeta*	6 g
Qin Jiao	*Gentiana*	6 g
Fang Feng	*Ledebouriella*	6 g
Chuan Xiong	*Ligusticum*	3 - 6 g
Man Jing Zi	*Vitex*	6 g
Chen Pi	*Citrus*	3 - 6 g
Sheng Jiang	*Zingiber*	3 - 6 g
Gan Cao	*Glycyrrhiza*	3 - 6 g

Wind cold damp (excess type) changing to heat which causes a common cold. This formula is also useful for sores, furuncles, and pus.

T thin white coat

P superficial, tight

JING FANG BAI DU SAN

Schizonepeta and Ledebouriella Powder to Overcome Pathogenic Influences

Extract Formula Name: Schizonepeta and Siler Formula

Jing Jie	*Schizonepeta*	3 - 6 g
Fang Feng	*Ledebouriellaa*	3 - 6 g
Chuan Xiong	*Ligusticum*	3 - 6 g
Qiang Huo	*Notopterygium*	3 - 6 g
Du Huo	*Angelica*	3 - 6 g
Chai Hu	*Bupleurum*	3 - 6 g
Fu Ling	*Poria*	3 - 6 g
Qian Hu	*Peucedanum*	3 - 6 g
Zhi Ke	*Citrus*	3 - 6 g
Jie Geng	*Platycodon*	3 - 6 g
Sheng Jiang	*Zingiber*	3 - 6 g
Gan Cao	*Glycyrrhiza*	2 - 4 g
[Bo He	*Mentha*	3 g]

Wind cold damp with pre-existing internal damp causing muscle aches; or external wind damp cold and internal heat causing intolerance to wind and cold, joint or body aches, lack of sweating, or thirst.

T normal color, or red, thin yellowish coat

P superficial, rapid, maybe slippery

JIU WEI QIANG HUO TANG

Nine-Ingredient Decoction with Notopterygium

Extract Formula Name: Chianghuo Combination

Qiang Huo	*Notopterygium*	3 - 6 g
Cang Zhu	*Atractylodes*	3 - 6 g
Xi Xin	*Asarum*	1 - 3 g
Fang Feng	*Ledebouriella*	3 - 6 g
Chuan Xiong	*Ligusticum*	3 - 6 g
Huang Qin	*Scutellaria*	3 - 9 g
Bai Zhi	*Angelica*	3 - 6 g
Sheng Di Huang	*Rehmannia*	3 - 9 g
Gan Cao	*Glycyrrhiza*	3 - 6 g

Wind cold with pre-existing damp causing wind cold edema, and a headache which feels as if there is a belt around the head.

T white coat

P superficial, maybe slippery

MA HUANG JIA ZHU TANG

Ephedra Decoction plus Atractylodes

Ma Huang	*Ephedra*	6 - 9 g
Xing Ren	*Prunus*	6 - 9 g
Gui Zhi	*Cinnamomum*	3 - 6 g
Gan Cao	*Glycyrrhiza*	3 - 6 g
Bai Zhu	*Atractylodes*	6 - 9 g

Wind cold causes facial edema and scanty urination. This formula is also useful for jaundice accompanied by taiyang symptoms.

T thin white coat

P superficial, tight

MA HUANG LIAN QIAO CHI XIAO DOU TANG

Ephedra, Forsythia, and Aduki Bean Decoction

Ma Huang	*Ephedra*	3 - 9 g
Lian Qiao	*Forsythia*	6 - 9 g
Chi Xiao Dou	*Phaseolus*	6 - 9 g
Sang Bai Pi	*Morus*	6 - 9 g
Xing Ren	*Prunus*	6 - 9 g
Sheng Jiang	*Zingiber*	3 - 6 g
Da Zao	*Ziziphus*	3 - 4 pc
Gan Cao	*Glycyrrhiza*	3 - 6 g

Wind cold (excess type) without sweating causing asthma or a common cold.

T thin white coat

P superficial, tight

✪ **Major Formula**

MA HUANG TANG

Ephedra Decoction

Extract Formula Name: Ma-Huang Combination

Ma Huang	*Ephedra*	6 - 9 g
Xing Ren	*Prunus*	6 - 9 g
Gui Zhi	*Cinnamomum*	6 - 9 g
Gan Cao	*Glycyrrhiza*	3 - 6 g

Wind cold damp with slight heat symptoms and fullness, nausea, joint pain, and a light cough.

T red tip, thin white coat

P superficial, maybe slightly rapid, slippery

MA XING YI GAN TANG

Ephedra, Apricot Kernel, Coix, and Licorice Decoction

Extract Formula Name: Ma-Huang and Coix Combination

Ma Huang	*Ephedra*	6 - 9 g
Xing Ren	*Prunus*	6 - 9 g
Yi Yi Ren	*Coix*	12 g
Gan Cao	*Glycyrrhiza*	3 - 6 g

Wind cold cough (excess type) causing body aches or nasal congestion with profuse white phlegm discharge. May be used in combination with 'Zhi Sou San - Stop Coughing Powder' to treat cough.

T thin white coat

P superficial, tight

SAN NIU TANG

Three-Unbinding Decoction

Extract Formula Name: Ma-Huang, Licorice and Apricot Seed Combination

Ma Huang	*Ephedra*	6 - 9 g
Xing Ren	*Prunus*	6 - 9 g
Gan Cao	*Glycyrrhiza*	3 - 6 g

Wind cold asthma with pre-existing phlegm and water (excess type) producing mild exterior symptoms such as dyspnea, wheezing with mild fever and chills.

T thick sticky white coat

P superficial, tight

SHE GAN MA HUANG TANG

Belamcanda and Ephedra Decoction

She Gan	*Belamcanda*	6 - 9 g
Ma Huang	*Ephedra*	6 - 9 g
Ban Xia	*Pinellia*	6 - 9 g
Zi Wan	*Aster*	6 - 9 g
Kuan Dong Hua	*Tussilago*	6 - 9 g
Wu Wei Zi	*Schisandra*	3 - 6 g
Xi Xin	*Asarum*	6 - 9 g
Sheng Jiang	*Zingiber*	9 - 12 g
Da Zao	*Ziziphus*	7 - 9 pc

Wind cold causing wheezing, cough, dyspnea, and tightness in the chest.

T thin white sticky coat

P superficial

SHEN MI TANG

Mysterious Decoction

Ma Huang	*Ephedra*	6 - 9 g
Xing Ren	*Prunus*	6 - 9 g
Hou Po	*Magnolia*	6 - 12 g
Chai Hu	*Bupleurum*	3 - 6 g
Zi Su Ye	*Perilla*	3 - 6 g
Chen Pi	*Citrus*	3 - 6 g
Gan Cao	*Glycyrrhiza*	3 - 6 g

Wind cold with internal heat causing lack of sweating, delirious speech, fever and chills, insomnia, bleeding in the upper parts, or fullness type headache.

T red, dry, yellow coat

P flooding, rapid

SHI GAO TANG

Gypsum Decoction

Shi Gao	*Gypsum*	15 - 35 g
Ma Huang	*Ephedra*	6 - 9 g
Huang Lian	*Coptis*	3 - 6 g
Huang Qin	*Scutellaria*	6 - 9 g
Zhi Zi	*Gardenia*	6 - 9 g
Huang Bai	*Phellodendron*	6 - 9 g
Dan Dou Chi	*Glycine*	6 - 9 g

Summer damp cold with mild fever and chills and profuse sweating.

T sticky white coat

P superficial

SHI WEI XIANG RU YIN

Ten-Ingredient Decoction with Elsholtzia

Extract Formula Name: Elsholtiza Ten Combination

Xiang Ru	*Elsholtzia*	6 - 9 g
Ren Shen	*Panax*	6 - 9 g
Bai Zhu	*Atractylodes*	3 - 6 g
Huang Qi	*Astragalus*	6 - 12 g
Chen Pi	*Citrus*	3 - 6 g
Bian Dou	*Dolichos*	6 - 9 g
Hou Po	*Magnolia*	6 - 12 g
Mu Gua	*Chaenomeles*	6 g
Fu Ling	*Poria*	6 - 9 g
Gan Cao	*Glycyrrhiza*	3 - 6 g

Wind cold with internal cold and damp and food stagnation affecting the middle jiao. This formula also treats five kinds of stagnation: qi, damp, blood, food, and cold. Symptoms include fever and chills without sweating and body aches.

T sticky white coat

P superficial, slow, or choppy

WU JI SAN

Five-Accumulation Powder

Extract Formula Name: Tang-Kuei and Magnolia Formula

Ma Huang	*Ephedra*	3 - 6 g
Gan Jiang	*Zingiber*	3 - 6 g
Hou Po	*Magnolia*	6 - 9 g
Cang Zhu	*Atractylodes*	3 - 9 g
Bai Zhi	*Angelica*	3 - 6 g
Rou Gui	*Cinnamomum*	3 g
Chuan Xiong	*Ligusticum*	3 - 6 g
Bai Shao Yao	*Paeonia*	6 - 9 g
Zhi Ke	*Citrus*	3 - 6 g
Dang Gui	*Angelica*	3 - 9 g
Fu Ling	*Poria*	6 - 9 g
Ban Xia	*Pinellia*	6 - 9 g
Chen Pi	*Citrus*	3 - 6 g
Jie Geng	*Platycodon*	6 - 9 g
Zhi Gan Cao	*Glycyrrhiza*	3 - 6 g

Pronounced wind cold with mild qi stagnation, or wind cold invasion during pregnancy.

T thin white coat

P superficial, tight

XIANG SU CONG CHI TANG

Cyperus, Perilla Leaf, Scallion, and Prepared Soybean Decoction

Zi Su Ye	*Perilla*	6 - 9 g
Xiang Fu	*Cyperus*	6 - 9 g
Cong Bai	*Allium*	2 - 4 pc
Dan Dou Chi	*Glycine*	9 - 12 g
Chen Pi	*Citrus*	3 - 6 g
Zhi Gan Cao	*Glycyrrhiza*	3 - 6 g

Wind cold with internal qi stagnation causing belching, decreased appetite, fever and chills, headache, absence of sweating and middle jiao fullness.

T thin white coat

P superficial

XIANG SU SAN

Cyperus and Perilla Leaf Powder

Extract Formula Name: Cyperus and Perilla Formula

Xiang Fu	*Cyperus*	6 - 9 g
Zi Su Ye	*Perilla*	6 - 9 g
Chen Pi	*Citrus*	3 - 6 g
Zhi Gan Cao	*Glycyrrhiza*	3 - 6 g

Wind cold with internal water accumulation causing profuse phlegm expectoration, bodyaches, or superficial edema.

T moist white coat

P superficial, tight

XIAO QING LONG TANG

Minor Blue Dragon Decoction

Extract Formula Name: Minor Blue Dragon Combination

Ma Huang	*Ephedra*	6 - 9 g
Gui Zhi	*Cinnamomum*	6 - 9 g
Xi Xin	*Asarum*	3 g
Wu Wei Zi	*Schisandra*	6 - 9 g
Gan Jiang	*Zingiber*	3 g
Bai Shao Yao	*Paeonia*	6 - 9 g
Ban Xia	*Pinellia*	6 - 9 g
Gan Cao	*Glycyrrhiza*	3 - 6 g

Wind cold causing nasal obstruction with white or clear profuse discharge.

T thin moist white coat

P superficial

XIN YI SAN

Magnolia Flower Powder

Extract Formula Name: Magnolia Flower Formula

Xin Yi Hua	*Magnolia*	6 - 9 g
Mu Tong	*Akebia*	6 - 9 g
Chuan Xiong	*Ligusticum*	3 - 9 g
Qiang Huo	*Notopterygium*	3 - 6 g
Xi Xin	*Asarum*	3 g
Gao Ben	*Ligusticum*	6 - 9 g
Fang Feng	*Ledebouriella*	6 - 9 g
Sheng Ma	*Cimicifuga*	3 - 6 g
Bai Zhi	*Angelica*	3 - 6 g
Gan Cao	*Glycyrrhiza*	3 - 6 g

Wind edema with fever and chills, or decreased urination.

T thin white coat

P superficial, slippery, or deep

YUE BI JIA ZHU TANG

Maidservant from Yue Decoction plus Atractylodes

Extract Formula Name: Atractylodes Combination

Ma Huang	*Ephedra*	6 - 9 g
Shi Gao	*Gypsum*	9 - 20 g
Bai Zhu	*Atractylodes*	6 - 9 g
Sheng Jiang	*Zingiber*	3 - 9 g
Da Zao	*Ziziphus*	3 - 7 pc
Gan Cao	*Glycyrrhiza*	3 - 6 g

Whole body edema due to wind causing wind intolerance, scanty urination, possible sweating, possible fever, or thirst.

T thin white coat

P superficial

YUE BI TANG

Maidservant from Yue Decoction

Extract Formula Name: Ma-Huang and Gypsum Combination

Ma Huang	*Ephedra*	6 - 15 g
Sheng Jiang	*Zingiber*	3 - 9 g
Shi Gao	*Gypsum*	15 - 30 g
Da Zao	*Ziziphus*	6 - 12 pc
Gan Cao	*Glycyrrhiza*	3 - 6 g

Cough due to wind with sputum. Mild exterior symptoms with persisting cough.

T thin white coat

P superficial

ZHI SOU SAN

Stop Coughing Powder

Extract Formula Name: Platycodon and Schizonepeta Formula

Zi Wan	*Aster*	6 - 9 g
Jing Jie	*Schizonepeta*	6 - 9 g
Bai Qian	*Cynanchum*	6 - 9 g
Jie Geng	*Platycodon*	6 - 9 g
Bai Bu	*Stemona*	6 - 9 g
Chen Pi	*Citrus*	3 - 6 g
Gan Cao	*Glycyrrhiza*	3 - 6 g

Wind Cold with Underlying Deficiency

Qi deficient patient gets evil qi invading taiyang, shaoyang, and yangming channels. This causes irritability, constipation, full chest, or heaviness.

T red, sticky coat

P rapid, wiry

☞ Da Huang - Rheum should be added during the last 3 minutes of the decoction process.

✘ Qian Dan - Minium is toxic and should be substituted with Dai Zhe Shi - Haematitum or Sheng Tie Luo - Frusta Ferri. Caution during pregnancy.

CHAI HU JIA LONG GU MU LI TANG

Bupleurum plus Dragon Bone and Oyster Shell Decoction

Extract Formula Name: Bupleurum and D.B. Combination

Chai Hu	Bupleurum	9 - 12 g
Huang Qin	Scutellaria	6 g
Ren Shen	Panax	6 g
Gui Zhi	Cinnamomum	3 - 6 g
Ban Xia	Pinellia	6 g
Fu Ling	Poria	6 g
Da Huang	Rheum	6 g
Long Gu	Os Draconis	3 - 6 g
Mu Li	Ostrea	3 - 6 g
Sheng Jiang	Zingiber	3 - 6 g
Da Zao	Ziziphus	3 - 6 pc
Qian Dan	Minium	1 - 4 g

Yin or blood deficient patient gets a wind cold or wind heat invasion. Symptoms include mild chills, weakness, headaches, and fever.

T pale or red, thin white coat

P thin, weak, rapid

CONG BAI QI WEI YIN

Scallion Decoction with Seven-Ingredients

Cong Bai	Allium	9 - 12 g
Dan Dou Chi	Glycine	6 - 9 g
Ge Gen	Pueraria	9 - 12 g
Sheng Di Huang	Rehmannia	9 - 15 g
Mai Men Dong	Ophiopogon	9 - 12 g
Sheng Jiang	Zingiber	3 - 9 g

Wind edema or wind damp with Spleen and wei qi deficiency causing sweating, urinary difficulty, or edema in the superficial layer.

T pale, thin white coat

P superficial

FANG JI HUANG QI TANG

Stephania and Astragalus Decoction

Extract Formula Name: Stephania and Astragalus Combination

Han Fang Ji	*Stephania*	9 - 12 g
Huang Qi	*Astragalus*	9 - 15 g
Bai Zhu	*Atractylodes*	6 - 9 g
Sheng Jiang	*Zingiber*	3 - 6 g
Da Zao	*Ziziphus*	3 - 4 pc
Gan Cao	*Glycyrrhiza*	3 - 6 g

Wind cold (deficiency type) with slight sweating, and the patient starts to have internal heat. The fever is greater than the chills.

T red tip, thin white coat

P superficial, forceful

GUI ZHI ER YUE BI YI TANG

Two-parts Cinnamon Twig Decoction with One-part Maidservant from Yeu's Decoction

Gui Zhi	*Cinnamomum*	3 - 6 g
Bai Shao Yao	*Paeonia*	3 - 6 g
Ma Huang	*Ephedra*	3 - 6 g
Shi Gao	*Gypsum*	3 - 6 g
Sheng Jiang	*Zingiber*	3 - 6 g
Da Zao	*Ziziphus*	3 - 4 pc
Gan Cao	*Glycyrrhiza*	3 - 6 g

Wind cold (deficiency type) with sweating and underlying yang deficiency leading to a common cold. Symptoms include body aches and mild chills.

T pale, wet

P slow, tight

GUI ZHI JIA FU ZI TANG

Cinnamon Twig Decoction plus Aconite

Extract Formula Name: Cinnamon, Hoelen and Aconite Combination

Gui Zhi	*Cinnamomum*	6 - 9 g
Bai Shao Yao	*Paeonia*	6 - 9 g
Sheng Jiang	*Zingiber*	3 - 6 g
Da Zao	*Ziziphus*	3 - 4 pc
Gan Cao	*Glycyrrhiza*	3 - 6 g
Fu Zi	*Aconitum*	1 - 6 g

Wind cold is lodged in the tai-yang channels which leads to severe upper body muscle pain and spasms.

T thin white coat

P superficial

GUI ZHI JIA GE GEN TANG

Cinnamon Twig Decoction plus Kudzu

Extract Formula Name: Cinnamon and Pueraria Combination

Gui Zhi	*Cinnamomum*	6 - 9 g
Bai Shao Yao	*Paeonia*	6 - 9 g
Ge Gen	*Pueraria*	9 - 12 g
Sheng Jiang	*Zingiber*	3 - 6 g
Da Zao	*Ziziphus*	3 - 4 pc
Gan Cao	*Glycyrrhiza*	3 - 6 g

Severe taiyin/taiyang disease with abdominal cramps as the main symptom.

T thin white coat

P superficial

GUI ZHI JIA SHAO YAO TANG

Cinnamon Twig Decoction plus Peony

Extract Formula Name: Cinnamon and Peony Combination

Gui Zhi	*Cinnamomum*	6 - 9 g
Bai Shao Yao	*Paeonia*	15 - 18 g
Sheng Jiang	*Zingiber*	3 - 6 g
Da Zao	*Ziziphus*	3 - 4 pc
Gan Cao	*Glycyrrhiza*	3 - 6 g

Mild taiyin with taiyang syndrome: wind cold with mild Spleen qi deficiency. The chills are predominant, and the patient experiences diarrhea with epigastric fullness.

T pale, thin white coat

P weak, may be superficial

GUI ZHI REN SHEN TANG

Cinnamon Twig and Ginseng Decoction

Extract Formula Name: Cinnamon and Ginseng Combination

Gui Zhi	*Cinnamomum*	9 - 12 g
Ren Shen	*Panax*	9 - 12 g
Gan Jiang	*Zingiber*	9 g
Bai Zhu	*Atractylodes*	9 g
Zhi Gan Cao	*Glycyrrhiza*	9 - 12 g

Wind cold (deficiency type) with sweating leading to a common cold.

T moist, thin white coat

P superficial, weak

✪ **Major Formula**

GUI ZHI TANG

Cinnamon Twig Decoction

Extract Formula Name: Cinnamon Combination

Gui Zhi	*Cinnamomum*	6 - 9 g
Bai Shao Yao	*Paeonia*	6 - 9 g
Sheng Jiang	*Zingiber*	3 - 6 g
Da Zao	*Ziziphus*	3 - 5 pc
Gan Cao	*Glycyrrhiza*	3 - 6 g

Wind cold (deficiency type) with internal fire: taiyang and yangming disorder. This causes sweating, chills, nasal congestion, and constipation with abdominal fullness.

T red, thin white or yellow coat

P superficial, rapid

✘ Caution during pregnancy.

HOU PO QI WU TANG

Seven-Substance Decoction with Magnolia Bark

Extract Formula Name: Magnolia 7 Combination

Hou Po	*Magnolia*	15 g
Da Huang	*Rheum*	9 g
Gui Zhi	*Cinnamomum*	6 g
Zhi Shi	*Citrus*	9 g
Sheng Jiang	*Zingiber*	12 g
Da Zao	*Ziziphus*	12 pc
Gan Cao	*Glycyrrhiza*	6 g

Mild yang deficiency with external wind cold without sweating. (shaoyin and taiyang disease). Symptoms include extreme chilliness with mild fever and severe fatigue.

T pale, white coat

P minute

MA HUANG FU ZI XI XIN TANG

Ephedra, Prepared Aconite, and Asarum Decoction

Extract Formula Name: Ma-Huang and Asarum Combination

Ma Huang	*Ephedra*	6 - 9 g
Fu Zi	*Aconitum*	3 - 6 g
Xi Xin	*Asarum*	3 - 6 g

Wind cold damp with pre-existing qi deficiency and mild heat which is just beginning. This causes high fever and chills, lack of sweating, tightness in the neck, or severe bodyaches.

T pale, swollen, teethmarks, sticky white coat

P slippery, superficial, slow, or soggy

REN SHEN BAI DU SAN

Ginseng Powder to Overcome Pathogenic Influences

Extract Formula Name: Ginseng and Mentha Formula

Chuan Xiong	*Ligusticum*	6 - 9 g
Du Huo	*Angelica*	6 - 9 g
Chai Hu	*Bupleurum*	6 - 9 g
Qiang Huo	*Notopterygium*	6 - 9 g
Qian Hu	*Peucedanum*	6 - 9 g
Ren Shen	*Panax*	6 - 9 g
Fu Ling	*Poria*	6 - 9 g
Zhi Ke	*Citrus*	6 - 9 g
Jie Geng	*Platycodon*	6 - 9 g
Gan Cao	*Glycyrrhiza*	3 - 6 g

Cold packs were used on a patient who had a common cold but also an underlying Spleen yang deficiency. Now the cold has moved into deeper layers and caused severe cold stagnation with water accumulation under the Heart. Symptoms include shortness of breath, watery sputum, angina, or stuffiness in the chest.

T pale, wet

P slow, slightly slippery

✘ Ba Dou - Croton is extremely toxic and should be used with caution. Do not use during pregnancy.

SAN WU BAI SAN

Three-White Herbs Powder

Jie Geng	*Platycodon*	3 - 6 g
Bei Mu	*Fritillaria*	6 - 12 g
Ba Dou	*Croton*	1 - 3 g

Wind cold with pre-existing qi and yang deficiency. Symptoms include fever and chills or cough with white and profuse phlegm expectoration.

T pale, swollen, teethmarks, white coat

P frail or superficial

SHEN SU YIN

Ginseng and Perilla Leaf Decoction

Extract Formula Name: Ginseng and Perilla Combination

Zhi Ke	*Citrus*	3 - 6 g
Ren Shen	*Panax*	6 - 9 g
Zi Su Ye	*Perilla*	6 - 9 g
Ge Gen	*Pueraria*	6 - 9 g
Qian Hu	*Peucedanum*	6 - 9 g
Fu Ling	*Poria*	6 - 9 g
Jie Geng	*Platycodon*	3 - 6 g
Mu Xiang	*Saussurea*	3 - 6 g
Ban Xia	*Pinellia*	6 - 9 g
Chen Pi	*Citrus*	3 - 6 g
Gan Cao	*Glycyrrhiza*	3 - 6 g
[Sheng Jiang	*Zingiber*	3 - 6 g]
[Da Zao	*Ziziphus*	3 - 6 pc]

Interior cold with yang deficiency and wind cold causing cold type hernia. Other symptoms include numb, cold hands and feet and body aches.

T pale, moist, white coat

P frail

✘ Do not take over a long period of time. Wu Tou - Aconitum is toxic.

WU TOU GUI ZHI TANG

Aconite and Cinnamon Twig Decoction

Extract Formula Name: Wu-tou and Cinnamon Combination

Gui Zhi	*Cinnamomum*	6 - 9 g
Wu Tou	*Aconitum*	3 - 6 g
Bai Shao Yao	*Paeonia*	6 - 9 g
Sheng Jiang	*Zingiber*	3 - 6 g
Da Zao	*Ziziphus*	3 - 5 pc
Gan Cao	*Glycyrrhiza*	3 - 6 g

Wind cold with internal damp causing a common cold without sweating, Stomach flu, heaviness in the head, cold intolerance, or nausea and vomiting.

T white sticky coat

P superficial

XIANG RU SAN

Elsholtzia Powder

Extract Formula Name: Elsholtzia Combination

Xiang Ru	*Elsholtzia*	9 - 12 g
Hou Po	*Magnolia*	9 - 12 g
Bian Dou	*Dolichos*	6 - 9 g

Qi/yang deficient patient with wind cold causing slight fever, lack of sweating, cold hands and feet, severe chills with a mild fever, and weakness.

T pale, thin white coat

P frail

ZAI ZAO SAN

Renewal Powder

Ren Shen	*Panax*	6 - 9 g
Huang Qi	*Astragalus*	6 - 12 g
Fu Zi	*Aconitum*	3 g
Xi Xin	*Asarum*	3 g
Gui Zhi	*Cinnamomum*	3 - 6 g
Chuan Xiong	*Ligusticum*	3 - 6 g
Qiang Huo	*Notopterygium*	3 - 6 g
Fang Feng	*Ledebouriella*	6 - 9 g
Sheng Jiang	*Zingiber*	3 - 6 g
Da Zao	*Ziziphus*	2 - 4 pc
Gan Cao	*Glycyrrhiza*	3 - 6 g

WIND HEAT INVASION

- fever greater than chills
- sore throat
- yellow nasal discharge
- body aches

T red tip, thin yellow or white coat

P superficial, rapid

Wind Heat

Wind heat causing thick nasal discharge with congestion, and frontal headache.

T yellow coat

P superficial, rapid

CANG ER ZI SAN

Xanthium Powder

Extract Formula Name: Xanthium Formula

Cang Er Zi	*Xanthium*	6 - 9 g
Xin Yi Hua	*Magnolia*	3 - 6 g
Bo He	*Mentha*	3 - 6 g
Bai Zhi	*Angelica*	6 - 9 g

Exterior wind cold or heat with internal heat which starts to go from the wei to the qi level into the yangming channel. Only mild exterior symptoms are present. Thirst, constipation, full and painful eye orbits, severe bodyaches, or restlessness are the main symptoms.

T red, dry, thin yellow coat

P superficial, slightly flooding, rapid

CHAI GE JIE JI TANG

Bupleurum and Kudzu Decoction to Release the Muscle Layer

Extract Formula Name: Bupleurum and Pueraria Combination

Chai Hu	*Bupleurum*	3 - 9 g
Ge Gen	*Pueraria*	9 - 12 g
Bai Zhi	*Angelica*	3 - 9 g
Shi Gao	*Gypsum*	6 - 15 g
Bai Shao Yao	*Paeonia*	6 - 9 g
Qiang Huo	*Notopterygium*	3 - 6 g
Huang Qin	*Scutellaria*	6 - 9 g
Jie Geng	*Platycodon*	3 - 6 g
Da Zao	*Ziziphus*	3 - 4 pc
Sheng Jiang	*Zingiber*	3 - 6 g
Gan Cao	*Glycyrrhiza*	3 - 6 g

Taiyang and shaoyang disease with joint congestion and intolerance to wind, or alternating fever and chills. Also useful for Liver overacting on Spleen.

T thin white coat

P possibly superficial

CHAI HU GUI ZHI TANG

Bupleurum and Cinnamon Twig Decoction

Extract Formula Name: Bupleurum and Cinnamon Combination

Gui Zhi	*Cinnamomum*	3 - 6 g
Chai Hu	*Bupleurum*	6 - 12 g
Ren Shen	*Panax*	3 - 6 g
Ban Xia	*Pinellia*	3 - 6 g
Huang Qin	*Scutellaria*	3 - 9 g
Bai Shao Yao	*Paeonia*	3 - 6 g
Sheng Jiang	*Zingiber*	3 - 6 g
Da Zao	*Ziziphus*	4 - 6 pc
Gan Cao	*Glycyrrhiza*	3 - 6 g

Wind heat with Lung heat leading to fever or soreness in the throat.

T red tip, white coat

P superficial, rapid

CONG BAI JIE GENG TANG

Scallion and Platycodon Decoction

Jie Geng	*Platycodon*	3 - 6 g
Cong Bai	*Allium*	9 - 12 g
Zhi Zi	*Gardenia*	6 - 9 g
Dan Dou Chi	*Glycine*	9 - 12 g
Lian Qiao	*Forsythia*	3 - 6 g
Bo He	*Mentha*	3 - 6 g
Dan Zhu Ye	*Lophatherum*	2 - 6 g
Gan Cao	*Glycyrrhiza*	3 - 6 g

Wind heat with internal heat: taiyang and yangming organ disease. The heat is severe. Symptoms include dark yellow urine, constipation, severe fever and chills, heat sensations in the body, sores and carbuncles, skin disorders, and a bitter taste.

T bright or dark red, dry, yellow coat

P flooding, rapid, wiry

☞ Ingredients should be ground into powder, then made into a pill with water. Take 6 g each time, twice a day.

✘ Do not use during pregnancy.

FANG FENG TONG SHENG SAN

Ledebouriella Powder that Sagely Unblocks

Extract Formula Name: Siler and Platycodon Formula

Fang Feng	*Ledebouriella*	9 - 15 g
Ma Huang	*Ephedra*	9 - 15 g
Da Huang	*Rheum*	9 - 15 g
Mang Xiao	*Mirabilitum*	9 - 15 g
Jing Jie	*Schizonepeta*	9 - 15 g
Bo He	*Mentha*	9 - 15 g
Zhi Zi	*Gardenia*	9 - 15 g
Hua Shi	*Talcum*	60 - 90 g
Shi Gao	*Gypsum*	15 - 30 g
Huang Qin	*Scutellaria*	15 - 30 g
Lian Qiao	*Forsythia*	9 - 15 g
Jie Geng	*Platycodon*	15 - 30 g
Dang Gui	*Angelica*	9 - 15 g
Bai Shao Yao	*Paeonia*	9 - 15 g
Chuan Xiong	*Ligusticum*	9 - 15 g
Bai Zhu	*Atractylodes*	9 - 15 g
Gan Cao	*Glycyrrhiza*	30 - 60 g

Wind heat with internal middle jiao heat and Large Intestine heat and damp causing dysentery: taiyang and yangming disease. Symptoms include fever, thirst, or burning anus.

T red, yellow coat

P rapid, slippery

GE GEN HUANG LIAN HUANG QIN TANG

Kudzu, Coptis, and Scutellaria Decoction

Extract Formula Name: Pueraria, Coptis and Scute Combination

Ge Gen	*Pueraria*	12 - 15 g
Huang Lian	*Coptis*	9 g
Huang Qin	*Scutellaria*	6 - 9 g
Gan Cao	*Glycyrrhiza*	3 - 6 g

Wind damp cold with damp heat causing epidemic influenza.

T pink or red, sticky white or yellow coat

P superficial, slippery

LIAN QIAO BAI DU SAN

Forsythia Powder to Overcome Pathogenic Influences

Lian Qiao	*Forsythia*	6 - 9 g
Jin Yin Hua	*Lonicera*	6 - 9 g
Fu Ling	*Poria*	6 - 9 g
Chuan Xiong	*Ligusticum*	3 - 9 g
Qiang Huo	*Notopterygium*	3 - 6 g
Du Huo	*Angelica*	6 - 9 g
Chai Hu	*Bupleurum*	6 - 9 g
Qian Hu	*Peucedanum*	6 - 9 g

Wind heat with fever, possible sweating, thirst, dyspnea, asthma: heat in the qi level.

T red tip or border, yellow coat

P rapid, flooding

MA XING SHI GAN TANG

Ephedra, Apricot Kernel, Gypsum, and Licorice Decoction

Extract Formula Name: Ma-Huang and Apricot Seed Combination

Ma Huang	*Ephedra*	6 - 15 g
Xing Ren	*Prunus*	6 - 9 g
Shi Gao	*Gypsum*	6 - 20 g
Gan Cao	*Glycyrrhiza*	3 - 6 g

Wind heat with toxin affecting the neck and head with swollen sore throat or glands, tonsillitis, or pharyngitis.

T red

P rapid

QIANG LAN TANG

Notopterygium and Isatis Root Decoction

Qiang Huo	*Notopterygium*	9 - 12 g
Ban Lan Gen	*Isatis*	12 - 20 g

Wind heat invasion leading to headaches.

T thin white coat

P superficial, rapid

QING KONG GAO

Clear Head Formula

Huang Qin	*Scutellaria*	6 - 9 g
Huang Lian	*Coptis*	6 - 9 g
Chuan Xiong	*Ligusticum*	12 - 15 g
Chai Hu	*Bupleurum*	6 - 9 g
Qiang Huo	*Notopterygium*	6 - 12 g
Fang Feng	*Ledebouriella*	6 - 12 g
Gan Cao	*Glycyrrhiza*	3 - 6 g
For frontal headaches add:		
Bai Zhi	*Angelica*	6 - 9 g
Ge Gen	*Pueraria*	6 - 9 g
Ma Huang	*Ephedra*	3 - 9 g
For occipital headaches add:		
Ma Huang	*Ephedra*	3 - 9 g
Qiang Huo	*Notopterygium*	6 - 9 g
For temple headaches add:		
Chai Hu	*Bupleurum*	6 - 9 g
Bai Shao Yao	*Paeonia*	6 - 9 g
For vertex headaches add:		
Man Jing Zi	*Vitex*	6 - 9 g
Gao Ben	*Ligusticum*	6 - 9 g

Wind heat with wind stroke causing paraplegia, or facial paralysis with severe heat symptoms.

T red, yellow coat

P rapid

✘ Caution during pregnancy.

QU FENG ZHI BAO DAN

Greatest Treasure Special Pill to Dispel Wind

Hua Shi	*Talcum*	12 - 15 g
Dang Gui	*Angelica*	9 - 12 g
Chuan Xiong	*Ligusticum*	9 g
Gan Cao	*Glycyrrhiza*	6 g
Fang Feng	*Ledebouriella*	6 - 9 g
Bai Shao Yao	*Paeonia*	6 - 9 g
Bai Zhu	*Atractylodes*	6 g
Du Huo	*Angelica*	6 g
Ren Shen	*Panax*	3 g
Qiang Huo	*Notopterygium*	3 - 6 g
Shu Di Huang	*Rehmannia*	6 g
Tian Ma	*Gastrodia*	6 g
Shi Gao	*Gypsum*	6 g
Huang Qin	*Scutellaria*	6 g
Jie Geng	*Platycodon*	3 g
Zhi Zi	*Gardenia*	1 - 3 g
Jing Jie	*Schizonepeta*	6 g
Bo He	*Mentha*	3 g
Da Huang	*Rheum*	6 g
Mang Xiao	*Mirabilitum*	6 g
Lian Qiao	*Forsythia*	3 - 6 g
Ma Huang	*Ephedra*	6 g
Huang Lian	*Coptis*	3 g
Huang Bai	*Phellodendron*	3 g
Xi Xin	*Asarum*	3 g
Quan Xie	*Buthus*	3 g

Wind heat causing coughing which is the first sign of the invasion. Symptoms include fever, thirst, or mild sweating.

T red tip

P superficial

SANG JU YIN

Mulberry Leaf and Chrysanthemum Decoction

Extract Formula Name: Morus and Chrysanthemum Combination

Sang Ye	*Morus*	6 - 9 g
Ju Hua	*Chrysanthemum*	3 g
Bo He	*Mentha*	3 g
Xing Ren	*Prunus*	6 - 9 g
Lu Gen	*Phragmites*	6 - 9 g
Jie Geng	*Platycodon*	3 - 6 g
Lian Qiao	*Forsythia*	3 - 6 g
Gan Cao	*Glycyrrhiza*	3 - 6 g

Wind heat and dryness attacks the Lungs. Symptoms include mild fever, dry or hacking cough with scanty sputum which is hard to expectorate.

T dry, thin white coat

P superficial, rapid

SANG XING TANG

Mulberry Leaf and Apricot Kernel Decoction

Extract Formula Name: Morus and Apricot Seed Combination

Sang Ye	*Morus*	3 - 6 g
Xing Ren	*Prunus*	4 - 6 g
Zhe Bei Mu	*Fritillaria*	3 - 6 g
Bei Sha Shen	*Glehnia*	6 - 9 g
Dan Dou Chi	*Glycine*	3 - 6 g
Zhi Zi	*Gardenia*	3 - 6 g
Li Pi	*Pyrus*	3 - 6 g

Wind heat causing measles and rashes. Symptoms include fever, chills, body aches, cough, or red eyes.

T red, dry

P superficial, rapid

SHENG MA GE GEN TANG

Cimicifuga and Kudzu Decoction

Extract Formula Name: Cimicifuga and Pueraria Combination

Sheng Ma	*Cimicifuga*	3 - 6 g
Chi Shao Yao	*Paeonia*	6 - 9 g
Ge Gen	*Pueraria*	3 - 6 g
Gan Cao	*Glycyrrhiza*	3 - 6 g

Wind heat and toxin causing measles, lack of sweating, cough, dark urine, or severe sore throat.

T red tip

P superficial, rapid

XUAN DU FA BIAO TANG

Dissipate Toxin and Release the Exterior Decoction

Sheng Ma	*Cimicifuga*	6 - 9 g
Ge Gen	*Pueraria*	6 - 9 g
Xing Ren	*Prunus*	6 - 9 g
Qian Hu	*Peucedanum*	6 - 9 g
Jie Geng	*Platycodon*	3 - 6 g
Bo He	*Mentha*	3 - 6 g
Fang Feng	*Ledebouriella*	3 - 6 g
Jing Jie	*Schizonepeta*	3 - 6 g
Lian Qiao	*Forsythia*	3 - 9 g
Niu Bang Zi	*Arctium*	3 - 6 g
Dan Zhu Ye	*Lophatherum*	3 - 6 g
Zhi Ke	*Citrus*	3 - 6 g
Mu Tong	*Akebia*	6 - 9 g
Gan Cao	*Glycyrrhiza*	3 - 6 g

Wind heat with strong internal heat causing fever or thirst.

T red, thin yellow coat

P rapid, superficial

YI WU CHAI GE JIE JI TANG

Bupleurum and Kudzu Decoction to Release the Muscle Layer from Medical Revelations

Chai Hu	*Bupleurum*	6 - 9 g
Ge Gen	*Pueraria*	6 - 9 g
Huang Qin	*Scutellaria*	6 - 9 g
Sheng Di Huang	*Rehmannia*	6 - 12 g
Mu Dan Pi	*Paeonia*	6 - 9 g
Zhe Bei Mu	*Fritillaria*	6 - 9 g
Chi Shao Yao	*Paeonia*	6 - 9 g
Zhi Mu	*Anemarrhena*	6 - 9 g
Gan Cao	*Glycyrrhiza*	3 - 6 g

Wind/toxic heat with damp and qi deficiency causing red, swollen sores or carbuncles.

T thin sticky white coat

P superficial

YIN QIAO BAI DU SAN

Honeysuckle and Forsythia Powder to Overcome Pathogenic Influences

Qiang Huo	*Notopterygium*	6 - 9 g
Chuan Xiong	*Ligusticum*	3 - 6 g
Du Huo	*Angelica*	3 - 6 g
Chai Hu	*Bupleurum*	6 - 9 g
Qian Hu	*Peucedanum*	6 - 9 g
Ren Shen	*Panax*	6 - 9 g
Jie Geng	*Platycodon*	3 - 6 g
Zhi Ke	*Citrus*	3 - 6 g
Fu Ling	*Poria*	3 - 6 g
Gan Cao	*Glycyrrhiza*	3 - 6 g
Jin Yin Hua	*Lonicera*	6 - 9 g
Lian Qiao	*Forsythia*	6 - 9 g

Wind/toxic heat causing a common cold, lack of sweating, rashes, sore throat, or throbbing headache.

T normal color or red tip, thin yellow coat

P superficial, rapid

✪ **Major Formula**

YIN QIAO SAN

Honeysuckle and Forsythia Powder

Extract Formula Name: Loniçera and Forsythia Formula

Jin Yin Hua	*Lonicera*	6 - 9 g
Lian Qiao	*Forsythia*	6 - 9 g
Niu Bang Zi	*Arctium*	6 - 9 g
Dan Dou Chi	*Glycine*	3 - 9 g
Bo He	*Mentha*	3 - 6 g
Jie Geng	*Platycodon*	3 - 6 g
Jing Jie	*Schizonepeta*	3 - 6 g
Dan Zhu Ye	*Lophatherum*	3 - 6 g
Lu Gen	*Phragmites*	3 - 9 g
Gan Cao	*Glycyrrhiza*	3 - 6 g

Cough due to wind with sputum. Mild exterior symptoms with persisting cough.

T thin white coat

P superficial

ZHI SOU SAN

Stop Coughing Powder

Extract Formula Name: Platycodon and Schizonepeta Formula

Zi Wan	*Aster*	6 - 9 g
Jing Jie	*Schizonepeta*	6 - 9 g
Bai Qian	*Cynanchum*	6 - 9 g
Jie Geng	*Platycodon*	6 - 9 g
Bai Bu	*Stemona*	6 - 9 g
Chen Pi	*Citrus*	3 - 6 g
Gan Cao	*Glycyrrhiza*	3 - 6 g

Wind Heat with Underlying Deficiency

Taiyang and shaoyang disease with joint congestion and intolerance to wind, or alternating fever and chills. Also useful for Liver overacting on Spleen.

T thin white coat

P possibly superficial

CHAI HU GUI ZHI TANG

Bupleurum and Cinnamon Twig Decoction

Extract Formula Name: Bupleurum and Cinnamon Combination

Gui Zhi	*Cinnamomum*	3 - 6 g
Chai Hu	*Bupleurum*	6 - 12 g
Ren Shen	*Panax*	3 - 6 g
Ban Xia	*Pinellia*	3 - 6 g
Huang Qin	*Scutellaria*	3 - 9 g
Bai Shao Yao	*Paeonia*	3 - 6 g
Sheng Jiang	*Zingiber*	3 - 6 g
Da Zao	*Ziziphus*	4 - 6 pc
Gan Cao	*Glycyrrhiza*	3 - 6 g

Wind heat common cold with pre-existing yin deficiency causing fever greater than chills, sore throat, dry mouth, night sweats, or bodyaches.

T red, narrow and thin, scanty coat

P rapid, thin

✪ **Major Formula**

JIA JIAN WEI ZHU TANG

Modified Polygonatum Odoratum Decoction

Yu Zhu	*Polygonatum*	6 - 9 g
Bai Wei	*Cynanchum*	3 - 6 g
Cong Bai	*Allium*	3 - 6 g
Dan Dou Chi	*Glycine*	9 - 12 g
Jie Geng	*Platycodon*	3 - 6 g
Da Zao	*Ziziphus*	2 - 5 pc
Gan Cao	*Glycyrrhiza*	3 - 6 g
Bo He	*Mentha*	3 - 6 g

Yin deficiency with wind cold which turns to heat and hides in the body, consuming more yin; or wind enters the body and consumes yin. Symptoms include night sweats, afternoon fever or heat, or blood-tinged sputum.

T red, dry, slight yellow coat

P weak, rapid

☞ Dissolve Bie Jia - Amyda first for about one hour, then decoct with the remaining herbs.

QIN JIAO BIE JIA SAN

Gentiana and Soft-shelled Turtle Shell Powder

Extract Formula Name: Chin-Chiu and T.S. Formula

Chai Hu	*Bupleurum*	6 - 9 g
Bie Jia	*Amyda*	6 - 12 g
Dang Gui	*Angelica*	6 - 9 g
Di Gu Pi	*Lycium*	6 - 9 g
Qin Jiao	*Gentiana*	6 - 9 g
Zhi Mu	*Anemarrhena*	6 - 12 g
[Wu Mei	*Prunus*	1 - 3 g]
[Qing Hao	*Artemisia*	1 - 3 g]

Wind heat with underlying mild yin deficiency. Symptoms include fever, sweating, five-palm heat, or night sweating.

T red

P superficial, slightly thin

WEI ZHU TANG

Polygonatum Odoratum Decoction

Yu Zhu	*Polygonatum*	6 - 9 g
Ma Huang	*Ephedra*	6 - 9 g
Cong Bai	*Allium*	3 - 6 g
Bai Wei	*Cynanchum*	6 - 9 g
Du Huo	*Angelica*	6 - 9 g
Chuan Xiong	*Ligusticum*	3 - 9 g
Xing Ren	*Prunus*	6 - 9 g
Shi Gao	*Gypsum*	12 - 15 g
Mu Xiang	*Saussurea*	3 - 6 g
Gan Cao	*Glycyrrhiza*	3 - 6 g

EXTERNAL DRYNESS ATTACKING THE LUNGS

- voice hoarseness
- dry skin and throat
- dry cough
- thirst with desire to drink

T dry

P empty

Lung heat with dryness and severe damage to the Lung yin as well as some wind symptoms. Manifestations include dry and itchy throat, full chest, or dry cough without phlegm.

T pink, dry, scanty coat

P weak or empty, rapid

☞ E Jiao - Equus should be dissolved at the end into the strained tea.

QING ZAO JIU FEI TANG

Eliminate Dryness and Rescue the Lungs Decoction

Extract Formula Name: Eriobotrya and Ophiopogon Combination

Sang Ye	*Morus*	6 - 9 g
Mai Men Dong	*Ophiopogon*	3 - 6 g
E Jiao	*Equus*	1 - 4 g
Ren Shen	*Panax*	6 - 9 g
Xing Ren	*Prunus*	3 - 6 g
Shi Gao	*Gypsum*	6 - 9 g
Pi Pa Ye	*Eriobotrya*	3 - 6 g
Gan Cao	*Glycyrrhiza*	3 - 6 g
Huo Ma Ren	*Cannabis*	3 - 6 g

Wind heat and dryness attacks the Lungs. Symptoms include mild fever, dry or hacking cough with scanty sputum which is hard to expectorate.

T dry, thin white coat

P superficial, rapid

SANG XING TANG

Mulberry Leaf and Apricot Kernel Decoction

Extract Formula Name: Morus and Apricot Seed Combination

Sang Ye	*Morus*	3 - 6 g
Xing Ren	*Prunus*	4 - 6 g
Zhe Bei Mu	*Fritillaria*	3 - 6 g
Bei Sha Shen	*Glehnia*	6 - 9 g
Dan Dou Chi	*Glycine*	3 - 6 g
Zhi Zi	*Gardenia*	3 - 6 g
Li Pi	*Pyrus*	3 - 6 g

Common cold with cold dryness affecting the Lungs. Symptoms include body aches, cough with white clear phlegm which is hard to expectorate, dryness but the patient has no desire to drink, and lack of sweating.

T dry white coat

P wiry

XING SU SAN

Apricot Kernel and Perilla Leaf Powder

Extract Formula Name: Apricot Seed and Perilla Formula

Zi Su Ye	*Perilla*	3 - 6 g
Xing Ren	*Prunus*	6 - 9 g
Qian Hu	*Peucedanum*	6 - 9 g
Zhi Ke	*Citrus*	3 - 6 g
Chen Pi	*Citrus*	3 - 6 g
Ban Xia	*Pinellia*	6 - 9 g
Fu Ling	*Poria*	6 - 9 g
Jie Geng	*Platycodon*	3 - 6 g
Sheng Jiang	*Zingiber*	3 - 6 g
Da Zao	*Ziziphus*	3 - 5 pc
Gan Cao	*Glycyrrhiza*	3 - 6 g

LUNG QI DEFICIENCY, WEI (DEFENSIVE) QI DEFICIENCY

- cough with watery expectoration
- frequent colds
- spontaneous day-time sweating
- weak cough

Lung qi deficiency without any heat symptoms causing cough, asthma, shortness of breath, or dyspnea.

T pale, thin white coat

P weak or frail

✪ **Major Formula**

BU FEI TANG

Tonify the Lungs Decoction

Extract Formula Name: Astragalus and Aster Combination

Huang Qi	*Astragalus*	12 - 20 g
Shu Di Huang	*Rehmannia*	12 - 20 g
Ren Shen	*Panax*	6 - 9 g
Zi Wan	*Aster*	6 - 9 g
Sang Bai Pi	*Morus*	6 - 12 g
Wu Wei Zi	*Schisandra*	6 - 9 g

Wind edema or wind damp with Spleen and wei qi deficiency causing sweating, urinary difficulty, or edema in the superficial layer.

T pale, thin white coat

P superficial

FANG JI HUANG QI TANG

Stephania and Astragalus Decoction

Extract Formula Name: Stephania and Astragalus Combination

Han Fang Ji	*Stephania*	9 - 12 g
Huang Qi	*Astragalus*	9 - 15 g
Bai Zhu	*Atractylodes*	6 - 9 g
Sheng Jiang	*Zingiber*	3 - 6 g
Da Zao	*Ziziphus*	3 - 4 pc
Gan Cao	*Glycyrrhiza*	3 - 6 g

Cold in the Lungs and Stomach causing Lung atrophy, cold extremities, or clear sputum.

T pale, moist

P weak, slow

GAN CAO GAN JIANG TANG

Licorice and Ginger Decoction

Extract Formula Name: Licorice and Ginger Combination

Zhi Gan Cao	*Glycyrrhiza*	9 - 12 g
Gan Jiang	*Zingiber*	6 - 9 g

Wei qi deficiency (defensive qi) due to Spleen qi/yang deficiency with qi stagnation symptoms. The patient experiences frequent colds or abdominal fullness.

T pale, maybe light purple

P weak

GUI ZHI LI ZHONG WAN

Cinnamon Twig with Regulate the Middle Pill

Gui Zhi	*Cinnamomum*	3 - 9 g
Gan Jiang	*Zingiber*	3 - 6 g
Bai Zhu	*Atractylodes*	6 - 9 g
Ren Shen	*Panax*	6 - 12 g
Gan Cao	*Glycyrrhiza*	3 - 6 g

Spleen/Stomach qi deficiency with cold and wei (defensive) qi deficiency; also useful for peptic ulcers and chronic allergies. Other symptoms include poor appetite or spontaneous sweating.

T pale, thin white coat

P weak, slow, thin, wiry

☞ Yi Tang - Saccharum Granorum should be added to the strained tea.

HUANG QI JIAN ZHONG TANG

Astragalus Decoction to Construct the Middle

Extract Formula Name: Astragalus Combination

Gui Zhi	*Cinnamomum*	9 g
Bai Shao Yao	*Paeonia*	18 g
Sheng Jiang	*Zingiber*	10 g
Da Zao	*Ziziphus*	3 - 6 pc
Gan Cao	*Glycyrrhiza*	6 g
Yi Tang	*Saccharum Granorum*	30 g
Huang Qi	*Astragalus*	9 g

Lung qi and yin deficiency resulting in cough and wheezing, and wei (defensive) qi deficiency.

T thin, scanty coat

P thin, rapid, weak

☞ E Jiao - Equus should be added at the end into the strained tea.

JIU XIAN SAN

Nine-Immortal Powder

Ren Shen	*Panax*	6 - 9 g
Wu Wei Zi	*Schisandra*	6 - 9 g
E Jiao	*Equus*	6 g
Bei Mu	*Fritillaria*	6 - 9 g
Kuan Dong Hua	*Tussilago*	6 - 9 g
Jie Geng	*Platycodon*	3 - 6 g
Ying Su Ke	*Papaver*	3 - 6 g
Wu Mei	*Prunus*	6 - 9 g
Sang Bai Pi	*Morus*	6 - 9 g
[Sheng Jiang	*Zingiber*	3 - 6 g]
[Da Zao	*Ziziphus*	3 g]

Qi and wei qi deficiency leading to spontaneous sweating which eventually injures the Heart yin. This leads to night sweating, insomnia, and palpitations.

T pale or red

P frail, thin

MU LI SAN

Oyster Shell Powder

Mu Li	*Ostrea*	15 - 30 g
Ma Huang Gen	*Ephredra*	3 - 9 g
Huang Qi	*Astragalus*	9 - 12 g
Fu Xiao Mai	*Triticum*	15 - 30 g

Lung qi deficiency damages Spleen qi which leads to damp accumulation with slight heat; or Lung qi deficiency with phlegm. Symptoms include wheezing, sticky yellow sputum, coughing of blood or pus, or heat in the chest.

T light purple, sticky white or yellow coat

P weak, superficial

REN SHEN GE JIE SAN

Ginseng and Gecko Powder

Ge Jie	*Gekko*	1 pair
Sang Bai Pi	*Morus*	6 - 9 g
Fu Ling	*Poria*	6 - 12 g
Xing Ren	*Prunus*	6 - 9 g
Chuan Bei Mu	*Fritillaria*	3 - 6 g
Ren Shen	*Panax*	6 - 12 g
Zhi Mu	*Anemarrhena*	6 - 9 g
Gan Cao	*Glycyrrhiza*	3 - 6 g

Lung/Kidney qi deficiency causing cough/asthma with wheezing. There are slightly more cold symptoms.

T pale, thin sticky white coat

P weak or frail

REN SHEN YANG YING TANG

Ginseng and Walnut Decoction

Extract Formula Name: Ginseng and Walnut Combination

Ren Shen	*Panax*	6 - 9 g
Hu Tao Ren	*Juglans*	3 - 6 pc
Sheng Jiang	*Zingiber*	3 - 6 pc
Da Zao	*Ziziphus*	3 pc

Spleen/Lung qi and blood deficiency with Heart yang deficiency, or ying level deficiency. The patient is easily startled, experiences shortness of breath, lack of taste sensation, insomnia, or palpitations. This formula is also useful for irregular periods or uterine bleeding.

T pale, swollen

P weak

REN SHEN YANG RONG WAN

Ginseng Decoction to Nourish the Nutritive Qi

Extract Formula Name: Ginseng Combination

Bai Shao Yao	*Paeonia*	9 - 15 g
Chen Pi	*Citrus*	3 - 6 g
Dang Gui	*Angelica*	3 - 9 g
Ren Shen	*Panax*	6 - 9 g
Huang Qi	*Astragalus*	6 - 12 g
Bai Zhu	*Atractylodes*	6 - 9 g
Shu Di Huang	*Rehmannia*	3 - 6 g
Wu Wei Zi	*Schisandra*	3 - 6 g
Fu Ling	*Poria*	3 - 6 g
Yuan Zhi	*Polygala*	2 - 6 g
Rou Gui	*Cinnamomum*	6 - 9 g
Gan Cao	*Glycyrrhiza*	3 - 6 g
[Da Zao	*Ziziphus*	2 pc]
[Gan Jiang	*Zingiber*	3 pc]

Lung/Kidney qi deficiency causing cough, asthma, and dyspnea.

T pale

P slow, weak

SHEN JIE SAN

Ginseng and Gecko Powder

Ren Shen	*Panax*	9 - 12 g
Ge Jie	*Gekko*	1 pair

Lung/Stomach qi deficiency with cough, expectoration of clear sputum, dry mouth, or thirst.

T pale, moist coat

P weak

SHENG JIANG GAN CAO TANG

Ginger and Licorice Decoction

Sheng Jiang	*Zingiber*	6 - 12 g
Ren Shen	*Panax*	6 - 9 g
Da Zao	*Ziziphus*	3 - 9 pc
Gan Cao	*Glycyrrhiza´*	6 - 12 g

Lung qi/yin deficiency with sweating and chronic cough producing scanty sputum which is hard to expectorate. This formula is also useful for palpitations, collapse, insomnia, or irregular pulse.

T pale or red

P weak or frail, slightly rapid

SHENG MAI SAN

Generate the Pulse Powder

Ginseng and Ophiopogon Formula

Ren Shen	*Panax*	9 - 15 g
Mai Men Dong	*Ophiopogon*	12 - 18 g
Wu Wei Zi	*Schisandra*	6 - 9 g

Lung/Spleen qi deficiency with qi sinking in the chest causing shortness of breath, dyspnea, or loose stools.

T pale, thin white coat

P deep, weak

SHENG XIAN TANG

Raise the Sinking Decoction

Huang Qi	*Astragalus*	15 - 20 g
Sheng Ma	*Cimicifuga*	3 - 6 g
Zhi Mu	*Anemarrhena*	6 - 9 g
Chai Hu	*Bupleurum*	3 - 9 g
Jie Geng	*Platycodon*	3 - 6 g

Lung/wei qi deficiency with sweating, frequent colds, aversion to wind, and weakness.

T pale

P weak, frail, or superficial

✪ **Major Formula**

YU PING FENG SAN

Jade Windscreen Powder

Extract Formula Name: Siler and Astragalus Formula

Fang Feng	*Ledebouriella*	6 - 9 g
Bai Zhu	*Atractylodes*	9 - 15 g
Huang Qi	*Astragalus*	6 - 20 g

LUNG YIN DEFICIENCY

- dry cough with scanty yellowish sputum which is hard to expectorate
- afternoon heat or fever
- thirst with dryness in the throat
- malar flush

T red, scanty coat

P empty, rapid

Lung/Kidney yin deficiency with cough and asthma, hemoptysis, tidal fever, or night sweats. This formula is also known as 'Mai Wei Di Huang Wan.'

T red, slight coat

P rapid, thin

BA XIAN CHANG SHOU WAN

Eight-Immortal Pill for Longevity

Shan Zhu Yu	Cornus	6 - 9 g
Shan Yao	Dioscorea	6 - 9 g
Sheng Di Huang	Rehmannia	6 - 12 g
Mu Dan Pi	Paeonia	6 - 9 g
Ze Xie	Alisma	6 - 9 g
Fu Ling	Poria	6 - 9 g
Wu Wei Zi	Schisandra	6 - 9 g
Mai Men Dong	Ophiopogon	6 - 9 g

Lung/Kidney yin deficiency with bleeding in the upper body due to false heat breaking the blood vessels; or chronic cough due to dryness in the throat.

T red, slight coat

P rapid, thin

✪ Major Formula

BAI HE GU JIN TANG

Lily Bulb Decoction to Preserve the Metal

Extract Formula Name: Lily Combination

Bai He	Lilium	3 - 12 g
Mai Men Dong	Ophiopogon	6 - 12 g
Sheng Di Huang	Rehmannia	6 - 12 g
Shu Di Huang	Rehmannia	6 - 12 g
Bei Mu	Fritillaria	3 - 6 g
Xuan Shen	Scrophularia	6 - 9 g
Dang Gui	Angelica	6 - 9 g
Bai Shao Yao	Paeonia	6 - 9 g
Jie Geng	Platycodon	3 - 6 g
Gan Cao	Glycyrrhiza	3 - 6 g

Upper jiao diabetes with heat: yangming channel syndrome with qi and yin deficiency causing severe sweating, fever, and thirst.

T red, dry yellow coat

P rapid, flooding, weak

☞ Decoct the first four herbs, then add the rice at the end. It will absorb the water to make a thick liquid.

BAI HU JIA REN SHEN TANG

White Tiger plus Ginseng Decoction

Extract Formula Name: Ginseng and Gypsum Combination

Shi Gao	*Gypsum*	15 - 20 g
Zhi Mu	*Anemarrhena*	9 - 12 g
Gan Cao	*Glycyrrhiza*	3 - 6 g
Ren Shen	*Panax*	3 - 9 g
Jing Mi	*Oryza*	9 - 12 g

Dryness in the Lungs with sticky phlegm and injury to the yin. The phlegm is very hard to expectorate. Other symptoms include wheezing and a very dry throat.

T red, dry, scanty coat

P empty, thin

BEI MU GUA LOU SAN

Fritillaria and Trichosanthes Fruit Powder

Chuan Bei Mu	*Fritillaria*	2 - 5 g
Gua Lou Ren	*Trichosanthes*	3 - 6 g
Fu Ling	*Poria*	6 - 9 g
Ju Hong	*Citrus*	3 - 6 g
Tian Hua Fen	*Trichosanthes*	3 - 6 g
Jie Geng	*Platycodon*	3 - 6 g

Lung yin deficiency produces false heat which burns the Lungs and causes dry cough with blood tinged sputum, tuberculosis, or bronchitis. There is wheezing, a scratchy throat, and slight thirst.

T red, slight, or no coat

P thin, rapid, or superficial

☞ E Jiao - Equus should be dissolved into the strained tea.

BU FEI E JIAO TANG

Tonify the Lungs Decoction with Ass-Hide Gelatin

E Jiao	*Equus*	6 - 9 g
Xing Ren	*Prunus*	6 - 9 g
Ma Dou Ling	*Aristolochia*	6 - 9 g
Jing Mi	*Oryza*	15 g
Niu Bang Zi	*Arctium*	6 - 9 g
Gan Cao	*Glycyrrhiza*	3 - 6 g

Lung/Kidney yin deficiency with bone steaming fever, cough with sticky phlegm, and five-palm heat.

T red, scanty coat

P thin, rapid

DA ZAO WAN

Great Creation Pill

Gui Ban	*Chinemys*	6 - 12 g
Huang Bai	*Phellodendron*	6 - 9 g
Zi He Che	*Placenta Hominis*	1 - 2 g
Huai Niu Xi	*Achyranthes*	6 - 9 g
Ren Shen	*Panax*	6 - 9 g
Du Zhong	*Eucommia*	6 - 9 g
Mai Men Dong	*Ophiopogon*	6 - 9 g
Tian Men Dong	*Asparagus*	6 - 9 g
Sheng Di Huang	*Rehmannia*	6 - 12 g

Lung yin deficiency with heat and bone-steaming fever, especially seen in children.

T red, slight or no coat

P rapid, thin

☞ Dissolve Bie Jia - Amyda first for about one hour, then decoct with the remaining herbs.

DI GU PI YIN

Lycium Root Bark Decoction

Di Gu Pi	*Lycium*	6 - 9 g
Zhi Mu	*Anemarrhena*	6 - 9 g
Bie Jia	*Amyda*	3 - 6 g
Ren Shen	*Panax*	3 - 9 g
Huang Qin	*Scutellaria*	6 - 9 g
Chai Hu	*Bupleurum*	6 - 9 g
Gan Cao	*Glycyrrhiza*	3 - 6 g
[Wu Mei	*Prunus*	1 - 3 g]
[Sheng Jiang	*Zingiber*	1 - 3 g]

Kidney/Lung qi/yin deficiency with wheezing, shortness of breath, or chronic cough. This formula is also known as 'Qi Wu Du Qi Wan'.

T red, slight coat

P thin, rapid

DU QI WAN

Capital Qi Pill

Extract Formula Name: Rehmannia and Schizandra Formula

Shan Zhu Yu	*Cornus*	6 - 9 g
Shan Yao	*Dioscorea*	6 - 9 g
Sheng Di Huang	*Rehmannia*	9 - 12 g
Fu Ling	*Poria*	6 - 9 g
Mu Dan Pi	*Paeonia*	6 - 9 g
Ze Xie	*Alisma*	6 - 9 g
Wu Wei Zi	*Schisandra*	6 - 9 g

Lung qi and yin deficiency with upper jiao diabetes. The main symptom is excessive thirst.

T red, thin yellow coat

P weak, thin, slightly rapid

ER DONG TANG

Ophiopogon and Asparagus Decoction

Mai Men Dong	*Ophiopogon*	12 - 15 g
Tian Men Dong	*Asparagus*	12 - 15 g
Tian Hua Fen	*Trichosanthes*	12 - 15 g
Huang Qin	*Scutellaria*	6 - 15 g
Zhi Mu	*Anemarrhena*	12 - 15 g
Gan Cao	*Glycyrrhiza*	3 - 6 g
Ren Shen	*Panax*	3 - 6 g

Lung/Kidney yin deficiency or jing deficiency with fire causing sweating, low back pain, slow mental and physical development in children, cough with scanty sticky blood-tinged phlegm, weight loss, or afternoon fever.

T red, slight yellow or no coat

P rapid, thin, or empty

HE CHE DA ZAO WAN

Pills of Human Placenta

Zi He Che	*Placenta Hominis*	9 - 30 g
Tian Men Dong	*Asparagus*	6 - 9 g
Mai Men Dong	*Ophiopogon*	6 - 9 g
Gui Ban	*Chinemys*	6 - 9 g
Shu Di Huang	*Rehmannia*	12 - 15 g
Huang Bai	*Phellodendron*	6 - 9 g
Du Zhong	*Eucommia*	6 - 9 g
Huai Niu Xi	*Achyranthes*	6 - 9 g

Kidney/Lung yin deficiency with Lung phlegm causing chronic bronchitis in the elderly, wheezing, or nausea.

T red, slight coat, or geographic

P thin, slightly rapid, slippery

JIN SHUI LIU JUN JIAN

Six-Gentlemen Decoction of Metal and Water

Chen Pi	*Citrus*	3 - 6 g
Ban Xia	*Pinellia*	6 - 9 g
Fu Ling	*Poria*	6 - 9 g
Gan Cao	*Glycyrrhiza*	3 - 6 g
Dang Gui	*Angelica*	6 - 9 g
Sheng Di Huang	*Rehmannia*	6 - 12 g
[Sheng Jiang	*Zingiber*	3 - 6 g]

Lung qi and yin deficiency resulting in cough and wheezing, and wei (defensive) qi deficiency.

T thin, scanty coat

P thin, rapid, weak

☞ E Jiao - Equus should be added at the end into the strained tea.

JIU XIAN SAN

Nine-Immortal Powder

Ren Shen	*Panax*	6 - 9 g
Wu Wei Zi	*Schisandra*	6 - 9 g
E Jiao	*Equus*	6 g
Bei Mu	*Fritillaria*	6 - 9 g
Kuan Dong Hua	*Tussilago*	6 - 9 g
Jie Geng	*Platycodon*	3 - 6 g
Ying Su Ke	*Papaver*	3 - 6 g
Wu Mei	*Prunus*	6 - 9 g
Sang Bai Pi	*Morus*	6 - 9 g
[Sheng Jiang	*Zingiber*	3 - 6 g]
[Da Zao	*Ziziphus*	3 g]

Liver fire attacking the Lung yin. This leads to thick blood-tinged phlegm, thirst, or bitter taste.

T red, cracked, sticky yellow coat

P wiry, rapid

KE XUE FANG

Coughing of Blood Formula

Zhi Zi	*Gardenia*	6 - 9 g
Gua Lou Ren	*Trichosanthes*	6 - 9 g
Qing Dai	*Indigo*	6 - 9 g
Fu Hai Shi	*Pumice*	6 - 9 g
He Zi	*Terminalia*	3 - 9 g

Stomach yin deficiency starts to produce heat which then burns Lung yin resulting in cough, wheezing, shortness of breath, or thirst.

T red, geographic spots, slight or no coat

P thin, rapid

MAI MEN DONG TANG

Ophiopogon Decoction

Extract Formula Name: Ophiopogon Combination

Mai Men Dong	*Ophiopogon*	6 - 12 g
Ren Shen	*Panax*	6 - 9 g
Ban Xia	*Pinellia*	6 - 9 g
Jing Mi	*Oryza*	9 - 12 g
Da Zao	*Ziziphus*	6 - 10 pc
Gan Cao	*Glycyrrhiza*	3 - 6 g

Yin deficiency with wind cold which turns to heat and hides in the body, consuming more yin; or wind enters the body and consumes yin. Symptoms include night sweats, afternoon fever or heat, or blood-tinged sputum.

T red, dry, slight yellow coat

P weak, rapid

☞ Dissolve Bie Jia - Amyda first for about one hour, then decoct with the remaining herbs.

QIN JIAO BIE JIA SAN

Gentiana and Soft-shelled Turtle Shell Powder

Extract Formula Name: Chin-Chiu and T.S. Formula

Chai Hu	*Bupleurum*	6 - 9 g
Bie Jia	*Amyda*	6 - 12 g
Dang Gui	*Angelica*	6 - 9 g
Di Gu Pi	*Lycium*	6 - 9 g
Qin Jiao	*Gentiana*	6 - 9 g
Zhi Mu	*Anemarrhena*	6 - 12 g
[Wu Mei	*Prunus*	1 - 3 g]
[Qing Hao	*Artemisia*	1 - 3 g]

Febrile disease causing low level chronic fever; or chronic disease damaged yin leading to later stages of febrile disease causing night sweats, AIDS, or tuberculosis.

T red, dry, scanty coat

P thin, rapid

☞ Bie Jia - Amyda should be soaked separately for 30 minutes to one hour, until it starts to dissolve; then soak the rest of the herbs. Qing Hao - Artemisia should be added at the end of the decoction process.

QING HAO BIE JIA TANG

Artemisia Annua and Soft-shelled Turtle Shell Decoction

Bie Jia	*Amyda*	9 - 12 g
Qing Hao	*Artemisia*	6 - 9 g
Mu Dan Pi	*Paeonja*	6 - 9 g
Sheng Di Huang	*Rehmannia*	6 - 12 g
Zhi Mu	*Anemarrhena*	6 - 9 g

Lung heat with dryness and severe damage to the Lung yin as well as some wind symptoms. Manifestations include dry and itchy throat, full chest, or dry cough without phlegm.

T pink, dry, scanty coat

P weak, or empty, rapid

☞ E Jiao - Equus should be dissolved at the end into the strained tea.

QING ZAO JIU FEI TANG

Eliminate Dryness and Rescue the Lungs Decoction

Extract Formula Name: Eriobotrya and Ophiopogon Combination

Sang Ye	*Morus*	6 - 9 g
Mai Men Dong	*Ophiopogon*	3 - 6 g
E Jiao	*Equus*	1 - 4 g
Ren Shen	*Panax*	6 - 9 g
Xing Ren	*Prunus*	3 - 6 g
Shi Gao	*Gypsum*	6 - 9 g
Pi Pa Ye	*Eriobotrya*	3 - 6 g
Gan Cao	*Glycyrrhiza*	3 - 6 g
Huo Ma Ren	*Cannabis*	3 - 6 g

Lung and Kidney yin deficiency with dryness in the Lungs causing chronic consumptive disease. Symptoms include thirst, night sweating, or scanty phlegm which is hard to expectorate.

T red, dry, scanty coat

P deep, thin, rapid

QONG YU SAN

Ginseng and Rehmannia Powder

Ren Shen	*Panax*	3 - 6 g
Sheng Di Huang	*Rehmannia*	15 - 30 g
Feng Mi	*Mel*	30 g
Fu Ling	*Poria*	15 - 30 g

Lung yin deficiency with false heat and Spleen qi deficiency causing cough with scanty sputum and fatigue.

T red, cracked, slight coat

P thin, rapid

☞ Dissolve Bie Jia - Amyda first for about one hour, then decoct with the remaining herbs.

REN SHEN HUANG QI SAN

Ginseng and Astragalus Powder

Ren Shen	*Panax*	6 - 12 g
Huang Qi	*Astragalus*	9 - 15 g
Fu Ling	*Poria*	6 - 9 g
Zhi Mu	*Anemarrhena*	6 - 9 g
Zi Wan	*Aster*	6 - 9 g
Sang Bai Pi	*Morus*	6 - 9 g
Qin Jiao	*Gentiana*	6 - 12 g
Jie Geng	*Platycodon*	3 - 6 g
Chai Hu	*Bupleurum*	6 - 9 g
Ban Xia	*Pinellia*	6 - 9 g
Di Gu Pi	*Lycium*	3 - 9 g
Sheng Di Huang	*Rehmannia*	6 - 15 g
Bie Jia	*Amyda*	6 - 12 g
Tian Men Dong	*Asparagus*	9 - 12 g
Chi Shao Yao	*Paeonia*	3 - 9 g
Gan Cao	*Glycyrrhiza*	3 - 6 g

Dryness damaged Lung and Stomach yin (wind is gone now) causing thirst, scanty sputum, and a persistent dry cough.

T red, slight coat

P rapid, weak

✪ Major Formula

SHA SHEN MAI MEN DONG TANG

Glehnia and Ophiopogon Decoction

Bei Sha Shen	*Glehnia*	6 - 15 g
Mai Men Dong	*Ophiopogon*	6 - 15 g
Sang Ye	*Morus*	3 - 9 g
Tian Hua Fen	*Trichosanthes*	6 - 9 g
Yu Zhu	*Polygonatum*	6 - 9 g
Bian Dou	*Dolichos*	3 - 9 g
Gan Cao	*Glycyrrhiza*	3 - 6 g

Lung qi/yin deficiency with sweating and chronic cough producing scanty sputum which is hard to expectorate. This formula is also useful for palpitations, collapse, insomnia, or irregular pulse.

T pale or red

P weak or frail, slightly rapid

SHENG MAI SAN

Generate the Pulse Powder

Ginseng and Ophiopogon Formula

Ren Shen	*Panax*	9 - 15 g
Mai Men Dong	*Ophiopogon*	12 - 18 g
Wu Wei Zi	*Schisandra*	6 - 9 g

Lung/Kidney yin deficiency with severe fire causing nosebleeds, or hemoptysis which occurs during or prior to the menses.

T red, cracks

P rapid, empty

SHUN JING TANG

Smooth the Menses Decoction

Shu Di Huang	*Rehmannia*	9 - 15 g
Mu Dan Pi	*Paeonia*	6 - 9 g
Dang Gui	*Angelica*	6 - 9 g
Bai Shao Yao	*Paeonia*	6 - 9 g
Bei Sha Shen	*Glehnia*	6 - 12 g
Jing Jie	*Schizonepeta*	6 - 9 g
Fu Ling	*Poria*	6 - 9 g

Diabetes manifesting mostly in the upper jiao. The main symptom is thirst.

T thin and narrow, slightly red, less coat than normal

P thin, slightly rapid

XIAO KE TANG

Wasting and Thirsting Decoction

Extract Formula Name: Rehmannia and Trichosanthes Formula

Ren Ru Zhi	*Lac Hominis*	50-200 cc
Huang Lian	*Coptis*	9-12 g
Tian Hua Fen	*Trichosanthes*	15-20 g
Sheng Di Huang	*Rehmannia*	12-15 g
Ou Jie	*Nelumbo*	9-20 g
Feng Mi	*Mel*	15-20 g
Sheng Jiang	*Zingiber*	6-9 g

Heat in the Lungs injuring the Lung yin and qi causing afternoon fever, wheezing, cough, or sticky, scanty phlegm.

T red, dry, yellow coat

P thin, rapid

XIE BAI SAN

Drain the White Powder

Extract Formula Name: Morus and Lycium Formula

Di Gu Pi	*Lycium*	20-30 g
Sang Bai Pi	*Morus*	20-30 g
Jing Mi	*Oryza*	15-25 g
Zhi Gan Cao	*Glycyrrhiza*	3-6 g

Lung yin deficiency leading to dryness and soreness in the throat causing dry cough with little or no phlegm.

T red, thin and narrow in size, less than normal coat

P thin, slightly rapid

XUAN MAI GAN JIE TANG

Scrophularia, Ophiopogon, Platycodon, and Licorice Decoction

Xuan Shen	*Scrophularia*	9-12 g
Mai Men Dong	*Ophiopogon*	6-9 g
Jie Geng	*Platycodon*	3-6 g
Gan Cao	*Glycyrrhiza*	3-6 g

Lung/Kidney yin deficiency with toxin causing diptheria, laryngitis, coarse breathing, or dry hacking cough.

T red, dry, yellow coat

P thin, rapid, or empty

YANG YIN QING FEI TANG

Nourish the Yin and Clear the Lungs Decoction

Sheng Di Huang	*Rehmannia*	6 - 12 g
Xuan Shen	*Scrophularia*	6 - 9 g
Bai Shao Yao	*Paeonia*	6 - 9 g
Mai Men Dong	*Ophiopogon*	6 - 12 g
Bo He	*Mentha*	3 - 6 g
Chuan Bei Mu	*Fritillaria*	3 - 6 g
Mu Dan Pi	*Paeonia*	6 - 9 g
Gan Cao	*Glycyrrhiza*	3 - 6 g

Kidney/Lung yin deficiency with heat and Lung consumption resulting in shortness of breath, dry cough, dry stools, dark scanty urine, or heat in the five centers.

T red, slight yellow or no coat

P rapid, weak, thin

☞ E Jiao - Equus should be dissolved at the end into the strained tea.

YUE HUA WAN

Moonlight Pill

Mai Men Dong	*Ophiopogon*	6 - 12 g
Tian Men Dong	*Asparagus*	6 - 12 g
Shu Di Huang	*Rehmannia*	6 - 12 g
Sheng Di Huang	*Rehmannia*	6 - 12 g
Bei Sha Shen	*Glehnia*	6 - 15 g
Bai Bu	*Stemona*	6 - 9 g
Chuan Bei Mu	*Fritillaria*	3 - 6 g
Shan Yao	*Dioscorea*	6 - 9 g
Fu Ling	*Poria*	6 - 9 g
Ju Hua	*Chrysanthemum*	6 - 9 g
Sang Ye	*Morus*	6 - 9 g
San Qi	*Panax*	9 - 12 g
E Jiao	*Equus*	6 - 9 g
Ta Gan	*Lutra*	6 - 9 g

PHLEGM DAMP IN THE LUNGS

- cough with profuse white sputum
- stuffy sensation in the chest
- shortness of breath

T thick sticky white coat

P slippery

(Lung) phlegm damp with cough or coma causing wind phlegm, dizziness, or hypertension.

T thick sticky coat

P slippery

✘ Tian Nan Xing - Arisaema is slightly toxic.

DAO TAN TANG

Guide Out Phlegm Decoction

Ban Xia	*Pinellia*	6 - 9 g
Chen Pi	*Citrus*	3 - 6 g
Fu Ling	*Poria*	6 - 9 g
Gan Cao	*Glycyrrhiza*	3 - 6 g
Zhi Shi	*Citrus*	3 - 6 g
Tian Nan Xing	*Arisaema*	1 - 3 g
Sheng Jiang	*Zingiber*	3 g

Cold phlegm in the Lungs with underlying Kidney yang deficiency. This produces cough with clear watery fluids, or shortness of breath.

T pale, thick sticky white coat

P frail or slippery

GUI LING WU WEI GAN CAO TANG

Cinnamon Twig, Poria, Schisandra, and Licorice Decoction

Gui Zhi	*Cinnamomum*	6 - 12 g
Fu Ling	*Poria*	6 - 12 g
Wu Wei Zi	*Schisandra*	9 - 15 g
Gan Cao	*Glycyrrhiza*	6 - 9 g

Phlegm in the Lungs with underlying Kidney yang deficiency. The Kidneys are unable to grasp Lung qi, so qi ascends to the chest causing fullness in chest and epigastrium. This is known as running piglet disorder. Symptoms also include wheezing, spontaneous sweating, and cold hands and feet.

T pale, sticky white coat

P minute

☞ Hei Xi - Plumbum and Liu Huang - Sulphur should both be dry fried. The remaining herbs are ground and made into pills with wine. Adults take 6 - 9 g per day, children take 2-3 g per day.

✘ To prevent lead poisoning, do not take longer than 3 days. Do not use during pregnancy.

HEI XI DAN

Lead Special Pill

Hei Xi	*Plumbum*	60 g
Liu Huang	*Sulphur*	60 g
Fu Zi	*Aconitum*	30 g
Rou Gui	*Cinnamomum*	60 g
Xiao Hui Xiang	*Foeniculum*	30 g
Rou Dou Kou	*Amomun*	30 g
Chen Xiang	*Aquilaria*	30 g
Yang Qi Shi	*Actinolitum*	30 g
Bu Gu Zhi	*Psoralea*	30 g
Mu Xiang	*Saussurea*	30 g
Chuan Lian Zi	*Melia*	30 g
Hu Lu Ba	*Trigonella*	30 g

Watery fluids in the Lungs and Spleen yang deficiency causing cough, wheezing, and a stuffy sensation in the chest.

T pale, sticky or slippery white coat

P slippery, wiry

LING GAN WU WEI JIANG XIN TANG

Poria, Licorice, Schisandra, Ginger, and Asarum Decoction

Fu Ling	*Poria*	6 - 12 g
Gan Cao	*Glycyrrhiza*	3 - 9 g
Wu Wei Zi	*Schisandra*	6 - 9 g
Gan Jiang	*Zingiber*	3 - 9 g
Xi Xin	*Asarum*	6 - 9 g

Spleen/Stomach yang deficiency causing phlegm accumulation which affects the Lungs; or taiyang disease was mistreated and guided into the Spleen leading to water accumulation. Symptoms include dyspnea, clear phlegm expectoration, and fullness in the chest and flanks.

T pale, slippery white coat

P slippery, weak, deep

LING GUI ZHU GAN TANG

Poria, Cinnamon Twig, Atractylodes, and Licorice Decoction

Extract Formula Name: Hoelen and Atractylodes Combination

Fu Ling	*Poria*	6 - 12 g
Gui Zhi	*Cinnamomum*	3 - 9 g
Bai Zhu	*Atractylodes*	6 - 9 g
Gan Cao	*Glycyrrhiza*	3 - 6 g

Cough and wheezing with sticky phlegm which is hard to bring up after a mild wind cold invasion.

T sticky white coat

P slippery, superficial

LIU AN JIAN

Six-Serenity Decoction

Ban Xia	*Pinellia*	6 - 9 g
Fu Ling	*Poria*	6 - 9 g
Chen Pi	*Citrus*	3 - 6 g
Gan Cao	*Glycyrrhiza*	3 - 6 g
Bai Jie Zi	*Brassica*	1 - 3 g
Xing Ren	*Prunus*	3 - 6 g
[*Sheng Jiang*	*Zingiber*	3 - 6 g]

Phlegm damp with migrating body pains, chills, or fever.

T slippery or sticky white coat

P deep, slippery

✘ Tian Nan Xing - Arisaema is slightly toxic, and should only be used in small amounts.

QING SHI HUA TAN TANG

Clear Dampness and Transform Phlegm Decoction

Extract Formula Name: Pinellia and Arisaema Combination

Ban Xia	*Pinellia*	6 - 9 g
Chen Pi	*Citrus*	3 - 6 g
Fu Ling	*Poria*	6 - 9 g
Gan Cao	*Glycyrrhiza*	3 - 6 g
Cang Zhu	*Atractylodes*	3 - 6 g
Tian Nan Xing	*Arisaema*	1 - 3 g
Qiang Huo	*Notopterygium*	3 g
Huang Qin	*Scutellaria*	3 - 6 g
Bai Zhi	*Angelica*	3 - 6 g
Bai Jie Zi	*Brassica*	1 - 3 g
Gan Jiang	*Zingiber*	3 - 6 g
Sheng Jiang	*Zingiber*	3 - 6 g

Phlegm damp cough with cold in the Lungs, or food stagnation. Symptoms include dyspnea with profuse phlegm expectoration, and poor appetite.

T sticky white coat

P slippery

SAN ZI YANG QIN TANG

Three-Seed Decoction to Nourish One's Parents

Zi Su Zi	*Perilla*	6 - 9 g
Lai Fu Zi	*Raphanus*	6 - 9 g
Bai Jie Zi	*Brassica*	3 - 9 g

Wind cold asthma with pre-existing phlegm and water (excess type) producing mild exterior symptoms such as dyspnea, wheezing with mild fever and chills.

T thick sticky white coat

P superficial, tight

SHE GAN MA HUANG TANG

Belamcanda and Ephedra Decoction

She Gan	*Belamcanda*	6 - 9 g
Ma Huang	*Ephedra*	6 - 9 g
Ban Xia	*Pinellia*	6 - 9 g
Zi Wan	*Aster*	6 - 9 g
Kuan Dong Hua	*Tussilago*	6 - 9 g
Wu Wei Zi	*Schisandra*	3 - 6 g
Xi Xin	*Asarum*	6 - 9 g
Sheng Jiang	*Zingiber*	9 - 12 g
Da Zao	*Ziziphus*	7 - 9 pc

Lung phlegm damp with underlying Kidney qi deficiency causing wheezing with profuse phlegm.

T sticky white coat

P weak, slippery

✪ **Major Formula**

SU ZI JIANG QI TANG

Perilla Fruit Decoction for Directing Qi Downward

Extract Formula Name: Perilla Fruit Combination

Zhi Gan Cao	*Glycyrrhiza*	6 g
Ban Xia	*Pinellia*	6 - 9 g
Zi Su Zi	*Perilla*	6 - 12 g
Dang Gui	*Angelica*	6 - 9 g
Hou Po	*Magnolia*	6 - 12 g
Qian Hu	*Peucedanum*	6 - 9 g
Rou Gui	*Cinnamomum*	3 g
[Sheng Jiang	*Zingiber*	1 - 3 g]
[Zi Su Ye	*Perilla*	3 - 6 g]
[Da Zao	*Ziziphus*	3 g]

Lung phlegm fluid causing eye/facial edema, cough or asthma, or Lung abscess with phlegm.

T sticky white coat

P slippery

TING LI DA ZAO XIE FEI TANG

Lepidium and Jujube Decoction to Drain the Lungs

Extract Formula Name: Lepidium and Jujube Combination

Ting Li Zi	*Lepidium*	6 - 9 g
Da Zao	*Ziziphus*	6 - 12 pc

Qi and blood stagnation causing chest pain with water/damp accumulation: Liver affects the Lungs. Symptoms include hypochondriac pain, possible coughing, or raspy voice.

T purple, thick sticky coat

P wiry

☞ Xuan Fu Hua - Inula should be wrapped in a cheesecloth.

XIANG FU XUAN FU HUA TANG

Cyperus and Inula Decoction

Xiang Fu	*Cyperus*	6 - 9 g
Xuan Fu Hua	*Inula*	6 - 9 g
Yi Yi Ren	*Coix*	9 - 15 g
Chen Pi	*Citrus*	3 - 6 g
Zi Su Zi	*Perilla*	6 - 9 g
Ban Xia	*Pinellia*	6 - 9 g
Fu Ling	*Poria*	6 - 9 g

Phlegm damp in the Lungs causing cough, wheezing, or shortness of breath. Phlegm expectoration may range from a clear to a thick white discharge.

T thin or thick white coat

P slippery

ZHI JIE ER CHEN TANG

Aurantium, Platycodon, and Two-Cured Decoction

Ban Xia	*Pinellia*	6 - 9 g
Chen Pi	*Citrus*	3 - 6 g
Fu Ling	*Poria*	6 - 9 g
Zhi Gan Cao	*Glycyrrhiza*	3 - 6 g
Zhi Ke	*Citrus*	3 - 9 g
Jie Geng	*Platycodon*	3 - 6 g

PHLEGM HEAT IN THE LUNGS

- barking cough with yellow or green expectoration
- shortness of breath
- heat sensation in the chest

T red, thick yellow sticky coat

P slippery, rapid

Water/heat accumulation in the chest and Lungs causing chest qi obstruction. Symptoms include stiff neck, and a full or suffocating sensation in the chest.

T red, sticky coat

P rapid, slippery

☞ Herbs should be made into 9 g pills with honey.

✘ Gan Sui - Euphorbia is toxic and should only be taken in small amounts. Do not use during pregnancy.

DA XIAN XIONG WAN

Major Sinking Into the Chest Pill

Da Huang	*Rheum*	25 g
Mang Xiao	*Mirabilitum*	17.5 g
Ting Li Zi	*Lepidium*	17.5 g
Xing Ren	*Prunus*	17.5 g
Gan Sui	*Euphorbia*	3 g

Wind cold in the exterior with phlegm heat in the interior causing cough and wheezing. The phlegm expectoration is thick and yellow.

T sticky yellow coat

P slippery, rapid

DING CHUAN TANG

Arrest Wheezing Decoction

Extract Formula Name: Ma-Huang and Ginkgo Combination

Bai Guo	*Gingko*	6 - 9 g
Ma Huang	*Ephedra*	6 - 9 g
Kuan Dong Hua	*Tussilago*	6 - 9 g
Zi Su Zi	*Perilla*	3 - 6 g
Xing Ren	*Prunus*	3 - 6 g
Ban Xia	*Pinellia*	6 - 9 g
Sang Bai Pi	*Morus*	6 - 9 g
Huang Qin	*Scutellaria*	6 - 9 g
Gan Cao	*Glycyrrhiza*	3 - 6 g

Phlegm heat in the Lungs; or dry cough with Kidney/Liver heat. The phlegm is hard to expectorate, or breathing is labored.

T red, sticky yellow coat

P rapid, slippery

GUA LOU ZHI SHI TANG

Trichosanthes Fruit and Immature Bitter Orange Decoction

Extract Formula Name: Trichosanthes and Chih-Shi Combination

Gua Lou Ren	*Trichosanthes*	3 - 6 g
Zhi Shi	*Citrus*	3 - 6 g
Zhe Bei Mu	*Fritillaria*	6 - 9 g
Fu Ling	*Poria*	6 - 9 g
Chen Pi	*Citrus*	3 - 6 g
Dang Gui	*Angelica*	3 - 9 g
Sha Ren	*Amomum*	3 - 6 g
Mu Xiang	*Saussurea*	3 - 6 g
Jie Geng	*Platycodon*	3 - 6 g
Zhi Zi	*Gardenia*	3 - 6 g
Huang Qin	*Scutellaria*	6 - 9 g
Zhu Ru	*Bambusa*	6 g
Gan Cao	*Glycyrrhiza*	3 - 6 g
Sheng Jiang	*Zingiber*	3 - 6 g
Zhu Li	*Bambusa*	1 - 3 g

Phlegm heat with damage to the Lung yin causing cough or asthma with thick yellow or green phlegm which is hard to expectorate, feelings of heat in the chest, tightness in the chest, or thirst without much desire to drink. This formula is useful for bronchitis.

T red, maybe geographic, dry, thick sticky yellow coat

P rapid, slippery, slightly thin

✪ **Major Formula**

QING JIN HUA TAN TANG

Clear Metal and Absorb Phlegm Decoction

Huang Qin	*Scutellaria*	6 - 12 g
Zhi Zi	*Gardenia*	3 - 6 g
Fu Ling	*Poria*	6 - 12 g
Zhe Bei Mu	*Fritillaria*	6 - 12 g
Jie Geng	*Platycodon*	3 - 6 g
Gua Lou	*Trichosanthes*	3 - 6 g
Zhi Mu	*Anemarrhena*	6 - 9 g
Sang Bei Pi	*Morus*	6 - 9 g
Mai Men Dong	*Ophiopogon*	6 - 9 g
Gan Cao	*Glycyrrhiza*	3 - 6 g

Phlegm heat cough causing yellow, sticky, phlegm expectoration or fullness in the chest. Symptoms include dyspnea, epigastric fullness, and nausea.

T red, sticky yellow coat

P rapid, slippery

✘ Dan Nan Xing - Arisaema is slightly toxic and should only be used in small amounts.

QING QI HUA TAN WAN

Clear the Qi and Transform Phlegm Pill

Ban Xia	*Pinellia*	6 - 9 g
Dan Nan Xing	*Arisaema*	1 - 3 g
Huang Qin	*Scutellaria*	6 - 9 g
Fu Ling	*Poria*	6 - 9 g
Gua Lou Ren	*Trichosanthes*	6 - 9 g
Chen Pi	*Citrus*	3 - 6 g
Zhi Shi	*Citrus*	3 - 6 g
Xing Ren	*Prunus*	3 - 9 g

Lung qi deficiency damages Spleen qi which leads to damp accumulation with slight heat; or Lung qi deficiency with phlegm. Symptoms include wheezing, sticky yellow sputum, coughing of blood or pus, or heat in the chest.

T light purple, sticky white or yellow coat

P weak, superficial

REN SHEN GE JIE SAN

Ginseng and Gecko Powder

Ge Jie	*Gekko*	1 pair
Sang Bai Pi	*Morus*	6 - 9 g
Fu Ling	*Poria*	6 - 12 g
Xing Ren	*Prunus*	6 - 9 g
Chuan Bei Mu	*Fritillaria*	3 - 6 g
Ren Shen	*Panax*	6 - 12 g
Zhi Mu	*Anemarrhena*	6 - 9 g
Gan Cao	*Glycyrrhiza*	3 - 6 g

Phlegm heat toxin and blood stagnation with pus causing Lung abscess, measles, whooping cough, cough with blood-streaked sputum, chest congestion, or low-grade fever.

T red, sticky yellow coat

P rapid, slippery

WEI JING TANG

Reed Decoction

Extract Formula Name: Phragmites Combination

Lu Gen	*Phragmitis*	40 - 60 g
Dong Gua Ren	*Benincasa*	15 - 25 g
Yi Yi Ren	*Coix*	15 - 20 g
Tao Ren	*Prunus*	6 - 9 g

Phlegm heat in the chest (Heart), or epigastrium (Stomach) leading to bronchitis, constipation, distending pain or pressure in the chest, numbness, or bitter taste.

T red, sticky yellow coat

P rapid, slippery

XIAO XIAN XIONG TANG

Minor Sinking Into the Chest Decoction

Extract Formula Name: Minor Trichosanthes Combination

Gua Lou	*Trichosanthes*	20 g
Huang Lian	*Coptis*	3 g
Ban Xia	*Pinellia*	6 - 9 g

HEART DISHARMONIES

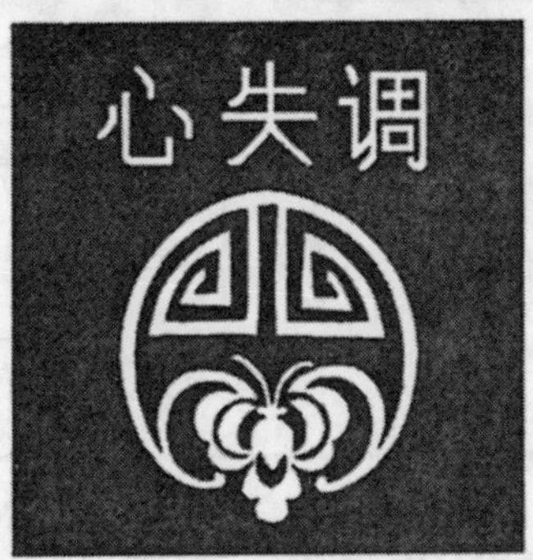

HEART QI DEFICIENCY

- pale face
- shortness of breath
- palpitations
- spontaneous sweating

T pale or normal color

P weak, or empty

This formula treats insomnia due to Heart and Gallbladder qi deficiency. This is commonly seen in children causing them to appear timid and scared of everything, fear ghosts and burglars, or not want to sleep alone. They sweat easily, especially in the hands and soles.

T pale or normal color, slightly swollen

P weak, thready, deep

AN SHEN DING ZHI TANG
Calm Spirit and Stop Fear Decoction

Ren Shen	*Panax*	9 - 12 g
Fu Ling	*Poria*	6 - 9 g
Fu Shen	*Poria*	6 - 9 g
Shi Chang Pu	*Acorus*	3 - 9 g
Long Gu	*Os Draconis*	6 - 9 g
Yuan Zhi	*Polygala*	6 - 9 g

Heart qi deficiency with disturbed shen causing anxiety, palpitations, forgetfulness, or fright.

T pale

P weak

✪ Major Formula

✘ Zhu Sha - Cinnabaris is toxic, and should only be used short-term.

DING ZHI WAN

Settle the Emotions Pill

Ren Shen	*Panax*	12 - 15 g
Fu Ling	*Poria*	6 - 9 g
Shi Chang Pu	*Acorus*	6 - 9 g
Yuan Zhi	*Polygala*	6 - 9 g
Fu Shen	*Poria*	9 - 12 g
Zhu Sha	*Cinnabaris*	6 - 9 g

After taiyang disease the patient develops Heart qi and yang deficiency; deficient type angina.

T pale

P weak

GUI ZHI GAN CAO TANG

Cinnamon Twig and Licorice Decoction

Gui Zhi	*Cinnamomum*	3 - 9 g
Gan Cao	*Glycyrrhiza*	3 - 6 g

Heart yang is not warmed by the Kidneys leading to water accumulation which rises upwards causing abdominal pain, angina, Stomach cramping, tingling sensation in the abdomen, (ben ten qi - running piglet sensation), or scanty urine.

T pale, wet, sticky white coat

P deep, weak, slightly slow

LING GUI ZAO GAN TANG

Poria, Cinnamon Twig, Jujube, and Licorice Decoction

Fu Ling	*Poria*	9 - 12 g
Gui Zhi	*Cinnamomum*	3 - 9 g
Da Zao	*Ziziphus*	3 - 4 pc
Gan Cao	*Glycyrrhiza*	3 - 6 g

Heart qi deficiency with Spleen qi deficiency leading to anxiety, insomnia, spontaneous sweating, or palpitations.

T pale, thin coating

P weak

✘ Zhu Sha - Cinnabaris is toxic, and should only be used short-term.

MIAO XIANG SAN

Marvelously Fragrant Powder

Ren Shen	*Panax*	6 - 12 g
Fu Ling	*Poria*	9 - 12 g
Fu Shen	*Poria*	9 - 12 g
Yuan Zhi	*Polygala*	9 - 12 g
Huang Qi	*Astragalus*	9 - 15 g
Shan Yao	*Dioscorea*	9 - 12 g
Mu Xiang	*Saussurea*	12 - 15 g
Jie Geng	*Platycodon*	1 - 3 g
Zhu Sha	*Cinnabaris*	1 - 3 g
She Xiang	*Moschus*	0.3 - 0.5 g
Gan Cao	*Glycyrrhiza*	3 - 6 g

Heart/Kidney qi/yin deficiency causing incontinence, spermatorrhea, frequent urination, and forgetfulness.

T pale or red

P weak, thin

SANG PIAO XIAO SAN

Mantis Egg-Case Powder

Extract Formula Name: Mantis Formula

Sang Piao Xiao	*Paratenodera*	9 - 12 g
Long Gu	*Os Draconis*	12 - 25 g
Fu Shen	*Poria*	9 - 12 g
Ren Shen	*Panax*	9 - 12 g
Shi Chang Pu	*Acorus*	6 - 9 g
Dang Gui	*Angelica*	6 - 9 g
Gui Ban	*Chinemys*	9 - 15 g
Yuan Zhi	*Polygala*	9 - 15 g

Heart/Gallbladder qi deficiency with edema in the extremities, tight chest, palpitations, anxiety, or timidity.

T pale

P weak

SHI WEI WEN DAN TANG

Ten-Ingredient Decoction to Warm the Gallbladder

Ban Xia	*Pinellia*	6 - 9 g
Chen Pi	*Citrus*	3 - 6 g
Zhi Shi	*Citrus*	6 g
Fu Ling	*Poria*	6 g
Ren Shen	*Panax*	3 - 6 g
Suan Zao Ren	*Ziziphus*	3 - 6 g
Shu Di Huang	*Rehmannia*	3 - 9 g
Wu Wei Zi	*Schisandra*	3 - 6 g
Yuan Zhi	*Polygala*	3 - 6 g
Zhi Gan Cao	*Glycyrrhiza*	3 g
Da Zao	*Ziziphus*	2 pc
Sheng Jiang	*Zingiber*	5 pc

Heart qi blood deficiency causing insomnia, anxiety, restlessness, and poor memory.

T pale

P weak, thin

YANG XIN TANG

Nourish the Heart Decoction

Extract Formula Name: Astragalus and Zizyphus Combination

Sheng Di Huang	*Rehmannia*	6 - 12 g
Shu Di Huang	*Rehmannia*	6 - 12 g
Dang Gui	*Angelica*	6 - 9 g
Ren Shen	*Panax*	6 - 12 g
Mai Men Dong	*Ophiopogon*	6 - 9 g
Suan Zao Ren	*Ziziphus*	6 - 9 g
Fu Shen	*Poria*	6 - 9 g
Bai Zi Ren	*Biota*	6 - 9 g
Wu Wei Zi	*Schisandra*	6 - 9 g
Gan Cao	*Glycyrrhiza*	3 - 6 g
[Lian Zi	*Nelumbo*	3 - 6 g]
[Deng Xin Cao	*Juncus*	3 - 6 g]

Heart qi/blood or yin deficiency causing arrhythmia, insomnia, pressure in the chest, coronary Heart disease, and anxiety.

T pale or red, thin white coat

P weak

☞ E Jiao - Equus should be dissolved into the strained tea.

ZHI GAN CAO TANG

Honey-Fried Licorice Decoction

Extract Formula Name: Baked Licorice Combination

Zhi Gan Cao	*Glycyrrhiza*	12 - 15 g
Sheng Di Huang	*Rehmannia*	30 g
Ren Shen	*Panax*	6 - 9 g
Gui Zhi	*Cinnamomum*	6 - 9 g
Huo Ma Ren	*Cannabis*	6 - 9 g
Mai Men Dong	*Ophiopogon*	9 g
E Jiao	*Equus*	6 g
Da Zao	*Ziziphus*	6 - 9 pc
Sheng Jiang	*Zingiber*	6 - 9 g

HEART YANG DEFICIENCY

- tightness in the chest
- palpitations
- feeling of cold or cold hands
- fatigue

T pale, light purple, swollen, moist

P deep, weak

Chest Bi: chest yang deficiency with mild cold and phlegm accumulation causing tightness in the chest, shortness of breath, palpitations, cough, or asthma.

T pale, light purple, wet, thick sticky white coat

P slow, slippery, wiry

✪ **Major Formula**

GUA LOU XIE BAI BAI JIU TANG

Trichonsanthes Fruit, Chinese Chive, and Wine Decoction

Extract Formula Name: Trichosanthes, Bakeri and White Wine Combination

Gua Lou	*Trichosanthes*	9 - 12 g
Xie Bai	*Allium*	9 - 12 g
Bai Jiu	*White Wine*	30 - 60 cc

Taiyang disease or inappropriate warming therapy causing Heart yang deficiency with yin deficiency. This leads to disturbed shen, restlessness, mania, sweating, palpitations, or insomnia.

T pale or red, thin white or yellowish coat

P weak, thin

GUI ZHI GAN CAO LONG GU MU LI TANG

Cinnamon Twig, Licorice, Dragon Bone, and Oyster Shell Decoction

Gui Zhi	*Cinnamomum*	3 - 6 g
Zhi Gan Cao	*Glycyrrhiza*	6 g
Long Gu	*Os Draconis*	6 - 15 g
Mu Li	*Ostrea*	6 - 15 g

After taiyang disease the patient develops Heart qi and yang deficiency; deficient type angina.

T pale

P weak

GUI ZHI GAN CAO TANG

Cinnamon Twig and Licorice Decoction

Gui Zhi	*Cinnamomum*	3 - 9 g
Gan Cao	*Glycyrrhiza*	3 - 6 g

A wind cold invasion has gone internally due to incorrect warming needle technique. Wind cold has heated up and is now trapped inside with a complication of internal water accumulation. This causes unspecific abdominal pain which bothers the Heart (also known as 'running piglet sensation' = ben ten qi). This is an external pathogen with internal water stagnation and cold.

T pale, wet, white coat

P slow, slightly slippery

GUI ZHI JIA ROU GUI TANG

Cinnamon Twig Decoction plus Cinnamon Bark

Gui Zhi	*Cinnamomum*	6 - 9 g
Bai Shao Yao	*Paeonia*	6 - 9 g
Sheng Jiang	*Zingiber*	3 - 6 g
Da Zao	*Ziziphus*	3 - 4 pc
Gan Cao	*Glycyrrhiza*	3 - 6 g
Rou Gui	*Cinnamomum*	3 - 9 g

Heart and Kidneys are not communicating. Kidney yang deficiency leads to Heart yang deficiency causing palpitations, cool limbs, or insomnia.

T pale, swollen, thin moist white coat

P deep, weak

JIAO TAI WAN

Grand Communication Pill

Extract Formula Name: Coptis and Cinnamon Formula

Huang Lian	*Coptis*	18 - 20 g
Rou Gui	*Cinnamomum*	3 - 6 g

Heart yang is not warmed by the Kidneys leading to water accumulation which rises upwards causing abdominal pain, angina, Stomach cramping, tingling sensation in the abdomen, (ben ten qi - running piglet sensation), or scanty urine.

T pale, wet, sticky white coat

P deep, weak, slightly slow

✪ Major Formula

LING GUI ZAO GAN TANG

Poria, Cinnamon Twig, Jujube, and Licorice Decoction

Fu Ling	*Poria*	9 - 12 g
Gui Zhi	*Cinnamomum*	3 - 9 g
Da Zao	*Ziziphus*	3 - 4 pc
Gan Cao	*Glycyrrhiza*	3 - 6 g

Spleen/Lung qi and blood deficiency with Heart yang deficiency, or ying level deficiency. The patient is easily startled, experiences shortness of breath, lack of taste sensation, insomnia, or palpitations. This formula is also useful for irregular periods or uterine bleeding.

T pale, swollen

P weak

REN SHEN YANG YING TANG

Ginseng Decoction to Nourish the Nutritive Qi

Extract Formula Name: Ginseng Combination

Bai Shao Yao	*Paeonia*	9 - 15 g
Chen Pi	*Citrus*	3 - 6 g
Dang Gui	*Angelica*	3 - 9 g
Ren Shen	*Panax*	6 - 9 g
Huang Qi	*Astragalus*	6 - 12 g
Bai Zhu	*Atractylodes*	6 - 9 g
Shu Di Huang	*Rehmannia*	3 - 6 g
Wu Wei Zi	*Schisandra*	3 - 6 g
Fu Ling	*Poria*	3 - 6 g
Yuan Zhi	*Polygala*	2 - 6 g
Rou Gui	*Cinnamomum*	6 - 9 g
Gan Cao	*Glycyrrhiza*	3 - 6 g
[Da Zao	*Ziziphus*	2 pc]
[Gan Jiang	*Zingiber*	3 pc]

HEART YIN DEFICIENCY

- insomnia with dream-disturbed sleep
- restlessness
- malarflush
- afternoon fever

T red, scanty coat, red tip

P thin, rapid, or empty

Kidney yin deficiency can't nourish the Heart which leads to Heart blood deficiency. Symptoms include insomnia, dizziness, poor memory, excessive dreaming, or night sweating.

T slightly red, or pale, scanty coat

P thin, rapid

BAI ZI YANG XIN WAN

Biota Seed Pill to Nourish the Heart

Bai Zi Ren	*Biota*	3 - 9 g
Mai Men Dong	*Ophiopogon*	6 - 9 g
Dang Gui	*Angelica*	6 - 12 g
Gou Qi Zi	*Lycium*	6 - 9 g
Xuan Shen	*Scrophularia*	6 - 12 g
Fu Shen	*Poria*	6 - 9 g
Shi Chang Pu	*Acorus*	6 - 9 g
Shu Di Huang	*Rehmannia*	12 - 15 g
Gan Cao	*Glycyrrhiza*	3 - 6 g

Mental disorder due to 1. Liver qi stagnation (use with Xiao Yao San); 2. Liver qi stagnation with fire burning the yin (use with Wen Dan Tang); 3. Yin deficiency with fire injuring the Heart.

T red, scanty coat

P thin, rapid

GAN MAI DA ZAO TANG

Licorice, Wheat, and Jujube Decoction

Extract Formula Name: Licorice and Jujube Combination

Gan Cao	*Glycyrrhiza*	9 - 12 g
Fu Xiao Mai	*Triticum*	9 - 15 g
Da Zao	*Ziziphus*	10 pc

Taiyang disease or inappropriate warming therapy causing Heart yang deficiency with yin deficiency. This leads to disturbed shen, restlessness, mania, sweating, palpitations, or insomnia.

T pale or red, thin white or yellowish coat

P weak, thin

GUI ZHI GAN CAO LONG GU MU LI TANG

Cinnamon Twig, Licorice, Dragon Bone, and Oyster Shell Decoction

Gui Zhi	*Cinnamomum*	3 - 6 g
Zhi Gan Cao	*Glycyrrhiza ,*	6 g
Long Gu	*Os Draconis*	6 - 15 g
Mu Li	*Ostrea*	6 - 15 g

Kidneys and Heart are not harmonizing accompanied with yin and yang deficiency. Symptoms include spermatorrhea, sexual dreams, or poor sleep.

T pale

P slow, hollow, weak

GUI ZHI JIA LONG GU MU LI TANG

Cinnamon Twig Decoction plus Dragon Bone and Oyster Shell

Extract Formula Name: Cinnamon and Dragon Bone Combination

Gui Zhi	*Cinnamomum*	6 - 9 g
Bai Shao Yao	*Paeonia*	6 - 9 g
Sheng Jiang	*Zingiber*	6 - 9 g
Da Zao	*Ziziphus*	4 - 12 pc
Mu Li	*Ostrea*	6 - 9 g
Long Gu	*Os Draconis*	6 - 9 g
Gan Cao	*Glycyrrhiza*	3 - 6 g

Heart/Kidney yin deficiency with fire after febrile disease leading to insomnia, palpitations, or tongue sores: shaoyin deficient heat syndrome.

T red, scanty coat

P rapid, thin

☞ E Jiao - Equus and egg yolks should be dissolved into the strained tea.

HUANG LIAN E JIAO TANG

Coptis and Ass-Hide Gelatin Decoction

Extract Formula Name: Coptis and Gelatin Combination

Huang Lian	*Coptis*	9 - 12 g
E Jiao	*Equus*	6 - 9 g
Huang Qin	*Scutellaria*	6 - 9 g
Bai Shao Yao	*Paeonia*	6 - 9 g
Ji Zi Huang	*Egg yolks*	2

1. Yin/blood deficiency with heat causing arrhythmia of the Heart. 2. High fever causing arrhythmia: yangming disease depleted yin which leads to an irregular Heart beat.

T red, scanty coat

P rapid, irregular

☞ E Jiao - Equus should be dissolved at the end into the strained tea.

JIA JIAN FU MAI TANG

Modified Restore-the-Pulse Decoction

Zhi Gan Cao	*Glycyrrhiza*	12 - 15 g
Bai Shao Yao	*Paeonia*	12 - 15 g
Mai Men Dong	*Ophiopogon*	9 - 12 g
Sheng Di Huang	*Rehmannia*	12 - 15 g
Huo Ma Ren	*Cannabis*	9 - 12 g
E Jiao	*Equus*	6 - 9 g

Qi and wei qi deficiency leading to spontaneous sweating which eventually injures the Heart yin. This leads to night sweating, insomnia, and palpitations.

T pale or red

P frail, thin

MU LI SAN

Oyster Shell Powder

Mu Li	*Ostrea*	15 - 30 g
Ma Huang Gen	*Ephredra*	3 - 9 g
Huang Qi	*Astragalus*	9 - 12 g
Fu Xiao Mai	*Triticum*	15 - 30 g

Heart yin/blood deficiency with false heat causing insomnia, poor memory, or restlessness.

T pale or red

P thin, rapid

✪ **Major Formula**

SUAN ZAO REN TANG

Sour Jujube Decoction

Extract Formula Name: Zizyphus Combination

Suan Zao Ren	*Ziziphus*	12 - 15 g
Fu Ling	*Poria*	6 - 9 g
Chuan Xiong	*Ligusticum*	3 - 9 g
Zhi Mu	*Anemarrhena*	6 - 12 g
Gan Cao	*Glycyrrhiza*	3 - 6 g

Heart/Kidney yin deficiency, Heart blood deficiency and false heat where Kidneys and Heart don't harmonize. This leads to insomnia, restlessness, palpitations, poor memory, or night sweats.

T red

P rapid, thin

✘ Zhu Sha - Cinnabaris is toxic and should only be used short-term.

✪ **Major Formula!**

TIAN WANG BU XIN DAN

Emperor of Heaven's Special Pill to Tonify the Heart

Extract Formula Name: Ginseng and Zizyphus Formula

Ren Shen	*Panax*	9 - 12 g
Mai Men Dong	*Ophiopogon*	6 - 12 g
Tian Men Dong	*Asparagus*	6 - 9 g
Xuan Shen	*Scrophularia*	6 - 9 g
Dan Shen	*Salvia*	6 - 12 g
Sheng Di Huang	*Rehmannia*	15 - 30 g
Fu Ling	*Poria*	6 - 9 g
Wu Wei Zi	*Schisandra*	6 - 9 g
Jie Geng	*Platycodon*	3 - 6 g
Yuan Zhi	*Polygala*	6 - 9 g
Bai Zi Ren	*Biota*	6 - 9 g
Dang Gui	*Angelica*	6 - 9 g
Suan Zao Ren	*Ziziphus*	6 - 12 g
Zhu Sha	*Cinnabaris*	1 - 3 g

Kidney and Liver yin/blood deficiency with fire which bothers the Heart. This causes Heart and Liver fire or Liver yang excess leading to excessive dreaming, insomnia, or outbursts of anger.

T red, cracks, thin or thick yellow coat

P rapid, wiry, thin

☞ Ingredients should be powdered, made into 9 - 12 g pills and taken three times a day. Xi Jiao - Rhinoceros should be substituted with Shui Niu Jiao - Bubalus.

ZHEN ZHU MU WAN

Mother-Of-Pearl Pill

Zhen Zhu Mu	*Pteria*	15 - 20 g
Ren Shen	*Panax*	9 - 12 g
Dang Gui	*Angelica*	6 - 12 g
Shu Di Huang	*Rehmannia*	9 - 12 g
Suan Zao Ren	*Ziziphus*	6 - 9 g
Bai Zi Ren	*Biota*	6 - 9 g
Fu Shen	*Poria*	6 - 9 g
Chen Xiang	*Aquilaria*	6 - 9 g
Xi Jiao	*Rhinoceros*	1 - 3 g

Heart qi/blood or yin deficiency causing arrhythmia, insomnia, pressure in the chest, coronary Heart disease, and anxiety.

T pale or red, thin white coat

P weak

☞ E Jiao - Equus should be dissolved into the strained tea.

ZHI GAN CAO TANG

Honey-Fried Licorice Decoction

Extract Formula Name: Baked Licorice Combination

Zhi Gan Cao	*Glycyrrhiza*	12 - 15 g
Sheng Di Huang	*Rehmannia*	30 g
Ren Shen	*Panax*	6 - 9 g
Gui Zhi	*Cinnamomum*	6 - 9 g
Huo Ma Ren	*Cannabis*	6 - 9 g
Mai Men Dong	*Ophiopogon*	9 g
E Jiao	*Equus*	6 g
Da Zao	*Ziziphus*	6 - 9 pc
Sheng Jiang	*Zingiber*	6 - 9 g

Heart fire with qi/blood/yin deficiency causing mental depression, heat in the chest, excessive dreaming, or palpitations. This formula acts as a sedative.

T red, thin coat

P rapid, thin

☞ Either grind all herbs and take 6 - 9 g twice a day; or decoct and add Zhu Sha - Cinnabaris at the end of the decoction process.

✘ Zhu Sha - Cinnabaris is toxic and should not be used over a long period of time.

ZHU SHA AN SHEN WAN

Cinnabaris Pill to Calm the Spirit

Extract Formula Name: Cinnabaris Formula

Zhu Sha	*Cinnabaris*	3 - 9 g
Huang Lian	*Coptis*	6 - 12 g
Dang Gui	*Angelica*	3 - 6 g
Sheng Di Huang	*Rehmannia*	3 - 6 g
Zhi Gan Cao	*Glycyrrhiza*	6 - 9 g

HEART PHLEGM ACCUMULATION

- stuffiness in the chest
- mental disorientation, or mania
- lethargy
- rattling sound in the throat

T thick sticky coat

P slippery

Severe Heart phlegm accumulation and qi stagnation with yang deficiency. Angina can be severe, and the patient experiences numbness radiating down the arm, shortness of breath: chest bi-syndrome.

T pale, light purple, wet, thick sticky white coat

P slippery

✪ **Major Formula**

GUA LOU XIE BAI BAN XIA TANG

Trichosanthes Fruit, Chinese Chive, and Pinellia Decoction

Extract Formula Name: Trichosanthes, Bakeri and Pinellia Combination

Gua Lou	*Trichosanthes*	9 - 12 g
Xie Bai	*Allium*	6 - 9 g
Ban Xia	*Pinellia*	9 - 12 g
Bai Jiu	*White Wine*	30 cc

Damp cold and phlegm causing sudden collapse, clenched jaw, or coma; or qi stagnation or damp cold leading to coldness in the chest and abdomen or chest pain, coma, or qi stagnation from an epidemic manifesting in fullness in the chest. The patient feels the urge to vomit or defecate but is unable to do so, which then leads to sudden loss of consciousness.

T pale

P slow, slippery

☞ The prescription is made into pills. Xi Jiao - Rhinoceros should be substituted with Shui Niu Jiao - Bubalus.

✘ Do not use during pregnancy. Zhu Sha - Cinnabaris is toxic, and should only be used short-term.

SU HE XIANG WAN

Liquid Styrax Pill

Extract Formula Name: Styrax Formula

Su He Xiang	*Liquidambar*	30 g
She Xiang	*Moschus*	60 g
Bing Pian	*Dryobalanops*	30 g
An Xi Xiang	*Styrax*	60 g
Ru Xiang	*Boswellia*	30 g
Tan Xiang	*Santalum*	60 g
Ding Xiang	*Eugenia*	60 g
Bi Ba	*Piper*	60 g
Xiang Fu	*Cyperus*	60 g
Xi Jiao	*Rhinoceros*	60 g
Bai Zhu	*Atractylodes*	60 g
He Zi	*Terminalia*	60 g
Zhu Sha	*Cinnabaris*	60 g
Mu Xiang	*Saussurea*	60 g
Chen Xiang	*Aquilaria*	60 g

Severe chest phlegm and qi stagnation leading to fullness, tightness, or cramping in the chest, with rebellious Stomach qi symptoms such as nausea and vomiting.

T purple, thick sticky white or yellowish coat

P slippery or wiry

ZHI SHI GUA LOU GUI ZHI TANG

Immature Bitter Orange, Trichosanthes Fruit, and Cinnamon Twig Decoction

Gua Lou Ren	*Trichosanthes*	6 - 12 g
Zhi Shi	*Citrus*	9 - 12 g
Xie Bai	*Allium*	9 - 12 g
Gui Zhi	*Cinnamomum*	3 - 6 g
Hou Po	*Magnolia*	12 - 15 g

HEART PHLEGM FIRE

- insomnia with dream-disturbed sleep
- mental restlessness
- muttering to oneself, or uncontrolled laughter
- speech impairment

T red, red tip, sticky yellow coat

P slippery, rapid

Phlegm fire obstructing the orifice causing mania, severe palpitations, cough with profuse phlegm, dizziness, wheezing, anxiety, bad dreams, or lumps in the neck.

T red, thick yellow sticky coat

P wiry, rapid, forceful

☞ Herbs should be made into 6 - 9 g pills. Adults take one pill one or two times a day.

✘ Do not use during pregnancy or post-partum.

GUN TAN WAN

Vaporize Phlegm Pill

Extract Formula Name: Lapis and Scute Formula

Da Huang	*Rheum*	200 - 240 g
Huang Qin	*Scutellaria*	200 - 240 g
Meng Shi	*Lapis Micae Seu Chloriti*	20 - 30 g
Chen Xiang	*Aquilaria*	9 - 15 g

Heart phlegm fire causing agitation, insomnia, mania, laughing or screaming without apparent reason, or severe head pain. There can be an underlying Liver qi stagnation and Spleen qi deficiency which further leads to phlegm stagnation..

T red, sticky yellow coat

P rapid, slippery, wiry

✘ Zhu Sha - Cinnabaris is toxic and should be used in small amounts. Do not use during pregnancy.

SHENG TIE LUO YIN

Iron Filings Decoction

Extract Formula Name: Iron Filings Combination

Sheng Tie Luo	*Frusta Ferri*	30 - 60 g
Dan Nan Xing	*Arisaema*	1 - 3 g
Zhe Bei Mu	*Fritillaria*	3 - 6 g
Mai Men Dong	*Ophiopogon*	6 - 9 g
Xuan Shen	*Scrophularia*	6 - 9 g
Tian Men Dong	*Asparagus*	6 - 9 g
Fu Shen	*Poria*	3 - 6 g
Fu Ling	*Poria*	3 - 6 g
Lian Qiao	*Forsythia*	3 - 6 g
Dan Shen	*Salvia*	3 - 6 g
Shi Chang Pu	*Acorus*	3 - 6 g
Gou Teng	*Uncaria*	3 - 6 g
Chen Pi	*Citrus*	3 - 6 g
Yuan Zhi	*Polygala*	3 - 6 g
Zhu Sha	*Cinnabaris*	0.5 g

HEART BLOOD DEFICIENCY

- pale face
- anxiety
- insomnia with dream-disturbed sleep
- dizziness

T pale, thin and narrow, dry

P thin

Heart blood and yin deficiency with Spleen qi deficiency leading to insomnia, decreased appetite, nightmares, irregular periods in women, or uterine bleeding which may manifest as beng lou – gushing or spotting. This formula is also useful for purpura due to Spleen qi/blood deficiency.

T pale, swollen, teethmarks, thin white coat

P weak, thin

✪ **Major Formula**

GUI PI TANG

Restore the Spleen Decoction

Extract Formula Name: Ginseng and Longan Combination

Ren Shen	*Panax*	6 - 9 g
Huang Qi	*Astralagus*	9 - 12 g
Fu Shen	*Poria*	6 - 9 g
Bai Zhu	*Atractylodes*	9 - 12 g
Long Yan Rou	*Euphoria*	9 - 12 g
Mu Xiang	*Saussurea*	3 - 6 g
Suan Zao Ren	*Zizyphus*	9 - 12 g
Dang Gui	*Angelica*	6 - 9 g
Yuan Zhi	*Polygala*	3 - 6 g
Gan Cao	*Glycyrrhiza*	3 - 6 g

1. Yin/blood deficiency with heat causing arrhythmia of the Heart. 2. High fever causing arrhythmia: yangming disease depleted yin which leads to an irregular Heart beat.

T red, scanty coat

P rapid, irregular

☞ E Jiao - Equus should be dissolved at the end into the strained tea.

JIA JIAN FU MAI TANG

Modified Restore-the-Pulse Decoction

Zhi Gan Cao	*Glycyrrhiza*	12 - 15 g
Bai Shao Yao	*Paeonia*	12 - 15 g
Mai Men Dong	*Ophiopogon*	9 - 12 g
Sheng Di Huang	*Rehmannia*	12 - 15 g
Huo Ma Ren	*Cannabis*	9 - 12 g
E Jiao	*Equus*	6 - 9 g

Heart qi blood deficiency causing insomnia, anxiety, restlessness, and poor memory.

T pale

P weak, thin

YANG XIN TANG

Nourish the Heart Decoction

Extract Formula Name: Astragalus and Zizyphus Combination

Sheng Di Huang	*Rehmannia*	6 - 12 g
Shu Di Huang	*Rehmannia*	6 - 12 g
Dang Gui	*Angelica*	6 - 9 g
Ren Shen	*Panax*	6 - 12 g
Mai Men Dong	*Ophiopogon*	6 - 9 g
Suan Zao Ren	*Ziziphus*	6 - 9 g
Fu Shen	*Poria*	6 - 9 g
Bai Zi Ren	*Biota*	6 - 9 g
Wu Wei Zi	*Schisandra*	6 - 9 g
Gan Cao	*Glycyrrhiza*	3 - 6 g
[Lian Zi	*Nelumbo*	3 - 6 g]
[Deng Xin Cao	*Juncus*	3 - 6 g]

Kidney and Liver yin/blood deficiency with fire which bothers the Heart. This causes Heart and Liver fire or Liver yang excess leading to excessive dreaming, insomnia, or outbursts of anger.

T red, cracks, thin or thick yellow coat

P rapid, wiry, thin

☞ Ingredients should be powdered, made into 9 - 12 g pills and taken three times a day. Xi Jiao - Rhinoceros should be substituted with Shui Niu Jiao - Bubalus.

ZHEN ZHU MU WAN

Mother-Of-Pearl Pill

Zhen Zhu Mu	*Pteria*	15 - 20 g
Ren Shen	*Panax*	9 - 12 g
Dang Gui	*Angelica*	6 - 12 g
Shu Di Huang	*Rehmannia*	9 - 12 g
Suan Zao Ren	*Ziziphus*	6 - 9 g
Bai Zi Ren	*Biota*	6 - 9 g
Fu Shen	*Poria*	6 - 9 g
Chen Xiang	*Aquilaria*	6 - 9 g
Xi Jiao	*Rhinoceros*	1 - 3 g

Heart qi/blood or yin deficiency causing arrhythmia, insomnia, pressure in the chest, coronary Heart disease, and anxiety.

T pale or red, thin white coat

P weak

☞ E Jiao - Equus should be dissolved into the strained tea.

ZHI GAN CAO TANG

Honey-Fried Licorice Decoction

Extract Formula Name: Baked Licorice Combination

Zhi Gan Cao	*Glycyrrhiza*	12 - 15 g
Sheng Di Huang	*Rehmannia*	30 g
Ren Shen	*Panax*	6 - 9 g
Gui Zhi	*Cinnamomum*	6 - 9 g
Huo Ma Ren	*Cannabis*	6 - 9 g
Mai Men Dong	*Ophiopogon*	9 g
E Jiao	*Equus*	6 g
Da Zao	*Ziziphus*	6 - 9 pc
Sheng Jiang	*Zingiber*	6 - 9 g

Heart fire with qi/blood/yin deficiency causing mental depression, heat in the chest, excessive dreaming, or palpitations. This formula acts as a sedative.

T red, thin coat

P rapid, thin

☞ Either grind all herbs and take 6 - 9 g twice a day; or decoct and add Zhu Sha - Cinnabaris at the end of the decoction process.

✘ Zhu Sha - Cinnabaris is toxic and should not be used over a long period of time.

ZHU SHA AN SHEN WAN

Cinnabaris Pill to Calm the Spirit

Extract Formula Name: Cinnabaris Formula

Zhu Sha	*Cinnabaris*	3 - 9 g
Huang Lian	*Coptis*	6 - 12 g
Dang Gui	*Angelica*	3 - 6 g
Sheng Di Huang	*Rehmannia*	3 - 6 g
Zhi Gan Cao	*Glycyrrhiza*	6 - 9 g

HEART BLOOD STAGNATION

- tightness in the chest
- pain in the chest which may radiate down the left arm
- cyanotic lips and nails
- cold extremities

T purple

P knotted

Qi stagnation in the upper and middle jiao with slow blood circulation causing intermittent chest pain, and epigastric or abdominal discomfort.

T purple

P choppy

DAN SHEN YIN

Salvia Decoction

Dan Shen	Salvia	30 g
Sha Ren	Amomum	5 g
Tan Xiang	Santalum	5 g

Severe Heart phlegm accumulation and qi stagnation with yang deficiency. Angina can be severe, and the patient experiences numbness radiating down the arm, shortness of breath: chest bi-syndrome.

T pale, light purple, wet, thick sticky white coat

P slippery

GUA LOU XIE BAI BAN XIA TANG

Trichosanthes Fruit, Chinese Chive, and Pinellia Decoction

Extract Formula Name: Trichosanthes, Bakeri and Pinellia Combination

Gua Lou	Trichosanthes	9 - 12 g
Xie Bai	Allium	6 - 9 g
Ban Xia	Pinellia	9 - 12 g
Bai Jiu	White Wine	30 cc

Blood stagnation in head, chest, and diaphragm causing angina, palpitations, insomnia, nightmares, or dysmenorrhea.

T purple or purple spots

P wiry

✘ Do not use during pregnancy.

✪ **Major Formula**

XUE FU ZHU YU TANG

Drive out Stasis in the Mansion of Blood Decoction

Extract Formula Name: Persica and Achyranthes Combination

Dang Gui	*Angelica*	6 - 9 g
Chuan Xiong	*Ligusticum*	3 - 9 g
Sheng Di Huang	*Rehmannia*	6 - 9 g
Chi Shao Yao	*Paeonia*	6 - 9 g
Tao Ren	*Prunus*	6 - 12 g
Hong Hua	*Carthamus*	6 - 9 g
Chuan Niu Xi	*Cyathula*	9 - 12 g
Jie Geng	*Platycodon*	3 - 6 g
Zhi Ke	*Citrus*	3 - 6 g
Chai Hu	*Bupleurum*	3 - 9 g
Gan Cao	*Glycyrrhiza*	3 - 6 g

HEART FIRE

- mental restlessness and agitation
- redness in the face
- mouth or tongue sores

T red, red tip, yellow coat

P forceful, rapid

Heart/Pericardium fire with toxic heat and fever which congeals into phlegm. This leads to delirium, coma, aphasia, or convulsions in children.

T dark red, sticky yellow coat

P rapid, forceful, wiry

☞ Herbs should be ground and made into 3 g pills. The adult dosage is one pill two to three times a day. Xi Jiao - Rhinoceros should be substituted with Shui Niu Jiao - Bubalus.

✘ Do not use during pregnancy. Do not take over a prolonged period of time. Note that Zhu Sha - Cinnabaris is toxic.

✪ **Major Formula**

AN GONG NIU HUANG WAN

Calm the Palace Pill with Cattle Gallstone

Extract Formula Name: Bos and Curcuma Formula

Niu Huang	*Bos*	25 - 30 g
Xi Jiao	*Rhinoceros*	25 - 30 g
She Xiang	*Moschus*	7.5 g
Huang Lian	*Coptis*	25 - 30 g
Zhi Zi	*Gardenia*	25 - 30 g
Huang Qin	*Scutellaria*	25 - 30 g
Bing Pian	*Dryobalanops*	7.5 g
Zhen Zhu Mu	*Pteria*	12 - 15 g
Yu Jin	*Curcuma*	25 - 30 g
Xiong Huang	*Realgar*	25 - 30 g
Zhu Sha	*Cinnabaris*	25 - 30 g

Heart fire and yang rising leading to severe insomnia, palpitations, hearing, or vision loss. The Kidneys and Heart don't harmonize.

T red, yellow coat

P rapid, maybe wiry

☞ Ingredients should be ground into powder, then made into pills with honey.

✘ Zhu Sha - Cinnabaris is toxic and should only be used short-term. Do not use during pregnancy.

CI ZHU WAN

Magnetite and Cinnabar Pill

Ci Shi	*Magnetitum*	60 g
Zhu Sha	*Cinnabaris*	30 g
Shen Qu	*Massa Fermentata*	120 g

Heart fire leading to Small Intestine fire, which in turn leads to Bladder damp heat causing hematuria, frequent urination, urinary retention, thirst, or tongue sores.

T bright red, sticky yellow coat

P rapid, wiry

DAO CHI SAN

Guide Out the Red Powder

Extract Formula Name: Rehmannia and Akebia Formula

Sheng Di Huang	*Rehmannia*	9 - 20 g
Dan Zhu Ye	*Lophatherum*	6 - 9 g
Mu Tong	*Akebia*	6 - 9 g
Gan Cao	*Glycyrrhiza*	3 - 6 g

Upper jiao heat with middle jiao cold usually caused by cold food which restricts Spleen qi. This leads to damp which then turns to heat. The heat rises upward and bothers the Heart causing thirst, restlessness, full/cold abdomen with pain, or nausea and vomiting.

T red or pale, red tip, thin sticky coat

P rapid, wiry

HUANG LIAN TANG

Coptis Decoction

Extract Formula Name: Coptis Combination

Huang Lian	*Coptis*	5 g
Gan Jiang	*Zingiber*	5 g
Gui Zhi	*Cinnamomum*	5 g
Ren Shen	*Panax*	3 g
Ban Xia	*Pinellia*	9 g
Da Zao	*Ziziphus*	9 - 12 pc
Gan Cao	*Glycyrrhiza*	6 g

Heart fire and excess heat leading to nose bleeding or premenstrual vomiting.

T red, yellow coat

P rapid, or empty

✘ Caution during pregnancy.

SAN HUANG SI WU TANG

Three-Yellow and Four-Substance Decoction

Shu Di Huang	*Rehmannia*	6 - 15 g
Bai Shao Yao	*Paeonia*	6 - 9 g
Chuan Xiong	*Ligusticum*	3 - 9 g
Dang Gui	*Angelica*	6 - 9 g
Huang Lian	*Coptis*	3 - 9 g
Da Huang	*Rheum*	6 - 12 g
Huang Qin	*Scutellaria*	6 - 9 g

Heart/Stomach fire with damp leading to fever, jaundice, fullness, alternating diarrhea or constipation, mouth and tongue sores, or carbuncles.

T dark red, yellow coat

P flooding, rapid

✘ Caution during pregnancy.

XIE XIN TANG

Drain the Epigastrium Decoction

Extract Formula Name: Coptis and Rhubarb Combination

Da Huang	*Rheum*	6 - 9 g
Huang Lian	*Coptis*	3 - 6 g
Huang Qin	*Scutellaria*	6 - 9 g

Heart fire with qi/blood/yin deficiency causing mental depression, heat in the chest, excessive dreaming, or palpitations. This formula acts as a sedative.

T red, thin coat

P rapid, thin

☞ Either grind all herbs and take 6 - 9 g twice a day; or decoct and add Zhu Sha - Cinnabaris at the end of the decoction process.

✘ Zhu Sha - Cinnabaris is toxic and should not be used over a long period of time.

ZHU SHA AN SHEN WAN

Cinnabaris Pill to Calm the Spirit

Extract Formula Name: Cinnabaris Formula

Zhu Sha	*Cinnabaris*	3 - 9 g
Huang Lian	*Coptis*	6 - 12 g
Dang Gui	*Angelica*	3 - 6 g
Sheng Di Huang	*Rehmannia*	3 - 6 g
Zhi Gan Cao	*Glycyrrhiza*	6 - 9 g

COLLAPSE OF YANG

- profuse and spontaneous sweating
- cyanotic lips
- shallow breathing
- palpitations

T purple or pale

P minute

Severe yang deficiency and cold causes the yang to be pushed superficially leading to superficial false yang symptoms. The patient gives the appearance that he/she will get better but in reality may die soon. Symptoms include diarrhea, low fever, or red face. Internal cold with superficial false heat: shaoyin syndrome.

T pale, red tip

P deep, faint

BAI TONG TANG

White Penetrating Decoction

Gan Jiang	*Zingiber*	3 - 6 g
Fu Zi	*Aconitum*	3 - 9 g
Cong Bai	*Allium*	3 - 6 g

Shock with severe sweating and qi loss after hemorrhaging or Heart failure.

T pale

P hollow or frail

DU SHEN TANG

Unaccompanied Ginseng Decoction

Ren Shen	*Panax*	30 g
[Da Zao	*Ziziphus*	3 - 6 g]

Kidney and Spleen yang deficiency with cold which has invaded all three yin channels (taiyin, shaoyin, and jueyin). Symptoms include shivering from cold, icy limbs and face, watery diarrhea, or cough with profuse saliva production.

T pale, wet, thin white moist coat

P minute or frail

☞ Remove She Xiang - Moschus, decoct the rest of the formula as usual, then add powdered Moschus to each dosage.

HUI YANG JIU JI TANG

Restore and Revive the Yang Decoction

Fu Zi	*Aconitum*	9 g
Rou Gui	*Cinnamomum*	3 - 6 g
Ren Shen	*Panax*	6 - 9 g
Gan Jiang	*Zingiber*	3 - 6 g
Fu Ling	*Poria*	6 - 9 g
Chen Pi	*Citrus*	3 - 6 g
Bai Zhu	*Atractylodes*	6 - 9 g
Wu Wei Zi	*Schisandra*	3 - 6 g
Ban Xia	*Pinellia*	6 - 9 g
Gan Cao	*Glycyrrhiza*	3 - 6 g
She Xiang	*Moschus*	0.3 g
[Sheng Jiang	*Zingiber*	1 - 3 g]

Severe yang and blood loss causing collapse and dehydration after sweating and diarrhea. The patient has cold extremities or chills.

T pale

P thin or hollow

SI NI JIA REN SHEN TANG

Frigid Extremities Decoction plus Ginseng

Extract Formula Name: G.L. and Aconite Combination with Ginseng

Fu Zi	*Aconitum*	6 - 9 g
Gan Jiang	*Zingiber*	3 - 6 g
Zhi Gan Cao	*Glycyrrhiza*	3 - 6 g
Ren Shen	*Panax*	6 - 9 g

Exterior cold has gone internally. qi and yang are very weak and Kidney/Spleen yang have been damaged. Symptoms include low blood pressure, cold limbs, shock, or sweating.

T pale, or purple, moist white coat

P minute

☞ The raw type of Aconite is used here since it is much warmer than the prepared kind. 6 - 12 g of honey are often added for detoxification. Fu Zi - Aconitum is soaked in 8 - 10 cups of boiling water for 30 minutes to one hour. The remaining herbs should be added during the last 25 minutes and decocted as usual.

✘ Fu Zi - Aconitum in its raw form is toxic and is intended for short-term use only.

✪ Major Formula

SI NI TANG

Frigid Extremities Decoction

Extract Formula Name: Aconite, Ginger and Licorice Combination

Fu Zi	*Aconitum*	9 - 15 g
Gan Jiang	*Zingiber*	6 - 12 g
Zhi Gan Cao	*Glycyrrhiza*	3 - 6 g

Shaoyin disease: severe yang deficiency with cold accumulation which causes false yang to be pushed to the exterior. The yang cannot stay in the interior causing icy limbs upon touch but no cold intolerance, flushed face, thirst without desire to drink, or a dry throat.

T pale, light purple, teethmarks, thin white coat

P slow, minute

TONG MAI SI NI TANG

Unblock the Pulse Decoction for Frigid Extremities

Extract Formula Name: Licorice, Aconite and Ginger Pulse Combination

Fu Zi	*Aconitum*	12 - 15 g
Gan Jiang	*Zingiber*	9 - 12 g
Gan Cao	*Glycyrrhiza*	3 - 6 g

SPLEEN DISHARMONIES

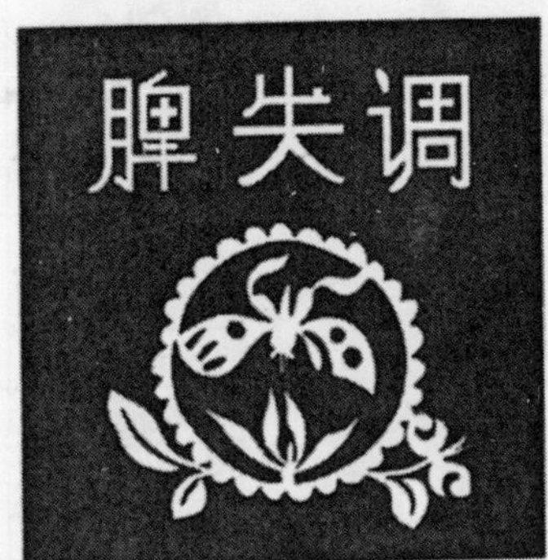

SPLEEN QI DEFICIENCY

- fatigue, especially after eating
- decreased appetite and lassitude
- pale or sallow complexion
- abdominal distention or fullness
- loose stools

T pale, swollen, teethmarks

P weak

Spleen qi deficiency causing morning sickness, a restless fetus, loose stools, or poor appetite.

T pale, swollen, white coat

P weak

BAO TAI ZI SHENG WAN

Protect the Fetus and Aid Life Pill

Ren Shen	*Panax*	6 - 9 g
Fu Ling	*Poria*	6 - 9 g
Bai Zhu	*Atractylodes*	6 - 9 g
Gan Cao	*Glycyrrhiza*	3 - 6 g
Lian Zi	*Nelumbo*	6 - 9 g
Bian Dou	*Dolichos*	6 - 9 g
Huo Xiang	*Agastache*	6 - 9 g
Bai Dou Kou	*Amomum*	3 - 6 g
Chen Pi	*Citrus*	3 - 6 g
Jie Geng	*Platycodon*	3 - 6 g
Shan Yao	*Dioscorea*	6 - 9 g
Yi Yi Ren	*Coix*	6 - 12 g
Ze Xie	*Alisma*	6 - 9 g
Mai Ya	*Hordeum*	12 - 20 g
Qian Shi	*Euryale*	6 - 9 g
Shan Zha	*Crataegus*	6 - 12 g
Huang Lian	*Coptis*	3 g

Spleen/Source qi deficiency resulting in low-grade fever, fatigue, or loose stools. Purpura due to qi/yang deficiency. Pediatric department: measles, chickenpox, or smallpox which turn to purpura, and may result in shock.

T pale, white coat

P weak

BAO YUAN TANG

Preserve the Basal Decoction

Extract Formula Name: Astragalus, Ginseng, and Cinnamon Combination

Ren Shen	*Panax*	6 - 9 g
Huang Qi	*Astragalus*	6 - 12 g
Rou Gui	*Cinnamomum*	6 - 9 g
Gan Cao	*Glycyrrhiza*	3 - 6 g

Spleen/Stomach qi deficiency where the Spleen qi is sinking, or the Spleen is not governing the blood. qi deficiency can lead to (morning) fever, early periods, weakness, diarrhea, or pallor.

T pale, swollen, teethmarks, thin white coat

P weak

BU ZHONG YI QI TANG

Tonify the Middle and Augment the Qi Decoction

Extract Formula Name: Ginseng and Astragalus Combination

Ren Shen	*Panax*	6 - 12 g
Huang Qi	*Astragalus*	9 - 15 g
Dang Gui	*Angelica*	6 - 9 g
Chen Pi	*Citrus*	3 - 6 g
Sheng Ma	*Cimicifuga*	3 - 6 g
Chai Hu	*Bupleurum*	3 - 9 g
Bai Zhu	*Atractylodes*	3 - 9 g
Zhi Gan Cao	*Glycyrrhiza*	3 - 6 g

Heat and cold in the middle jiao with Spleen/Stomach qi deficiency, and cold predominance. The patient experiences mild middle jiao qi stagnation symptoms such as fullness or bloating.

T thin yellow coat

P weak, slightly wiry

GAN CAO XIE XIN TANG

Licorice Decoction to Drain the Epigastrium

Extract Formula Name: Pinellia and Licorice Combination

Ban Xia	*Pinellia*	6 - 9 g
Huang Qin	*Scutellaria*	9 - 12 g
Zhi Gan Cao	*Glycyrrhiza*	12 - 15 g
Gan Jiang	*Zingiber*	9 - 12 g
Ren Shen	*Panax*	9 - 12 g
Huang Lian	*Coptis*	3 - 6 g
Da Zao	*Ziziphus*	9 - 15 pc

Spleen/Stomach qi deficiency and cold causing vomiting during pregnancy.

T pale, thin white coat

P weak

GAN JIANG REN SHEN BAN XIA WAN

Ginger, Ginseng, and Pinellia Pill

Extract Formula Name: G.P. and Ginseng Formula

Gan Jiang	*Zingiber*	3 g
Ren Shen	*Panax*	3 g
Ban Xia	*Pinellia*	6 g
[Sheng Jiang	*Zingiber*	1 - 3 g]

Heart blood and yin deficiency with Spleen qi deficiency leading to insomnia, decreased appetite, nightmares, irregular periods in women, or uterine bleeding which may manifest as beng lou – gushing or spotting. This formula is also useful for purpura due to Spleen qi/blood deficiency.

T pale, swollen, teethmarks, thin white coat

P weak, thin

GUI PI TANG

Restore the Spleen Decoction

Extract Formula Name: Ginseng and Longan Combination

Ren Shen	*Panax*	6 - 9 g
Huang Qi	*Astralagus*	9 - 12 g
Fu Shen	*Poria*	6 - 9 g
Bai Zhu	*Atractylodes*	9 - 12 g
Long Yan Rou	*Euphoria*	9 - 12 g
Mu Xiang	*Saussurea*	3 - 6 g
Suan Zao Ren	*Ziziphus*	9 - 12 g
Dang Gui	*Angelica*	6 - 9 g
Yuan Zhi	*Polygala*	3 - 6 g
Gan Cao	*Glycyrrhiza*	3 - 6 g

Severe taiyin/taiyang disease with abdominal cramps as the main symptom.

T thin white coat

P superficial

GUI ZHI JIA SHAO YAO TANG

Cinnamon Twig Decoction plus Peony

Extract Formula Name: Cinnamon and Peony Combination

Gui Zhi	*Cinnamomum*	6 - 9 g
Bai Shao Yao	*Paeonia*	15 - 18 g
Sheng Jiang	*Zingiber*	3 - 6 g
Da Zao	*Ziziphus*	3 - 4 pc
Gan Cao	*Glycyrrhiza*	3 - 6 g

Mild taiyin with taiyang syndrome: wind cold with mild Spleen qi deficiency. The chills are predominant, and the patient experiences diarrhea with epigastric fullness.

T pale, thin white coat

P weak, maybe superficial

GUI ZHI REN SHEN TANG

Cinnamon Twig and Ginseng Decoction

Extract Formula Name: Cinnamon and Ginseng Combination

Gui Zhi	*Cinnamomum*	9 - 12 g
Ren Shen	*Panax*	9 - 12 g
Gan Jiang	*Zingiber*	9 g
Bai Zhu	*Atractylodes*	9 g
Zhi Gan Cao	*Glycyrrhiza*	9 - 12 g

Spleen qi deficiency with preexisting taiyang syndrome but no direct exterior symptoms are present anymore. Symptoms include epigastric distention, vomiting, or poor appetite.

T pale, thin white coat

P weak

HOU PO SHENG JIANG BAN XIA TANG

Magnolia Bark, Ginger, and Pinellia Decoction

Extract Formula Name: Magnolia-Five Combination

Hou Po	*Magnolia*	6 - 12 g
Sheng Jiang	*Zingiber*	3 - 6 g
Ban Xia	*Pinellia*	6 - 9 g
Ren Shen	*Panax*	6 - 9 g
Gan Cao	*Glycyrrhiza*	3 - 6 g

Spleen/Stomach qi deficiency with cold and wei (defensive) qi deficiency; also useful for peptic ulcers and chronic allergies. Other symptoms include poor appetite or spontaneous sweating.

T pale, thin white coat

P weak, slow, thin, wiry

☞ Yi Tang - Saccharum Granorum is dissolved into the strained decoction.

HUANG QI JIAN ZHONG TANG

Astragalus Decoction to Construct the Middle

Extract Formula Name: Astragalus Combination

Gui Zhi	*Cinnamomum*	9 g
Bai Shao Yao	*Paeonia*	18 g
Sheng Jiang	*Zingiber*	10 g
Da Zao	*Ziziphus*	3 - 6 pc
Gan Cao	*Glycyrrhiza*	6 g
Yi Tang	*Saccharum Granorum*	30 g
Huang Qi	*Astragalus*	9 g

Spleen qi deficiency during pregnancy with lethargy, spotting, or low back pain.

T pale, swollen, teethmarks, thin white coat

P weak, thin

☞ E Jiao - Equus should be added at the end to the strained tea.

JIA JIAN BU ZHONG YI QI TANG

Modified Tonify the Middle and Augment the Qi Decoction

Ren Shen	*Panax*	6 - 9 g
Huang Qi	*Astragalus*	6 - 12 g
Chen Pi	*Citrus*	3 - 6 g
Bai Zhu	*Atractylodes*	3 - 9 g
Sheng Ma	*Cimicifuga*	3 - 6 g
Chai Hu	*Bupleurum*	3 - 9 g
E Jiao	*Equus*	3 - 9 g
Ai Ye	*Artemisia*	3 - 9 g
Gan Cao	*Glycyrrhiza*	3 - 6 g

Spleen qi deficiency causing severe uterine bleeding which is pale in color, or early or irregular periods. The Spleen qi is sinking causing a restless fetus.

T pale, swollen, teethmarks, thin white coat

P weak

JU YUAN JIAN

Lift the Source Decoction

Ren Shen	Panax	6 - 9 g
Huang Qi	Astragalus	9 - 12 g
Sheng Ma	Cimicifuga	3 - 6 g
Bai Zhu	Atractylodes	3 - 6 g
Gan Cao	Glycyrrhiza	3 - 6 g

Spleen/Stomach qi deficiency with mild damp symptoms including decreased appetite, middle jiao distention, or nausea and vomiting.

T pale, thin sticky coat

P weak, slightly slippery

LIU JUN ZI TANG

Six-Gentlemen Decoction

Extract Formula Name: Six Major Herbs Combination

Ren Shen	Panax	6 - 9 g
Bai Zhu	Atractylodes	6 - 9 g
Fu Ling	Poria	6 - 9 g
Chen Pi	Citrus	3 - 6 g
Ban Xia	Pinellia	6 - 9 g
Gan Cao	Glycyrrhiza	3 - 6 g

Heart qi deficiency with Spleen qi deficiency leading to anxiety, insomnia, spontaneous sweating, or palpitations.

T pale, thin coating

P weak

✘ Zhu Sha - Cinnabaris is toxic, and should only be used short-term.

MIAO XIANG SAN

Marvelously Fragrant Powder

Ren Shen	Panax	6 - 12 g
Fu Ling	Poria	9 - 12 g
Fu Shen	Poria	9 - 12 g
Yuan Zhi	Polygala	9 - 12 g
Huang Qi	Astragalus	9 - 15 g
Shan Yao	Dioscorea	9 - 12 g
Mu Xiang	Saussurea	12 - 15 g
Jie Geng	Platycodon	1 - 3 g
Zhu Sha	Cinnabaris	1 - 3 g
She Xiang	Moschus	0.3 - 0.5 g
Gan Cao	Glycyrrhiza	3 - 6 g

Spleen/Stomach qi deficiency causing diarrhea and vomiting with extreme thirst due to depletion of fluids. Commonly used in the pediatric department.

T pale, swollen, teethmarks, thin white coat

P weak

QI WEI BAI ZHU SAN

Seven-Ingredient Powder with Atractylodes Macrocephala

Ren Shen	*Panax*	6-9 g
Bai Zhu	*Atractylodes*	3-9 g
Mu Xiang	*Saussurea*	3-9 g
Fu Ling	*Poria*	6-9 g
Huo Xiang Ye	*Agastache*	9-15 g
Ge Gen	*Pueraria*	9-15 g
Gan Cao	*Glycyrrhiza*	3-6 g

Spleen qi deficiency causing thin, clear or reddish leukorrhea, with low back pain.

T pale, thin white coat

P deep, thin, slippery

QING DAI TANG

Clear Discharge Decoction

Shan Yao	*Dioscorea*	9-30 g
Mu Li	*Ostrea*	9-15 g
Long Gu	*Os Draconis*	9-15 g
Qian Cao Gen	*Rubia*	6-9 g
Hai Piao Xiao	*Sepia*	9-12 g

Lung yin deficiency with false heat and Spleen qi deficiency causing cough with scanty sputum and fatigue.

T red, cracked, slight coat

P thin, rapid

☞ Dissolve Bie Jia - Amyda for about one hour, then decoct with the remaining herbs.

REN SHEN HUANG QI SAN

Ginseng and Astragalus Powder

Ren Shen	*Panax*	6 - 12 g
Huang Qi	*Astragalus*	9 - 15 g
Fu Ling	*Poria*	6 - 9 g
Zhi Mu	*Anemarrhena*	6 - 9 g
Zi Wan	*Aster*	6 - 9 g
Sang Bai Pi	*Morus*	6 - 9 g
Qin Jiao	*Gentiana*	6 - 12 g
Jie Geng	*Platycodon*	3 - 6 g
Chai Hu	*Bupleurum*	6 - 9 g
Ban Xia	*Pinellia*	6 - 9 g
Di Gu Pi	*Lycium*	3 - 9 g
Sheng Di Huang	*Rehmannia*	6 - 15 g
Bie Jia	*Amyda*	6 - 12 g
Tian Men Dong	*Asparagus*	9 - 12 g
Chi Shao Yao	*Paeonia*	3 - 9 g
Gan Cao	*Glycyrrhiza*	3 - 6 g

Spleen qi deficiency with damp leading to diarrhea and irregular periods. Other symptoms include weight loss, fatigue, poor appetite, or pale face.

T pale, white coat

P weak or thin

SHEN LING BAI ZHU SAN

Ginseng, Poria, and Atractylodes Powder

Extract Formula Name: Ginseng and Atractylodes Formula

Ren Shen	*Panax*	9 - 15 g
Fu Ling	*Poria*	9 - 12 g
Bai Zhu	*Atractylodes*	3 - 9 g
Gan Cao	*Glycyrrhiza*	6 - 9 g
Lian Zi	*Nelumbo*	3 - 9 g
Yi Yi Ren	*Coix*	6 - 15 g
Shan Yao	*Dioscorea*	9 - 15 g
Bian Dou	*Dolichos*	6 - 9 g
Jie Geng	*Platycodon*	3 - 6 g
Sha Ren	*Amomum*	3 g

Spleen/Kidney qi and yang deficiency causing edema which manifests mostly in the lower body. Other symptoms include cold limbs, poor appetite, decreased urination, or heaviness.

T pale, sticky coat

P deep, slow, maybe thin

SHI PI YIN

Bolster the Spleen Decoction

Extract Formula Name: Magnolia and Atractylodes Combination

Fu Zi	*Aconitum*	6 - 9 g
Bai Zhu	*Atractylodes*	6 - 9 g
Mu Gua	*Chaenomeles*	6 - 9 g
Hou Po	*Magnolia*	6 - 12 g
Gan Jiang	*Zingiber*	6 - 9 g
Mu Xiang	*Saussurea*	6 - 9 g
Fu Ling	*Poria*	6 - 9 g
Da Fu Pi	*Areca*	3 - 6 g
Cao Guo	*Amomum*	3 - 6 g
Zhi Gan Cao	*Glycyrrhiza*	3 - 6 g
[Da Zao	*Ziziphus*	1 - 3 pc]
[Sheng Jiang	*Zingiber*	3 - 6 g]

Stomach/Spleen qi deficiency. This is the basic prescription for building qi. Symptoms include poor appetite, loose bowel movements, or lethargy.

T pale, thin white coat

P weak, deep

✪ Major Formula

SI JUN ZI TANG

Four-Gentlemen Decoction

Extract Formula Name: Four Major Herbs Combination

Ren Shen	*Panax*	6 - 9 g
Bai Zhu	*Atractylodes*	3 - 9 g
Fu Ling	*Poria*	6 - 9 g
Gan Cao	*Glycyrrhiza*	3 - 6 g

Spleen qi deficiency with Liver qi stagnation causing leukorrhea. The discharge is thin, watery, or white. Other symptoms include loose stools, poor appetite, and possible irritability.

T pale, light purple, swollen, sticky white coat

P slippery, slow

WAN DAI TANG

End Discharge Decoction

Bai Zhu	*Atractylodes*	20 - 30 g
Cang Zhu	*Atractylodes*	3 - 6 g
Shan Yao	*Dioscorea*	20 - 30 g
Chen Pi	*Citrus*	3 - 6 g
Bai Shao Yao	*Paeonia*	6 - 12 g
Chai Hu	*Bupleurum*	3 - 6 g
Jing Jie	*Schizonepeta*	6 - 9 g
Che Qian Zi	*Plantago*	6 - 9 g
Ren Shen	*Panax*	6 - 9 g
Gan Cao	*Glycyrrhiza*	3 - 6 g

Spleen Qi deficiency with mild Qi stagnation and damp in the middle jiao. Symptoms include fullness in the epigastrium or abdomen, gas, loose stools, or epigastric pain.

T pale or light purple, swollen, teethmarks, white coat

P weak

WU WEI YI GONG SAN

Five-Herbs, an Exceptionally Effective Powder

Ren Shen	*Panax*	6 - 9 g
Fu Ling	*Poria*	6 - 9 g
Bai Zhu	*Atractylodes*	3 - 9 g
Gan Cao	*Glycyrrhiza*	3 - 6 g
Chen Pi	*Citrus*	3 - 6 g
[Da Zao	*Ziziphus*	3 - 6 g]
[Sheng Jiang	*Zingiber*	3 - 6 g]

Diarrhea due to Spleen qi deficiency with damp and Stomach heat causing dysentery with mucous and possible bleeding.

T sticky yellow coat

P slippery, rapid

XIANG LIAN WAN

Aucklandia and Coptis Pill

Extract Formula Name: Saussurea and Coptis Formula

Mu Xiang	*Saussurea*	6 - 9 g
Huang Lian	*Coptis*	3 - 6 g
Wu Zhu Yu	*Evodia*	3 - 12 g

1. Chronic Spleen qi deficiency with chronic cold evil qi leading to qi and blood deficiency. The main symptom is abdominal spasms. 2. Liver qi stagnation or Liver overacting on Spleen. In the latter two instances the dosage of 'Bai Shao Yao - Paeonia' should be increased.

T pale or light purple, thin white coat

P weak or slightly wiry

☞ Yi Tang - Saccharum Granorum should be added to the strained tea.

XIAO JIAN ZHONG TANG

Minor Construct the Middle Decoction

Extract Formula Name: Minor Cinnamon and Peony Combination

Yi Tang	*Saccharum Granorum*	15 - 30 g
Gui Zhi	*Cinnamomum*	3 - 9 g
Bai Shao Yao	*Paeonia*	6 - 9 g
Sheng Jiang	*Zingiber*	6 - 9 g
Da Zao	*Ziziphus*	3 - 5 pc
Zhi Gan Cao	*Glycyrrhiza*	3 - 6 g

Spleen qi with yin deficiency and heat accumulation causing constipation, or hardness and fullness in the abdomen.

T cracked, thin dry yellowish coat

P weak, thin, deep

XIN JIA HÜANG LONG TANG

Newly-Augmented Yellow Dragon Decoction

Sheng Di Huang	*Rehmannia*	6 - 15 g
Ren Shen	*Panax*	6 - 9 g
Da Huang	*Rheum*	6 - 9 g
Mang Xiao	*Mirabilitum*	3 - 5 g
Mai Men Dong	*Ophiopogon*	9 - 15 g
Dang Gui	*Angelica*	6 - 9 g
Xuan Shen	*Scrophularia*	9 - 15 g
Gan Cao	*Glycyrrhiza*	3 - 6 g
Hai Shen	*Strichopus*	1 - 2 g

Spleen qi deficiency with middle jiao qi stagnation and diarrhea, or malnutrition in children.

T pale, light purple, white coat

P weak, thin

YI HUANG SAN

Benefit the Yellow Powder

Chen Pi	*Citrus*	30 g
Qing Pi	*Citrus*	15 g
Ding Xiang	*Eugenia*	3 - 6 g
He Zi	*Terminalia*	15 g
Zhi Gan Cao	*Glycyrrhiza*	15 g

Spleen qi deficiency causing damp which heats up. This leads to heat type leukorrhea with a fishy smell or delayed periods from qi and blood deficiency.

T pale, thin sticky yellow or white coat

P slippery, weak

YI HUANG TANG

Change Yellow (Discharge) Decoction

Shan Yao	Dioscorea	9 - 30 g
Huang Bai	Phellodendron	6 - 9 g
Qian Shi	Euryale	9 - 30 g
Bai Guo	Gingko	6 - 10 pc
Che Qian Zi	Plantago	3 - 6 g

Chronic middle jiao deficiency leading to visual disturbance and hearing loss or tinnitus.

T pale, white coat

P weak

YI QI CONG MING TANG

Augment the Qi and Increase Acuity Decoction

Extract Formula Name: Ginseng, Astragalus and Pueraria Combination

Ren Shen	Panax	6 - 12 g
Huang Qi	Astragalus	6 - 12 g
Zhi Gan Cao	Glycyrrhiza	6 - 12 g
Man Jing Zi	Vitex	6 - 9 g
Bai Shao Yao	Paeonia	3 - 9 g
Huang Bai	Phellodendron	3 - 9 g
Ge Gen	Pueraria	6 - 9 g
Sheng Ma	Cimicifuga	3 - 6 g

Chronic Spleen qi deficiency causing qi stagnation. The qi stagnation gives rise to cold and heat symptoms in the middle jiao. This in turn damages the Spleen and Stomach again causing distention in the epigastrium and abdomen, or alternating constipation and diarrhea.

T pale, thin yellowish coat

P wiry

ZHI SHI XIAO PI WAN

Immature Bitter Orange Pill to Reduce Focal Distention

Zhi Shi	*Citrus*	6 - 12 g
Hou Po	*Magnolia*	6 - 15 g
Ban Xia	*Pinellia*	6 - 9 g
Huang Lian	*Coptis*	9 - 15 g
Fu Ling	*Poria*	6 - 9 g
Bai Zhu	*Atractylodes*	3 - 9 g
Ren Shen	*Panax*	6 - 9 g
Gan Jiang	*Zingiber*	3 - 6
Mai Ya	*Hordeum*	3 - 9 g
Zhi Gan Cao	*Glycyrrhiza*	3 - 6 g

1. Chronic food stagnation with severe Spleen qi deficiency.
2. Severe acute food stagnation with mild Spleen qi deficiency. Symptoms include epigastric and abdominal distention, loose stools, and poor appetite.

T sticky coat

P wiry

ZHI ZHU WAN

Immature Bitter Orange and Atractylodes Pill

Bai Zhu	*Atractylodes*	9 - 15 g
Zhi Shi	*Citrus*	6 - 12 g

Severe abdominal distention (pi man - fullness, firmness) due to Spleen qi deficiency, or qi stagnation with damp and heat. Symptoms include constipation, or odorous diarrhea, thirst, yellow urine, or fever.

T sticky yellow coat

P wiry, rapid

ZHONG MAN FEN XIAO WAN

Separate and Reduce Fullness in the Middle Pill

Hou Po	*Magnolia*	9 - 18 g
Jiang Huang	*Curcuma*	6 g
Zhi Shi	*Citrus*	9 - 12 g
Ban Xia	*Pinellia*	6 - 12 g
Ren Shen	*Panax*	3 g
Zhi Mu	*Anemarrhena*	6 - 9 g
Gan Jiang	*Zingiber*	3 - 6 g
Huang Lian	*Coptis*	3 - 9 g
Huang Qin	*Scutellaria*	9 - 15 g
Bai Zhu	*Atractylodes*	6 g
Ze Xie	*Alisma*	6 g
Sha Ren	*Amomum*	3 - 6 g
Chen Pi	*Citrus*	3 - 6 g
Fu Ling	*Poria*	6 - 9 g
Zhu Ling	*Polyporus*	3 - 6 g
Zhi Gan Cao	*Glycyrrhiza*	3 - 6 g

SPLEEN QI AND BLOOD DEFICIENCY

- fatigue
- decreased appetite
- dizziness
- blurry vision
- loose stools

T pale

P weak, thin

Spleen qi and blood deficiency. Symptoms include dizziness, sallow complexion, chronic emaciation, mild fever, shortness of breath, or fatigue.

T pale, thin white coat

P thin, weak

✪ Major Formula

BA ZHEN TANG

Eight-Treasure Decoction

Extract Formula Name: Tang-kuei and Ginseng Eight Combination

Ren Shen	*Panax*	6 - 9 g
Bai Zhu	*Atractylodes*	3 - 9 g
Fu Ling	*Poria*	6 - 9 g
Gan Cao	*Glycyrrhiza*	3 - 6 g
Dang Gui	*Angelica*	6 - 12 g
Chuan Xiong	*Ligusticum*	3 - 6 g
Shu Di Huang	*Rehmannia*	6 - 15 g
Bai Shao Yao	*Paeonia*	6 - 9 g
[Da Zao	*Ziziphus*	2 - 3 pc]
[Sheng Jiang	*Zingiber*	2 - 6 g]

Qi and blood deficiency with blood stagnation. This formula is for a restless fetus, infertility, irregular periods, poor appetite, weakness, or fatigue.

T pale, thin white coat

P weak, maybe wiry

BA ZHEN YI MU WAN

Eight-Treasure Pill to Benefit Mothers

Shu Di Huang	*Rehmannia*	6 - 15 g
Chuan Xiong	*Ligusticum*	3 - 9 g
Dang Gui	*Angelica*	6 - 9 g
Bai Shao Yao	*Paeonia*	6 - 12 g
Ren Shen	*Panax*	6 - 12 g
Bai Zhu	*Atractylodes*	3 - 9 g
Fu Ling	*Poria*	6 - 9 g
Yi Mu Cao	*Leonurus*	6 - 18 g
Gan Cao	*Glycyrrhiza*	3 - 6 g

Spleen/Stomach qi deficiency where the Spleen qi is sinking, or the Spleen is not governing the blood. qi deficiency can lead to (morning) fever, early periods, weakness, diarrhea, or pallor.

T pale, swollen, teethmarks, thin white coat

P weak

BU ZHONG YI QI TANG

Tonify the Middle and Augment the Qi Decoction

Extract Formula Name: Ginseng and Astragalus Combination

Ren Shen	*Panax*	6 - 12 g
Huang Qi	*Astragalus*	9 - 15 g
Dang Gui	*Angelica*	6 - 9 g
Chen Pi	*Citrus*	3 - 6 g
Sheng Ma	*Cimicifuga*	3 - 6 g
Chai Hu	*Bupleurum*	3 - 9 g
Bai Zhu	*Atractylodes*	3 - 9 g
Zhi Gan Cao	*Glycyrrhiza*	3 - 6 g

Post-partum abdominal pain of the deficiency type after qi and blood loss from giving birth.

T pale

P frail

☞ E Jiao - Equus should be added to the strained tea.

CHANG NING TANG

Intestinal Serenity Decoction

Shu Di Huang	*Rehmannia*	6 - 12 g
Dang Gui	*Angelica*	6 - 12 g
Mai Men Dong	*Ophiopogon*	6 - 9 g
Ren Shen	*Panax*	6 - 9 g
Xu Duan	*Dipsacus*	6 - 9 g
Rou Gui	*Cinnamomum*	3 g
E Jiao	*Equus*	6 - 9 g
Shan Yao	*Dioscorea*	6 - 9 g
Gan Cao	*Glycyrrhiza*	3 - 6 g

Kidney yin and Spleen qi/blood deficiency causing uterine prolapse with low back pain, night urination, or hearing loss and tinnitus.

T red or pale

P frail

DA BU YUAN JIAN

Great Tonify the Basal Decoction

Ren Shen	*Panax*	6 - 12 g
Shu Di Huang	*Rehmannia*	9 - 25 g
Shan Yao	*Dioscorea*	6 - 9 g
Shan Zhu Yu	*Cornus*	3 - 6 g
Gou Qi Zi	*Lycium*	6 - 9 g
Dang Gui	*Angelica*	6 - 9 g
Du Zhong	*Eucommia*	6 - 9 g
Gan Cao	*Glycyrrhiza*	3 - 6 g

Qi/blood deficiency with bleeding, fever, heat feelings in the muscles, thirst with a desire for warm liquids, or irregular periods.

T pale, thin coat

P empty

DANG GUI BU XUE TANG

Dang Gui Decoction to Tonify the Blood

Extract Formula Name: Tang-Kuei and Astragalus Combination

Huang Qi	*Astragalus*	30 g
Dang Gui	*Angelica*	6 g

Spleen qi and blood deficiency with slight cold leading to spasm pain or post-partum emaciation.

T pale, white coat

P weak

☞ Yi Tang - Saccharum Granorum should be added to the strained tea.

DANG GUI JIAN ZHONG TANG

Dang Gui Decoction to Construct the Middle

Extract Formula Name: Tang-Kuei, Cinnamon and Peony Combination

Yi Tang	*Saccharum Granorum*	6 - 20 g
Gui Zhi	*Cinnamomum*	3 - 9 g
Bai Shao Yao	*Paeonia*	6 - 9 g
Sheng Jiang	*Zingiber*	3 - 6 g
Da Zao	*Ziziphus*	3 - 6 pc
Gan Cao	*Glycyrrhiza*	3 - 6 g
Dang Gui	*Angelica*	6 - 9 g

Spleen qi and blood deficiency with yin deficiency and restless fetus. This prescription can be taken as a preventative during pregnancy.

T pale or red

P thin, weak

DANG GUI SAN

Dang Gui Powder

Extract Formula Name: Tang-Kuei Formula

Dang Gui	*Angelica*	6 - 12 g
Huang Qin	*Scutellaria*	6 - 12 g
Chuan Xiong	*Ligusticum*	3 g
Bai Zhu	*Atractylodes*	3 - 9 g
Bai Shao Yao	*Paeonia*	6 - 9 g

Liver overacting on Spleen causing mild cramping in the abdomen with Liver blood deficiency and some damp accumulation. Symptoms include urinary retention and lower body edema. This is often seen during pregnancy.

T pale, orange color on the sides

P weak, thin, or slightly wiry

DANG GUI SHAO YAO SAN

Dang Gui and Peony Powder

Extract Formula Name: Tang-Kuei and Peony Formula

Dang Gui	*Angelica*	6 - 9 g
Bai Shao Yao	*Paeonia*	3 - 9 g
Bai Zhu	*Atractylodes*	3 - 9 g
Fu Ling	*Poria*	6 - 9 g
Chuan Xiong	*Ligusticum*	3 - 6 g
Ze Xie	*Alisma*	6 - 9 g

Blood deficiency with external cold after childbirth. This leads to spasms or hernia pain which are both relieved by pressure.

T pale

P deep, wiry, weak

☞ This formula should be prepared as a stew with eight cups of water. Simmer until it is reduced to three to four cups.

DANG GUI SHENG JIANG YANG ROU TANG

Mutton Stew with Dang Gui and Fresh Ginger Decoction

Dang Gui	*Angelica*	9 - 12 g
Sheng Jiang	*Zingiber*	9 - 15 g
Yang Rou	*Mutton*	40 - 50 g

Blood and yin deficient patient with cold evil qi which leads to obstruction of the channels which causes pain. This is known as jueyin syndrome in which the patient feels cold subjectively but not to the touch. Raynaud's disease.

T pale, white coat

P deep, thin, or minute

DANG GUI SI NI TANG

Dang Gui Decoction for Frigid Extremities

Extract Formula Name: Tang-Kuei and Jujube Combination

Dang Gui	*Angelica*	6 - 12 g
Gui Zhi	*Cinnamomum*	3 - 9 g
Bai Shao Yao	*Paeonia*	6 - 9 g
Mu Tong	*Akebia*	6 - 9 g
Xi Xin	*Asarum*	3 - 6 g
Da Zao	*Ziziphus*	3 - 5 pc
Gan Cao	*Glycyrrhiza*	3 - 6 g

Blood deficiency with yang deficiency and cold causing coldness in the uterus with dysmenorrhea. The blood is scanty, pale, and watery. The patient experiences severe cramping upon menstrual onset.

T pale, light purple, some cracks, thin white coat

P slow, thin, weak

GUI FU SI WU TANG

Cinnamon Bark, Aconite, and Four-Substance Decoction

Sheng Di Huang	*Rehmannia*	6 - 12 g
Dang Gui	*Angelica*	6 - 9 g
Chuan Xiong	*Ligusticum*	3 - 9 g
Bai Shao Yao	*Paeonia*	6 - 9 g
Rou Gui	*Cinnamomum*	3 - 9 g
Fu Zi	*Aconitum*	1 - 6 g

Heart blood and yin deficiency with Spleen qi deficiency leading to insomnia, decreased appetite, nightmares, irregular periods in women, or uterine bleeding which may manifest as beng loú – gushing or spotting. This formula is also useful for purpura due to Spleen qi/blood deficiency.

T pale, swollen, teethmarks, thin white coat

P weak, thin

GUI PI TANG

Restore the Spleen Decoction

Extract Formula Name: Ginseng and Longan Combination

Ren Shen	Panax	6 - 9 g
Huang Qi	Astralagus	9 - 12 g
Fu Shen	Poria	6 - 9 g
Bai Zhu	Atractylodes	9 - 12 g
Long Yan Rou	Euphoria	9 - 12 g
Mu Xiang	Saussurea	3 - 6 g
Suan Zao Ren	Ziziphus	9 - 12 g
Dang Gui	Angelica	6 - 9 g
Yuan Zhi	Polygala	3 - 6 g
Gan Cao	Glycyrrhiza	3 - 6 g

Blood deficiency giving rise to internal wind which then leads to tendon or muscle spasms, itchy skin rashes, or blurry vision.

T pale, quivery

P weak, maybe superficial

GUI XIONG SI WU TANG

Altered Four-Substance Decoction

Shu Di Huang	Rehmannia	9 - 15 g
Chuan Xiong	Ligusticum	3 - 9 g
Bai Shao Yao	Paeonia	6 - 9 g
Dang Gui	Angelica	6 - 9 g
Fang Feng	Ledebouriella	9 - 15 g
Bai Zhu	Atractylodes	6 - 9 g
Huai Niu Xi	Achyranthes	6 - 12 g
Tian Men Dong	Asparagus	9 - 12 g

Chronic malaria has depleted Liver blood and Spleen qi and blood. The patient experiences alternating fever and chills which are aggravated with only mild stress.

T pale

P empty

HE REN YIN

Polygonum Multiflorum Root and Ginseng Decoction

He Shou Wu	*Polygonum*	9 - 20 g
Ren Shen	*Panax*	9 - 12 g
Chen Pi	*Citrus*	3 - 9 g
Dang Gui	*Angelica*	3 - 9 g
Wei Jiang	*Zingiber*	3 - 12 g

Yin/blood deficiency causing constipation with dry stools; or excess heat causing constipation.

T red, dry yellow coat

P rapid, thin, or empty

✘ Do not use during pregnancy.

MA ZI REN WAN

Hemp Seed Pill

Extract Formula Name: Apricot Seed and Linum Formula

Huo Ma Ren	*Cannabis*	6 - 12 g
Da Huang	*Rheum*	6 - 9 g
Xing Ren	*Prunus*	6 - 9 g
Zhi Shi	*Citrus*	3 - 6 g
Bai Shao Yao	*Paeonia*	6 - 9 g
Hou Po	*Magnolia*	6 - 12 g

Blood deficiency with deficient or excess heat causing purple menstrual blood, early periods, or thick leukorrhea with tidal fever.

T pale

P rapid, thin, weak

QIN LIAN SI WU TANG

Four-Substance Decoction with Scutellaria and Coptis

Huang Qin	*Scutellaria*	6 - 9 g
Huang Lian	*Coptis*	3 - 6 g
Chuan Xiong	*Ligusticum*	3 - 6 g
Bai Shao Yao	*Paeonia*	6 - 9 g
Dang Gui	*Angelica*	6 - 9 g
Mai Men Dong	*Ophiopogon*	6 - 9 g
Sheng Di Huang	*Rehmannia*	9 - 12 g

Spleen/Lung qi and blood deficiency with Heart yang deficiency, or ying level deficiency. The patient is easily startled, experiences shortness of breath, lack of taste sensation, insomnia, or palpitations. This formula is also useful for irregular periods or uterine bleeding.

T pale, swollen

P weak

REN SHEN YANG YING TANG

Ginseng Decoction to Nourish the Nutritive Qi

Extract Formula Name: Ginseng Combination

Bai Shao Yao	*Paeonia*	9 - 15 g
Chen Pi	*Citrus*	3 - 6 g
Dang Gui	*Angelica*	3 - 9 g
Ren Shen	*Panax*	6 - 9 g
Huang Qi	*Astragalus*	6 - 12 g
Bai Zhu	*Atractylodes*	6 - 9 g
Shu Di Huang	*Rehmannia*	3 - 6 g
Wu Wei Zi	*Schisandra*	3 - 6 g
Fu Ling	*Poria*	3 - 6 g
Yuan Zhi	*Polygala*	2 - 6 g
Rou Gui	*Cinnamomum*	6 - 9 g
Gan Cao	*Glycyrrhiza*	3 - 6 g
[Da Zao	*Ziziphus*	2 pc]
[Gan Jiang	*Zingiber*	3 pc]

Constipation due to yin/blood deficiency. This is commonly seen in the elderly, or after giving birth.

T red or pale, dry

P thin

RUN CHANG WAN I

Moisten the Intestines Pill from Master Shen's Book

Huo Ma Ren	*Cannabis*	9 - 15 g
Dang Gui	*Angelica*	9 - 12 g
Sheng Di Huang	*Rehmannia*	6 - 9 g
Tao Ren	*Prunus*	6 - 9 g
Zhi Ke	*Citrus*	6 - 9 g

Wind heat invading the intestines and damaging the Spleen and Stomach qi. Severe constipation with blood deficiency which may lead to wind, or blood stagnation.

T pale or purple

P thin or choppy

RUN CHANG WAN II

Moisten the Intestines Pill from Discussion of the Spleen and Stomach

Da Huang	*Rheum*	9 - 12 g
Tao Ren	*Prunus*	15 - 25 g
Huo Ma Ren	*Cannabis*	15 - 30 g
Dang Gui Wei	*Angelica*	6 - 12 g
Qiang Huo	*Notopterygium*	6 - 9 g

Severe qi deficiency with yang and blood deficiency and cold symptoms. Irregular menstruation with a pale and watery flow, dizziness, pale or sallow face, cold limbs, or chills.

T pale, wet, thin white coat

P deep, weak, thready

SHAN HE YIN

Mountain and River Decoction

Shu Di Huang	*Rehmannia*	15 - 25 g
Dang Gui	*Angelica*	6 - 9 g
Bai Shao Yao	*Paeonia*	6 - 9 g
Chuan Xiong	*Ligusticum*	3 - 9 g
Rou Gui	*Cinnamomum*	3 - 9 g
Huang Qi	*Astragalus*	6 - 15 g

Spleen qi/blood deficiency causing slow blood circulation with deficiency type abdominal pain during menstruation, or bleeding sores.

T pale, light purple, thin white coat

P thin, weak

SHENG YU TANG

Sage-like Healing Decoction

Shu Di Huang	*Rehmannia*	15 - 25 g
Ren Shen	*Panax*	12 - 15 g
Dang Gui	*Angelica*	12 - 15 g
Huang Qi	*Astragalus*	15 - 20 g
Chuan Xiong	*Ligusticum*	6 - 9 g
Bai Shao Yao	*Paeonia*	15 - 20 g

Qi/yang/blood deficiency. Symptoms include poor appetite, general malaise, mild cold symptoms, severe deficiency, rashes, dysmenorrhea, uterine bleeding, or post-partum deficiency.

T pale, thin white coat

P weak, thin, deep

SHI QUAN DA BU TANG

All-Inclusive Great Tonifying Decoction

Extract Formula Name: Ginseng and Tang-Kuei Ten Combination

Ren Shen	*Panax*	6 - 9 g
Fu Ling	*Poria*	9 - 12 g
Bai Zhu	*Atractylodes*	9 - 12 g
Gan Cao	*Glycyrrhiza*	3 - 6 g
Dang Gui	*Angelica*	12 - 15 g
Shu Di Huang	*Rehmannia*	15 - 20 g
Bai Shao Yao	*Paeonia*	12 - 15 g
Chuan Xiong	*Ligusticum*	3 - 9 g
Rou Gui	*Cinnamomum*	6 - 9 g
Huang Qi	*Astragalus*	15 - 20 g
[Da Zao	*Ziziphus*	1 - 3 g]
[Sheng Jiang	*Zingiber*	3 - 6 g]

Blood deficiency with blood stagnation. Symptoms include irregular menstruation, dysmenorrhea, dizziness, or pale or purple fingernails.

T pale or purple

P thin or choppy

✪ Major Formula

SI WU TANG

Four-Substance Decoction

Extract Formula Name: Tang-Kuei Four Combination

Shu Di Huang	*Rehmannia*	6 - 12 g
Chuan Xiong	*Ligusticum*	3 - 9 g
Dang Gui	*Angelica*	6 - 9 g
Bai Shao Yao	*Paeonia*	6 - 9 g

Spleen qi/blood deficiency during pregnancy causing restless fetus, or use formula if the woman has a history of miscarriage or infertility.

T pale, thin white coat

P weak, thin, slippery

TAI SHAN PAN SHI SAN

Powder that Gives the Stability of Mount Tai

Ren Shen	*Panax*	6 - 9 g
Huang Qi	*Astragalus*	12 - 15 g
Shu Di Huang	*Rehmannia*	9 - 12 g
Chuan Xiong	*Ligusticum*	3 - 6 g
Bai Zhu	*Atractylodes*	9 - 12 g
Sha Ren	*Amomum*	1 - 3 g
Huang Qin	*Scutellaria*	6 - 9 g
Xu Duan	*Dipsacus*	3 - 6 g
Bai Shao Yao	*Paeonia*	6 - 9 g
Zhi Gan Cao	*Glycyrrhiza*	3 - 6 g
Nuo Mi	*Glutinous Oryza*	3 - 6 g

Mild blood deficiency with severe blood stagnation causing early periods or dysmenorrhea.

T pale or purple

P choppy or wiry

✘ Do not use during pregnancy.

TAO HONG SI WU TANG

Four-Substance Decoction with Safflower and Peach Pit

Shu Di Huang	*Rehmannia*	6 - 12 g
Bai Shao Yao	*Paeonia*	6 - 9 g
Chuan Xiong	*Ligusticum*	3 - 6 g
Dang Gui	*Angelica*	6 - 9 g
Tao Ren	*Prunus*	3 - 9 g
Hong Hua	*Carthamus*	3 - 6 g

Boils/carbuncles with pus and qi and blood deficiency. The pus stays trapped under the skin.

T pale

P weak

✘ Do not use during pregnancy.

TOU NONG SAN

Discharge Pus Powder

Huang Qi	*Astragalus*	15 g
Chuan Xiong	*Ligusticum*	3 - 9 g
Dang Gui	*Angelica*	6 - 9 g
Chuan Shan Jia	*Manis*	1 - 3 g
Zao Jiao Ci	*Gleditsia*	3 - 6 g

Blood deficiency causing constipation.

T pale

P weak, thin

WU REN WAN

Five-Seed Pill

Xing Ren	*Prunus*	9 - 20 g
Bai Zi Ren	*Biota*	3 - 6 g
Tao Ren	*Prunus*	9 - 15 g
Yu Li Ren	*Prunus*	3 - 6 g
Sha Ren	*Amomum*	3 - 6 g

Qi and blood deficiency with qi/blood and phlegm stagnation causing masses on the neck, breasts, or axilla areas.

T pale or purple

P weak or choppy

XIANG BEI YANG YING TANG

Cyperus and Fritillaria Decoction to Nourish the Nutritive Qi

Ren Shen	*Panax*	6 - 9 g
Bai Zhu	*Atractylodes*	3 - 6 g
Fu Ling	*Poria*	6 - 9 g
Chuan Xiong	*Ligusticum*	3 - 6 g
Chen Pi	*Citrus*	3 - 6 g
Dang Gui	*Angelica*	6 - 9 g
Xiang Fu	*Cyperus*	6 - 9 g
Shu Di Huang	*Rehmannia*	6 - 12 g
Bei Mu	*Fritillaria*	3 - 6 g
Bai Shao Yao	*Paeonia*	6 - 9 g
Jie Geng	*Platycodon*	3 - 6 g
Da Zao	*Ziziphus*	3 - 6 pc
Sheng Jiang	*Zingiber*	3 - 6 g
Gan Cao	*Glycyrrhiza*	1 - 3 g

Blood deficiency with interior excess heat causing constipation; or blood stagnation with excess heat resulting in amenorrhea.

T red or purple, yellow coat

P rapid

✘ Do not use during pregnancy.

YU ZHU SAN

Jade Candle Powder

Chuan Xiong	*Ligusticum*	3 - 9 g
Shu Di Huang	*Rehmannia*	6 - 12 g
Dang Gui	*Angelica*	6 - 9 g
Bai Shao Yao	*Paeonia*	6 - 9 g
Da Huang	*Rheum*	6 - 9 g
Mang Xiao	*Mirabilitum*	3 - 6 g
Gan Cao	*Glycyrrhiza*	3 - 6 g

SPLEEN QI DEFICIENCY WITH DAMP

Please see under Jin Ye (Body Fluid) Disharmonies

SPLEEN YANG DEFICIENCY WITH COLD

- no appetite
- cold extremities
- sallow or pale complexion
- coldness and pain in the epigastrium
- watery stools with undigested food

T pale, swollen, moist, teeth marks

P deep, slow, weak

Spleen yang deficiency with cold, qi, and blood stagnation causing epigastric or abdominal pain which is better with food.

T pale, swollen, teethmarks, wet, light or dark purple

P slow, frail

AN ZHONG SAN

Calm the Middle Powder

Extract Formula Name: Cardamon and Fennel Formula

Gui Zhi	*Cinnamomum*	3 - 9 g
Mu Li	*Ostrea*	3 - 9 g
Yan Hu Suo	*Corydalis*	6 - 9 g
Gao Liang Jiang	*Alpinia*	3 g
Xiao Hui Xiang	*Foeniculum*	3 - 9 g
Sha Ren	*Amomum*	3 g
Gan Cao	*Glycyrrhiza*	3 - 6 g
[Fu Ling	*Poria*	3-6 g]

Cold accumulation or yang deficiency in the abdomen leading to constipation with cramping pain. The qi stagnates and heats up which can cause a mild fever. Other symptoms include cold extremities and chills.

T normal or pale, white coat

P wiry or tight, deep

☞ Fu Zi - Aconitum should be powdered. Da Huang - Rheum should be added during the last 3 - 5 minutes of the decoction process.

✘ Do not use during pregnancy.

DA HUANG FU ZI TANG

Rhubarb and Aconite Decoction

Extract Formula Name: Rhubarb and Aconite Combination

Da Huang	*Rheum*	6 - 9 g
Fu Zi	*Aconitum*	6 g
Xi Xin	*Asarum*	3 - 6 g

Spleen yang deficiency with cold stagnation causing severe cramping pain, borborygmus, or possible vomiting.

T pale, light purple, swollen, moist white coat

P wiry or slow, deep

☞ Yi Tang - Saccharum Granorum is added to the strained tea.

DA JIAN ZHONG TANG

Major Construct the Middle Decoction

Extract Formula Name: Major Zanthoxylum Combination

Chuan Jiao	*Zanthoxylum*	3 - 6 g
Ren Shen	*Panax*	6 - 9 g
Gan Jiang	*Zingiber*	3 - 6 g
Yi Tang	*Saccharum Granorum*	20 g

Spleen/Kidney yang deficiency causing dawn diarrhea with middle jiao qi stagnation symptoms such as excruciating abdominal pain and severe fullness feelings.

T pale, swollen, teethmarks, light purple, white coat

P deep, weak, or slippery

DAN LIAO SI SHEN WAN

Four-Miracle Pill from the Tranquil Hut

Bu Gu Zhi	*Psoralea*	6 - 12 g
Xiao Hui Xiang	*Foeniculum*	3 - 9 g
Rou Dou Kou	*Myristica*	9 - 12 g
Mu Xiang	*Saussurea*	3 - 6 g

Spleen qi and blood deficiency with slight cold leading to spasm pain or post-partum emaciation.

T pale, white coat

P weak

☞ Yi Tang - Saccharum Granorum is added to the strained tea.

DANG GUI JIAN ZHONG TANG

Dang Gui Decoction to Construct the Middle

Extract Formula Name: Tang-Kuei, Cinnamon and Peony Combination

Yi Tang	*Saccharum Granorum*	6 - 20 g
Gui Zhi	*Cinnamomum*	3 - 9 g
Bai Shao Yao	*Paeonia*	6 - 9 g
Sheng Jiang	*Zingiber*	3 - 6 g
Da Zao	*Ziziphus*	3 - 6 pc
Gan Cao	*Glycyrrhiza*	3 - 6 g
Dang Gui	*Angelica*	6 - 9 g

Longstanding cold with blood and yang deficiency leading to diarrhea, nausea and vomiting, or abdominal cramps.

T pale, swollen, teethmarks, wet, white coat

P slow, frail

DANG GUI SI NI JIA WU ZHU YU SHENG JIANG TANG

Dang Gui Decoction for Frigid Extremities plus Evodia and Fresh Ginger

Extract Formula Name: Tang-Kuei, Evodia and Ginger Combination

Dang Gui	*Angelica*	6 - 9 g
Gui Zhi	*Cinnamomum*	3 - 9 g
Xi Xin	*Asarum*	3 - 6 g
Bai Shao Yao	*Paeonia*	6 - 9 g
Mu Tong	*Akebia*	6 - 9 g
Wu Zhu Yu	*Evodia*	3 - 6 g
Da Zao	*Ziziphus*	25 pc
Sheng Jiang	*Zingiber*	4 pc
Gan Cao	*Glycyrrhiza*	3 - 6 g

Blood and yin deficient patient with cold evil qi which leads to obstruction of the channels which causes pain. This is known as jueyin syndrome in which the patient feels cold subjectively but not to the touch. Raynaud's disease.

T pale, white coat

P deep, thin, or minute

DANG GUI SI NI TANG

Dang Gui Decoction for Frigid Extremities

Extract Formula Name: Tang-Kuei and Jujube Combination

Dang Gui	*Angelica*	6 - 12 g
Gui Zhi	*Cinnamomum*	3 - 9 g
Bai Shao Yao	*Paeonia*	6 - 9 g
Mu Tong	*Akebia*	6 - 9 g
Xi Xin	*Asarum*	3 - 6 g
Da Zao	*Ziziphus*	3 - 5 pc
Gan Cao	*Glycyrrhiza*	3 - 6 g

Spleen/Stomach qi yang deficiency resulting in hiccups, belching, and vomiting, and symptoms of coldness in the middle jiao.

T pale, thin coat

P weak, deep, maybe slow

✘ Contraindicated during pregnancy

DING XIANG SHI DI TANG

Clove and Kaki Decoction

Extract Formula Name: Clove and Kaki Combination

Ding Xiang	*Eugenia*	6-9 g
Shi Di	*Diospyrós*	6-9 g
Ren Shen	*Panax*	3-9 g
Sheng Jiang	*Zingiber*	3-6 g

Spleen yang deficiency with a painful abdomen and watery vomiting.

T pale, swollen, teethmarks, white coat

P weak, deep, slow

DING YU LI ZHONG TANG

Clove and Evodia Decoction to Regulate the Middle

Ren Shen	*Panax*	6-9 g
Bai Zhu	*Atractylodes*	3-9 g
Gan Jiang	*Zingiber*	3-9 g
Wu Zhu Yu	*Evodia*	3-9 g
Ding Xiang	*Eugenia*	3-9 g
Zhi Gan Gao	*Glycyrrhiza*	3-6 g

Stomach/Spleen yang deficiency causing watery diarrhea and epigastric pain. Severe cold symptoms such as cold limbs and vomiting of clear fluids.

T pale, swollen, teethmarks, white coat

P minute

✪ Major Formula

FU ZI LI ZHONG WAN

Prepared Aconite Pill to Regulate the Middle

Extract Formula Name: Aconite, Ginseng, and Ginger Combination

Fu Zi	*Aconitum*	6-9 g
Ren Shen	*Panax*	3-9 g
Bai Zhu	*Atractylodes*	3-9 g
Gan Jiang	*Zingiber*	3-9 g
Zhi Gan Cao	*Glycyrrhiza*	3-6 g

Stomach and Spleen yang deficiency with wei qi deficiency and internal heat and damp. Symtoms include loose stools, sweating, or cold hands and feet.

T pale or red, white or yellow sticky coat

P deep, weak, thin, or rapid

✘ Caution during pregnancy.

FU ZI XIE XIN TANG

Aconite Decoction to Drain the Epigastrium

Fu Zi	*Aconitum*	3 - 6 g
Da Huang	*Rheum*	6 - 9 g
Huang Qin	*Scutellaria*	3 - 6 g
Huang Lian	*Coptis*	3 - 6 g

Spleen/Stomach qi deficiency and cold causing vomiting during pregnancy.

T pale, thin white coat

P weak

GAN JIANG REN SHEN BAN XIA WAN

Ginger, Ginseng, and Pinellia Pill

Extract Formula Name: G.P. and Ginseng Formula

Gan Jiang	*Zingiber*	3 g
Ren Shen	*Panax*	3 g
Ban Xia	*Pinellia*	6 g
[Sheng Jiang	*Zingiber*	1 - 3 g]

Cold in the middle jiao resulting in loose stools or watery nonodorous diarrhea, cold extremities, or a desire for warm drinks.

T pale, light purple, thin white or wet coat

P slow, weak, or tight

GAO LIANG JIANG WAN

Galanga Pill

Gao Liang Jiang	*Alpinia*	3 - 6 g
Bi Ba	*Piper*	3 - 9 g

Spleen/Kidney yang deficiency causing watery diarrhea with undigested food, spasms in hands and feet, fatigue, and spontanous severe sweating.

T pale, swollen, teethmarks, wet, white coat

P minute

GU ZHEN TANG

Stabilize the True Decoction

Fu Zi	*Aconitum*	6 - 9 g
Ren Shen	*Panax*	6 - 9 g
Bai Zhu	*Atractylodes*	6 - 9 g
Fu Ling	*Poria*	6 - 9 g
Huang Qi	*Astragalus*	6 - 15 g
Shan Yao	*Dioscorea*	6 - 9 g
Rou Gui	*Cinnamomum*	3 - 9 g
Gan Cao	*Glycyrrhiza*	3 - 6 g
[Sheng Jiang	*Zingiber*	3 - 6 g]
[Da Zao	*Ziziphus*	1 - 2 pc]

Severe cold stagnation with Spleen/Kidney yang deficiency causing coldness in the face, cramping pain in the center, or dawn diarrhea.

T pale, purple, wet coat

P slow, tight

GUI FU LI ZHONG TANG

Cinnamon and Prepared Aconite Decoction to Regulate the Middle

Ren Shen	*Panax*	10 - 15 g
Bai Zhu	*Atractylodes*	6 - 9 g
Gan Jiang	*Zingiber*	6 - 9 g
Gan Cao	*Glycyrrhiza*	3 - 6 g
Fu Zi	*Aconitum*	3 - 6 g
Rou Gui	*Cinnamomum*	3 - 9 g

Wei qi deficiency (defensive qi) due to Spleen qi/yang deficiency with qi stagnation symptoms. The patient experiences frequent colds or abdominal fullness.

T pale, maybe light purple

P weak

GUI ZHI LI ZHONG WAN

Cinnamon Twig with Regulate the Middle Pill

Gui Zhi	*Cinnamomum*	3 - 9 g
Gan Jiang	*Zingiber*	3 - 6 g
Bai Zhu	*Atractylodes*	6 - 9 g
Ren Shen	*Panax*	6 - 12 g
Gan Cao	*Glycyrrhiza*	3 - 6 g

Cold in the Spleen/Stomach after ingestion of cold food with damp and qi stagnation in the center. Symptoms include lack of appetite, loose stools, or nausea and vomiting.

T pale, sticky white coat

P weak, deep, or tight

HOU PO WEN ZHONG TANG

Magnolia Bark Decoction for Warming the Middle

Extract Formula Name: Magnolia and Saussurea Combination

Hou Po	*Magnolia*	30 g
Gan Jiang	*Zingiber*	2 g
Mu Xiang	*Saussurea*	15 g
Chen Pi	*Citrus*	30 g
Fu Ling	*Poria*	15 g
Cao Dou Kou	*Alpinia*	15 g
Zhi Gan Cao	*Glycyrrhiza*	15 g
[Sheng Jiang	*Zingiber*	3 g]

Upper jiao heat with middle jiao cold usually caused by cold food which restricts Spleen qi. This leads to damp which then turns to heat. The heat rises upward and bothers the Heart causing thirst, restlessness, full/cold abdomen with pain, or nausea and vomiting.

T red or pale, red tip, thin sticky coat

P rapid, wiry

HUANG LIAN TANG

Coptis Decoction

Extract Formula Name: Coptis Combination

Huang Lian	*Coptis*	5 g
Gan Jiang	*Zingiber*	5 g
Gui Zhi	*Cinnamomum*	5 g
Ren Shen	*Panax*	3 g
Ban Xia	*Pinellia*	9 g
Da Zao	*Ziziphus*	9 - 12 pc
Gan Cao	*Glycyrrhiza*	6 g

Qi/yang/blood deficiency with bleeding where the Spleen is not governing blood causing melena, hematemesis, or uterine bleeding which is pale in color.

T pale, thin white coat

P deep, thin, weak

☞ Fu Long Gan - Terra Flava Usta should be cooked 30 minutes prior to adding the remaining herbs. E Jiao - Equus should be added to the strained tea.

HUANG TU TANG

Yellow Earth Decoction

Extract Formula Name: Fu-lung-kan Combination

Fu Long Gan	*Terra Flava Usta*	30 g
E Jiao	*Equus*	9 g
Sheng Di Huang	*Rehmannia*	9 g
Fu Zi	*Aconitum*	9 g
Huang Qin	*Scutellaria*	9 g
Bai Zhu	*Atractylodes*	9 g
Gan Cao	*Glycyrrhiza*	9 g

Kidney and Spleen yang deficiency with cold which has invaded all three yin channels (taiyin, shaoyin, and jueyin). Symptoms include shivering from cold, icy limbs and face, watery diarrhea, or cough with profuse saliva production.

T pale, wet, thin white moist coat

P minute or frail

☞ Remove She Xiang - Moschus, decoct the rest of the formula as usual, then add powdered Moschus to each dosage.

HUI YANG JIU JI TANG

Restore and Revive the Yang Decoction

Fu Zi	Aconitum	9 g
Rou Gui	Cinnamomum	3 - 6 g
Ren Shen	Panax	6 - 9 g
Gan Jiang	Zingiber	3 - 6 g
Fu Ling	Poria	6 - 9 g
Chen Pi	Citrus	3 - 6 g
Bai Zhu	Atractylodes	6 - 9 g
Wu Wei Zi	Schisandra	3 - 6 g
Ban Xia	Pinellia	6 - 9 g
Gan Cao	Glycyrrhiza	3 - 6 g
She Xiang	Moschus	0.3 g
[Sheng Jiang	Zingiber	1 - 3 g]

Spleen yang deficiency with cold and phlegm. Cough or vomiting with clear sputum, and decreased appetite.

T pale, moist white coat

P deep, slow, slippery

LI ZHONG HUA TAN WAN

Regulate the Middle and Transform Phlegm Pill

Ren Shen	Panax	6 - 9 g
Fu Ling	Poria	6 - 9 g
Bai Zhu	Atractylodes	3 - 9 g
Gan Jiang	Zingiber	3 - 9 g
Ban Xia	Pinellia	6 - 9 g
Gan Cao	Glycyrrhiza	3 - 6 g

Middle jiao qi/yang deficiency resulting in loss of appetite, absence of thirst, watery diarrhea with undigested food, or cold or painful limbs.

T pale, swollen, teethmarks, white coat

P deep, weak

✪ Major Formula

LI ZHONG WAN

Regulate the Middle Pill

Extract Formula Name: Ginseng and Ginger Combination

Ren Shen	*Panax*	6 - 9 g
Gan Jiang	*Zingiber*	6 - 9 g
Bai Zhu	*Atractylodes*	6 - 9 g
Gan Cao	*Glycyrrhiza*	3 - 6 g

Liver qi stagnation with cold in the Stomach causing abdominal pain which is relieved by warmth. The Formula is also useful for dysmenorrhea.

T pale, white coat

P weak, slow, or wiry

LIANG FU WAN

Galanga and Cyperus Pill

Extract Formula Name: Galanga and Cyperus Formula

Gao Liang Jiang	*Alpinia*	6 - 9 g
Xiang Fu	*Cyperus*	6 - 9 g

Watery fluids in the Lungs and Spleen yang deficiency causing cough, wheezing, and a stuffy sensation in the chest.

T pale, sticky or slippery white coat

P slippery, wiry

LING GAN WU WEI JIANG XIN TANG

Poria, Licorice, Schisandra, Ginger, and Asarum Decoction

Fu Ling	*Poria*	6 - 12 g
Gan Cao	*Glycyrrhiza*	3 - 9 g
Wu Wei Zi	*Schisandra*	6 - 9 g
Gan Jiang	*Zingiber*	3 - 9 g
Xi Xin	*Asarum*	6 - 9 g

Spleen/Stomach yang deficiency causing phlegm accumulation which affects the Lungs; or taiyang disease was mistreated and guided into the Spleen leading to water accumulation. Symptoms include dyspnea, clear phlegm expectoration, and fullness in the chest and flanks.

T pale, slippery white coat

P slippery, weak, deep

LING GUI ZHU GAN TANG

Poria, Cinnamon Twig, Atractylodes, and Licorice Decoction

Extract Formula Name: Hoelen and Atractylodes Combination

Fu Ling	*Poria*	6 - 12 g
Gui Zhi	*Cinnamomum*	3 - 9 g
Bai Zhu	*Atractylodes*	6 - 9 g
Gan Cao	*Glycyrrhiza*	3 - 6 g

Sudden cold stagnation and cold food obstructing the Stomach and Large Intestines completely. This causes sudden, severe pain and bowel obstruction.

T pale

P tight, deep

☞ The herbs should be powdered and adults should take 1 g doses with warm water.

✘ Ba Dou - Croton is a toxic herb that should be used with extreme caution. Do not use during pregnancy.

SAN WU BEI JI WAN

Three-Substance Pill for Emergencies

Extract Formula Name: Rhubarb, Ginger and Croton Formula

Da Huang	*Rheum*	30 g
Ba Dou	*Croton*	30 g
Gan Jiang	*Zingiber*	30 g

Severe qi deficiency with yang and blood deficiency and cold symptoms. Irregular menstruation with a pale and watery flow, dizziness, pale or sallow face, cold limbs, or chills.

T pale, wet, thin white coat

P deep, weak, thready

SHAN HE YIN

Mountain and River Decoction

Shu Di Huang	*Rehmannia*	15 - 25 g
Dang Gui	*Angelica*	6 - 9 g
Bai Shao Yao	*Paeonia*	6 - 9 g
Chuan Xiong	*Ligusticum*	3 - 9 g
Rou Gui	*Cinnamomum*	3 - 9 g
Huang Qi	*Astragalus*	6 - 15 g

Spleen/Kidney qi and yang deficiency causing edema which manifests mostly in the lower body. Other symptoms include cold limbs, poor appetite, decreased urination, or heaviness.

T pale, sticky coat

P deep, slow, maybe thin

SHI PI YIN

Bolster the Spleen Decoction

Extract Brion Name: Magnolia and Atractylodes Combination

Fu Zi	*Aconitum*	6 - 9 g
Bai Zhu	*Atractylodes*	6 - 9 g
Mu Gua	*Chaenomeles*	6 - 9 g
Hou Po	*Magnolia*	6 - 12 g
Gan Jiang	*Zingiber*	6 - 9 g
Mu Xiang	*Saussurea*	6 - 9 g
Fu Ling	*Poria*	6 - 9 g
Da Fu Pi	*Areca*	3 - 6 g
Cao Guo	*Amomum*	3 - 6 g
Zhi Gan Cao	*Glycyrrhiza*	3 - 6 g
[Da Zao	*Ziziphus*	1 - 3 pc]
[Sheng Jiang	*Zingiber*	3 - 6 g]

Exterior cold has gone internally. qi and yang are very weak and Kidney/Spleen yang have been damaged. Symptoms include low blood pressure, cold limbs, shock, or sweating.

T pale, or purple, moist white coat

P minute

☞ The raw type of Aconite is used here since it is much warmer than the prepared kind. 6 - 12 g of honey are often added for detoxification. Fu Zi - Aconitum is soaked in 8 - 10 cups of boiling water for 30 minutes to one hour. The remaining herbs should be added during the last 25 minutes and decocted as usual.

✘ Fu Zi - Aconitum in its raw form is toxic and is intended for short-term use only.

SI NI TANG

Frigid Extremities Decoction

Extract Formula Name: Aconite, Ginger and Licorice Combination

Fu Zi	*Aconitum*	9 - 15 g
Gan Jiang	*Zingiber*	6 - 12 g
Zhi Gan Cao	*Glycyrrhiza*	3 - 6 g

Kidney/Spleen yang deficiency leading to dawn diarrhea.

T pale, white coat

P deep, weak, slow

SI SHEN WAN

Four-Miracle Pill

Extract Formula Name: Psoralea and Myristica Formula

Bu Gu Zhi	*Psoralea*	12 - 18 g
Rou Dou Kou	*Myristica*	6 - 9 g
Wu Zhu Yu	*Evodia*	3 - 6 g
Wu Wei Zi	*Schisandra*	6 - 9 g
[Sheng Jiang	*Zingiber*	3 - 6 g]
[Da Zao	*Ziziphus*	3 - 5 pc]

Kidney and Spleen yang deficiency which developed after a chronic damp heat dysentery causing damp cold. This obstructs the Large Intestines, manifesting as dark blood in the stools with pus.

T pale

P minute

☞ Ingredients should be ground into a powder.

TAO HUA TANG

Peach Blossom Decoction

Extract Formula Name: Kaolin and Oryza Combination

Chi Shi Zhi	*Halloysitum Rubrum*	20 - 30 g
Jing Mi	*Oryza*	20 - 30 g
Gan Jiang	*Zingiber*	6 - 9 g

Spleen yang deficiency causing constipation or diarrhea with pain. Dysentery with pus or blood.

T pale, swollen, teethmarks, white coat

P deep, weak, thin, or wiry

☞ Da Huang - Rheum should be added during the last 3 - 5 minutes of the decoction process.

✘ Do not use during pregnancy.

WEN PI TANG

Warm the Spleen Decoction

Da Huang	*Rheum*	6 - 12 g
Gan Jiang	*Zingiber*	3 - 9 g
Ren Shen	*Panax*	6 - 9 g
Fu Zi	*Aconitum*	6 - 9 g
Gan Cao	*Glycyrrhiza*	3 - 9 g

Spleen qi deficiency with cold which restricts the Liver and Stomach. This results in tight abdominal pain, cold in the middle and lower jiao, vomiting, or acid regurgitation; or cold causes vertex headaches via the Liver channel. This Liver qi stagnation is not due to emotional reasons but is caused by cold.

T pale, purplish, moist white coat

P slow, or wiry, thin

WU ZHU YU TANG

Evodia Decoction

Extract Formula Name: Evodia Combination

Wu Zhu Yu	*Evodia*	3 - 6 g
Ren Shen	*Panax*	6 - 9 g
Sheng Jiang	*Zingiber*	12 - 20 g
Da Zao	*Ziziphus*	6 - 12 pc

Spleen qi and yang deficiency with damp and water accumulation causing loose stools with undigested food.

T pale, swollen, teethmarks, white sticky coat

P weak, deep, or frail

XIAO BAN XIA TANG

Minor Pinellia Decoction

Ban Xia	*Pinellia*	6 - 9 g
Sheng Jiang	*Zingiber*	3 - 6 g

1. Chronic Spleen qi deficiency with chronic cold evil qi leading to qi and blood deficiency. The main symptom is abdominal spasms. 2. Liver qi stagnation or Liver overacting on Spleen. In the latter two instances the dosage of 'Bai Shao Yao - Paeonia' should be increased.

T pale or light purple, thin white coat

P weak or slightly wiry

☞ Yi Tang - Saccharum Granorum should be added to the strained tea.

XIAO JIAN ZHONG TANG

Minor Construct the Middle Decoction

Extract Formula Name: Minor Cinnamon and Peony Combination

Yi Tang	*Saccharum Granorum*	15 - 30 g
Gui Zhi	*Cinnamomum*	3 - 9 g
Bai Shao Yao	*Paeonia*	6 - 9 g
Sheng Jiang	*Zingiber*	6 - 9 g
Da Zao	*Ziziphus*	3 - 5 pc
Zhi Gan Cao	*Glycyrrhiza*	3 - 6 g

Cold damp has entered the Spleen leading to water accumulation and Spleen yang deficiency. This causes damp in the middle jiao which bothers the Gallbladder so the bile cannot circulate properly. This manifests as yin-type jaundice.

T pale, white coat

P weak, deep

YIN CHEN ZHU FU TANG

Artemisia Yinchenhao, Atractylodes and Prepared Aconite Decoction

Extract Formula Name: Capillaris, Atractylodes and Aconite Combination

Yin Chen Hao	*Artemisia*	3 - 6 g
Gan Jiang	*Zingiber*	3 - 6 g
Bai Zhu	*Atractylodes*	6 - 9 g
Rou Gui	*Cinnamomum*	1 - 3 g
Fu Zi	*Aconitum*	1 - 3 g
Zhi Gan Cao	*Glycyrrhiza*	3 - 6 g

Chronic diarrhea has depleted Spleen and Kidney yang causing prolapse of the rectum or bowel incontinence.

T pale, white coat

P deep, slow

ZHEN REN YANG ZANG TANG

True Man's Decoction to Nourish the Organs

Ren Shen	*Panax*	6 - 9 g
Rou Gui	*Cinnamomum*	3 g
Bai Zhu	*Atractylodes*	6 - 12 g
He Zi	*Terminalia*	6 - 9 g
Rou Dou Kou	*Myristica*	9 - 12 g
Ying Su Ke	*Papaver*	6 - 15 g
Mu Xiang	*Saussurea*	3 - 9 g
Dang Gui	*Angelica*	6 - 15 g
Bai Shao Yao	*Paeonia*	9 - 12 g
Zhi Gan Cao	*Glycyrrhiza*	3- 6 g

Spleen/Kidney qi and yang deficient patient suffers easily from wind cold with internal water accumulation, or experiences urinary difficulty, diarrhea, or edema.

T pale, swollen, teethmarks, moist, thin white coat

P frail or minute

ZHEN WU TANG

True Warrior Decoction

Extract Formula Name: Vitality Combination

Fu Zi	*Aconitum*	6 - 9 g
Bai Zhu	*Atractylodes*	6 - 9 g
Bai Shao Yao	*Paeonia*	6 - 9 g
Fu Ling	*Poria*	6 - 9 g
Sheng Jiang	*Zingiber*	6 - 9 g

Spleen yang deficiency with middle jiao qi stagnation causing fullness and distention.

T pale, light purple, swollen, teethmarks, white coat

P weak, deep

ZHI SHI LI ZHONG WAN

Immature Bitter Orange Pill to Regulate the Middle

Zhi Shi	*Citrus*	6 - 9 g
Ren Shen	*Panax*	6 - 9 g
Gan Jiang	*Zingiber*	3 - 9 g
Bai Zhu	*Atractylodes*	6 - 9 g
Fu Ling	*Poria*	6 - 9 g
Gan Cao	*Glycyrrhiza*	3 - 6 g

Joint pain due to cold damp and Spleen yang deficiency.

T pale, sticky white coat

P deep, slippery, thin

☞ Grind herbs into a powder and administer as a draft with 4 - 8 pieces of Sheng Jiang - Zingiber.

ZHU FU TANG

Atractylodes and Prepared Aconite Decoction

Bai Zhu	*Atractylodes*	90 - 120 g
Fu Zi	*Aconitum*	30 - 45 g
Gan Cao	*Glycyrrhiza*	30 - 45 g
[Sheng Jiang	*Zingiber*	4 - 8 pc]

SPLEEN QI SINKING

- bearing down sensation
- prolapses of any kind

T pale

P weak

Spleen/Stomach qi deficiency where the Spleen qi is sinking, or the Spleen is not governing the blood. qi deficiency can lead to (morning) fever, early periods, weakness, diarrhea, or pallor.

T pale, swollen, teethmarks, thin white coat

P weak

✪ Major Formula

BU ZHONG YI QI TANG

Tonify the Middle and Augment the Qi Decoction

Extract Formula Name: Ginseng and Astragalus Combination

Ren Shen	*Panax*	6 - 12 g
Huang Qi	*Astragalus*	9 - 15 g
Dang Gui	*Angelica*	6 - 9 g
Chen Pi	*Citrus*	3 - 6 g
Sheng Ma	*Cimicifuga*	3 - 6 g
Chai Hu	*Bupleurum*	3 - 9 g
Bai Zhu	*Atractylodes*	3 - 9 g
Zhi Gan Cao	*Glycyrrhiza*	3 - 6 g

Kidney yin and Spleen qi/blood deficiency causing uterine prolapse with low back pain, night urination, or hearing loss and tinnitus.

T red or pale

P frail

DA BU YUAN JIAN

Great Tonify the Basal Decoction

Ren Shen	*Panax*	6 - 12 g
Shu Di Huang	*Rehmannia*	9 - 25 g
Shan Yao	*Dioscorea*	6 - 9 g
Shan Zhu Yu	*Cornus*	3 - 6 g
Gou Qi Zi	*Lycium*	6 - 9 g
Dang Gui	*Angelica*	6 - 9 g
Du Zhong	*Eucommia*	6 - 9 g
Gan Cao	*Glycyrrhiza*	3 - 6 g

Spleen qi deficiency during pregnancy with lethargy, spotting, or low back pain.

T pale, swollen, teethmarks, thin white coat

P weak, thin

☞ E Jiao - Equus should be added at the end to the strained tea.

JIA JIAN BU ZHONG YI QI TANG

Modified Tonify the Middle and Augment the Qi Decoction

Ren Shen	*Panax*	6 - 9 g
Huang Qi	*Astragalus*	6 - 12 g
Chen Pi	*Citrus*	3 - 6 g
Bai Zhu	*Atractylodes*	3 - 9 g
Sheng Ma	*Cimicifuga*	3 - 6 g
Chai Hu	*Bupleurum*	3 - 9 g
E Jiao	*Equus*	3 - 9 g
Ai Ye	*Artemisia*	3 - 9 g
Gan Cao	*Glycyrrhiza*	3 - 6 g

Spleen qi deficiency causing severe uterine bleeding which is pale in color, or early or irregular periods. The Spleen qi is sinking causing a restless fetus.

T pale, swollen, teethmarks, thin white coat

P weak

JU YUAN JIAN

Lift the Source Decoction

Ren Shen	Panax	6 - 9 g
Huang Qi	Astragalus	9 - 12 g
Sheng Ma	Cimicifuga	3 - 6 g
Bai Zhu	Atractylodes	3 - 6 g
Gan Cao	Glycyrrhiza	3 - 6 g

Spleen qi deficiency with qi sinking in the chest causing shortness of breath, dyspnea, or loose stools.

T pale, thin white coat

P deep, weak

SHENG XIAN TANG

Raise the Sinking Decoction

Huang Qi	*Astragalus*	15 - 20 g
Sheng Ma	*Cimicifuga*	3 - 6 g
Zhi Mu	*Anemarrhena*	6 - 9 g
Chai Hu	*Bupleurum*	3 - 9 g
Jie Geng	*Platycodon*	3 - 6 g

Chronic diarrhea has depleted Spleen and Kidney yang causing prolapse of the rectum or bowel incontinence.

T pale, white coat

P deep, slow

ZHEN REN YANG ZANG TANG

True Man's Decoction to Nourish the Organs

Ren Shen	Panax	6 - 9 g
Rou Gui	Cinnamomum	3 g
Bai Zhu	Atractylodes	6 - 12 g
He Zi	Terminalia	6 - 9 g
Rou Dou Kou	Myristica	9 - 12 g
Ying Su Ke	Papaver	6 - 15 g
Mu Xiang	Saussurea	3 - 9 g
Dang Gui	Angelica	6 - 15 g
Bai Shao Yao	Paeonia	9 - 12 g
Zhi Gan Cao	Glycyrrhiza	3- 6 g

SPLEEN NOT CONTROLLING THE BLOOD

- bleeding under the skin (purpura)
- uterine bleeding
- bruising

T pale

P weak, thin

Spleen is cold and deficient, and fails to govern the blood. This leads to bleeding in the upper body. Liver yang rising symptoms usually accompany this symptom picture.

T pale, thin white coat

P slow, weak

BAI YE TANG

Biota Twig Decoction

Ce Bai Ye	Biota	6 - 9 g
Pao Jiang	Zingiber	6 - 9 g
Ai Ye	Artemisia	9 - 15 g

Spleen/Stomach qi deficiency where the Spleen qi is sinking, or the Spleen is not governing the blood. Qi deficiency can lead to (morning) fever, early periods, weakness, diarrhea, or pallor.

T pale, swollen, teethmarks, thin white coat

P weak

BU ZHONG YI QI TANG

Tonify the Middle and Augment the Qi Decoction

Extract Formula Name: Ginseng and Astragalus Combination

Ren Shen	*Panax*	6 - 12 g
Huang Qi	*Astragalus*	9 - 15 g
Dang Gui	*Angelica*	6 - 9 g
Chen Pi	*Citrus*	3 - 6 g
Sheng Ma	*Cimicifuga*	3 - 6 g
Chai Hu	*Bupleurum*	3 - 9 g
Bai Zhu	*Atractylodes*	3 - 9 g
Zhi Gan Cao	*Glycyrrhiza*	3 - 6 g

Qi/blood deficiency with bleeding, fever, heat feelings in the muscles, thirst with a desire for warm liquids, or irregular periods.

T pale, thin coat

P empty

DANG GUI BU XUE TANG

Dang Gui Decoction to Tonify the Blood

Extract Formula Name: Tang-Kuei and Astragalus Combination

Huang Qi	*Astragalus*	30 g
Dang Gui	*Angelica*	6 g

Spleen qi deficiency leading to uncontrolled menstrual bleeding which is pale and watery (ben lou syndrome).

T pale, swollen, teethmarks, thin coat

P hollow or thin, deep, weak

GU BEN ZHI BENG TANG

Stabilize the Root and Stop Excessive Uterine Bleeding Decoction

Shu Di Huang	*Rehmannia*	6 - 20 g
Bai Zhu	*Atractylodes*	6 - 15 g
Huang Qi	*Astragalus*	6 - 15 g
Dang Gui	*Angelica*	6 - 9 g
Ren Shen	*Panax*	6 - 9 g
Pao Jiang	*Zingiber*	3 - 6 g

Heart blood and yin deficiency with Spleen qi deficiency leading to insomnia, decreased appetite, nightmares, irregular periods in women, or uterine bleeding which may manifest as beng lou – gushing or spotting. This formula is also useful for purpura due to Spleen qi/blood deficiency.

T pale, swollen, teethmarks, thin white coat

P weak, thin

✪ Major Formula

GUI PI TANG

Restore the Spleen Decoction

Extract Formula Name: Ginseng and Longan Combination

Ren Shen	*Panax*	6 - 9 g
Huang Qi	*Astralagus*	9 - 12 g
Fu Shen	*Poria*	6 - 9 g
Bai Zhu	*Atractylodes*	9 - 12 g
Long Yan Rou	*Euphoria*	9 - 12 g
Mu Xiang	*Saussurea*	3 - 6 g
Suan Zao Ren	*Zizyphus*	9 - 12 g
Dang Gui	*Angelica*	6 - 9 g
Yuan Zhi	*Polygala*	3 - 6 g
Gan Cao	*Glycyrrhiza*	3 - 6 g

Qi/yang/blood deficiency with bleeding where the Spleen is not governing blood causing melena, hematemesis, or uterine bleeding which is pale in color.

T pale, thin white coat

P deep, thin, weak

☞ Fu Long Gan - Terra Flava Usta should be cooked 30 minutes prior to adding the remaining herbs. E Jiao - Equus should be added to the strained tea.

HUANG TU TANG

Yellow Earth Decoction

Extract Formula Name: Fu-lung-kan Combination

Fu Long Gan	*Terra Flava Usta*	30 g
E Jiao	*Equus*	9 g
Sheng Di Huang	*Rehmannia*	9 g
Fu Zi	*Aconitum*	9 g
Huang Qin	*Scutellaria*	9 g
Bai Zhu	*Atractylodes*	9 g
Gan Cao	*Glycyrrhiza*	9 g

Spleen qi deficiency during pregnancy with lethargy, spotting, or low back pain.

T pale, swollen, teethmarks, thin white coat

P weak, thin

☞ E Jiao - Equus should be added at the end to the strained tea.

JIA JIAN BU ZHONG YI QI TANG

Modified Tonify the Middle and Augment the Qi Decoction

Ren Shen	Panax	6 - 9 g
Huang Qi	Astragalus	6 - 12 g
Chen Pi	Citrus	3 - 6 g
Bai Zhu	Atractylodes	3 - 9 g
Sheng Ma	Cimicifuga	3 - 6 g
Chai Hu	Bupleurum	3 - 9 g
E Jiao	Equus	3 - 9 g
Ai Ye	Artemisia	3 - 9 g
Gan Cao	Glycyrrhiza	3 - 6 g

Spleen qi deficiency causing severe uterine bleeding which is pale in color, or early or irregular periods. The Spleen qi is sinking causing a restless fetus.

T pale, swollen, teethmarks, thin white coat

P weak

JU YUAN JIAN

Lift the Source Decoction

Ren Shen	Panax	6 - 9 g
Huang Qi	Astragalus	9 - 12 g
Sheng Ma	Cimicifuga	3 - 6 g
Bai Zhu	Atractylodes	3 - 6 g
Gan Cao	Glycyrrhiza	3 - 6 g

STOMACH DISHARMONIES

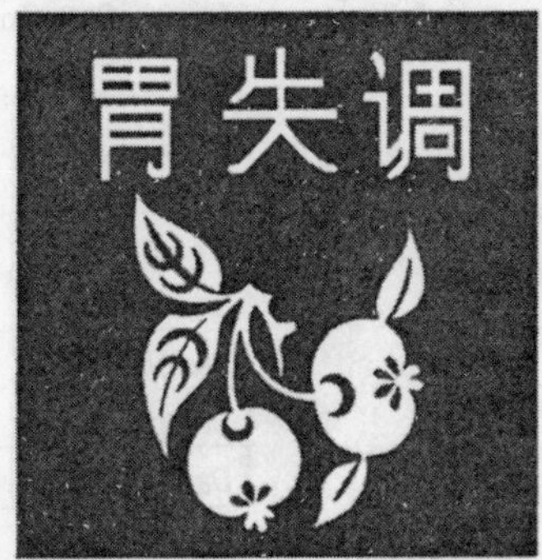

STOMACH AND SPLEEN QI DEFICIENCY

- epigastric discomfort
- hiccups or nausea
- decreased appetite
- loose stools

T pale

P weak

Spleen/Stomach qi yang deficiency resulting in hiccups, belching, and vomiting, and symptoms of coldness in the middle jiao.

T pale, thin coat

P weak, deep, maybe slow

✘ Contraindicated during pregnancy

DING XIANG SHI DI TANG

Clove and Kaki Decoction

Extract Formula Name: Clove and Kaki Combination

Ding Xiang	*Eugenia*	6 - 9 g
Shi Di	*Diospyros*	6 - 9 g
Ren Shen	*Panax*	3 - 9 g
Sheng Jiang	*Zingiber*	3 - 6 g

Heat and cold in the middle jiao with Spleen/Stomach qi deficiency, and cold predominance. The patient experiences mild middle jiao qi stagnation symptoms such as fullness or bloating.

T thin yellow coat

P weak, slightly wiry

GAN CAO XIE XIN TANG

Licorice Decoction to Drain the Epigastrium

Extract Formula Name: Pinellia and Licorice Combination

Ban Xia	*Pinellia*	6 - 9 g
Huang Qin	*Scutellaria*	9 - 12 g
Zhi Gan Cao	*Glycyrrhiza*	12 - 15 g
Gan Jiang	*Zingiber*	9 - 12 g
Ren Shen	*Panax*	9 - 12 g
Huang Lian	*Coptis*	3 - 6 g
Da Zao	*Ziziphus*	9 - 15 pc

Spleen/Stomach qi deficiency and cold causing vomiting during pregnancy.

T pale, thin white coat

P weak

GAN JIANG REN SHEN BAN XIA WAN

Ginger, Ginseng, and Pinellia Pill

Extract Formula Name: G.P. and Ginseng Formula

Gan Jiang	*Zingiber*	3 g
Ren Shen	*Panax*	3 g
Ban Xia	*Pinellia*	6 g
[Sheng Jiang	*Zingiber*	1 - 3 g]

Spleen/Stomach qi deficiency with cold and wei (defensive) qi deficiency; also useful for peptic ulcers and chronic allergies. Other symptoms include poor appetite or spontaneous sweating.

T pale, thin white coat

P weak, slow, thin, wiry

☞ Yi Tang - Saccharum Granorum is added to the strained tea.

HUANG QI JIAN ZHONG TANG

Astragalus Decoction to Construct the Middle

Extract Formula Name: Astragalus Combination

Gui Zhi	*Cinnamomum*	9 g
Bai Shao Yao	*Paeonia*	18 g
Sheng Jiang	*Zingiber*	10 g
Da Zao	*Ziziphus*	3 - 6 pc
Gan Cao	*Glycyrrhiza*	6 g
Yi Tang	*Saccharum Granorum*	30 g
Huang Qi	*Astragalus*	9 g

Heat in the Stomach with qi and yin deficiency and rebellious Stomach qi causing thirst, vomiting, loss of appetite, nausea, or hiccups.

T red

P thin, rapid, weak

JU PI ZHU RU TANG I

Tangerine Peel and Bamboo Shaving Decoction

Extract Formula Name: Aurantium and Bamboo Combination

Chen Pi	*Citrus*	6 - 12 g
Ren Shen	*Panax*	6 - 9 g
Zhu Ru	*Bambusa*	6 - 12 g
Da Zao	*Ziziphus*	3 - 6 pc
Sheng Jiang	*Zingiber*	3 - 9 g
Gan Cao	*Glycyrrhiza*	3 - 6 g

Wind heat invading the intestines and damaging the Spleen and Stomach qi. Severe constipation with blood deficiency which may lead to wind, or blood stagnation.

T pale or purple

P thin or choppy

RUN CHANG WAN II

Moisten the Intestines Pill from Discussion of the Spleen and Stomach

Da Huang	*Rheum*	9 - 12 g
Tao Ren	*Prunus*	15 - 25 g
Huo Ma Ren	*Cannabis*	15 - 30 g
Dang Gui Wei	*Angelica*	6 - 12 g
Qiang Huo	*Notopterygium*	6 - 9 g

Lung/Stomach qi deficiency with cough, expectoration of clear sputum, dry mouth, or thirst.

T pale, moist coat

P weak

SHENG JIANG GAN CAO TANG

Ginger and Licorice Decoction

Sheng Jiang	*Zingiber*	6 - 12 g
Ren Shen	*Panax*	6 - 9 g
Da Zao	*Ziziphus*	3 - 9 pc
Gan Cao	*Glycyrrhiza*	6 - 12 g

Stomach/Spleen qi deficiency. This is the basic prescription for building qi. Symptoms include poor appetite, loose bowel movements, or lethargy.

T pale, thin white coat

P weak, deep

✪ Major Formula

SI JUN ZI TANG

Four-Gentlemen Decoction

Extract Formula Name: Four Major Herbs Combination

Ren Shen	*Panax*	6 - 9 g
Bai Zhu	*Atractylodes*	3 - 9 g
Fu Ling	*Poria*	6 - 9 g
Gan Cao	*Glycyrrhiza*	3 - 6 g

Phlegm accumulation with Stomach qi deficiency causing hiccups, fullness, or nausea and vomiting.

T pale, white sticky coat

P frail, slippery, or wiry

☞ Xuan Fu Hua - Inula should be wrapped in a cheese cloth for decoction.

XUAN FU DAI ZHE TANG

Inula and Hematite Decoction

Extract Formula Name: Inula and Hematite Combination

Xuan Fu Hua	*Inula*	6 - 9 g
Dai Zhe Shi	*Haematitum*	6 - 12 g
Ren Shen	*Panax*	6 - 9 g
Ban Xia	*Pinellia*	6 - 9 g
Da Zao	*Ziziphus*	3 - 6 pc
Sheng Jiang	*Zingiber*	6 - 9 g
Zhi Gan Cao	*Glycyrrhiza*	3 - 6 g

Chronic Spleen qi deficiency causing qi stagnation. The qi stagnation gives rise to cold and heat symptoms in the middle jiao. This in turn damages the Spleen and Stomach again causing distention in the epigastrium and abdomen, or alternating constipation and diarrhea.

T pale, thin yellowish coat

P wiry

ZHI SHI XIAO PI WAN

Immature Bitter Orange Pill to Reduce Focal Distention

Zhi Shi	*Citrus*	6 - 12 g
Hou Po	*Magnolia*	6 - 15 g
Ban Xia	*Pinellia*	6 - 9 g
Huang Lian	*Coptis*	9 - 15 g
Fu Ling	*Poria*	6 - 9 g
Bai Zhu	*Atractylodes*	3 - 9 g
Ren Shen	*Panax*	6 - 9 g
Gan Jiang	*Zingiber*	3 - 6
Mai Ya	*Hordeum*	3 - 9 g
Zhi Gan Cao	*Glycyrrhiza*	3 - 6 g

QI AND BLOOD STAGNATION IN THE STOMACH

- stabbing pain which gets worse after eating
- melena
- hematemesis

T purple

P wiry or choppy

Intestinal abscess or acute appendicitis due to heat and blood stagnation causing mass formation in the lower right quadrant with pain.

T yellow sticky coat

P rapid, slippery

☞ Da Huang - Rheum should be added during the last 3 - 5 minutes of the decoction process. Mang Xiao - Mirabilitum should be added to the strained tea..

✘ Do not use with appendicitis during pregnancy.

DA HUANG MU DAN TANG

Rhubarb and Moutan Decoction

Extract Formula Name: Rhubarb and Moutan Combination

Da Huang	*Rheum*	6 - 12 g
Mang Xiao	*Mirabilitum*	6 - 12 g
Dong Gua Ren	*Benincasa*	12 - 20 g
Tao Ren	*Prunus*	9 - 12 g
Mu Dan Pi	*Paeonia*	6 - 9 g

Yin and blood deficiency with blood stagnation causing emaciation, no appetite, amenorrhea, tidal fever, or abdominal distention.

T red, pale, purple or purple spots

P thin, choppy

✘ Do not use during pregnancy.

DA HUANG ZHE CHONG WAN

Rhubarb and Eupolyphaga Pill

Da Huang	*Rheum*	12 - 18 g
Tu Bie Chong	*Eupolyphaga*	3 g
Xing Ren	*Prunus*	3 - 6 g
Gan Qi	*Sinica*	3 g
Sheng Di Huang	*Rehmannia*	12 - 18 g
Bai Shao Yao	*Paeonia*	6 - 12 g
Meng Chong	*Tabanus*	3 - 6 g
Qi Cao	*Holotrichia*	3 - 6 g
Tao Ren	*Prunus*	6 - 9 g
Shui Zhi	*Hirudo*	3 - 6 g
Huang Qin	*Scutellaria*	6 g
Gan Cao	*Glycyrrhiza*	3 - 6 g

Spleen/Kidney yang deficiency causing dawn diarrhea with middle jiao qi stagnation symptoms such as excruciating abdominal pain and severe fullness feelings.

T pale, swollen, teethmarks, light purple, white coat

P deep, weak, or slippery

DAN LIAO SI SHEN WAN

Four-Miracle Pill from the Tranquil Hut

Bu Gu Zhi	*Psoralea*	6 - 12 g
Xiao Hui Xiang	*Foeniculum*	3 - 9 g
Rou Dou Kou	*Myristica*	9 - 12 g
Mu Xiang	*Saussurea*	3 - 6 g

Qi stagnation in the upper and middle jiao with slow blood circulation causing intermittent chest pain, and epigastric or abdominal discomfort.

T purple

P choppy

DAN SHEN YIN

Salvia Decoction

Dan Shen	*Salvia*	30 g
Sha Ren	*Amomum*	5 g
Tan Xiang	*Santalum*	5 g

Heat and cold in the middle jiao with Spleen/Stomach qi deficiency, and cold predominance. The patient experiences mild middle jiao qi stagnation symptoms such as fullness or bloating.

T thin yellow coat

P weak, slightly wiry

GAN CAO XIE XIN TANG

Licorice Decoction to Drain the Epigastrium

Extract Formula Name: Pinellia and Licorice Combination

Ban Xia	*Pinellia*	6 - 9 g
Huang Qin	*Scutellaria*	9 - 12 g
Zhi Gan Cao	*Glycyrrhiza*	12 - 15 g
Gan Jiang	*Zingiber*	9 - 12 g
Ren Shen	*Panax*	9 - 12 g
Huang Lian	*Coptis*	3 - 6 g
Da Zao	*Ziziphus*	9 - 15 pc

Qi/blood stagnation under the diaphragm and epigastrium, or masses in the abdomen or epigastrium.

T purple

P wiry or choppy

✘ Do not use during pregnancy.

✪ Major Formula

GE XIA ZHU YU TANG

Drive Out Blood Stasis Below the Diaphragm Decoction

Extract Formula Name: Persica and Carthamus Combination

Dang Gui	*Angelica*	6 - 9 g
Chuan Xiong	*Ligusticum*	6 - 9 g
Tao Ren	*Prunus*	6 - 9 g
Hong Hua	*Carthamus*	3 - 6 g
Mu Dan Pi	*Paeonia*	6 - 9 g
Chi Shao Yao	*Paeonia*	6 - 9 g
Yan Hu Suo	*Corydalis*	3 - 6 g
Xiang Fu	*Cyperus*	3 - 9 g
Zhi Ke	*Citrus*	3 - 6 g
Wu Ling Zhi	*Trogopterus*	6 - 9 g
Wu Yao	*Lindera*	3 - 6 g
Gan Cao	*Glycyrrhiza*	6 - 9 g

Cold in the Spleen/Stomach after ingestion of cold food with damp and qi stagnation in the center. Symptoms include lack of appetite, loose stools, or nausea and vomiting.

T pale, sticky white coat

P weak, deep, or tight

HOU PO WEN ZHONG TANG

Magnolia Bark Decoction for Warming the Middle

Extract Formula Name: Magnolia and Saussurea Combination

Hou Po	*Magnolia*	30 g
Gan Jiang	*Zingiber*	2 g
Mu Xiang	*Saussurea*	15 g
Chen Pi	*Citrus*	30 g
Fu Ling	*Poria*	15 g
Cao Dou Kou	*Alpinia*	15 g
Zhi Gan Cao	*Glycyrrhiza*	15 g
[Sheng Jiang	*Zingiber*	3 g]

Wind cold and damp accumulation, with qi stagnation in the middle jiao causing diarrhea, nausea, vomiting, headache, or fever and chills.

T white sticky coat

P soggy or slippery

☞ All ingredients should be ground into a powder. Take 6 g two to three times a day.

HUO XIANG ZHENG QI SAN

Agastache Powder to Rectify the Qi

Extract Formula Name: Agastache Formula

Huo Xiang	*Agastache*	9 g
Hou Po	*Magnolia*	6 - 9 g
Bai Zhi	*Angelica*	3 - 6 g
Zi Su Ye	*Perilla*	3 - 6 g
Chen Pi	*Citrus*	6 g
Bai Zhu	*Atractylodes*	6 g
Fu Ling	*Poria*	3 - 6 g
Ban Xia	*Pinellia*	6 g
Da Fu Pi	*Areca*	3 - 6 g
Jie Geng	*Platycodon*	6 g
Gan Cao	*Glycyrrhiza*	6 - 9 g
[Da Zao	*Ziziphus*	1 - 3 g]
[Sheng Jiang	*Zingiber*	3 - 6 g]

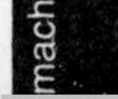

Yangming organ syndrome in the abdomen (pi man zao shi - glomus, fullness, dryness, excess) with blood stasis causing acute yang jaundice, Gallbladder infection, intestinal obstruction, possible palpable mass, or nausea and vomiting.

T very red, maybe purplish, dry, rough surface, yellow/brown coat

P flooding, rapid

☞ Da Huang - Rheum should be added during the last 3 - 5 minutes of the decoction process. Mang Xiao - Mirabilitum should be dissolved into the strained tea.

✘ Do not use during pregnancy.

JIA JIAN CHENG QI TANG

Modified Order the Qi Decoction

Da Huang	*Rheum*	9 - 12 g
Mang Xiao	*Mirabilitum*	6 - 9 g
Hou Po	*Magnolia*	9 - 12 g
Zhi Shi	*Citrus* ′	6 g
Tao Ren	*Prunus*	9 - 15 g
Bai Shao Yao	*Paeonia*	9 - 15 g
Lai Fu Zi	*Raphanus*	6 - 12 g

Food stagnation with severe heat, qi, damp, and blood stagnation causing fullness, belching with sour taste, dysentery, or severe abdominal pain.

T forceful, rapid

P thick sticky yellow coat

✘ Do not use during pregnancy.

MU XIANG BING LANG WAN

Aucklandia and Betel Nut Pill

Mu Xiang	*Saussurea*	3 - 9 g
Bing Lang	*Areca*	3 - 9 g
Xiang Fu	*Cyperus*	3 - 9 g
Qing Pi	*Citrus*	3 - 6 g
Da Huang	*Rheum*	9 - 12 g
Qian Niu Zi	*Pharbitis*	9 - 18 g
E Zhu	*Curcuma*	3 - 9 g
Huang Bai	*Phellodendron*	6 - 12 g
Huang Lian	*Coptis*	3 - 9 g
[Sheng Jiang	*Zingiber*	3 - 6 g]

Stomach/Spleen deficiency with cold damp and middle jiao qi stagnation causing fullness and distention.

T thick sticky white coat

P slippery

PING WEI SAN

Calm the Stomach Powder

Extract Formula Name: Magnolia and Ginger Formula

Hou Po	*Magnolia*	6 - 12 g
Cang Zhu	*Atractylodes*	9 - 15 g
Chen Pi	*Citrus*	6 - 12 g
Gan Cao	*Glycyrrhiza*	3 - 6 g
[Da Zao	*Ziziphus*	3 - 6 pc]
[Sheng Jiang	*Zingiber*	3 - 6 g]

Stomach

Qi and blood stagnation with cold causing pain and discomfort in the Stomach and abdomen.

T dark purple

P wiry or choppy

✘ Do not use during pregnancy.

SHOU NIAN SAN

Pinch Powder

Wu Ling Zhi	*Trogopterus*	15 g
Yan Hu Suo	*Corydalis*	15 g
Mo Yao	*Commiphora*	15 g
Cao Guo	*Amomum*	15 g

Blood stagnation with fire in the lower jiao causing constipation, sudden abdominal pain, dysmenorrhea, intestinal obstruction, or melena. In severe cases this may lead to restlessness, or even delirium.

T purple

P choppy or forceful

☞ Da Huang - Rheum should be added during the last 3 - 5 minutes of the decoction process. Mang Xiao - Mirabilitum should be added to the strained tea.

✘ Do not use during pregnancy.

TAO HE CHENG QI TANG

Peach Pit Decoction to Order the Qi

Extract Formula Name: Prunus and Rhubarb Combination

Tao Ren	*Prunus*	9 - 15 g
Gui Zhi	*Cinnamomum*	6 - 9 g
Mang Xiao	*Mirabilitum*	3 - 6 g
Da Huang	*Rheum*	9 - 12 g
Gan Cao	*Glycyrrhiza*	3 - 6 g

Spleen/Stomach qi deficiency with qi stagnation and cold damp in the middle jiao causing abdominal fullness or morning sickness.

T pale, light purple, swollen, sticky white coat

P slippery, weak

XIANG SHA LIU JUN ZI TANG

Six-Gentlemen Decoction with Aucklandia and Amomum

Extract Formula Name: Saussurea and Cardamon Combination

Ren Shen	*Panax*	6 - 9 g
Fu Ling	*Poria*	6 - 9 g
Bai Zhu	*Atractylodes*	3 - 9 g
Chen Pi	*Citrus*	3 - 6 g
Ban Xia	*Pinellia*	6 - 9 g
Sha Ren	*Amomum*	3 g
Mu Xiang	*Saussurea*	3 - 6 g
Zhi Gan Cao	*Glycyrrhiza*	3 - 6 g

Excess fire with qi stagnation causing fullness, possible palpable mass, or constipation. This is a mild yangming organ disease.

T red, thin sticky yellow coat

P rapid, slightly forceful

✘ Do not use during pregnancy.

XIAO CHENG QI TANG

Minor Order the Qi Decoction

Extract Formula Name: Minor Rhubarb Combination

Da Huang	*Rheum*	9 - 12 g
Zhi Shi	*Citrus*	6 g
Hou Po	*Magnolia*	6 - 12 g

Spleen qi deficiency with middle jiao qi stagnation and diarrhea, or malnutrition in children.

T pale, light purple, white coat

P weak, thin

YI HUANG SAN

Benefit the Yellow Powder

Chen Pi	*Citrus*	30 g
Qing Pi	*Citrus*	15 g
Ding Xiang	*Eugenia*	3 - 6 g
He Zi	*Terminalia*	15 g
Zhi Gan Cao	*Glycyrrhiza*	15 g

Chronic Spleen qi deficiency causing qi stagnation. The qi stagnation gives rise to cold and heat symptoms in the middle jiao. This in turn damages the Spleen and Stomach again causing distention in the epigastrium and abdomen, or alternating constipation and diarrhea.

T pale, thin yellowish coat

P wiry

ZHI SHI XIAO PI WAN

Immature Bitter Orange Pill to Reduce Focal Distention

Zhi Shi	*Citrus*	6 - 12 g
Hou Po	*Magnolia*	6 - 15 g
Ban Xia	*Pinellia*	6 - 9 g
Huang Lian	*Coptis*	9 - 15 g
Fu Ling	*Poria*	6 - 9 g
Bai Zhu	*Atractylodes*	3 - 9 g
Ren Shen	*Panax*	6 - 9 g
Gan Jiang	*Zingiber*	3 - 6
Mai Ya	*Hordeum*	3 - 9 g
Zhi Gan Cao	*Glycyrrhiza*	3 - 6 g

Severe abdominal distention (pi man - fullness, firmness) due to Spleen qi deficiency, or qi stagnation with damp and heat. Symptoms include constipation, or odorous diarrhea, thirst, yellow urine, or fever.

T sticky yellow coat

P wiry, rapid

ZHONG MAN FEN XIAO WAN

Separate and Reduce Fullness in the Middle Pill

Hou Po	*Magnolia*	9 - 18 g
Jiang Huang	*Curcuma*	6 g
Zhi Shi	*Citrus*	9 - 12 g
Ban Xia	*Pinellia*	6 - 12 g
Ren Shen	*Panax*	3 g
Zhi Mu	*Anemarrhena*	6 - 9 g
Gan Jiang	*Zingiber*	3 - 6 g
Huang Lian	*Coptis*	3 - 9 g
Huang Qin	*Scutellaria*	9 - 15 g
Bai Zhu	*Atractylodes*	6 g
Ze Xie	*Alisma*	6 g
Sha Ren	*Amomum*	3 - 6 g
Chen Pi	*Citrus*	3 - 6 g
Fu Ling	*Poria*	6 - 9 g
Zhu Ling	*Polyporus*	3 - 6 g
Zhi Gan Cao	*Glycyrrhiza*	3 - 6 g

Stomach

FOOD OR PHLEGM STAGNATION IN THE STOMACH

- bad breath
- fullness and distention worse with eating and better with vomiting
- nausea
- sour regurgitation, or belching

T thick sticky coat

P forceful, slippery

Disharmony between Stomach and Intestines which leads to failure to descend qi which, subsequently, leads to food, damp, or water accumulation (or heat and cold accumulation in the Stomach). This is known as glomus and fullness (pi man). Symptoms include epigastric fullness, gurgling, reflux or loose stools.

T yellow sticky coat

P wiry, rapid

BAN XIA XIE XIN TANG

Pinellia Decoction to Drain the Epigastrium

Extract Formula Name: Pinellia Combination

Ban Xia	*Pinellia*	6 - 12 g
Huang Qin	*Scutellaria*	6 - 9 g
Huang Lian	*Coptis*	3 - 6 g
Gan Jiang	*Zingiber*	3 - 6 g
Ren Shen	*Panax*	6 - 9 g
Da Zao	*Ziziphus*	3 - 5 pc
Gan Cao	*Glycyrrhiza*	3 - 6 g

Food stagnation with indigestion, nausea and vomiting, fullness, diarrhea, foul belching, or no appetite.

T white yellow or sticky yellow coat

P slippery

✪ Major Formula

BAO HE WAN

Preserve Harmony Pill

Extract Formula Name: Citrus and Crataegus Formula

Lai Fu Zi	*Raphanus*	6 - 9 g
Lian Qiao	*Forsythia*	3 - 9 g
Shan Zha	*Crataegus*	6 - 12 g
Shen Qu	*Massa Fermentata*	6 - 12 g
Fu Ling	*Poria*	6 - 9 g
Ban Xia	*Pinellia*	6 - 9 g
Chen Pi	*Citrus*	3 - 6 g

Basic formula for phlegm amd damp accumulation from Stomach and Spleen qi deficiency. Symptoms include nausea and vomiting, or epigastric distention.

T sticky coat

P slippery

ER CHEN TANG

Two-Cured Decoction

Extract Formula Name: Citrus and Pinellia Combination

Ban Xia	*Pinellia*	6-9 g
Chen Pi	*Citrus*	3-6 g
Fu Ling	*Poria*	6-9 g
Gan Cao	*Glycyrrhiza*	3-6 g
[Sheng Jiang	*Zingiber*	3-6 g]
[Da Zao	*Ziziphus*	3 pc]

Damp/water accumulation in the middle jiao causing abdominal fullness, ascites, or scanty urination.

T sticky white coat

P slippery

FEN XIAO TANG

Separate and Reduce Decoction

Extract Formula Name: Hoelen and Alisma Combination

Cang Zhu	*Atractylodes*	3-6 g
Bai Zhu	*Atractylodes*	3-6 g
Hou Po	*Magnolia*	6-9 g
Fu Ling	*Poria*	6-9 g
Chen Pi	*Citrus*	3-6 g
Zhu Ling	*Polyporus*	3-6 g
Deng Xin Cao	*Juncus*	1 pc
Ze Xie	*Alisma*	3-6 g
Xiang Fu	*Cyperus*	3-6 g
Mu Xiang	*Saussurea*	3-6 g
Zhi Shi	*Citrus*	3-6 g
Sha Ren	*Amomum*	1-3 g
Da Fu Pi	*Areca*	3-6 g
Sheng Jiang	*Zingiber*	3-6 g

1. Food stagnation, or overconsumption of alcohol has damaged the Spleen and now there is more cold stagnation in the middle jiao. The Spleen is very weak, and now produces more damp. 2. Alcohol poisoning with Spleen qi deficiency, damp and cold accumulation in the middle jiao. 3. Spleen qi deficiency with an abdominal mass or firmness (pi man).

T pale, swollen, teethmarks, white sticky coat

P deep, slippery, weak

GE HUA JIE XING TANG

Pueraria Flower Decoction

Ren Shen	*Panax*	6 - 9 g
Bai Zhu	*Atractylodes*	6 - 9 g
Fu Ling	*Poria*	9 - 12 g
Gan Cao	*Glycyrrhiza*	3 - 6 g
Chen Pi	*Citrus*	3 - 6 g
Mu Xiang	*Saussurea*	6 - 9 g
Sha Ren	*Amomum*	3 - 6 g
Ze Xie	*Alisma*	3 - 9 g
Zhu Ling	*Polyporus*	3 - 9 g
Qing Pi	*Citrus*	3 - 6 g
Shen Qu	*Massa Fermentata*	6- 15 g
Ge Hua	*Pueraria*	6 - 15 g
Bai Dou Kou	*Amomum*	3 - 6 g

Phlegm or food stagnation in the chest/diaphragm/upper epigastrium area. This formula will relieve the stagnation by causing vomiting.

T sticky coat

P slippery, somewhat superficial in the first (cun) position.

☞ Decoct for only 5 - 10 minutes or make into a paste with 10 g of Dan Dou Chi - Glycine.

✘ This formula will cause vomiting. Do not use during pregnancy.

GUA DI SAN

Melon Pedicle Powder

Extract Formula Name: Melon Pedicle Formula

Gua Di	*Cucumis*	1 - 3 g
Chi Xiao Dou	*Phaseolus*	1 - 3 g

Food stagnation damaged the Spleen leading to qi/damp/food stagnation which starts to create some heat. Symptoms include indigestion or borborygmus.

T sticky yellow coat

P slippery, weak

JIAN PI WAN

Strengthen the Spleen Pill

Ren Shen	*Panax*	6 - 12 g
Bai Zhu	*Atractylodes*	9 - 15 g
Fu Ling	*Poria*	9 - 12 g
Shen Qu	*Massa Fermentata*	9 - 12 g
Shan Yao	*Dioscorea*	6 - 9 g
Shan Zha	*Crataegus*	6 - 9 g
Mu Xiang	*Saussurea*	3 g
Mai Ya	*Hordeum*	6 - 9 g
Huang Lian	*Coptis*	3 g
Rou Dou Kou	*Myristica*	3 - 9 g
Sha Ren	*Amomum*	3 - 6 g
Chen Pi	*Citrus*	3 - 6 g
Gan Cao	*Glycyrrhiza*	3 g

Food stagnation with severe heat, qi, damp, and blood stagnation causing fullness, belching with sour taste, dysentery, or severe abdominal pain.

T forceful, rapid

P thick sticky yellow coat

✘ Do not use during pregnancy.

MU XIANG BING LANG WAN

Aucklandia and Betel Nut Pill

Mu Xiang	*Saussurea*	3 - 9 g
Bing Lang	*Areca*	3 - 9 g
Xiang Fu	*Cyperus*	3 - 9 g
Qing Pi	*Citrus*	3 - 6 g
Da Huang	*Rheum*	9 - 12 g
Qian Niu Zi	*Pharbitis*	9 - 18 g
E Zhu	*Curcuma*	3 - 9 g
Huang Bai	*Phellodendron*	6 - 12 g
Huang Lian	*Coptis*	3 - 9 g
[Sheng Jiang	*Zingiber*	3 - 6 g]

Food stagnation causing damp and heat. This leads to diarrhea which is usually incomplete, or tenesmus with a painful rectum.

T red, thick sticky coat

P slippery, rapid

✘ Do not use during pregnancy.

MU XIANG DAO ZHI WAN

Aucklandia to Guide Out Stagnation Pill

Zhi Shi	*Citrus*	6 - 15 g
Da Huang	*Rheum*	6 - 12 g
Huang Qin	*Scutellaria*	6 - 9 g
Huang Lian	*Coptis*	6 g
Fu Ling	*Poria*	6 - 9 g
Shen Qu	*Massa Fermentata*	6 - 15 g
Bai Zhu	*Atractylodes*	3 - 9 g
Ze Xie	*Alisma*	6 - 9 g
Mu Xiang	*Saussurea*	6 - 9 g
Bing Lang	*Areca*	6 - 9 g

Phlegm damp cough with cold in the Lungs or food stagnation. Symptoms include dyspnea with profuse phlegm expectoration, and poor appetite.

T sticky white coat

P slippery

SAN ZI YANG QIN TANG

Three-Seed Decoction to Nourish One's Parents

Zi Su Zi	*Perilla*	6 - 9 g
Lai Fu Zi	*Raphanus*	6 - 9 g
Bai Jie Zi	*Brassica*	3 - 9 g

Water accumulation with heat, damp and qi stagnation; or Stomach deficiency with food stagnation and water. Symptoms include diarrhea, borborygmus, or epigastric distention.

T red, sticky yellow coat

P slippery, rapid

SHENG JIANG XIE XIN TANG

Fresh Ginger Decoction to Drain the Epigastrium

Extract Formula Name: Pinellia and Ginger Combination

Sheng Jiang	*Zingiber*	9 - 12 g
Ban Xia	*Pinellia*	6 - 9 g
Ren Shen	*Panax*	6 - 12 g
Gan Jiang	*Zingiber*	3 - 6 g
Huang Qin	*Scutellaria*	6 - 9 g
Huang Lian	*Coptis*	3 - 6 g
Da Zao	*Ziziphus*	6 - 10 pc
Gan Cao	*Glycyrrhiza*	3 - 6 g

Stomach phlegm heat causing palpitations, insomnia, dizziness, bitter taste, or fullness in the chest.

T sticky yellow coat

P rapid, slippery

SHI YI WEI WEN DAN TANG

Eleven-Ingredient Decoction to Warm the Gallbladder

Chen Pi	*Citrus*	6 g
Ban Xia	*Pinellia*	6 - 9 g
Fu Ling	*Poria*	6 - 12 g
Gan Cao	*Glycyrrhiza*	3 - 6 g
Zhu Ru	*Bambusa*	6 - 12 g
Zhi Shi	*Citrus*	3 - 6 g
Shi Chang Pu	*Acorus*	6 - 9 g
Huang Lian	*Coptis*	3 - 6 g
Yuan Zhi	*Polygala*	3 - 6 g
Zhen Zhu Mu	*Pteria*	12 - 25 g
Ye Jiao Teng	*Polygonum*	12 - 25 g

Chronic water accumulation in the chest and hypochondrium causing cough and shortness of breath.

T white sticky coat

P deep, wiry

☞ Grind ingredients into a powder and take in 0.7 g doses in the morning with a warm tea made from ten pieces of Da Zao - Ziziphus. Between five and six bowel movements are expected after each dose.

✘ Do not use during pregnancy or in weak patients. Gan Sui - Euphorbia is toxic.

SHI ZAO TANG

Ten-Jujube Decoction

Extract Formula Name: Jujube Combination

Gan Sui	*Euphorbia*	6 g
Yuan Hua	*Daphne*	6 g
Jing Da Ji	*Euphorbia*	6 g

Liver and Stomach imbalance with phlegm accumulation and Gallbladder heat. Symptoms include fullness in the chest, bitter taste, thirst without desire to drink, or vomiting. In severe cases, mental confusion or a rattly throat may be seen.

T red, sticky yellow coat

P rapid, slippery and/or wiry

WEN DAN TANG

Warm the Gallbladder Decoction

Extract Formula Name: Hoelen and Bamboo Combination

Ban Xia	*Pinellia*	6 - 9 g
Chen Pi	*Citrus*	9 - 12 g
Fu Ling	*Poria*	6 - 12 g
Zhi Shi	*Citrus*	3 - 6 g
Zhu Ru	*Bambusa*	6 g
Sheng Jiang	*Zingiber*	3 - 6 g
Gan Cao	*Glycyrrhiza*	3 - 6 g
Da Zao	*Ziziphus*	2 pc

Food stagnation with abdominal fullness, pain, or disgust at food.

T thick sticky coat

P slippery

XIANG SHA PING WEI SAN

Cyperus and Amomum Powder to Calm the Stomach

Xiang Fu	*Cyperus*	6 g
Sha Ren	*Amomum*	3 - 6 g
Cang Zhu	*Atractylodes*	6 - 12 g
Shan Zha	*Crataegus*	6 - 9 g
Chen Pi	*Citrus*	3 - 6 g
Bai Shao Yao	*Paeonia*	6 - 9 g
Zhi Ke	*Citrus*	3 - 6 g
Mai Ya	*Hordeum*	6 - 12 g
Sheng Jiang	*Zingiber*	3 - 6 g
Gan Cao	*Glycyrrhiza*	3 - 6 g

Infant with food stagnation, vomiting, or poor digestion.

T sticky coat

P wiry

☞ Herbs should be powdered and mixed with glutinous rice.

XIAO RU WAN

Reduce Infantile Stagnation Pill

Xiang Fu	*Cyperus*	30 - 60 g
Shen Qu	*Massa Fermentata*	15 - 30 g
Mai Ya	*Hordeum*	15 - 30 g
Zhi Gan Cao	*Glycyrrhiza*	9 - 15 g
Chen Pi	*Citrus*	9 - 15 g
Sha Ren	*Amomum*	15 - 30 g

Phlegm accumulation with Stomach qi deficiency causing hiccups, fullness, or nausea and vomiting.

T pale, white sticky coat

P frail, slippery, or wiry

☞ Xuan Fu Hua - Inula should be wrapped in a cheese cloth for decoction.

XUAN FU DAI ZHE TANG

Inula and Hematite Decoction

Extract Formula Name: Inula and Hematite Combination

Xuan Fu Hua	*Inula*	6 - 9 g
Dai Zhe Shi	*Haematitum*	6 - 12 g
Ren Shen	*Panax*	6 - 9 g
Ban Xia	*Pinellia*	6 - 9 g
Da Zao	*Ziziphus*	3 - 6 pc
Sheng Jiang	*Zingiber*	6 - 9 g
Zhi Gan Cao	*Glycyrrhiza*	3 - 6 g

Stagnations of all kinds (qi, blood, food, damp, etc.). Symptoms include epigastric or chest fullness, nausea and vomiting, or poor appetite.

T depends on particular syndrome involved

P depends on particular syndrome involved

YUE JU WAN

Escape Restraint Pill

Chuan Xiong	*Ligusticum*	3 - 9 g
Cang Zhu	*Atractylodes*	3 - 9 g
Zhi Zi	*Gardenia*	3 - 9 g
Xiang Fu	*Cyperus*	3 - 9 g
Shen Qu	*Massa Fermentata*	3 - 9 g

Food stagnation in the middle jiao with damp and heat accumulation: cold and heat in the middle jiao with Spleen deficiency. Symptoms include fullness with pain, odorous diarrhea, mucus, tenesmus, gas, or constipation.

T red, red sides, rough, thick sticky yellow coat

P slippery, rapid, forceful

✘ Caution during pregnancy.

ZHI SHI DAO ZHI WAN

Immature Bitter Orange Pill to Guide Out Stagnation

Extract Formula Name: Chih-shih and Rhubarb Formula

Zhi Shi	*Citrus*	9 - 15 g
Shen Qu	*Massa Fermentata*	9 - 15 g
Da Huang	*Rheum*	15 - 25 g
Huang Qin	*Scutellaria*	6 - 9 g
Huang Lian	*Coptis*	6 - 9 g
Fu Ling	*Poria*	6 - 9 g
Ze Xie	*Alisma*	6 - 9 g
Bai Zhu	*Atractylodes*	6 - 9 g

Chronic Spleen qi deficiency causing qi stagnation. The qi stagnation gives rise to cold and heat symptoms in the middle jiao. This in turn damages the Spleen and Stomach again causing distention in the epigastrium and abdomen, or alternating constipation and diarrhea.

T pale, thin yellowish coat

P wiry

ZHI SHI XIAO PI WAN

Immature Bitter Orange Pill to Reduce Focal Distention

Zhi Shi	*Citrus*	6 - 12 g
Hou Po	*Magnolia*	6 - 15 g
Ban Xia	*Pinellia*	6 - 9 g
Huang Lian	*Coptis*	9 - 15 g
Fu Ling	*Poria*	6 - 9 g
Bai Zhu	*Atractylodes*	3 - 9 g
Ren Shen	*Panax*	6 - 9 g
Gan Jiang	*Zingiber*	3 - 6
Mai Ya	*Hordeum*	3 - 9 g
Zhi Gan Cao	*Glycyrrhiza*	3 - 6 g

1. Chronic food stagnation with severe Spleen qi deficiency.
2. Severe acute food stagnation with mild Spleen qi deficiency. Symptoms include epigastric and abdominal distention, loose stools, and poor appetite.

T sticky coat

P wiry

ZHI ZHU WAN

Immature Bitter Orange and Atractylodes Pill

Bai Zhu	*Atractylodes*	9 - 15 g
Zhi Shi	*Citrus*	6 - 12 g

Damp heat accumulation in the middle jiao. There is more damp than heat causing fullness in the abdomen, thirst without desire to drink, or immediate fullness upon eating or drinking. This formula is also useful for yang jaundice.

T red, thick sticky coat

P slippery, rapid

ZHONG JIAO XIAN BI TANG

Middle Jiao and Clear Damp Decoction

Xing Ren	*Prunus*	3 - 6 g
Yi Yi Ren	*Coix*	9 - 12 g
Hua Shi	*Talcum*	6 g
Dou Juan	*Glycine*	9 g
Zhi Zi	*Gardenia*	6 - 9 g
Lian Qiao	*Forsythia*	6 g
Ban Xia	*Pinellia*	6 - 9 g
Han Fang Ji	*Stephania*	6 - 9 g
Can Sha	*Bombyx*	3 - 6 g
Shan Zha	*Crataegus*	3 - 9 g
Bian Dou	*Dolichos*	6 - 9 g

COLD OR YANG DEFICIENCY IN THE STOMACH

- **if cold:** acute sharp pain in the epigastrium with a preference for warmth
- vomiting of clear fluid
- any cool fluid is immediately vomited
- **if yang deficiency:** the epigastric pain is better with eating, pressure, and/or warmth
- cold extremities

T pale, moist, thick white coat

P deep, slow, tight

Disharmony between Stomach and Intestines which leads to failure to descend qi which, subsequently, leads to food, damp, or water accumulation (or heat and cold accumulation in the Stomach). This is known as glomus and fullness (pi man). Symptoms include epigastric fullness, gurgling, reflux or loose stools.

T yellow sticky coat

P wiry, rapid

BAN XIA XIE XIN TANG

Pinellia Decoction to Drain the Epigastrium

Extract Formula Name: Pinellia Combination

Ban Xia	*Pinellia*	6 - 12 g
Huang Qin	*Scutellaria*	6 - 9 g
Huang Lian	*Coptis*	3 - 6 g
Gan Jiang	*Zingiber*	3 - 6 g
Ren Shen	*Panax*	6 - 9 g
Da Zao	*Ziziphus*	3 - 5 pc
Gan Cao	*Glycyrrhiza*	3 - 6 g

Cold accumulation or yang deficiency in the abdomen leading to constipation with cramping pain. The qi stagnates and heats up which can cause a mild fever. Other symptoms include cold extremities and chills.

T normal or pale, white coat

P wiry or tight, deep

☞ Fu Zi - Aconitum should be powdered. Da Huang - Rheum should be added during the last 3 - 5 minutes of the decoction process.

✘ Do not use during pregnancy.

DA HUANG FU ZI TANG

Rhubarb and Aconite Decoction

Extract Formula Name: Rhubarb and Aconite Combination

Da Huang	*Rheum*	6 - 9 g
Fu Zi	*Aconitum*	6 g
Xi Xin	*Asarum*	3 - 6 g

Spleen yang deficiency with cold stagnation causing severe cramping pain, borborygmus, or possible vomiting.

T pale, light purple, swollen, moist white coat

P wiry or slow, deep

☞ Yi Tang - Saccharum Granorum is added to the strained tea.

DA JIAN ZHONG TANG

Major Construct the Middle Decoction

Extract Formula Name: Major Zanthoxylum Combination

Chuan Jiao	*Zanthoxylum*	3 - 6 g
Ren Shen	*Panax*	6 - 9 g
Gan Jiang	*Zingiber*	3 - 6 g
Yi Tang	*Saccharum Granorum*	20 g

Spleen qi and blood deficiency with slight cold leading to spasm pain or post-partum emaciation.

T pale, white coat

P weak

☞ Yi Tang - Saccharum Granorum is added to the strained tea.

DANG GUI JIAN ZHONG TANG

Dang Gui Decoction to Construct the Middle

Extract Formula Name: Tang-Kuei, Cinnamon and Peony Combination

Yi Tang	*Saccharum Granorum*	6 - 20 g
Gui Zhi	*Cinnamomum*	3 - 9 g
Bai Shao Yao	*Paeonia*	6 - 9 g
Sheng Jiang	*Zingiber*	3 - 6 g
Da Zao	*Ziziphus*	3 - 6 pc
Gan Cao	*Glycyrrhiza*	3 - 6 g
Dang Gui	*Angelica*	6 - 9 g

Longstanding cold with blood and yang deficiency leading to diarrhea, nausea and vomiting, or abdominal cramps.

T pale, swollen, teethmarks, wet, white coat

P slow, frail

DANG GUI SI NI JIA WU ZHU YU SHENG JIANG TANG

Dang Gui Decoction for Frigid Extremities plus Evodia and Fresh Ginger

Extract Formula Name: Tang-Kuei, Evodia and Ginger Combination

Dang Gui	*Angelica*	6 - 9 g
Gui Zhi	*Cinnamomum*	3 - 9 g
Xi Xin	*Asarum*	3 - 6 g
Bai Shao Yao	*Paeonia*	6 - 9 g
Mu Tong	*Akebia*	6 - 9 g
Wu Zhu Yu	*Evodia*	3 - 6 g
Da Zao	*Ziziphus*	25 pc
Sheng Jiang	*Zingiber*	4 pc
Gan Cao	*Glycyrrhiza*	3 - 6 g

Spleen/Stomach qi yang deficiency resulting in hiccups, belching, and vomiting, and symptoms of coldness in the middle jiao.

T pale, thin coat

P weak, deep, maybe slow

✘ Do not use during pregnancy

DING XIANG SHI DI TANG

Clove and Kaki Decoction

Extract Formula Name: Clove and Kaki Combination

Ding Xiang	*Eugenia*	6 - 9 g
Shi Di	*Diospyros*	6 - 9 g
Ren Shen	*Panax*	3 - 9 g
Sheng Jiang	*Zingiber*	3 - 6 g

Stomach/Spleen yang deficiency causing watery diarrhea and epigastric pain. Severe cold symptoms such as cold limbs and vomiting of clear fluids.

T pale, swollen, teethmarks, white coat

P minute

✪ **Major Formula**

FU ZI LI ZHONG WAN

Prepared Aconite Pill to Regulate the Middle

Extract Formula Name: Aconite, Ginseng, and Ginger Combination

Fu Zi	*Aconitum*	6 - 9 g
Ren Shen	*Panax*	3 - 9 g
Bai Zhu	*Atractylodes*	3 - 9 g
Gan Jiang	*Zingiber*	3 - 9 g
Zhi Gan Cao	*Glycyrrhiza*	3 - 6 g

Stomach and Spleen yang deficiency with wei qi deficiency and internal heat and damp. Symtoms include loose stools, sweating, or cold hands and feet.

T pale or red, white or yellow sticky coat

P deep, weak, thin, or rapid

✘ Caution during pregnancy.

FU ZI XIE XIN TANG

Aconite Decoction to Drain the Epigastrium

Fu Zi	*Aconitum*	3 - 6 g
Da Huang	*Rheum*	6 - 9 g
Huang Qin	*Scutellaria*	3 - 6 g
Huang Lian	*Coptis*	3 - 6 g

Cold in the Lungs and Stomach causing Lung atrophy, cold extremities, or clear sputum.

T pale, moist

P weak, slow

GAN CAO GAN JIANG TANG

Licorice and Ginger Decoction

Extract Formula Name: Licorice and Ginger Combination

Zhi Gan Cao	*Glycyrrhiza*	9 - 12 g
Gan Jiang	*Zingiber*	6 - 9 g

Heat and cold in the middle jiao with Spleen/Stomach qi deficiency, and cold predominance. The patient experiences mild middle jiao qi stagnation symptoms such as fullness or bloating.

T thin yellow coat

P weak, slightly wiry

GAN CAO XIE XIN TANG

Licorice Decoction to Drain the Epigastrium

Extract Formula Name: Pinellia and Licorice Combination

Ban Xia	*Pinellia*	6 - 9 g
Huang Qin	*Scutellaria*	9 - 12 g
Zhi Gan Cao	*Glycyrrhiza*	12 - 15 g
Gan Jiang	*Zingiber*	9 - 12 g
Ren Shen	*Panax*	9 - 12 g
Huang Lian	*Coptis*	3 - 6 g
Da Zao	*Ziziphus*	9 - 15 pc

Severe cold stagnation with Spleen/Kidney yang deficiency causing coldness in the face, cramping pain in the center, or dawn diarrhea.

T pale, purple, wet coat

P slow, tight

GUI FU LI ZHONG TANG

Cinnamon and Prepared Aconite Decoction to Regulate the Middle

Ren Shen	*Panax*	10 - 15 g
Bai Zhu	*Atractylodes*	6 - 9 g
Gan Jiang	*Zingiber*	6 - 9 g
Gan Cao	*Glycyrrhiza*	3 - 6 g
Fu Zi	*Aconitum*	3 - 6 g
Rou Gui	*Cinnamomum*	3 - 9 g

Upper jiao heat with middle jiao cold usually caused by cold food which restricts Spleen qi. This leads to damp which then turns to heat. The heat rises upward and bothers the Heart causing thirst, restlessness, full/cold abdomen with pain, or nausea and vomiting.

T red or pale, red tip, thin sticky coat

P rapid, wiry

HUANG LIAN TANG

Coptis Decoction

Extract Formula Name: Coptis Combination

Huang Lian	*Coptis*	5 g
Gan Jiang	*Zingiber*	5 g
Gui Zhi	*Cinnamomum*	5 g
Ren Shen	*Panax*	3 g
Ban Xia	*Pinellia*	9 g
Da Zao	*Ziziphus*	9 - 12 pc
Gan Cao	*Glycyrrhiza*	6 g

Wind cold and damp accumulation, with qi stagnation in the middle jiao causing diarrhea, nausea, vomiting, headache, or fever and chills.

T white sticky coat

P soggy or slippery

☞ All ingredients should be ground into a powder. Take 6 g two to three times a day.

HUO XIANG ZHENG QI SAN

Agastache Powder to Rectify the Qi

Extract Formula Name: Agastache Formula

Huo Xiang	*Agastache*	9 g
Hou Po	*Magnolia*	6 - 9 g
Bai Zhi	*Angelica*	3 - 6 g
Zi Su Ye	*Perilla*	3 - 6 g
Chen Pi	*Citrus*	6 g
Bai Zhu	*Atractylodes*	6 g
Fu Ling	*Poria*	3 - 6 g
Ban Xia	*Pinellia*	6 g
Da Fu Pi	*Areca*	3 - 6 g
Jie Geng	*Platycodon*	6 g
Gan Cao	*Glycyrrhiza*	6 - 9 g
[Da Zao	*Ziziphus*	1 - 3 g]
[Sheng Jiang	*Zingiber*	3 - 6 g]

Cold in the Stomach causing rebellious qi which leads to nausea, vomiting, or diarrhea.

T pale, white coat

P weak, slow

JU PI TANG

Tangerine Peel Decoction

Chen Pi	*Citrus*	9 - 12 g
Sheng Jiang	*Zingiber*	6 - 9 g

Middle jiao qi/yang deficiency resulting in loss of appetite, absence of thirst, watery diarrhea with undigested food, or cold or painful limbs.

T pale, swollen, teethmarks, white coat

P deep, weak

LI ZHONG WAN

Regulate the Middle Pill

Extract Formula Name: Ginseng and Ginger Combination

Ren Shen	*Panax*	6 - 9 g
Gan Jiang	*Zingiber*	6 - 9 g
Bai Zhu	*Atractylodes*	6 - 9 g
Gan Cao	*Glycyrrhiza*	3 - 6 g

Liver qi stagnation with cold in the Stomach causing abdominal pain which is relieved by warmth. The Formula is also useful for dysmenorrhea.

T pale, white coat

P weak, slow, or wiry

LIANG FU WAN

Galanga and Cyperus Pill

Extract Formula Name: Galanga and Cyperus Formula

Gao Liang Jiang	*Alpinia*	6 - 9 g
Xiang Fu	*Cyperus*	6 - 9 g

Sudden cold stagnation and cold food obstructing the Stomach and Large Intestines completely. This causes sudden, severe pain and bowel obstruction.

T pale

P tight, deep

☞ The herbs should be powdered and adults should take 1 g doses with warm water.

✘ Ba Dou - Croton is a toxic herb that should be used with extreme caution. Do not use during pregnancy.

SAN WU BEI JI WAN

Three-Substance Pill for Emergencies

Extract Formula Name: Rhubarb, Ginger and Croton Formula

Da Huang	*Rheum*	30 g
Ba Dou	*Croton*	30 g
Gan Jiang	*Zingiber*	30 g

Stomach deficiency with cold causing hiccups, vomiting, chronic belching, or fullness in the chest.

T pale

P weak

SHI DI TANG

Persimmon Calyx Decoction

Extract Formula Name: Kaki Combination

Shi Di	*Diospyros*	3 - 9 g
Ding Xiang	*Eugenia*	3 - 6 g
Sheng Jiang	*Zingiber*	3 - 9 g

Spleen qi deficiency with cold which restricts the Liver and Stomach. This results in tight abdominal pain, cold in the middle and lower jiao, vomiting, or acid regurgitation; or cold causes vertex headaches via the Liver channel. This Liver qi stagnation is not due to emotional reasons but is caused by cold.

T pale, purplish, moist white coat

P slow, or wiry, thin

WU ZHU YU TANG

Evodia Decoction

Extract Formula Name: Evodia Combination

Wu Zhu Yu	*Evodia*	3 - 6 g
Ren Shen	*Panax*	6 - 9 g
Sheng Jiang	*Zingiber*	12 - 20 g
Da Zao	*Ziziphus*	6 - 12 pc

Wind cold with internal qi stagnation causing belching, decreased appetite fever and chills, headache, absence of sweating and middle jiao fullness.

T thin white coat

P superficial

XIANG SU SAN

Cyperus and Perilla Leaf Powder

Extract Formula Name: Cyperus and Perilla Formula

Xiang Fu	*Cyperus*	6 - 9 g
Zi Su Ye	*Perilla*	6 - 9 g
Chen Pi	*Citrus*	3 - 6 g
Zhi Gan Cao	*Glycyrrhiza*	3 - 6 g

1. Chronic Spleen qi deficiency with chronic cold evil qi leading to qi and blood deficiency. The main symptom is abdominal spasms. 2. Liver qi stagnation or Liver overacting on Spleen. In the latter two instances the dosage of 'Bai Shao Yao - Paeonia' should be increased.

T pale or light purple, thin white coat

P weak or slightly wiry

☞ Yi Tang - Saccharum Granorum should be added to the strained tea.

XIAO JIAN ZHONG TANG

Minor Construct the Middle Decoction

Extract Formula Name: Minor Cinnamon and Peony Combination

Yi Tang	*Saccharum Granorum*	15 - 30 g
Gui Zhi	*Cinnamomum*	3 - 9 g
Bai Shao Yao	*Paeonia*	6 - 9 g
Sheng Jiang	*Zingiber*	6 - 9 g
Da Zao	*Ziziphus*	3 - 5 pc
Zhi Gan Cao	*Glycyrrhiza*	3 - 6 g

STOMACH YIN DEFICIENCY

- constipation with dry stools
- afternoon heat
- thirst
- increased appetite

T red, geographic, scanty coat

P empty, or thin, rapid

Yangming channel disease, damp stagnation and yin deficiency leading to mouth sores, swollen, red gums with pus, bad breath, sore throat, or eye disorders.

T thick sticky yellow coat

P rapid, slippery, thin

GAN LU YIN

Sweet Dew Decoction

Extract Formula Name: Sweet Combination

Shu Di Huang	*Rehmannia*	6 - 9 g
Sheng Di Huang	*Rehmannia*	6 - 9 g
Huang Qin	*Scutellaria*	6 - 9 g
Zhi Ke	*Citrus*	3 - 6 g
Mai Men Dong	*Ophiopogon*	6 - 9 g
Tian Men Dong	*Asparagus*	6 - 9 g
Pi Pa Ye	*Eriobotrya*	12 - 18 g
Yin Chen Hao	*Artemisia*	6 - 9 g
Shi Hu	*Dendrobium*	6 - 9 g
Gan Cao	*Glycyrrhiza*	3 - 6 g

Epistaxis or hematemesis during menses due to Stomach deficiency and rebellious qi.

T pale

P weak, thin

JIA WEI MAI MEN DONG TANG

Augmented Ophiopogon Decoction

Mai Men Dong	*Ophiopogon*	9 - 15 g
Shan Yao	*Dioscorea*	9 - 12 g
Ren Shen	*Panax*	9 - 12 g
Dan Shen	*Salvia*	9 - 12 g
Ban Xia	*Pinellia*	6 - 9 g
Bai Shao Yao	*Paeonia*	6 - 9 g
Tao Ren	*Prunus*	3 - 6 g
Da Zao	*Ziziphus*	3 - 5 pc
Gan Cao	*Glycyrrhiza*	3 - 6 g

Heat in the Stomach with qi and yin deficiency and rebellious Stomach qi causing thirst, vomiting, loss of appetite, nausea, or hiccups.

T red

P thin, rapid, weak

JU PI ZHU RU TANG I

Tangerine Peel and Bamboo Shaving Decoction

Extract Formula Name: Aurantium and Bamboo Combination

Chen Pi	*Citrus*	6 - 12 g
Ren Shen	*Panax*	6 - 9 g
Zhu Ru	*Bambusa*	6 - 12 g
Da Zao	*Ziziphus*	3 - 6 pc
Sheng Jiang	*Zingiber*	3 - 9 g
Gan Cao	*Glycyrrhiza*	3 - 6 g

Stomach heat with qi and yin deficiency causing severe thirst, nausea and vomiting, or decreased appetite.

T red, thin yellow coat

P thin, weak, slightly rapid

JU PI ZHU RU TANG II

Tangerine Peel and Bamboo Shavings Decoction from Formulas to Aid the Living

Zhu Ru	*Bambusa*	6 - 9 g
Ban Xia	*Pinellia*	6 - 9 g
Chi Fu Ling	*Poria*	6 - 9 g
Ren Shen	*Panax*	3 - 6 g
Pi Pa Ye	*Eriobotrya*	6 - 9 g
Chen Pi	*Citrus*	3 - 6 g
Mai Men Dong	*Ophiopogon*	6 - 9 g
Zhi Gan Cao	*Glycyrrhiza*	3 - 6 g
[Sheng Jiang	*Zingiber*	3 - 6 pc]

Yin/blood deficiency causing constipation with dry stools; or excess heat causing constipation.

T red, dry yellow coat

P rapid, thin, or empty

✗ Do not use during pregnancy.

MA ZI REN WAN

Hemp Seed Pill

Extract Formula Name: Apricot Seed and Linum Formula

Huo Ma Ren	*Cannabis*	6 - 12 g
Da Huang	*Rheum*	6 - 9 g
Xing Ren	*Prunus*	6 - 9 g
Zhi Shi	*Citrus*	3 - 6 g
Bai Shao Yao	*Paeonia*	6 - 9 g
Hou Po	*Magnolia*	6 - 12 g

Stomach yin deficiency starts to produce heat which then burns Lung yin resulting in cough, wheezing, shortness of breath, or thirst.

T red, geographic spots, slight or no coat

P thin, rapid

MAI MEN DONG TANG

Ophiopogon Decoction

Extract Formula Name: Ophiopogon Combination

Mai Men Dong	*Ophiopogon*	6 - 12 g
Ren Shen	*Panax*	6 - 9 g
Ban Xia	*Pinellia*	6 - 9 g
Jing Mi	*Oryza*	9 - 12 g
Da Zao	*Ziziphus*	6 - 10 pc
Gan Cao	*Glycyrrhiza*	3 - 6 g

Blood deficiency causing constipation.

T pale

P weak, thin

WU REN WAN

Five-Seed Pill

Xing Ren	*Prunus*	9 - 20 g
Bai Zi Ren	*Biota*	3 - 6 g
Tao Ren	*Prunus*	9 - 15 g
Yu Li Ren	*Prunus*	3 - 6 g
Sha Ren	*Amomum*	3 - 6 g

Spleen qi with yin deficiency and heat accumulation causing constipation, or hardness and fullness in the abdomen.

T cracked, thin dry yellowish coat

P weak, thin, deep

XIN JIA HUANG LONG TANG

Newly-Augmented Yellow Dragon Decoction

Sheng Di Huang	*Rehmannia*	6 - 15 g
Ren Shen	*Panax*	6 - 9 g
Da Huang	*Rheum*	6 - 9 g
Mang Xiao	*Mirabilitum*	3 - 5 g
Mai Men Dong	*Ophiopogon*	9 - 15 g
Dang Gui	*Angelica*	6 - 9 g
Xuan Shen	*Scrophularia*	9 - 15 g
Gan Cao	*Glycyrrhiza*	3 - 6 g
Hai Shen	*Strichopus*	1 - 2 g

Stomach heat causing hiccups.

T red

P rapid

☞ 6 - 9 g of ginger juice should be added to the tea.

XIN ZHI JU PI ZHU RU TANG

Newly-Formulated Tangerine Peel and Bamboo Shavings Decoction

Zhu Ru	*Bambusa*	6 - 9 g
Chen Pi	*Citrus*	3 - 9 g
Shi Di	*Diospyros*	6 - 9 g
Sheng Jiang Zhi	*Zingiber*	6 - 9 g

Stomach yin deficiency due to febrile disease or Liver fire. Symptoms include bleeding gums, increased appetite, and thirst.

T slightly red, dry, scanty yellowish coat

P thin

YI WEI TANG

Benefit the Stomach Decoction

Extract Formula Name: Glehnia and Ophiopogon Combination

Sheng Di Huang	*Rehmannia*	9 - 15 g
Mai Men Dong	*Ophiopogon*	9 - 15 g
Bei Sha Shen	*Glehnia*	6 - 12 g
Yu Zhu	*Polygonatum*	3 - 6 g
Bing Tang	*Rock candy*	1 - 3 g

Stomach fire has damaged Stomach yin causing bleeding gums, frontal headache, aching teeth, or excess hunger.

T red, geographic, scanty yellow coat

P rapid, empty, thin

✪ Major Formula

YU NU JIAN

Jade Woman Decoction

Extract Formula Name: Rehmannia and Gypsum Combination

Shi Gao	*Gypsum*	6 - 15 g
Zhi Mu	*Anemarrhena*	9 - 15 g
Mai Men Dong	*Ophiopogon*	6 - 15 g
Shu Di Huang	*Rehmannia*	12 - 15 g
Huai Niu Xi	*Achyranthes*	9 - 15 g

Middle jiao diabetes (xiao ke) leading to hunger as the key symptom due to Stomach yin deficiency.

T red, scanty coat

P thin, slightly rapid

YU QUAN WAN

Jade Spring Pill

Tian Hua Fen	*Trichosanthes*	6 - 9 g
Ren Shen	*Panax*	6 - 9 g
Fu Ling	*Poria*	6 - 9 g
Huang Qi	*Astragalus*	6 - 12 g
Zi Su Zi	*Perilla*	3 - 9 g
Mai Men Dong	*Ophiopogon*	6 - 12 g
Gan Cao	*Glycyrrhiza*	3 - 6 g

Diabetes due to Kidney and Stomach yin deficiency with qi deficiency causing thirst and frequent, profuse urination.

T red, dry

P weak, thin

YU YE TANG

Jade Fluid Decoction

Shan Yao	*Dioscorea*	15 - 30 g
Tian Hua Fen	*Trichosanthes*	6 - 9 g
Huang Qi	*Astragalus*	9 - 15 g
Ji Nei Jin	*Gallus*	3 - 6 g
Zhi Mu	*Anemarrhena*	12 - 18 g
Wu Wei Zi	*Schisandra*	6 - 9 g
Ge Gen	*Pueraria*	2 - 5 g

Yin deficiency with dryness and heat in the yangming leading to constipation.

T red, dry yellow coat

P rapid, thin, wiry

☞ Da Huang - Rheum should be added during the last 3 minutes of the cooking process. Mang Xiao - Mirabilitum should be added to the strained tea.

✘ Do not use during pregnancy.

ZENG YE CHENG QI TANG

Increase the Fluids and Order the Qi Decoction

Xuan Shen	*Scrophularia*	15 - 25 g
Sheng Di Huang	*Rehmannia*	15 - 20 g
Mai Men Dong	*Ophiopogon*	15 - 20 g
Mang Xiao	*Mirabilitum*	3 - 6 g
Da Huang	*Rheum*	6 - 9 g

Yin deficiency with dryness and heat in the yangming leading to constipation.

T red, dry, scanty yellow coat

P thin, rapid, weak

ZENG YE TANG

Increase the Fluids Decoction

Extract Formula Name: Scrophularia and Ophiopogon Combination

Xuan Shen	*Scrophularia*	15 - 25 g
Sheng Di Huang	*Rehmannia*	15 - 20 g
Mai Men Dong	*Ophiopogon*	15 - 20 g

Qi level heat damaged the qi and yin. Now there is residual heat and a mild fever, dry mouth, and irritability.

T red

P rapid, weak, thin

ZHU YE SHI GAO TANG

Lophatherum and Gypsum Decoction

Extract Formula Name: Bamboo Leaves and Gypsum Combination

Dan Zhu Ye	*Lophatherum*	6 - 15 g
Shi Gao	*Gypsum*	20 - 30 g
Ban Xia	*Pinellia*	6 - 9 g
Ren Shen	*Panax*	3 - 6 g
Zhi Gan Cao	*Glycyrrhiza*	3 - 6 g
Jing Mi	*Oryza*	9 - 15 g
Mai Men Dong	*Ophiopogon*	12 - 15 g

STOMACH FIRE

- burning epigastric pain
- ravenous appetite
- gum bleeding
- mouth sores and bad breath

T red, thick yellow coat

P forceful, rapid

Toxic heat in the yangming channel causing dysentery, or pus or blood in the stools.

T red, yellow coat

P wiry, rapid, rolling

BAI TOU WENG TANG

Pulsatilla Decoction

Extract Formula Name: Anemone Combination

Bai Tou Weng	*Pulsatilla*	20 - 40 g
Huang Bai	*Phellodendron*	9 - 12 g
Qin Pi	*Fraxinus*	9 - 15 g
Huang Lian	*Coptis*	6 - 9 g

Intestinal abscess or acute appendicitis due to heat and blood stagnation causing mass formation in the lower right quadrant with pain.

T yellow sticky coat

P rapid, slippery

☞ Da Huang - Rheum should be added during the last 3 - 5 minutes of the decoction process. Mang Xiao - Mirabilitum should be added to the strained tea..

✘ Do not use with appendicitis during pregnancy.

DA HUANG MU DAN TANG

Rhubarb and Moutan Decoction

Extract Formula Name: Rhubarb and Moutan Combination

Da Huang	*Rheum*	6 - 12 g
Mang Xiao	*Mirabilitum*	6 - 12 g
Dong Gua Ren	*Benincasa*	12 - 20 g
Tao Ren	*Prunus*	9 - 12 g
Mu Dan Pi	*Paeonia*	6 - 9 g

Heat in the middle and upper jiao with fullness as the main symptom (pi-syndrome from pi man zhao shi - firmness, fullness, dryness, excess). Symptoms include nausea and vomiting, possible hematemesis, red face, palpitations, diarrhea, or bleeding in the upper body.

T red, yellow coat

P rapid

✘ Do not use during pregnancy.

DA HUANG XIE XIN TANG

Rhubarb to Drain the Epigastrium Decoction

Da Huang	*Rheum*	6 - 12 g
Huang Lian	*Coptis*	3 - 9 g

Wind heat with internal heat: taiyang and yangming organ disease. The heat is severe. Symptoms include dark yellow urine, constipation, severe fever and chills, heat sensations in the body, skin disorders, and a bitter taste.

T bright or dark red, dry, yellow coat

P flooding, rapid, wiry

☞ Ingredients should be ground into powder, then made into a pill with water. Take 6 g each time, twice a day.

✘ Do not use during pregnancy.

FANG FENG TONG SHENG SAN

Ledebouriella Powder that Sagely Unblocks

Extract Formula Name: Siler and Platycodon Formula

Fang Feng	*Ledebouriella*	9 - 15 g
Ma Huang	*Ephedra*	9 - 15 g
Da Huang	*Rheum*	9 - 15 g
Mang Xiao	*Mirabilitum*	9 - 15 g
Jing Jie	*Schizonepeta*	9 - 15 g
Bo He	*Mentha*	9 - 15 g
Zhi Zi	*Gardenia*	9 - 15 g
Hua Shi	*Talcum*	60 - 90 g
Shi Gao	*Gypsum*	15 - 30 g
Huang Qin	*Scutellaria*	15 - 30 g
Lian Qiao	*Forsythia*	9 - 15 g
Jie Geng	*Platycodon*	15 - 30 g
Dang Gui	*Angelica*	9 - 15 g
Bai Shao Yao	*Paeonia*	9 - 15 g
Chuan Xiong	*Ligusticum*	9 - 15 g
Bai Zhu	*Atractylodes*	9 - 15 g
Gan Cao	*Glycyrrhiza*	30 - 60 g

Wind heat with internal middle jiao heat and Large Intestine heat and damp causing dysentery: taiyang and yangming disease. Symptoms include fever, thirst, or burning anus.

T red, yellow coat

P rapid, slippery

GE GEN HUANG LIAN HUANG QIN TANG

Kudzu, Coptis, and Scutellaria Decoction

Extract Formula Name: Pueraria, Coptis and Scute Combination

Ge Gen	*Pueraria*	12 - 15 g
Huang Lian	*Coptis*	9 g
Huang Qin	*Scutellaria*	6 - 9 g
Gan Cao	*Glycyrrhiza*	3 - 6 g

Fire in the upper/middle jiao (chest/diaphragm) causing thirst, red lips, epistaxis, redness in the face, dark yellow urine, constipation, or delirium.

T red, dry yellow coat

P rapid

✘ Do not use during pregnancy.

LIANG GE SAN

Cool the Diaphragm Powder

Extract Formula Name: Forsythia and Rhubarb Formula

Da Huang	*Rheum*	6 - 9 g
Mang Xiao	*Mirabilitum*	6 - 9 g
Zhi Zi	*Gardenia*	3 - 6 g
Huang Qin	*Scutellaria*	6 - 9 g
Bo He	*Mentha*	3 - 6 g
Lian Qiao	*Forsythia*	9 - 12 g
Gan Cao	*Glycyrrhiza*	3 - 6 g
[Dan Zhu Ye	*Lophatherum*	3 - 6 g]

Yin/blood deficiency causing constipation with dry stools; or excess heat causing constipation.

T red, dry yellow coat

P rapid, thin, or empty

✘ Do not use during pregnancy.

MA ZI REN WAN

Hemp Seed Pill

Extract Formula Name: Apricot Seed and Linum Formula

Huo Ma Ren	*Cannabis*	6 - 12 g
Da Huang	*Rheum*	6 - 9 g
Xing Ren	*Prunus*	6 - 9 g
Zhi Shi	*Citrus*	3 - 6 g
Bai Shao Yao	*Paeonia*	6 - 9 g
Hou Po	*Magnolia*	6 - 12 g

Liver and Stomach fire causing dizziness, bad breath, anger outbursts, oral sores or ulcers, or constipation.

T red, sticky yellow coat

P rapid, wiry, forceful

☞ Niu Huang - Bos should be added at the end of the decoction process. Bing Pian - Dryobalanops and Xiong Huang - Realgar should be powdered prior to the decoction. This prescription is available in prepared form.

✘ Do not use during pregnancy

NIU HUANG JIE DU PIEN

Antiphlogistic Pills with Bos Calculus

Niu Huang	*Bos*	3 - 6 g
Xiong Huang	*Realgar*	3 - 6 g
Da Huang	*Rheum*	6 - 9 g
Jie Geng	*Platycodon*	3 - 6 g
Bing Pian	*Dryobalanops*	3 - 6 g
Shi Gao	*Gypsum*	9 - 15 g
Huang Qin	*Scutellaria*	6 - 9 g
Gan Cao	*Glycyrrhiza*	3 - 6 g

Yangming channel disease/Stomach fire causing bleeding gums, toothache, soreness in the tongue, headaches, or red eyes.

T red, dry

P rapid, flooding

✪ Major Formula

QING WEI SAN

Clear the Stomach Powder

Extract Formula Name: Coptis and Rehmannia Formula

Huang Lian	*Coptis*	3 - 6 g
Sheng Di Huang	*Rehmannia*	9 - 12 g
Mu Dan Pi	*Paeonia*	9 - 12 g
Dang Gui Shen	*Angelica*	9 - 12 g
Sheng Ma	*Cimicifuga*	9 - 15 g

Severe Stomach fire causing gum problems, ravenous appetite, or foul breath.

T red, sticky yellow coat

P wiry, forceful, rapid

QING WEI TANG

Clear the Stomach Decoction

Shi Gao	*Gypsum*	12 - 15 g
Sheng Di Huang	*Rehmannia*	6 - 12 g
Huang Qin	*Scutellaria*	6 - 9 g
Huang Lian	*Coptis*	6 g
Mu Dan Pi	*Paeonia*	6 - 9 g
Sheng Ma	*Cimicifuga*	3 - 6 g

Qi stagnation with fire causing acute pancreatitis. The patient will vomit immediately after food or liquid intake, and experiences epigastric discomfort. Acute pancreatitis can cause shock or sudden death.

T red, thin yellow coat

P rapid, wiry

☞ Mu Xiang - Saussurea and Da Huang - Rheum should be added near the end of decoction process. Mang Xiao - Mirabilitum should be added to the strained tea.

✘ Do not use during pregnancy.

QING YI TANG

Clear the Pancreas Decoction

Chai Hu	*Bupleurum*	6 - 15 g
Bai Shao Yao	*Paeonia*	6 - 15 g
Huang Qin	*Scutellaria*	9 - 12 g
Yan Hu Suo	*Corydalis*	6 - 9 g
Da Huang	*Rheum*	9 - 15 g
Mu Xiang	*Saussurea*	6 - 9 g
Hu Huang Lian	*Picrorhiza*	6 - 9 g
Mang Xiao	*Mirabilitum*	6 - 9 g

Liver and Stomach fire causing any kind of sudden bleeding disorder. The fire heats up the blood leading to hematemesis, epistaxis, or hemoptysis.

T dark red, yellow coat

P rapid, forceful, wiry

☞ The herbs should be partially charred prior to the decoction process.

✘ Caution during pregnancy.

SHI HUI SAN

Ten Partially-Charred Substance Powder

Xiao Ji	*Cephalanoplos*	9 - 15 g
Da Ji	*Cirsium*	9 - 12 g
Ce Bai Ye	*Biota*	9 - 12 g
Qian Cao Gen	*Rubia*	9 - 12 g
Da Huang	*Rheum*	9 - 12 g
He Ye	*Nelumbo*	9 - 12 g
Zhi Zi	*Gardenia*	6 - 12 g
Bai Mao Gen	*Imperata*	9 - 12 g
Zong Lu Pi	*Trachycarpus*	6 - 9 g
Mu Dan Pi	*Paeonia*	6 - 9 g

Diarrhea due to Spleen qi deficiency with damp and Stomach heat causing dysentery with mucous and possible bleeding.

T sticky yellow coat

P slippery, rapid

XIANG LIAN WAN

Aucklandia and Coptis Pill

Extract Formula Name: Saussurea and Coptis Formula

Mu Xiang	*Saussurea*	6 - 9 g
Huang Lian	*Coptis*	3 - 6 g
Wu Zhu Yu	*Evodia*	3 - 12 g

Stomach

Fire or heat hiding in the Spleen due to overeating leading to thirst, ravenous hunger, mouth sores, the tongues of infants hang out of the mouth, or drooling. Seen in the pediatric department.

T red, dry, yellow coat

P rapid

XIE HUANG SAN

Drain the Yellow Powder

Extract Formula Name: Siler and Licorice Formula

Shi Gao	*Gypsum*	12 - 15 g
Fang Feng	*Ledebouriella*	12 - 15 g
Huo Xiang	*Agastache*	3 - 6 g
Zhi Zi	*Gardenia*	1 - 3 g
Gan Cao	*Glycyrrhiza*	6 - 12 g

Heart/Stomach fire with damp leading to fever, jaundice, fullness, alternating diarrhea or constipation, mouth and tongue sores, or carbuncles.

T dark red, yellow coat

P flooding, rapid

✘ Caution during pregnancy.

XIE XIN TANG

Drain the Epigastrium Decoction

Extract Formula Name: Coptis and Rhubarb Combination

Da Huang	*Rheum*	6 - 9 g
Huang Lian	*Coptis*	3 - 6 g
Huang Qin	*Scutellaria*	6 - 9 g

Stomach fire has damaged Stomach yin causing bleeding gums, frontal headache, aching teeth, or excess hunger.

T red, geographic, scanty yellow coat

P rapid, empty, thin

✪ Major Formula

YU NU JIAN

Jade Woman Decoction

Extract Formula Name: Rehmannia and Gypsum Combination

Shi Gao	*Gypsum*	6 - 15 g
Zhi Mu	*Anemarrhena*	9 - 15 g
Mai Men Dong	*Ophiopogon*	6 - 15 g
Shu Di Huang	*Rehmannia*	12 - 15 g
Huai Niu Xi	*Achyranthes*	9 - 15 g

Heat in the center after incorrect purging therapy causing irritability, fever, or abdominal discomfort.

T red

P rapid, forceful

ZHI ZI GAN JIANG TANG

Gardenia and Ginger Decoction

Zhi Zi	*Gardenia*	3 - 9 g
Gan Jiang	*Zingiber*	3 - 6 g

Fullness or bloating in the epigastrium or abdomen with heat after strong purging therapy.

T red

P slightly rapid, weak

ZHI ZI HOU PO TANG

Gardenia and Magnolia Bark Decoction

Zhi Zi	*Gardenia*	6 - 12 g
Hou Po	*Magnolia*	6 - 12 g
Zhi Shi	*Citrus*	3 - 9 g

Liver qi stagnation causing Liver fire which burns the Stomach. This leads to vomiting or belching, ulcers due to heat, gas, sour or bitter regurgitation. This is a Liver/Stomach imbalance.

T red, dry, yellow coat

P rapid, wiry

☞ This formula may also be prepared as a powder with ten times the dosage.

ZUO JIN WAN

Left Metal Pill

Extract Formula Name: Coptis and Evodia Formula

Huang Lian	*Coptis*	12 - 18 g
Wu Zhu Yu	*Evodia*	1 - 4 g

PARASITES IN THE DIGESTIVE TRACT

- diarrhea
- occasional worms in the stools
- abdominal discomfort

T unremarkable

P unremarkable

Pediatric roundworms causing stagnation of qi/food in the middle jiao with Spleen deficiency and deficiency type heat. Symptoms include fever, vision disturbances, abdominal distention, or emaciation.

T pale

P frail

☞ Herbs should be ground into a fine powder and taken in the morning in 3 g doses together with pork broth.

BU DAI WAN

Cloth Sack Pill

Ye Ming Sha	*Vespertilio*	60 g
Wu Yi	*Ulmus*	60 g
Shi Jun Zi	*Quisqualis*	60 g
Lu Hui	*Aloe*	9 - 15 g
Ren Shen	*Panax*	9 - 15 g
Fu Ling	*Poria*	9 - 15 g
Bai Zhu	*Atractylodes*	9 - 15 g
Gan Cao	*Glycyrrhiza*	9 - 15 g

Upper right quadrant pain or mass due to roundworms in the biliary tract, also useful for tapeworms, pinworms, and fasciolopsis.

T depends on syndrome involved

P depends on syndrome involved

DAN DAO QU HUI TANG

Drive Roundworms from the Biliary Tract Decoction

Bing Lang	*Areca*	20 - 30 g
Ku Lian Gen Pi	*Melia*	9 - 15 g
Mu Xiang	*Saussurea*	6 - 9 g
Shi Jun Zi	*Quisqualis*	9 - 15 g
Zhi Ke	*Citrus*	3 - 6 g
Yu Jin	*Curcuma*	6 - 9 g

Worm infestation in the Large Intestines causing indigestion and Large Intestine function disorder with Spleen qi deficiency and Stomach heat. Symptoms include malnutrition in children, ascaris, tapeworms, nausea or vomiting after eating, or low grade fever.

T red

P weak, rapid

☞ Herbs should be powdered and made into pills with pig gall. Adults take 3 g doses on an empty stomach. The dosage is decreased in children.

FEI ER WAN

Fat Baby Pill

Huang Lian	*Coptis*	300 g
Shen Qu	*Massa Fermentata*	300 g
Shi Jun Zi	*Quisqualis*	150 g
Mai Ya	*Hordeum*	150 g
Rou Dou Kou	*Myristica*	150 g
Bing Lang	*Areca*	120 g
Mu Xiang	*Saussurea*	60 g

Intestinal parasites with recurring abdominal pain (roundworms, pinworms, etc.).

T depends on syndrome involved

P depends on syndrome involved

☞ Powder herbs and make into pills with wheat dough. For adults the dosage should be 6 g daily in the morning. Small children should only take 1.5 g per day.

✘ Qian Dan - Minium is toxic, and should be administered with caution. Do not use during pregnancy.

HUA CHONG WAN I

Dissolve Parasites Pills

Bing Lang	*Areca*	1500 g
Qian Dan	*Minium*	1500 g
He Shi	*Carpesium*	1500 g
Ku Lian Gen Pi	*Melia*	1500 g
Ming Fan	*Alumen*	370 g

Intestinal parasites with recurring abdominal pain (roundworms, pinworms, etc.). This prescription is somewhat stronger than the previous formula.

T depends on syndrome involved

P depends on syndrome involved

✘ Qian Dan - Minium is toxic and should be administered with caution. Do not use during pregnancy.

HUA CHONG WAN II

Dissolve Parasites Pill from the Analytic Collection

Bing Lang	*Areca*	15 g
Qian Dan	*Minium*	15 g
He Shi	*Carpesium*	15 g
Ku Lian Gen Pi	*Melia*	15 g
Ming Fan	*Alumen*	3.5 g
Shi Jun Zi	*Quisqualis*	3.5 g
Wu Yi	*Ulmus*	3.5 g

Spleen/Stomach deficiency with cold and roundworms causing loose, watery stools.

T pale, white coat

P weak

LI ZHONG AN HUI TANG

Regulate the Middle and Calm Roundworms Decoction

Ren Shen	*Panax*	6 - 9 g
Fu Ling	*Poria*	6 - 9 g
Bai Zhu	*Atractylodes*	3 - 6 g
Gan Jiang	*Zingiber*	3 - 6 g
Chuan Jiao	*Zanthoxylum*	6 - 9 g
Wu Mei	*Prunus*	6 - 9 g

Roundworms with severe heat in the Liver and Stomach causing irritability.

T red, yellow coat

P rapid

LIAN MEI AN HUI TANG

Picrorhiza and Mume Decoction to Calm Roundworms

Chuan Jiao	*Zanthoxylum*	1 - 2 g
Hu Huang Lian	*Picrorhiza*	2 - 3 g
Wu Mei	*Prunus*	3 - 6 g
Bing Lang	*Areca*	6 - 9 g
Lei Wan	*Omphalia*	6 - 9 g
Huang Bai	*Phellodendron*	2 - 3 g

This prescription will cause diarrhea which contains tapeworms about five hours after ingestion.

T depends on syndrome involved

P depends on syndrome involved

☞ Nan Gua Zi - Cucurbita should be taken first. Take Bing Lang - Areca as a decocted tea about 2 hours later.

✘ Do not use during pregnancy.

QU TIAO TANG

Expel Tapeworms Decoction

Nan Gua Zi	*Cucurbita*	60 g
Bing Lang	*Areca*	30 g

Trichomonas due to damp. External wash only!

T not important

P not important

☞ Herbs should be ground into a powder, then prepared as a draft.

✘ For external use only.

SHE CHUANG ZI SAN

Cnidium Powder

She Chuang Zi	*Cnidium*	9 - 15 g
Bai Bu	*Stemona*	9 - 15 g
Chuan Jiao	*Zanthoxylum*	9 - 15 g
Ming Fan	*Alumen*	9 - 15 g
Ku Shen	*Sophora*	9 - 15 g

1. Roundworms have migrated upward due to cold in the Large Intestines to the warmth of the epigastrium/chest. 2. Large Intestine cold and Stomach heat: mixed syndrome - jueyin syndrome.

T pale

P weak

☞ Wu Mei - Prunus should be soaked in vinegar for 12 hours.

WU MEI WAN

Mume Pill

Extract Formula Name: Mume Formula

Wu Mei	*Prunus*	20 - 25 g
Xi Xin	*Asarum*	1 - 3 g
Chuan Jiao	*Zanthoxylum*	1 - 3 g
Gan Jiang	*Zingiber*	12 - 15 g
Fu Zi	*Aconitum*	6 - 9 g
Huang Lian	*Coptis*	9 - 12 g
Huang Bai	*Phellodendron*	6 - 9 g
Gui Zhi	*Cinnamomum*	3 - 9 g
Dang Gui	*Angelica*	6 - 9 g
Ren Shen	*Panax*	6 - 9 g

EMETICS

- nausea and vomiting

T depends on the involved syndrome

P depends on the involved syndrome

Phlegm or food stagnation in the chest/diaphragm/upper epigastrium area. This formula will relieve the stagnation by causing vomiting.

T sticky coat

P slippery, somewhat superficial in the first (cun) position.

☞ Decoct for only 5 - 10 minutes or make into a paste with 10 g of Dan Dou Chi - Glycine.

✘ This formula will cause vomiting. Do not use during pregnancy.

GUA DI SAN

Melon Pedicle Powder

Extract Formula Name: Melon Pedicle Formula

Gua Di	*Cucumis*	1 - 3 g
Chi Xiao Dou	*Phaseolus*	1 - 3 g

Pre-existing phlegm or damp accumulation with shaoyang disease leading to malaria. There is a slight possibility that this formula can cause vomiting.

T thick sticky white coat

P superficial, slippery, wiry

✘ Note that Chang Shan - Dichroa is an emetic. The formula may cause vomiting.

JIE NUE QI BAO YIN

Seven-Treasure Decoction to Check Malarial Conditions

Chang Shan	*Dichroa*	3 - 5 g
Bing Lang	*Areca*	3 g
Chen Pi	*Citrus*	3 g
Hou Po	*Magnolia*	3 g
Cao Guo	*Amomum*	3 g
Qing Pi	*Citrus*	3 g
Gan Cao	*Glycyrrhiza*	3 g

Wind stroke with phlegm accumulation causing hemiplegia, facial paralysis, aphasia, or seizures from wind phlegm.

T sticky coat

P slippery, forceful

☞ Herbs should be ground into a powder and then taken as a draft. The actual dosage of Li Lu - Veratrum depends on the constitution of the patient.

✘ This formula causes vomiting.

SAN SHENG SAN

Three-Sage Powder

Gua Di	*Cucumis*	100 - 150 g
Li Lu	*Veratrum*	6 - 25 g
Fang Feng	*Ledebouriella*	100 - 150 g

Heat in the chest and Lungs due to taiyang disease; or lingering qi level heat manifesting in the yangming channel layer. In some patients this formula will induce vomiting, after which the symptoms will disappear.

T red, especially the tip, yellow coat

P rapid, forceful, superficial

✘ This prescription can cause vomiting.

ZHI ZI DOU CHI TANG

Gardenia and Prepared Soybean Decoction

Zhi Zi	*Gardenia*	6 - 9 g
Dan Dou Chi	*Glycine*	6 - 9 g

Li Lu	Veratrum	[illegible]
[illegible]	[illegible]	[illegible]
[illegible]	[illegible]	[illegible]

Wind stroke with phlegm [illegible] facial paralysis, aphasia, or [illegible] from wind phlegm.

T sticky coat

P slippery, forceful

Li Lu should be ground into a powder, and then taken as a draft. The actual dosage of Li Lu – Veratrum depends on the constitution of the patient.

This formula causes vomiting.

ZHI ZI DOU CHI TANG

Gardenia and Prepared Soybean Decoction

Zhi Zi	Gardenia	9–15 g
Dan Dou Chi	[illegible]	9–15 g

Heat in the chest and Lungs due to lingering disease or lingering [illegible] level heat manifesting in the [illegible] layer. In some patients this formula will induce vomiting, after which the symptoms will disappear.

T red, especially the tip, yellow coat

P rapid, forceful, superficial

This prescription can cause vomiting.

BAN XIA HOU PO TANG

Pinellia and Magnolia Bark Decoction

Ban Xia	Pinellia	[illegible]
Hou Po	Magnolia	[illegible]
[illegible]	[illegible]	[illegible]
[illegible]	[illegible]	[illegible]
[illegible]	[illegible]	[illegible]

Phlegm [illegible] causing hysteria, plum pit qi, or depression

T light [illegible] sticky white or yellowish coat

P slippery [illegible]

Major Formulas

LIVER DISHARMONIES

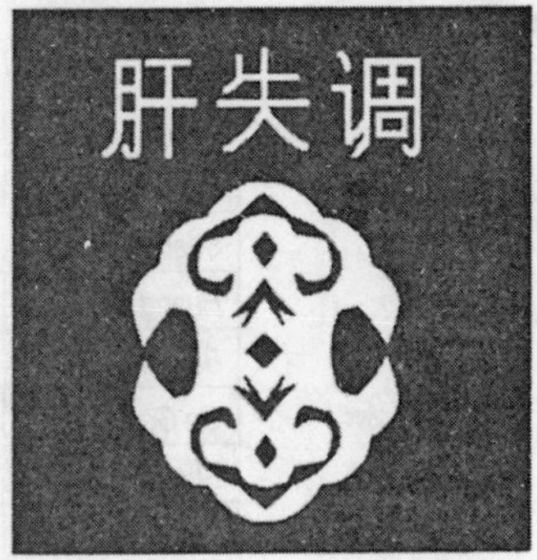

LIVER QI STAGNATION

- irritability and sighing
- hypochondriac distention
- depression or moodswings
- belching and abdominal distention

T light purple

P wiry

Phlegm and Liver qi stagnation causing hysteria, plumpit qi, or depression.

T light purple, sticky white or yellowish coat

P slippery or wiry

✪ Major Formula

BAN XIA HOU PO TANG

Pinellia and Magnolia Bark Decoction

Extract Formula Name: Pinellia and Magnolia Combination

Ban Xia	*Pinellia*	6 - 9 g
Hou Po	*Magnolia*	6 - 15 g
Zi Su Ye	*Perilla*	3 - 6 g
Fu Ling	*Poria*	6 - 9 g
Sheng Jiang	*Zingiber*	9 - 12 g

Liver qi stagnation with false heat rising which affects the Heart and causes a tingling sensation in the epigastrium and chest (running piglet sensation).

T red sides, thin yellowish coat

P wiry, rapid

BEN TUN TANG

Running Piglet Decoction

Chuan Xiong	*Ligusticum*	6 g
Dang Gui	*Angelica*	6 - 9 g
Bai Shao Yao	*Paeonia*	6 - 12 g
Sheng Di Huang	*Rehmannia*	6 - 12 g
Huang Qin	*Scutellaria*	6 - 9 g
Ban Xia	*Pinellia*	9 - 12 g
Ge Gen	*Pueraria*	9 g
Sheng Jiang	*Zingiber*	3 - 6 g
Sang Bai Pi	*Morus*	6 - 9 g

Liver qi and mild blood stagnation causing dysmenorrhea or premenstrual syndrome.

T purple

P wiry

CHAI HU SU GAN SAN

Bupleurum Powder to Spread the Liver

Extract Formula Name: Bupleurum and Cyperus Combination

Chai Hu	*Bupleurum*	6 - 9 g
Chuan Xiong	*Ligusticum*	3 - 6 g
Xiang Fu	*Cyperus*	3 - 6 g
Bai Shao Yao	*Paeonia*	6 - 9 g
Zhi Ke	*Citrus*	3 - 6 g
Gan Cao	*Glycyrrhiza*	3 - 6 g
Chen Pi	*Citrus*	6 - 9 g

Early phase of appendicitis with Liver qi and blood stagnation symptoms.

T purple

P wiry

DAN HUANG SI NI SAN

Moutan and Phellodendron Powder for Frigid Extremitis

Chai Hu	*Bupleurum*	6 - 12 g
Bai Shao Yao	*Paeonia*	30 - 60 g
Huang Bai	*Phellodendron*	6 - 12 g
Mu Dan Pi	*Paeonia*	6 - 12 g
Zhi Shi	*Citrus*	3 - 12 g
Gan Cao	*Glycyrrhiza*	3 - 12 g

Liver/Spleen disharmony with heat. Symptoms include irregular menstruation, red or bloodshot eyes, or irritability.

T red sides, light purple, thin white coat

P wiry, rapid

DAN ZHI XIAO YAO SAN (JIA WEI XIAO YAO SAN)

Moutan, Gardenia, and Rambling Powder

Extract Formula Name: Bupleurum and Peony Formula

Mu Dan Pi	*Paeonia*	6 - 9 g
Zhi Zi	*Gardenia*	3 - 6 g
Chai Hu	*Bupleurum*	6 - 9 g
Bo He	*Mentha*	3 - 6 g
Dang Gui	*Angelica*	6 - 9 g
Bai Shao Yao	*Paeonia*	6 - 9 g
Bai Zhu	*Atractylodes*	3 - 9 g
Fu Ling	*Poria*	6 - 9 g
Gan Cao	*Glycyrrhiza*	3 - 6 g
[Sheng Jiang	*Zingiber*	3 - 6 g]

Liver qi stagnation with cold in the Liver channel causing a hernia.

T pale, light purple

P wiry

DAO QI TANG

Conduct the Qi Decoction

Mu Xiang	*Saussurea*	3 - 9 g
Chuan Lian Zi	*Melia*	9 - 12 g
Wu Zhu Yu	*Evodia*	3 - 6 g
Xiao Hui Xiang	*Foeniculum*	3 - 6 g

Mental disorder due to 1. Liver qi stagnation (use with Xiao Yao San); 2. Liver qi stagnation with fire burning the yin (use with Wen Dan Tang); 3. Yin deficiency with fire injuring the Heart.

T red, scanty coat

P thin, rapid

GAN MAI DA ZAO TANG

Licorice, Wheat, and Jujube Decoction

Extract Formula Name: Licorice and Jujube Combination

Gan Cao	*Glycyrrhiza*	9 - 12 g
Fu Xiao Mai	*Triticum*	9 - 15 g
Da Zao	*Ziziphus*	10 pc

Liver qi stagnation with blood deficiency causing delayed periods with clots.

T pale, purple

P choppy, wiry

GUO QI YIN

Delayed Menstruation Decoction

Shu Di Huang	*Rehmannia*	6 - 9 g
Dang Gui	*Angelica*	6 - 9 g
Bai Shao Yao	*Paeonia*	6 - 9 g
Chuan Xiong	*Ligusticum*	3 - 6 g
Hong Hua	*Carthamus*	3 - 6 g
Tao Ren	*Prunus*	3 - 6 g
Xiang Fu	*Cyperus*	3 - 6 g
Mu Tong	*Akebia*	3 - 6 g
E Zhu	*Curcuma*	3 - 6 g
Rou Gui	*Cinnamomum*	1 - 3 g
Gan Cao	*Glycyrrhiza*	3 - 6 g

Phlegm accumulation causing hardenings; or Liver qi stagnation leading to goiter or cancer.

T sticky coat

P slippery, wiry

HAI ZAO YU HU TANG

Sargassum Decoction for the Jade Flask

Hai Zao	*Sargassum*	3 - 6 g
Kun Bu	*Laminaria*	3 - 6 g
Hai Dai	*Ecklonia*	1.5 g
Du Huo	*Angelica*	3 - 6 g
Lian Qiao	*Forsythia*	3 - 6 g
Zhe Bei Mu	*Fritillaria*	3 - 6 g
Chuan Xiong	*Ligusticum*	3 - 6 g
Ban Xia	*Pinellia*	3 - 6 g
Dang Gui	*Angelica*	3 - 6 g
Chen Pi	*Citrus*	3 - 6 g
Qing Pi	*Citrus*	3 - 6 g
Gan Cao	*Glycyrrhiza*	3 - 6 g

Liver qi stagnation with heat causing hypochrondriac or abdominal pain and irritability.

T red sides, yellow coat

P wiry, rapid

☞ Grind into a powder and take 9 g each time.

JIN LING ZI SAN

Melia Toosandan Powder

Extract Formula Name: Melia and Corydalis Formula

Chuan Lian Zi	*Melia*	30 g
Yan Hu Suo	*Corydalis*	30 g

Liver qi stagnation with cold in the Stomach causing abdominal pain which is relieved by warmth. The formula is also useful for dysmenorrhea.

T pale, white coat

P weak, slow, or wiry

LIANG FU WAN

Galanga and Cyperus Pill

Extract Formula Name: Galanga and Cyperus Formula

Gao Liang Jiang	*Alpinia*	6 - 9 g
Xiang Fu	*Cyperus*	6 - 9 g

Kidney qi/yang deficiency causing qi/cold stagnation in the Liver channel. Symptoms include hernia, nodules in the lower jiao, impotence, or cold uterus with cramps prior to menses.

T pale, purple

P wiry or tight

NUAN GAN JIAN

Warm the Liver Decoction

Dang Gui	*Angelica*	6 - 9 g
Gou Qi Zi	*Lycium*	6 - 9 g
Wu Yao	*Lindera*	3 - 6 g
Chen Xiang	*Aquilaria*	3 - 6 g
Fu Ling	*Poria*	6 - 9 g
Rou Gui	*Cinnamomum*	3 - 6 g
Xiao Hui Xiang	*Foeniculum*	3 - 6 g
Sheng Jiang	*Zingiber*	3 - 6 g

Excess fire cholecystitis with Liver qi and damp stagnation causing alternating fever and chills or severe hypochondriac pain.

T deep red, sticky yellow coat

P wiry, slippery, rapid, or flooding

☞ Mang Xiao - Mirabilitum should be dissolved into the strained tea. Da Huang - Rheum should be added within the last 3 - 5 minutes of the decoction process.

✘ Do not use during pregnancy

QING DAN XIE HUO TANG

Clear the Gallbladder and Drain Fire Decoction

Chai Hu	*Bupleurum*	9 - 15 g
Ban Xia	*Pinellia*	6 - 9 g
Yin Chen Hao	*Artemisia*	15 - 25 g
Long Dan Cao	*Gentiana*	6 - 9 g
Yu Jin	*Curcuma*	6 - 9 g
Da Huang	*Rheum*	6 - 9 g
Huang Qin	*Scutellaria*	6 - 15 g
Zhi Zi	*Gardenia*	6 - 9 g
Mang Xiao	*Mirabilitum*	6 - 9 g
Mu Xiang	*Saussurea*	3 - 6 g

Qi stagnation with fire causing acute pancreatitis. The patient will vomit immediately after food or liquid intake, and experiences epigastric discomfort. Acute pancreatitis can cause shock or sudden death.

T red, thin yellow coat

P rapid, wiry

☞ Mu Xiang - Saussurea and Da Huang - Rheum should be added near the end of decoction process. Mang Xiao - Mirabilitum should be added to the strained tea.

✘ Do not use during pregnancy.

QING YI TANG

Clear the Pancreas Decoction

Chai Hu	*Bupleurum*	6 - 15 g
Bai Shao Yao	*Paeonia*	6 - 15 g
Huang Qin	*Scutellaria*	9 - 12 g
Yan Hu Suo	*Corydalis*	6 - 9 g
Da Huang	*Rheum*	9 - 15 g
Mu Xiang	*Saussurea*	6 - 9 g
Hu Huang Lian	*Picrorhiza*	6 - 9 g
Mang Xiao	*Mirabilitum*	6 - 9 g

Pain in the lower legs due to blood or yin deficiency, or spasmodic abdominal pain.

T red or pale

P weak, thin

SHAO YAO GAN CAO TANG

Peony and Licorice Decoction

Extract Formula Name: Peony and Licorice Combination

Bai Shao Yao	*Paeonia*	15 - 30 g
ZhiGan Cao	*Glycyrrhiza*	12 - 20 g

Liver overacting on the Lungs or Stomach leading to wheezing, shortness of breath, or epigastric distention respectively.

T light purple, thin coat

P wiry

SI MO TANG

Four-Milled Herb Decoction

Ren Shen	*Panax*	6 - 9 g
Chen Xiang	*Aquilaria*	3 - 6 g
Wu Yao	*Lindera*	3 - 6 g
Bing Lang	*Areca*	6 - 9 g

Liver overacting on Spleen with mild heat. This is the basic prescription for this syndrome.

T light purple, thin coat

P wiry, slightly wiry

✪ Major Formula

SI NI SAN

Frigid Extremities Powder

Extract Formula Name: Bupleurum and Chih-Shih Formula

Chai Hu	*Bupleurum*	6 - 9 g
Zhi Shi	*Citrus*	6 - 9 g
Bai Shao Yao	*Paeonia*	3 - 9 g
Zhi Gan Cao	*Glycyrrhiza*	3 - 6 g

Liver overacting on Stomach with pain, depression, fullness, regurgitation, and indigestion.

T white or yellow coat

P wiry

SU GAN WAN

Liver Soothing Pills

Chai Hu	*Bupleurum*	6 - 9 g
Bai Shao Yao	*Paeonia*	6 - 9 g
Fu Ling	*Poria*	6 - 9 g
Yan Hu Suo	*Corydalis*	3 - 6 g
Hou Po	*Magnolia*	6 - 12 g
Jiang Huang	*Curcuma*	6 - 9 g
Chen Xiang	*Aquilaria*	3 - 6 g
Chen Pi	*Citrus*	3 - 6 g
Zhi Ke	*Citrus*	3 - 6 g
Mu Xiang	*Saussurea*	3 - 6 g
Sha Ren	*Amomum*	3 - 6 g
Chuan Lian Zi	*Melia*	6 - 12 g
Bai Dou Kou	*Amomum*	3 - 6 g

External cold causing stagnation in the Liver channel. This leads to testicle pain and swelling in men, or to clear leukorrhea in women.

T pale, purple, thin white coat

P slow, wiry, or tight

☞ Ba Dou - Croton and Chuan Lian Zi - Melia should be dry fried for 5 - 10 minutes. Discard Ba Dou, then decoct as usual. This way the effect of Chuan Lian Zi is to actually warm the Liver channel.

TIAN TAI WU YAO SAN

Top-Quality Lindera Powder

Wu Yao	*Lindera*	6 - 9 g
Xiao Hui Xiang	*Foeniculum*	3 - 6 g
Gao Liang Jiang	*Alpinia*	3 - 6 g
Mu Xiang	*Saussurea*	3 - 6 g
Qing Pi	*Citrus*	3 - 6 g
Chuan Lian Zi	*Melia*	6 - 9 g
Bing Lang	*Areca*	6 - 9 g
Ba Dou	*Croton*	6 - 15 g

Liver qi stagnation causing severe acute hearing loss from emotional upset.

T light purple, thin white coat

P wiry

✘ Caution during pregnancy.

TONG QI SAN

Unblock the Qi Powder

Xiang Fu	*Cyperus*	6 - 9 g
Chai Hu	*Bupleurum*	6 - 9 g
Chuan Xiong	*Ligusticum*	3 - 9 g

Liver qi stagnation causes constipation. The bowel movements are often incomplete and have a thin and long shape. The person has an urge but can only discharge gas.

T light purple

P wiry

✘ Do not use during pregnancy.

WU MAO SAN

Five-Powder Formula

Wu Yao	*Lindera*	3 - 6 g
Mu Xiang	*Saussurea*	6 - 9 g
Zhi Shi	*Prunus*	6 - 9 g
Da Huang	*Rheum*	9 - 15 g
Chen Xiang	*Aquilaria*	6 - 9 g
Bing Lang	*Areca*	6 - 9 g

Liver qi stagnation causing late periods, irritability, premenstrual syndrome, or distention in the urinary tract.

T light purple, thin coat

P wiry

WU YAO TANG

Lindera Decoction

Wu Yao	*Lindera*	3 - 6 g
Dang Gui	*Angelica*	6 - 9 g
Xiang Fu	*Cyperus*	3 - 9 g
Mu Xiang	*Saussurea*	3 - 9 g
Gan Cao	*Zingiber*	3 - 6 g

Liver qi stagnation manifesting mostly as irregular periods. Menstruation is sometimes early or sometimes late, and the patient experiences severe premenstrual syndrome, cramping prior to the onset of bleeding, or breast distention.

T light purple, thin coat

P wiry

XIANG WU SAN

Cyperus and Lindera Powder

Xiang Fu	*Cyperus*	6 - 12 g
Wu Yao	*Lindera*	3 - 9 g
Chai Hu	*Bupleurum*	6 - 9 g
Bai Zhu	*Atractylodes*	3 - 9 g
Bai Shao Yao	*Paeonia*	6 - 9 g
Dang Gui	*Angelica*	6 - 9 g
Fu Ling	*Poria*	6 - 9 g

1. Chronic Spleen qi deficiency with chronic cold evil qi leading to qi and blood deficiency. The main symptom is abdominal spasms. 2. Liver qi stagnation or Liver overacting on Spleen. In the latter two instances the dosage of 'Bai Shao Yao - Paeonia' should be increased.

T pale or light purple, thin white coat

P weak or slightly wiry

☞ Yi Tang - Saccharum Granorum should be added to the strained tea.

XIAO JIAN ZHONG TANG

Minor Construct the Middle Decoction

Extract Formula Name: Minor Cinnamon and Peony Combination

Yi Tang	*Saccharum Granorum*	15 - 30 g
Gui Zhi	*Cinnamomum*	3 - 9 g
Bai Shao Yao	*Paeonia*	6 - 9 g
Sheng Jiang	*Zingiber*	6 - 9 g
Da Zao	*Ziziphus*	3 - 5 pc
Zhi Gan Cao	*Glycyrrhiza*	3 - 6 g

Liver/Spleen disharmony with blood deficiency: decreased appetite, irregular menstruation, pain in the flanks, or breast distention.

T light purple, pale, thin white coat

P wiry

✪ Major Formula

XIAO YAO SAN

Rambling Powder

Extract Formula Name: Bupleurum and Tang-Kuei Powder

Chai Hu	*Bupleurum*	6 - 9 g
Dang Gui	*Angelica*	6 - 9 g
Bai Zhu	*Atractylodes*	3 - 9 g
Bai Shao Yao	*Paeonia*	6 - 9 g
Fu Ling	*Poria*	6 - 9 g
Bo He	*Mentha*	3 - 6 g
Gan Cao	*Glycyrrhiza*	3 - 6 g
Sheng Jiang	*Zingiber*	3 - 6 g

Liver qi stagnation produces heat which consumes Kidney and Liver yin, or Liver overacts on the Spleen and Stomach causing emotional upset, nausea, belching with sour taste, hiatal hernia, or epigastric or abdominal pain; or Liver yin cannot nourish the tendons and ligaments producing heel or posterior hip pain.

T red, dry

P thin, wiry

YI GUAN JIAN

Linking Decoction

Extract Formula Name: Glehnia and Rehmannia Combination

Sheng Di Huang	*Rehmannia*	15 - 30 g
Gou Qi Zi	*Lycium*	6 - 15 g
Dang Gui	*Angelica*	6 - 12 g
Bei Sha Shen	*Glehnia*	6 - 9 g
Mai Men Dong	*Ophiopogon*	6 - 9 g
Chuan Lian Zi	*Melia*	3 - 6 g

Stagnations of all kinds (qi, blood, food, damp, etc.). Symptoms include epigastric or chest fullness, nausea and vomiting, or poor appetite.

T depends on particular syndrome involved

P depends on particular syndrome involved

YUE JU WAN

Escape Restraint Pill

Chuan Xiong	*Ligusticum*	3 - 9 g
Cang Zhu	*Atractylodes*	3 - 9 g
Zhi Zi	*Gardenia*	3 - 9 g
Xiang Fu	*Cyperus*	3 - 9 g
Shen Qu	*Massa Fermentata*	3 - 9 g

LIVER BLOOD STAGNATION

- menstrual clots
- dysmenorrhea with clots
- sharp localized pains

T purple, or purple spots

P wiry

Liver

Qi and blood deficiency with blood stagnation. This formula is for a restless fetus, infertility, irregular periods, poor appetite, weakness, or fatigue.

T pale, thin white coat

P weak, maybe wiry

BA ZHEN YI MU WAN

Eight-Treasure Pill to Benefit Mothers

Shu Di Huang	*Rehmannia*	6 - 15 g
Chuan Xiong	*Ligusticum*	3 - 9 g
Dang Gui	*Angelica*	6 - 9 g
Bai Shao Yao	*Paeonia*	6 - 12 g
Ren Shen	*Panax*	6 - 12 g
Bai Zhu	*Atractylodes*	3 - 9 g
Fu Ling	*Poria*	6 - 9 g
Yi Mu Cao	*Leonurus*	6 - 18 g
Gan Cao	*Glycyrrhiza*	3 - 6 g

Qi and blood stagnation with qi deficiency and blockage in the channels leading to wind stroke, hemiplegia, and atrophy in the lower limbs. The patient has difficulty walking.

T purple, thin white coat

P wiry, weak, slow

BU YANG HUAN WU TANG

Tonify the Yang to Restore Five-tenths Decoction

Extract Formula Name: Astragalus and Peony Combination

Huang Qi	*Astragalus*	60 - 120 g
Chuan Xiong	*Ligusticum*	3 - 6 g
Chi Shao Yao	*Paeonia*	3 - 6 g
Dang Gui Wei	*Angelica*	6 - 9 g
Hong Hua	*Carthamus*	3 - 6 g
Tao Ren	*Prunus*	3 - 6 g
Di Long	*Pheretima*	3 - 6 g

Liver qi and mild blood stagnation causing dysmenorrhea or premenstrual syndrome.

T purple

P wiry

✪ Major Formula

CHAI HU SU GAN SAN

Bupleurum Powder to Spread the Liver

Extrac Formula Name: Bupleurum and Cyperus Combination

Chai Hu	*Bupleurum*	6 - 9 g
Chuan Xiong	*Ligusticum*	3 - 6 g
Xiang Fu	*Cyperus*	3 - 6 g
Bai Shao Yao	*Paeonia*	6 - 9 g
Zhi Ke	*Citrus*	3 - 6 g
Gan Cao	*Glycyrrhiza*	3 - 6 g
Chen Pi	*Citrus*	6 - 9 g

Early phase of appendicitis with Liver qi and blood stagnation symptoms.

T purple

P wiry

DAN HUANG SI NI SAN

Moutan and Phellodendron Powder for Frigid Extremitis

Chai Hu	*Bupleurum*	6 - 12 g
Bai Shao Yao	*Paeonia*	30 - 60 g
Huang Bai	*Phellodendron*	6 - 12 g
Mu Dan Pi	*Paeonia*	6 - 12 g
Zhi Shi	*Citrus*	3 - 12 g
Gan Cao	*Glycyrrhiza*	3 - 12 g

Qi/blood stagnation under the diaphragm and epigastrium, or masses in the abdomen or epigastrium.

T purple

P wiry or choppy

✘ Do not use during pregnancy.

GE XIA ZHU YU TANG

Drive Out Blood Stasis Below the Diaphragm Decoction

Extract Formula Name: Persica and Carthamus Combination

Dang Gui	*Angelica*	6 - 9 g
Chuan Xiong	*Ligusticum*	6 - 9 g
Tao Ren	*Prunus*	6 - 9 g
Hong Hua	*Carthamus*	3 - 6 g
Mu Dan Pi	*Paeonia*	6 - 9 g
Chi Shao Yao	*Paeonia*	6 - 9 g
Yan Hu Suo	*Corydalis*	3 - 6 g
Xiang Fu	*Cyperus*	3 - 9 g
Zhi Ke	*Citrus*	3 - 6 g
Wu Ling Zhi	*Trogopterus*	6 - 9 g
Wu Yao	*Lindera*	3 - 6 g
Gan Cao	*Glycyrrhiza*	6 - 9 g

Blood and phlegm stagnation in the uterus leading to masses or lumps, amenorrhea, dysmenorrhea, or restless fetus.

T purple, sticky coat

P wiry, slippery, choppy

GUI ZHI FU LING WAN

Cinnamon Twig and Poria Pill

Extract Formula Name: Cinnamon and Hoelen Formula

Gui Zhi	*Cinnamomum*	6 - 12 g
Fu Ling	*Poria*	6 - 12 g
Mu Dan Pi	*Paeonia*	6 - 12 g
Tao Ren	*Prunus*	6 - 12 g
Chi Shao Yao	*Paeonia*	9 - 12 g

Qi and blood stagnation causing dysmenorrhea, clots, low back pain, or headaches prior to menses.

T purple

P wiry, choppy

✘ Do not use during pregnancy.

HONG HUA TAO REN JIAN

Carthamus and Peach Seed Decoction

Hong Hua	*Carthamus*	6 - 9 g
Tao Ren	*Prunus*	6 - 9 g
Chi Shao Yao	*Paeonia*	6 - 9 g
Dang Gui	*Angelica*	6 - 9 g
Chuan Xiong	*Ligusticum*	3 - 9 g
Sheng Di Huang	*Rehmannia*	6 - 12 g
Dan Shen	*Salvia*	6 - 9 g
Xiang Fu	*Cyperus*	6 - 9 g
Qing Pi	*Citrus*	3 - 6 g
Yan Hu Suo	*Corydalis*	6 - 9 g

Qi/blood stagnation causing delayed periods with clotty bleeding, and breast distention.

T normal, or purple

P wiry or choppy

JIA WEI WU YAO TANG

Augmented Lindera Decoction

Wu Yao	*Lindera*	10 g
Xiang Fu	*Cyperus*	10 g
Yan Hu Suo	*Corydalis*	10 g
Sha Ren	*Amomum*	10 g
Bing Lang	*Areca*	10 g
Mu Xiang	*Saussurea*	10 g
Gan Cao	*Glycyrrhiza*	10 g
[Sheng Jiang	*Zingiber*	1 - 3 g]

Qi/blood stagnation from external or internal injury of all kinds causing pain and bleeding.

T purple

P wiry or choppy

☞ Powder herbs and take in a 0.2 - 1.5 g dosage internally. For external use mix herbs with wine.

✘ Do not use during pregnancy. Zhu Sha - Cinnabaris is toxic, and should only be used short-term.

QI LI SAN

Seven-Thousandths of a Tael Powder

Extract Formula Name: Musk and Catechu Formula

Xue Jie	*Dracaena*	30 g
Ru Xiang	*Boswellia*	3 - 6 g
Hong Hua	*Carthamus*	3 - 6 g
Mo Yao	*Commiphora*	3 - 6 g
Er Cha	*Acacia*	6 - 9 g
Zhu Sha	*Cinnabaris*	3 - 5 g
She Xiang	*Moschus*	0.5 g
Bing Pian	*Dryobalanops*	0.5 g

Blood and cold stagnation in the lower jiao with mass formation, blood clots, and dysmenorrhea. This formula is also useful for liver cirrhosis.

T pale, purple

P wiry or choppy

✘ Do not use during pregnancy.

SHAO FU ZHU YU TANG

Drive Out Blood Stasis in the Lower Abdomen Decoction

Extract Formula Name: Cnidium and Bulrush Combination

Yan Hu Suo	*Corydalis*	3 - 6 g
Dang Gui	*Angelica*	6 - 9 g
Mo Yao	*Commiphora*	3 - 6 g
Rou Gui	*Cinnamomum*	3 - 6 g
Xiao Hui Xiang	*Foeniculum*	1.5 - 3 g
Gan Jiang	*Zingiber*	3 - 6 g
Pu Huang	*Typha*	6 - 9 g
Chi Shao Yao	*Paeonia*	6 - 9 g
Wu Ling Zhi	*Trogopterus*	6 - 9 g
Chuan Xiong	*Ligusticum*	3 - 9 g

Qi and blood stagnation in the channels causing pain in the extremities or muscles.

T purple

P wiry

SHEN TONG ZHU YU TANG

Drive Out Blood Stasis from a Painful Body Decoction

Chuan Xiong	*Ligusticum*	3 - 9 g
Tao Ren	*Prunus*	6 - 9 g
Hong Hua	*Carthamus*	6 - 9 g
Qin Jiao	*Gentiana*	6 - 9 g
Qiang Huo	*Notopterygium*	3 - 6 g
Dang Gui	*Angelica*	6 - 9 g
Chuan Niu Xi	*Cyathula*	6 - 12 g
Mo Yao	*Commiphora*	6 - 9 g
Wu Ling Zhi	*Trogopterus*	6 - 9 g
Di Long	*Pheretima*	6 - 9 g
Xiang Fu	*Cyperus*	3 - 6 g
Gan Cao	*Glycyrrhiza*	3 - 6 g

Post-partum retention of lochia due to blood and cold stagnation.

T pale, purple

P choppy

☞ Add yellow wine to the decoction.

SHENG HUA TANG

Generation and Transformation Decoction

Extract Formula Name: Tang-Kuei and Ginger Combination

Dang Gui	*Angelica*	15 - 28 g
Tao Ren	*Prunus*	6 - 9 g
Pao Jiang	*Zingiber*	3 - 6 g
Chuan Xiong	*Ligusticum*	6 - 9 g
Gan Cao	*Glycyrrhiza*	3 - 6 g

Post-partum blood (lochia) retention with dark clots and severe abdominal pain. The stagnation is in the Chong and Ren channels.

T purple

P wiry

✘ Do not use during pregnancy.

SHI XIAO SAN

Sudden Smile Powder

Extract Formula Name: Pteropus and Bulrush Formula

Pu Huang	*Typha*	6 - 12 g
Wu Ling Zhi	*Trogopterus*	6 - 9 g

Lower body wind cold damp bi-syndrome with blood stagnation causing low back pain, muscle aches, sciatica, or hemiplegia.

T purple

P wiry, slippery

✘ Do not use during pregnancy.

SHU JING HUO XUE TANG

Relax the Channels and Invigorate the Blood Decoction

Extract Formula Name: Clematis and Stephania Combination

Bai Shao Yao	*Paeonia*	6 - 9 g
Chuan Xiong	*Ligusticum*	3 - 9 g
Sheng Di Huang	*Rehmannia*	6 - 9 g
Dang Gui	*Angelica*	6 - 9 g
Cang Zhu	*Atractylodes*	3 - 6 g
Fu Ling	*Poria*	6 - 9 g
Long Dan Cao	*Gentiana*	6 - 9 g
Tao Ren	*Prunus*	3 - 6 g
Wei Ling Xian	*Clematis*	3 - 6 g
Huai Niu Xi	*Achyranthes*	6 - 9 g
Qiang Huo	*Notopterygium*	3 - 6 g
Chen Pi	*Citrus*	3 - 6 g
Fang Feng	*Ledebouriella*	6 - 9 g
Han Fang Ji	*Stephania*	6 - 9 g
Bai Zhi	*Angelica*	3 - 6 g
Sheng Jiang	*Zingiber*	3 - 6 g
Gan Cao	*Glycyrrhiza*	3 - 6 g

Blood deficiency with blood stagnation. Symptoms include irregular menstruation, dysmenorrhea, dizziness, or pale or purple fingernails.

T pale or purple

P thin or choppy

✪ **Major Formula**

SI WU TANG

Four-Substance Decoction

Extract Formula Name: Tang-Kuei Four Combination

Shu Di Huang	*Rehmannia*	6 - 12 g
Chuan Xiong	*Ligusticum*	3 - 9 g
Dang Gui	*Angelica*	6 - 9 g
Bai Shao Yao	*Paeonia*	6 - 9 g

Mild blood deficiency with severe blood stagnation causing early periods or dysmenorrhea.

T pale or purple

P choppy or wiry

✘ Do not use during pregnancy.

TAO HONG SI WU TANG

Four-Substance Decoction with Safflower and Peach Pit

Shu Di Huang	*Rehmannia*	6 - 12 g
Bai Shao Yao	*Paeonia*	6 - 9 g
Chuan Xiong	*Ligusticum*	3 - 6 g
Dang Gui	*Angelica*	6 - 9 g
Tao Ren	*Prunus*	3 - 9 g
Hong Hua	*Carthamus*	3 - 6 g

Blood stagnation in the head, face, and neck area leading to migraines or cyanotic lips.

T purple or purple spots

P wiry or choppy

☞ Decoct all herbs except She Xiang - Moschus for 15 minutes. Add 230 cc of rice wine and let cook for another 5 - 10 minutes, then add powdered She Xiang - Moschus and dissolve into the tea.

✘ Do not use during pregnancy.

TONG QIAO HUO XUE TANG

Unblock the Orifices and Invigorate the Blood Decoction

Extract Formula Name: Persica and Cnidium Combination

Hong Hua	*Carthamus*	6 - 9 g
Tao Ren	*Prunus*	6 - 9 g
Chuan Xiong	*Ligusticum*	3 - 9 g
Chi Shao Yao	*Paeonia*	6 - 9 g
Cong Bai	*Allium*	3 - 6 g
She Xiang	*Moschus*	0.1 - 0.3 g
Da Zao	*Ziziphus*	3 - 6 pc
Sheng Jiang	*Zingiber*	3 - 6 g

Qi and blood deficiency with qi/blood and phlegm stagnation causing masses on the neck, breasts, or axilla areas.

T pale or purple

P weak or choppy

XIANG BEI YANG YING TANG

Cyperus and Fritillaria Decoction to Nourish the Nutritive Qi

Ren Shen	*Panax*	6 - 9 g
Bai Zhu	*Atractylodes*	3 - 6 g
Fu Ling	*Poria*	6 - 9 g
Chuan Xiong	*Ligusticum*	3 - 6 g
Chen Pi	*Citrus*	3 - 6 g
Dang Gui	*Angelica*	6 - 9 g
Xiang Fu	*Cyperus*	6 - 9 g
Shu Di Huang	*Rehmannia*	6 - 12 g
Bei Mu	*Fritillaria*	3 - 6 g
Bai Shao Yao	*Paeonia*	6 - 9 g
Jie Geng	*Platycodon*	3 - 6 g
Da Zao	*Ziziphus*	3 - 6 pc
Sheng Jiang	*Zingiber*	3 - 6 g
Gan Cao	*Glycyrrhiza*	1 - 3 g

Qi and blood stagnation causing chest pain with water/damp accumulation: Liver affects the Lungs. Symptoms include hypochondriac pain, possible coughing, or raspy voice.

T purple, thick sticky coat

P wiry

☞ Xuan Fu Hua - Inula should be wrapped in a cheesecloth.

XIANG FU XUAN FU HUA TANG

Cyperus and Inula Decoction

Xiang Fu	*Cyperus*	6 - 9 g
Xuan Fu Hua	*Inula*	6 - 9 g
Yi Yi Ren	*Coix*	9 - 15 g
Chen Pi	*Citrus*	3 - 6 g
Zi Su Zi	*Perilla*	6 - 9 g
Ban Xia	*Pinellia*	6 - 9 g
Fu Ling	*Poria*	6 - 9 g

Blood stagnation in head, chest, and diaphragm causing angina, palpitations, insomnia, nightmares, or dysmenorrhea.

T purple or purple spots

P wiry

✘ Do not use during pregnancy.

XUE FU ZHU YU TANG

Drive out Stasis in the Mansion of Blood Decoction

Extract Formula Name: Persica and Achyranthes Combination

Dang Gui	*Angelica*	6 - 9 g
Chuan Xiong	*Ligusticum*	3 - 9 g
Sheng Di Huang	*Rehmannia*	6 - 9 g
Chi Shao Yao	*Paeonia*	6 - 9 g
Tao Ren	*Prunus*	6 - 12 g
Hong Hua	*Carthamus*	6 - 9 g
Chuan Niu Xi	*Cyathula*	9 - 12 g
Jie Geng	*Platycodon*	3 - 6 g
Zhi Ke	*Citrus*	3 - 6 g
Chai Hu	*Bupleurum*	3 - 9 g
Gan Cao	*Glycyrrhiza*	3 - 6 g

Blood stagnation with abdominal pain, severe spasms, and irregular periods.

T purple, or purple spots

P choppy, wiry

✘ Do not use during pregnancy.

YAN HU SUO TANG

Corydalis Decoction

Yan Hu Suo	*Corydalis*	30 - 45 g
Chi Shao Yao	*Paeonia*	9 - 15 g
Rou Gui	*Cinnamomum*	9 - 15 g
Ru Xiang	*Boswellia*	60 - 90 g
Mo Yao	*Commiphora*	60 - 90 g
Jiang Huang	*Curcuma*	60 - 90 g
Dang Gui	*Angelica*	9 - 15 g
Mu Xiang	*Saussurea*	60 - 90 g
Pu Huang	*Typha*	9 - 15 g
Gan Cao	*Glycyrrhiza*	6 - 9 g
[Sheng Jiang	*Zingiber*	3 - 6 g]

Stagnations of all kinds (qi, blood, food, damp, etc.). Symptoms include epigastric or chest fullness, nausea and vomiting, or poor appetite.

T depends on particular syndrome involved

P depends on particular syndrome involved

YUE JU WAN

Escape Restraint Pill

Chuan Xiong	*Ligusticum*	3 - 9 g
Cang Zhu	*Atractylodes*	3 - 9 g
Zhi Zi	*Gardenia*	3 - 9 g
Xiang Fu	*Cyperus*	3 - 9 g
Shen Qu	*Massa Fermentata*	3 - 9 g

Deficient cold with blood stagnation causing uterine bleeding with pain which is better with the passage of clots.

T pale, dark purple

P choppy or wiry

☞ The first seven ingredients (which may be calcined) should be ground and made into 9 - 12 g pills with glutinous rice and water. The pills should be coated with Zhu Sha - Cinnabaris. One pill per day with wine is the recommeded dosage.

✘ Do not use during pregnancy. Zhu Sha - Cinnabaris is toxic and should therefore not be taken long-term.

ZHEN LING DAN

Rouse the Spirits Special Pill

Zi Shi Ying	*Fluoritum*	60 g
Yu Liang Shi	*Limonite*	60 g
Dai Zhe Shi	*Haematitum*	60 g
Wu Ling Zhi	*Trogopterus*	30 g
Ru Xiang	*Boswellia*	30 g
Chi Shi Zhi	*Halloysitum Rubrum*	60 g
Mo Yao	*Commiphora*	30 g
Zhu Sha	*Cinnabaris*	15 g

Localized swellings which are about to ulcerate with underlying qi deficiency and mild blood stagnation. Swellings are mildly painful and warm.

T pale, light purple

P weak

✘ Caution during pregnancy.

ZHONG HE TANG

Middle-Heartening Decoction

Ren Shen	*Panax*	6 - 9 g
Huang Qi	*Astragalus*	6 g
Dang Gui	*Angelica*	6 - 9 g
Fu Ling	*Poria*	6 - 9 g
Chuan Xiong	*Ligusticum*	3 - 6 g
Bai Zhu	*Atractylodes*	3 - 6 g
Bai Zhi	*Angelica*	3 - 6 g
Chen Pi	*Citrus*	6 g
Ru Xiang	*Boswellia*	3 - 6 g
Jin Yin Hua	*Lonicera*	3 - 6 g
Zao Jiao Ci	*Gleditsia*	3 g
Mo Yao	*Commiphora*	3 g
Gan Cao	*Glycyrrhiza*	3 g

LIVER OVERACTING ON SPLEEN OR STOMACH

- alternating diarrhea and constipation
- incomplete bowel movements
- gas and abdominal bloating
- belching or acid regurgitation
- irritability or emotional upset
- fatigue

T pale, or light purple

P wiry

Weak Spleen is overacted by the Liver, or congested Liver overacts on the Spleen. The qi deficiency is greater than the qi stagnation.

T pale or light purple, thin white coat

P weak or wiry

CHAI SHAO LIU JUN ZI TANG

Bupleurum, Peony, and Six-Gentlemen Decoction

Extract Formula Name: Bupleurum, Paeonia and Six Major Herbs Combination

Ren Shen	*Panax*	6 - 9 g
Fu Ling	*Poria*	6 - 9 g
Bai Zhu	*Atractylodes*	3 - 9 g
Chen Pi	*Citrus*	3 - 6 g
Ban Xia	*Pinellia*	6 - 9 g
Bai Shao Yao	*Paeonia*	6 - 9 g
Chai Hu	*Bupleurum*	6 - 9 g
Gan Cao	*Glycyrrhiza*	3 - 6 g

Liver/Spleen disharmony with heat. Symptoms include irregular menstruation, red or bloodshot eyes, or irritability.

T red sides, light purple, thin white coat

P wiry, rapid

DAN ZHI XIAO YAO SAN (JIA WEI XIAO YAO SAN)

Moutan, Gardenia, and Rambling Powder

Extract Formula Name: Bupleurum and Peony Formula

Mu Dan Pi	*Paeonia*	6 - 9 g
Zhi Zi	*Gardenia*	3 - 6 g
Chai Hu	*Bupleurum*	6 - 9 g
Bo He	*Mentha*	3 - 6 g
Dang Gui	*Angelica*	6 - 9 g
Bai Shao Yao	*Paeonia*	6 - 9 g
Bai Zhu	*Atractylodes*	3 - 9 g
Fu Ling	*Poria*	6 - 9 g
Gan Cao	*Glycyrrhiza*	3 - 6 g
[Sheng Jiang	*Zingiber*	3 - 6 g]

Liver overacting on Spleen causing mild cramping in the abdomen with Liver blood deficiency and some damp accumulation. Symptoms include urinary retention and lower body edema. This is often seen during pregnancy.

T pale, orange color on the sides

P weak, thin, or slightly wiry

DANG GUI SHAO YAO SAN

Dang Gui and Peony Powder

Extract Formula Name: Tang-Kuei and Peony Formula

Dang Gui	*Angelica*	6 - 9 g
Bai Shao Yao	*Paeonia*	3 - 9 g
Bai Zhu	*Atractylodes*	3 - 9 g
Fu Ling	*Poria*	6 - 9 g
Chuan Xiong	*Ligusticum*	3 - 6 g
Ze Xie	*Alisma*	6 - 9 g

Liver/Spleen disharmony with severe blood deficiency. This leads to dysmenorrhea and uterine bleeding.

T pale, thin white coat

P frail or wiry

HEI XIAO YAO SAN

Black Rambling Powder

Bai Zhu	*Atractylodes*	6 - 9 g
Di Huang	*Rehmannia*	6 - 15 g
Fu Ling	*Poria*	6 - 9 g
Chai Hu	*Bupleurum*	6 - 9 g
Bai Shao Yao	*Paeonia*	6 - 9 g
Dang Gui	*Angelica*	6 - 9 g
Gan Cao	*Glycyrrhiza*	3 - 6 g
[Bo He	*Mentha*	3 - 6 g]
[Sheng Jiang	*Zingiber*	3 - 6 g]

Liver overacting on the Stomach leading to constipation, belching, and abdominal pain.

T light purple, thin white coat

P wiry

✘ Caution during pregnancy

LIU MO TANG

Six-Milled Herb Decoction

Bing Lang	*Areca*	6 - 9 g
Wu Yao	*Lindera*	3 g
Chen Xiang	*Aquilaria*	3 - 6 g
Mu Xiang	*Saussurea*	3 - 6 g
Zhi Ke	*Citrus*	3 - 6 g
Da Huang	*Rheum*	6 - 9 g

Liver qi stagnation overacting on Spleen. This leads to damp which in turn heats up and then causes red leukorrhea. Or, the Liver fails to store the blood which also manifests as red leukorrhea.

T purple or pale

P wiry, or weak, thin

☞ E Jiao - Equus should be dissolved into the strained tea.

QING GAN ZHI LIN TANG

Clear Liver and Stop Leukorrhea Decoction

Bai Shao Yao	*Paeonia*	30 g
Dang Gui	*Angelica*	30 g
Shu Di Huang	*Rehmannia*	15 g
E Jiao	*Equus*	9 g
Mu Dan Pi	*Paeonia*	9 g
Huang Bai	*Phellodendron*	6 g
Huai Niu Xi	*Achyranthes*	6 g
Xiang Fu	*Cyperus*	3 g
Da Zao	*Ziziphus*	7 - 10 pc
no pinyin name	*Small Black beans*	30 g

Severe Liver qi/blood stagnation with Spleen qi/blood deficiency causing severe flank pain, and chronic hepatitis. The prescription also treats early stage liver cirrhosis.

T purple, thin coat

P wiry

SHU GAN LI PI TANG

Spread the Liver and Regulate the Spleen Decoction

Chai Hu	*Bupleurum*	9 - 12 g
Bai Zhu	*Atractylodes*	3 - 9 g
Dang Shen	*Codonopsis*	9 - 15 g
He Shou Wu	*Polygonum*	6 - 12 g
Dan Shen	*Salvia*	9 - 12 g
Xiang Fu	*Cyperus*	6 - 9 g
Ze Xie	*Alisma*	6 - 9 g
San Qi	*Panax*	3 g

Liver overacting on the Lungs or Stomach leading to wheezing, shortness of breath, or epigastric distention respectively.

T light purple, thin coat

P wiry

SI MO TANG

Four-Milled Herb Decoction

Ren Shen	*Panax*	6 - 9 g
Chen Xiang	*Aquilaria*	3 - 6 g
Wu Yao	*Lindera*	3 - 6 g
Bing Lang	*Areca*	6 - 9 g

Liver overacting on Spleen with mild heat. This is the basic prescription for this syndrome.

T light purple, thin coat

P wiry, slightly wiry

✪ Major Formula

SI NI SAN

Frigid Extremities Powder

Extract Formula Name: Bupleurum and Chih-Shih Formula

Chai Hu	*Bupleurum*	6 - 9 g
Zhi Shi	*Citrus*	6 - 9 g
Bai Shao Yao	*Paeonia*	3 - 9 g
Zhi Gan Cao	*Glycyrrhiza*	3 - 6 g

Liver overacting on Stomach with pain, depression, fullness, regurgitation, and indigestion.

T white or yellow coat

P wiry

SU GAN WAN

Liver Soothing Pills

Chai Hu	*Bupleurum*	6 - 9 g
Bai Shao Yao	*Paeonia*	6 - 9 g
Fu Ling	*Poria*	6 - 9 g
Yan Hu Suo	*Corydalis*	3 - 6 g
Hou Po	*Magnolia*	6 - 12 g
Jiang Huang	*Curcuma*	6 - 9 g
Chen Xiang	*Aquilaria*	3 - 6 g
Chen Pi	*Citrus*	3 - 6 g
Zhi Ke	*Citrus*	3 - 6 g
Mu Xiang	*Saussurea*	3 - 6 g
Sha Ren	*Amomum*	3 - 6 g
Chuan Lian Zi	*Melia*	6 - 12 g
Bai Dou Kou	*Amomum*	3 - 6 g

Liver/Spleen disharmony causing diarrhea and gurgling sounds in the abdomen.

T light purple, thin white coat

P wiry, thin, slow

TONG XIE YAO FANG

Important Formula for Painful Diarrhea

Extract Formula Name: Siler and Atractylodes Formula

Bai Shao Yao	*Paeonia*	9 - 12 g
Bai Zhu	*Atractylodes*	12 - 15 g
Fang Feng	*Ledebouriella*	6 - 9 g
Chen Pi	*Citrus*	6 - 9 g

Liver/Spleen disharmony leading to epigastric aches, acid regurgitation, diarrhea, or hot dysentery.

T light purple, thin coat

P wiry

☞ Herbs should be made into pills with flour.

WU JI WAN

Fifth and Sixth Heavenly Stem Pill

Huang Lian	*Coptis*	20 g
Bai Shao Yao	*Paeonia*	20 g
Wu Zhu Yu	*Evodia*	20 g

Wandering epigastric/abdominal pain after an attack of anger. There are no qi deficiency signs or symptoms.

T thin coat

P wiry

WU MO YIN ZI

Five-Milled Herb Decoction

Bing Lang	*Areca*	6 - 9 g
Zhi Shi	*Citrus*	6 - 9 g
Mu Xiang	*Saussurea*	6 - 9 g
Chen Xiang	*Aquilaria*	3 - 6 g
Wu Yao	*Lindera*	3 - 6 g

1. Chronic Spleen qi deficiency with chronic cold evil qi leading to qi and blood deficiency. The main symptom is abdominal spasms. 2. Liver qi stagnation or Liver overacting on Spleen. In the latter two instances the dosage of 'Bai Shao Yao - Paeonia' should be increased.

T pale or light purple, thin white coat

P weak or slightly wiry

☞ Yi Tang - Saccharum Granorum should be added to the strained tea.

XIAO JIAN ZHONG TANG

Minor Construct the Middle Decoction

Extract Formula Name: Minor Cinnamon and Peony Combination

Yi Tang	*Saccharum Granorum*	15 - 30 g
Gui Zhi	*Cinnamomum*	3 - 9 g
Bai Shao Yao	*Paeonia*	6 - 9 g
Sheng Jiang	*Zingiber*	6 - 9 g
Da Zao	*Ziziphus*	3 - 5 pc
Zhi Gan Cao	*Glycyrrhiza*	3 - 6 g

Liver/Spleen disharmony with blood deficiency: decreased appetite, irregular menstruation, pain in the flanks, or breast distention.

T light purple, pale, thin white coat

P wiry

✪ Major Formula

XIAO YAO SAN

Rambling Powder

Extract Formula Name: Bupleurum and Tang-Kuei Powder

Chai Hu	*Bupleurum*	6 - 9 g
Dang Gui	*Angelica*	6 - 9 g
Bai Zhu	*Atractylodes*	3 - 9 g
Bai Shao Yao	*Paeonia*	6 - 9 g
Fu Ling	*Poria*	6 - 9 g
Bo He	*Mentha*	3 - 6 g
Gan Cao	*Glycyrrhiza*	3 - 6 g
Sheng Jiang	*Zingiber*	3 - 6 g

Liver/Spleen disharmony with false heat due to Liver yin deficiency in children with chronic deficiency problems leading to spasms, seizures, hysteria, and being scared at night.

T red sides, light purple, thin yellowish coat

P wiry, slightly rapid, thin

YI GAN SAN

Restrain the Liver Powder

Extract Formula Name: Bupleurum Formula

Dang Gui	*Angelica*	6 - 9 g
Fu Ling	*Poria*	6 - 9 g
Bai Zhu	*Atractylodes*	6 - 9 g
Gou Teng	*Uncaria*	6 - 9 g
Chai Hu	*Bupleurum*	6 - 9 g
Chuan Xiong	*Ligusticum*	3 - 9 g
Gan Cao	*Glycyrrhiza*	3 - 6 g
[Chen Pi	*Citrus*	3 - 6 g]
[Ban Xia	*Pinellia*	6 - 9 g]

Liver

Liver qi stagnation causing Liver fire which burns the Stomach. This leads to vomiting or belching, ulcers due to heat, gas, sour or bitter regurgitation. This is a Liver/Stomach imbalance.

T red, dry, yellow coat

P rapid, wiry

☞ This formula may also be prepared as a powder with ten times the dosage.

ZUO JIN WAN

Left Metal Pill

Extract Formula Name: Coptis and Evodia Formula

Huang Lian	*Coptis*	12 - 18 g
Wu Zhu Yu	*Evodia*	1 - 4 g

LIVER YIN DEFICIENCY

- red, dry or blood shot eyes
- poor night vision
- malarflush and afternoon heat
- early but scanty menstruation

T red sides, scanty coat

P thin, rapid, wiry, or empty

Kidney/Liver yin deficiency with blood deficiency causing post-partum sweating, or night sweats.

T red, thin yellow coat

P thin, rapid

BA WEI DI HUANG WAN

Eight-Ingredient Pill with Rehmannia

Sheng Di Huang	*Rehmannia*	6 - 12 g
Shan Zhu Yu	*Cornus*	6 - 9 g
Shan Yao	*Dioscorea*	6 - 9 g
Fu Ling	*Poria*	6 - 9 g
Ze Xie	*Alisma*	6 - 9 g
Mu Dan Pi	*Paeonia*	6 - 9 g
Wu Wei Zi	*Schisandra*	6 - 9 g
Huang Qi	*Astragalus*	9 - 15 g

Liver blood/yin deficiency causing blurred vision, red and dry eyes, and muscle twitches.

T red, thin yellow coat

P thin, wiry, slightly rapid

BU GAN TANG

Tonify the Liver Decoction

Shu Di Huang	*Rehmannia*	9 - 20 g
Dang Gui	*Angelica*	6 - 12 g
Bai Shao Yao	*Paeonia*	6 - 12 g
Mu Gua	*Chaenomeles*	6 - 9 g
Suan Zao Ren	*Ziziphus*	6 - 9 g
Chuan Xiong	*Ligusticum*	3 - 9 g
Gan Cao	*Glycyrrhiza*	3 - 6 g
Mai Men Dong	*Ophiopogon*	6 - 9 g

Purpura due to yin deficiency with heat. Strong false fire due to Kidney and Liver yin deficiency which leads to tidal fever and night sweats.

T red, thin yellow coat or no coat

P rapid, thin, or empty

DA BU YIN WAN

Great Tonify the Yin Pill

Shu Di Huang	*Rehmannia*	6 - 12 g
Gui Ban	*Chinemys*	6 - 12 g
Huang Bai	*Phellodendron*	6 - 9 g
Zhi Mu	*Anemarrhena*	6 - 9 g

Liver wind due to Liver yin deficiency causing spasms and twitches.

T dark red, scanty yellow coat

P thin, wiry, rapid

☞ E Jiao - Equus should be added to the strained tea. Bie Jia - Amyda, Mu Li - Ostrea, and Gui Ban - Chinemys should all be crushed or powdered, and cooked 45 minutes prior to the other herbs. The egg-yolks are boiled hard, then made into a soft mass and mixed into the tea.

DA DING FENG ZHU

Major Arrest Wind Pearl

Ji Zi Huang	*Egg Yolk*	2
Wu Wei Zi	*Schisandra*	6 - 9 g
E Jiao	*Equus*	6 - 9 g
Bai Shao Yao	*Paeonia*	9 - 15 g
Mai Men Dong	*Ophiopogon*	9 - 15 g
Huo Ma Ren	*Cannabis*	3 - 6 g
Sheng Di Huang	*Rehmannia*	9 - 15 g
Bie Jia	*Amyda*	6 - 12 g
Gui Ban	*Chinemys*	6 - 12 g
Mu Li	*Ostrea*	6 - 12 g
Gan Cao	*Glycyrrhiza*	6 - 12 g

Kidney and Liver yin deficiency causing irregular menses, scanty menstrual flow, tinnitus, dizziness, or night sweating.

T red, scanty coat

P thin, rapid

DANG GUI DI HUANG YIN

Dang Gui and Rehmannia Decoction

Dang Gui	*Angelica*	6 - 9 g
Shu Di Huang	*Rehmannia*	6 - 12 g
Huai Niu Xi	*Achyranthes*	6 - 9 g
Shan Yao	*Dioscorea*	6 - 9 g
Du Zhong	*Eucommia*	6 - 9 g
Shan Zhu Yu	*Cornus*	6 - 9 g
Zhi Gan Cao	*Glycyrrhiza*	3 - 6 g

Liver/Kidney yin deficiency causing weakness in the low back and knees, or atrophy; or Liver cannot store the soul (hun) causing insomnia or bad dreams.

T red, dry, scanty coat

P thin, rapid

☞ Equal amounts of both herbs should be used.

ER ZHI WAN

Two-Ultimate Pill

Han Lian Cao	*Eclipta*	10 g
Nu Zhen Zi	*Ligustrum*	10 g

Liver qi stagnation with heat causing uterine bleeding which depletes yin (ben lou syndrome).

T red, no coat

P thin, rapid

GU JING WAN

Stabilize the Menses Pill

Extract Formula Name: Tortoise Shell and Scute Combination

Gui Ban	*Chinemys*	15 - 30 g
Chun Pi	*Ailanthus*	6 - 12 g
Bai Shao Yao	*Paeonia*	15 - 30 g
Huang Bai	*Phellodendron*	6 - 9 g
Huang Qin	*Scutellaria*	15 - 30 g
Xiang Fu	*Cyperus*	3 - 6 g

Kidney qi deficiency with Kidney/Liver yin deficiency causing amenorrhea, or back and knee pain.

T pale or red, thin white or scanty coat

P weak, maybe thin especially in the left chi (third) position

GUI SHEN TANG

Comeback Kidney Decoction

Shu Di Huang	*Rehmannia*	6 - 15 g
Shan Yao	*Dioscorea*	9 - 15 g
Shan Zhu Yu	*Cornus*	9 - 12 g
Gou Qi Zi	*Lycium*	9 - 15 g
Dang Gui	*Angelica*	9 - 12 g
Du Zhong	*Eucommia*	6 - 12 g
Fu Ling	*Poria*	6 - 12 g
Tu Si Zi	*Cuscuta*	9 - 12 g

Kidney and Liver yin deficiency causing bone bi-syndrome or wei syndrome. Deficient yin cannot nourish tendons and false heat burns tendons and muscles. This leads to atrophy, joint swelling, or deformities. The pain tends to be more fixed.

T red, scanty coat

P thin, rapid, weak

☞ All ingredients should be ground up as powder. Take 10 g each time, twice a day.

HU QIAN WAN

Hidden Tiger Pill

Extract Formula Name: Tiger Bone and Tortoise Shell Formula

Gui Ban	*Chinemys*	120 g
Huang Bai	*Phellodendron*	150 g
Shu Di Huang	*Rehmannia*	60 g
Zhi Mu	*Anemarrhena*	60 g
Bai Shao Yao	*Paeonia*	60 g
Suo Yang	*Cynomorium*	45 g
Hu Gu	*Panthera*	30 g
Chen Pi	*Citrus*	60 g
Gan Jiang	*Zingiber*	15 g

Liver yin deficiency with yang/wind rising causing palpitations, hypertension, or restlessness.

T red, thin yellow coat

P thin, rapid, slightly wiry

JIAN LING TANG

Construct Roof Tiles Decoction

Huai Niu Xi	*Achyranthes*	30 g
Shan Yao	*Dioscorea*	30 g
Long Gu	*Os Draconis*	18 g
Mu Li	*Ostrea*	18 g
Dai Zhi Shi	*Haematitum*	24 g
Sheng Di Huang	*Rehmannia*	18 g
Bai Zi Ren	*Biota*	12 g
Bai Shao Yao	*Paeonia*	12 g

Kidney and Liver yin deficiency, yang deficiency, or jing deficiency causing spermatorrhea, tinnitus, or impotence.

T pale or red, thin white coat

P thin, weak

JIN SUO GU JING WAN

Metal Lock Pill to Stabilize the Essence

Extract Formula Name: Lotus Stamen Formula

Qian Shi	*Euryale*	6 - 12 g
Sha Yuan Ji Li	*Astragalus*	6 - 12 g
Long Gu	*Os Draconis*	6 - 9 g
Mu Li	*Ostrea*	6 - 9 g
Lian Xu	*Nelumbo*	6 - 9 g
Lian Zi	*Nelumbo*	9 - 15 g

Basic prescription for Kidney/Liver yin deficiency with mild damp. This can cause dry, flaky, pale red rashes, excess sexual activity, or sweating. In women it may lead to irregular menses or night sweating and afternoon heat.

T red, thin yellow coat, or scanty coat

P rapid, thin

✪ **Major Formula**

LIU WEI DI HUANG WAN

Six-Ingredient Pill with Rehmannia

Extract Formula Name: Rehmannia Six Formula

Shan Zhu Yu	*Cornus*	6 - 9 g
Shan Yao	*Dioscorea*	6 - 9 g
Sheng Di Huang	*Rehmannia*	6 - 12 g
Fu Ling	*Poria*	6 - 9 g
Ze Xie	*Alisma*	6 - 9 g
Mu Dan Pi	*Paeonia*	6 - 9 g

Kidney and Liver yin deficiency with yang rising causing vision disturbances, dry red eyes, or blurry vision.

T red, scanty yellow coat

P thin, rapid

MING MU DI HUANG WAN

Improve Vision Pill with Rehmannia

Shu Di Huang	*Rehmannia*	9 - 20 g
Sheng Di Huang	*Rehmannia*	9 - 15 g
Mu Dan Pi	*Paeonia*	6 - 9 g
Shan Yao	*Dioscorea*	6 - 9 g
Shan Zhu Yu	*Cornus*	6 - 9 g
Ze Xie	*Alisma*	6 - 9 g
Dang Gui	*Angelica*	6 - 9 g
Fu Shen	*Poria*	6 - 9 g
Chai Hu	*Bupleurum*	6 - 9 g
Wu Wei Zi	*Schisandra*	6 - 9 g

Hemorrhage in the eye due to trauma with underlying yin deficiency symptoms. Other symptoms include tinnitus, malar flush, or night sweating.

T dark red, scanty yellow coat

P thin, rapid, wiry

☞ Zhi Zi - Gardenia should be charcoaled to increase the stop bleeding effect. E Jiao - Equus should be added to the strained decoction.

NING XUE TANG

Quiet the Blood Decoction

Han Lian Cao	*Eclipta*	9 - 15 g
Xian He Cao	*Agrimonia*	9 - 15 g
Zhi Zi Tan	*Gardenia*	6 - 9 g
Sheng Di Huang	*Rehmannia*	9 - 15 g
Bai Lian	*Ampelopsis*	3 - 6 g
E Jiao	*Equus*	9 - 15 g
Bai Mao Gen	*Imperata*	9 - 15 g
Bai Shao Yao	*Paeonia*	9 - 15 g
Ce Bai Ye	*Biota*	9 - 15 g
Bai Ji	*Bletilla*	6 - 9 g

Liver blood/yin deficiency with Kidney qi deficiency causing early greying, hairloss, poor teeth, and seminal emissions.

T pale

P thin, weak

QI BAO MEI RAN DAN

Seven-Treasure Special Pill for Beautiful Whiskers

He Shou Wu	*Polygonum*	6 - 9 g
Huai Niu Xi	*Achyranthes*	6 - 12 g
Fu Ling	*Poria*	6 - 9 g
Tu Si Zi	*Cuscuta*	6 - 9 g
Gou Qi Zi	*Lycium*	6 - 9 g
Bu Gu Zhi	*Psoralea*	6 - 9 g
Dang Gui	*Angelica*	6 - 9 g

Kidney and Liver yin deficiency with eye disturbances.

T red, scanty yellow coat

P thin, rapid

QI JU DI HUANG WAN

Lycium Fruit, Chrysanthemum, and Rehmannia Pill

Extract Formula Name: Lycium, Chrysanthemum and Rehmannia Formula

Shu Di Huang	*Rehmannia*	6 - 12 g
Shan Yao	*Dioscorea*	6 - 9 g
Shan Zhu Yu	*Cornus*	6 - 9 g
Mu Dan Pi	*Paeonia*	6 - 9 g
Fu Ling	*Poria*	6 - 9 g
Ze Xie	*Alisma*	6 - 9 g
Gou Qi Zi	*Lycium*	6 - 12 g
Ju Hua	*Chrysanthemum*	6 - 9 g

Liver wind or yang rising due to yin or blood deficiency. Symptoms include spasms, vertigo, or heat in the palms, soles, and chest.

T dark red, dry, or geographic

P thin, rapid, wiry

☞ E Jiao - Equus should be dissoved at the end into the strained tea.

✘ Caution during pregnancy.

SAN JIA FU MAI TANG

Three-Shell Decoction to Restore the Pulse

Zhi Gan Cao	*Glycyrrhiza*	9 - 15 g
Bai Shao Yao	*Paeonia*	9 - 15 g
Sheng Di Huang	*Rehmannia*	9 - 15 g
E Jiao	*Equus*	6 - 9 g
Bie Jia	*Amyda*	9 - 20 g
Gui Ban	*Chinemys*	15 - 30 g
Huo Ma Ren	*Cannabis*	6 - 9 g
Mu Li	*Ostrea*	9 - 15 g
Mai Men Dong	*Ophiopogon*	9 - 15 g

Kidney and Liver yin deficiency with blood deficiency and wind damp. This leads to blurry vision, cough, constipation, or bi-syndrome.

T red, scanty yellow coat

P thin

☞ Herbs should be formed into 9 g pills. Adults take one pill two times a day.

SANG MA WAN

Mulberry Leaf and Sesame Seed Pill

Sang Ye	*Morus*	250 - 300 g
Hei Zhi Ma	*Sesamum*	100 - 120 g
Feng Mi	*Mel*	250 - 300 g

Kidney/Liver yin deficiency with yang rising causing blurry vision, photophobia, excessive tearing, poor night vision, early stage catarract, or blood-shot eyes.

T red, thin and narrow in size, maybe cracked, scanty coat

P thin, rapid

☞ Xi Jiao - Rhinoceros should be substituted with Shui Niu Jiao - Bubalus.

SHI HU YE GUANG WAN

Dendrobium Pill for Night Vision

Tian Men Dong	*Asparagus*	6-9 g
Fu Ling	*Poria*	6 - 9 g
Ren Shen	*Panax*	6 - 9 g
Shu Di Huang	*Rehmannia*	12 - 15 g
Mai Men Dong	*Ophiopogon*	6 - 9 g
Tu Si Zi	*Cuscuta*	3 - 9 g
Ju Hua	*Chrysanthemum*	3 - 6 g
Xing Ren	*Prunus*	3 - 6 g
Jue Ming Zi	*Cassia*	6 - 9 g
Gou Qi Zi	*Lycium*	6 - 9 g
Shan Yao	*Dioscorea*	6 - 12 g
Wu Wei Zi	*Schisandra*	6 - 9 g
Huai Niu Xi	*Achyranthes*	6 - 12 g
Bai Ji Li	*Tribulus*	6 - 9 g
Chuan Xiong	*Ligusticum*	3 - 6 g
Rou Cong Rong	*Cistanche*	3 - 6 g
Shi Hu	*Dendrobium*	6 - 12 g
Zhi Ke	*Citrus*	3 - 6 g
Qing Xiang Zi	*Celosia*	3 - 9 g
Xi Jiao	*Rhinoceros*	1 - 3 g
Huang Lian	*Coptis*	3 - 6 g
Fang Feng	*Ledebouriella*	6 - 9 g
Ling Yang Jiao	*Saiga*	1 - 3 g
Gan Cao	*Glycyrrhiza*	3 - 6 g

Liver yin deficiency with yang or wind rising causing headaches, hypertension, tinnitus, or dizziness.

T red

P thin, rapid, wiry

TIAN MA GOU TENG YIN

Gastrodia and Uncaria Decoction

Extract Formula Name: Gastrodia and Uncaria Combination

Tian Ma	*Gastrodia*	9 - 12 g
Gou Teng	*Uncaria*	9 - 15 g
Chuan Niu Xi	*Cyathula*	9 - 12 g
Huang Qin	*Scutellaria*	6 - 9 g
Shi Jue Ming	*Haliotis*	15 - 25 g
Zhi Zi	*Gardenia*	3 - 6 g
Yi Mu Cao	*Leonurus*	6 - 12 g
Ye Jiao Teng	*Polygonum*	9 - 20 g
Du Zhong	*Eucommia*	6 - 12 g
Sang Ji Sheng	*Loranthus*	6 - 20 g
Fu Shen	*Poria*	6 - 12 g

Kidney and Liver yin deficiency causing amenorrhea, cold feeling in the abdomen, retarded growth in puberty, or clear leukorrhea.

T pale or slightly red

P weak, thin

☞ E Jiao - Equus should be added at the end to the strained tea.

TIAO GAN TANG

Regulating the Liver Decoction

Shan Yao	*Dioscorea*	9 - 12 g
E Jiao	*Equus*	6 - 12 g
Ba Ji Tian	*Morinda*	6 - 9 g
Dang Gui	*Angelica*	6 - 9 g
Ze Lan	*Lycopus*	6 - 12 g
Shan Zhu Yu	*Cornus*	6 - 9 g
Bai Shao Yao	*Paeonia*	6 - 9 g
Dan Shen	*Salvia*	6 - 9 g
Gan Cao	*Glycyrrhiza*	3 - 6 g

Liver

Liver qi stagnation produces heat which consumes Kidney and Liver yin, or Liver overacts on the Spleen and Stomach causing emotional upset, nausea, belching with sour taste, hiatal hernia, or epigastric or abdominal pain; or Liver yin cannot nourish the tendons and ligaments producing heel or posterior hip pain.

T red, dry

P thin, wiry

✪ Major Formula

YI GUAN JIAN

Linking Decoction

Extract Formula Name: Glehnia and Rehmannia Combination

Sheng Di Huang	*Rehmannia*	15 - 30 g
Gou Qi Zi	*Lycium*	6 - 15 g
Dang Gui	*Angelica*	6 - 12 g
Bei Sha Shen	*Glehnia*	6 - 9 g
Mai Men Dong	*Ophiopogon*	6 - 9 g
Chuan Lian Zi	*Melia*	3 - 6 g

Kidney and Liver yin/blood deficiency with fire which bothers the Heart. This causes Heart and Liver fire or Liver yang excess leading to excessive dreaming, insomnia, or outbursts of anger.

T red, cracks, thin or thick yellow coat

P rapid, wiry, thin

☞ Ingredients should be powdered, made into 9 - 12 g pills and taken three times a day. Xi Jiao - Rhinoceros should be substituted with Shui Niu Jiao - Bubalus.

ZHEN ZHU MU WAN

Mother-Of-Pearl Pill

Zhen Zhu Mu	*Pteria*	15 - 20 g
Ren Shen	*Panax*	9 - 12 g
Dang Gui	*Angelica*	6 - 12 g
Shu Di Huang	*Rehmannia*	9 - 12 g
Suan Zao Ren	*Ziziphus*	6 - 9 g
Bai Zi Ren	*Biota*	6 - 9 g
Fu Shen	*Poria*	6 - 9 g
Chen Xiang	*Aquilaria*	6 - 9 g
Xi Jiao	*Rhinoceros*	1 - 3 g

Kidney and Liver yin deficiency with damp stagnation. This causes poor vision, blurry vision, or dry eyes.

T red, sticky yellowish coat

P thin, weak

ZHU JING WAN

Preserve Vistas Pill

Tu Si Zi	*Cuscuta*	9 - 15 g
Shu Di Huang	*Rehmannia*	9 - 12 g
Che Qian Zi	*Plantago*	6 - 9 g

Kidney and Liver yin deficiency with false heat and bone steaming fever, lumbago, involuntary emissions, night sweats, or impotence. Stronger than 'Zuo Gui Yin'.

T red, scanty coat

P thin, rapid, or empty

ZUO GUI WAN

Restore the Left [Kidney] Pill

Extract Formula Name: Achyranthes and Rehmannia Formula

Shu Di Huang	*Rehmannia*	9 - 25 g
Gou Qi Zi	*Lycium*	9 - 12 g
Chuan Niu Xi	*Cyathula*	9 - 12 g
Shan Yao	*Dioscorea*	9 - 12 g
Shan Zhu Yu	*Cornus*	9 - 12 g
Lu Jiao Jiao	*Cervus*	9 - 12 g
Tu Si Zi	*Cuscuta*	9 - 12 g
Gui Ban	*Chinemys*	9 - 12 g

LIVER BLOOD DEFICIENCY

- blurry vision or spots in front of the eyes
- dizziness
- delayed, scanty and short menstruation
- soft or brittle nails

T pale, or orangy sides

P thin, weak, or choppy

Qi and blood deficiency with blood stagnation. This formula is for a restless fetus, infertility, irregular periods, poor appetite, weakness, or fatigue.

T pale, thin white coat

P weak, maybe wiry

BA ZHEN YI MU WAN

Eight-Treasure Pill to Benefit Mothers

Shu Di Huang	*Rehmannia*	6 - 15 g
Chuan Xiong	*Ligusticum*	3 - 9 g
Dang Gui	*Angelica*	6 - 9 g
Bai Shao Yao	*Paeonia*	6 - 12 g
Ren Shen	*Panax*	6 - 12 g
Bai Zhu	*Atractylodes*	3 - 9 g
Fu Ling	*Poria*	6 - 9 g
Yi Mu Cao	*Leonurus*	6 - 18 g
Gan Cao	*Glycyrrhiza*	3 - 6 g

Liver blood/yin deficiency causing blurred vision, red and dry eyes, and muscle twitches.

T red, thin yellow coat

P thin, wiry, slightly rapid

BU GAN TANG

Tonify the Liver Decoction

Shu Di Huang	*Rehmannia*	9 - 20 g
Dang Gui	*Angelica*	6 - 12 g
Bai Shao Yao	*Paeonia*	6 - 12 g
Mu Gua	*Chaenomeles*	6 - 9 g
Suan Zao Ren	*Ziziphus*	6 - 9 g
Chuan Xiong	*Ligusticum*	3 - 9 g
Gan Cao	*Glycyrrhiza*	3 - 6 g
Mai Men Dong	*Ophiopogon*	6 - 9 g

Kidney yin and Spleen qi/blood deficiency causing uterine prolapse with low back pain, night urination, or hearing loss and tinnitus.

T red or pale

P frail

DA BU YUAN JIAN

Great Tonify the Basal Decoction

Ren Shen	*Panax*	6 - 12 g
Shu Di Huang	*Rehmannia*	9 - 25 g
Shan Yao	*Dioscorea*	6 - 9 g
Shan Zhu Yu	*Cornus*	3 - 6 g
Gou Qi Zi	*Lycium*	6 - 9 g
Dang Gui	*Angelica*	6 - 9 g
Du Zhong	*Eucommia*	6 - 9 g
Gan Cao	*Glycyrrhiza*	3 - 6 g

Liver overacting on Spleen causing mild cramping in the abdomen with Liver blood deficiency and some damp accumulation. Symptoms include urinary retention and lower body edema. This is often seen during pregnancy.

T pale, orange color on the sides

P weak, thin, or slightly wiry

DANG GUI SHAO YAO SAN

Dang Gui and Peony Powder

Extract Formula Name: Tang-Kuei and Peony Formula

Dang Gui	*Angelica*	6 - 9 g
Bai Shao Yao	*Paeonia*	3 - 9 g
Bai Zhu	*Atractylodes*	3 - 9 g
Fu Ling	*Poria*	6 - 9 g
Chuan Xiong	*Ligusticum*	3 - 6 g
Ze Xie	*Alisma*	6 - 9 g

Blood deficiency with external cold after childbirth. This leads to spasms or hernia pain which are both relieved by pressure.

T pale

P deep, wiry, weak

☞ This formula should be prepared as a stew with eight cups of water. Simmer until it is reduced to three to four cups.

DANG GUI SHENG JIANG YANG ROU TANG

Mutton Stew with Dang Gui and Fresh Ginger Decoction

Dang Gui	*Angelica*	9 - 12 g
Sheng Jiang	*Zingiber*	9 - 15 g
Yang Rou	*Mutton*	40 - 50 g

Blood deficiency with yang deficiency and cold causing coldness in the uterus with dysmenorrhea. The blood is scanty, pale, and watery. The patient experiences severe cramping upon menstrual onset.

T pale, light purple, some cracks, thin white coat

P slow, thin, weak

GUI FU SI WU TANG

Cinnamon Bark, Aconite, and Four-Substance Decoction

Sheng Di Huang	*Rehmannia*	6 - 12 g
Dang Gui	*Angelica*	6 - 9 g
Chuan Xiong	*Ligusticum*	3 - 9 g
Bai Shao Yao	*Paeonia*	6 - 9 g
Rou Gui	*Cinnamomum*	3 - 9 g
Fu Zi	*Aconitum*	1 - 6 g

Weakness in the extremities with difficulty walking and muscle atrophy due to blood deficiency and damp stagnation.

T pale, sticky coat

P thin, slippery

JIA WEI SI WU TANG

Augmented Four-Substance Decoction

Dang Gui	*Angelica*	6 - 9 g
Huang Bai	*Phellodendron*	6 - 9 g
Mai Men Dong	*Ophiopogon*	6 - 9 g
Shu Di Huang	*Rehmannia*	9 - 12 g
Cang Zhu	*Atractylodes*	3 - 9 g
Du Zhong	*Eucommia*	3 - 6 g
Bai Shao Yao	*Paeonia*	3 - 9 g
Ren Shen	*Panax*	3 g
Wu Wei Zi	*Schisandra*	3 - 6 g
Zhi Mu	*Anemarrhena*	6 - 9 g
Huai Niu Xi	*Achyranthes*	3 - 9 g
Huang Lian	*Coptis*	3 g
Chuan Xiong	*Ligusticum*	3 - 6 g

Chong and Ren imbalance with blood deficiency causing restless fetus, pale post-partum bleeding, abdominal pain, a weak low back, or a cold uterus.

T pale

P frail, slow

☞ E Jiao - Equus should be dissolved at the end into the strained tea.

JIAO AI TANG

Ass-Hide Equus and Mugwort Decoction

Extract Formula Name: Tang-kuei and Equus Combination

E Jiao	*Equus*	6 - 9 g
Ai Ye	*Artemisia*	6 - 9 g
Dang Gui	*Angelica*	6 - 9 g
Sheng Di Huang	*Rehmannia*	18 g
Bai Shao Yao	*Paeonia*	12 g
Chuan Xiong	*Ligusticum*	6 g
Gan Cao	*Glycyrrhiza*	3 - 6 g

Liver blood/yin deficiency with Kidney qi deficiency causing early greying, hairloss, poor teeth, and seminal emissions.

T pale

P thin, weak

QI BAO MEI RAN DAN

Seven-Treasure Special Pill for Beautiful Whiskers

He Shou Wu	*Polygonum*	6 - 9 g
Huai Niu Xi	*Achyranthes*	6 - 12 g
Fu Ling	*Poria*	6 - 9 g
Tu Si Zi	*Cuscuta*	6 - 9 g
Gou Qi Zi	*Lycium*	6 - 9 g
Bu Gu Zhi	*Psoralea*	6 - 9 g
Dang Gui	*Angelica*	6 - 9 g

Liver wind or yang rising due to yin or blood deficiency. Symptoms include spasms, vertigo, or heat in the palms, soles, and chest.

T dark red, dry, or geographic

P thin, rapid, wiry

☞ E Jiao - Equus should be dissoved at the end into the strained tea.

✘ Caution during pregnancy.

SAN JIA FU MAI TANG

Three-Shell Decoction to Restore the Pulse

Zhi Gan Cao	*Glycyrrhiza*	9 - 15 g
Bai Shao Yao	*Paeonia*	9 - 15 g
Sheng Di Huang	*Rehmańnia*	9 - 15 g
E Jiao	*Equus*	6 - 9 g
Bie Jia	*Amyda*	9 - 20 g
Gui Ban	*Chinemys*	15 - 30 g
Huo Ma Ren	*Cannabis*	6 - 9 g
Mu Li	*Ostrea*	9 - 15 g
Mai Men Dong	*Ophiopogon*	9 - 15 g

Qi/yang/blood deficiency. Symptoms include poor appetite, general malaise, mild cold symptoms, severe deficiency, rashes, dysmenorrhea, uterine bleeding, or post-partum deficiency.

T pale, thin white coat

P weak, thin, deep

SHI QUAN DA BU TANG

All-Inclusive Great Tonifying Decoction

Extract Formula Name: Ginseng and Tang-Kuei Ten Combination

Ren Shen	*Panax*	6 - 9 g
Fu Ling	*Poria*	9 - 12 g
Bai Zhu	*Atractylodes*	9 - 12 g
Gan Cao	*Glycyrrhiza*	3 - 6 g
Dang Gui	*Angelica*	12 - 15 g
Shu Di Huang	*Rehmannia*	15 - 20 g
Bai Shao Yao	*Paeonia*	12 - 15 g
Chuan Xiong	*Ligusticum*	3 - 9 g
Rou Gui	*Cinnamomum*	6 - 9 g
Huang Qi	*Astragalus*	15 - 20 g
[Da Zao	*Ziziphus*	1 - 3 g]
[Sheng Jiang	*Zingiber*	3 - 6 g]

Blood deficiency with blood stagnation. Symptoms include irregular menstruation, dysmenorrhea, dizziness, or pale or purple fingernails.

T pale or purple

P thin or choppy

✪ Major Formula

SI WU TANG

Four-Substance Decoction

Extract Formula Name: Tang-Kuei Four Combination

Shu Di Huang	*Rehmannia*	6 - 12 g
Chuan Xiong	*Ligusticum*	3 - 9 g
Dang Gui	*Angelica*	6 - 9 g
Bai Shao Yao	*Paeonia*	6 - 9 g

Blood deficiency which gives rise to wind. This causes an itchy rash which is dry and pale red.

T pale or purple

P thin

SI WU XIAO FENG YIN

Eliminate Wind Decoction with the Four-Substances

Sheng Di Huang	*Rehmannia*	6 - 9 g
Dang Gui	*Angelica*	6 - 9 g
Chi Shao Yao	*Paeonia*	3 - 6 g
Chuan Xiong	*Ligusticum*	3 - 6 g
Jing Jie	*Schizonepeta*	3 - 6 g
Fang Feng	*Ledebouriella*	3 - 6 g
Bai Xian Pi	*Dictamnus*	3 - 6 g
Bo He	*Mentha*	3 - 6 g
Chai Hu	*Bupleurum*	2 g
Du Huo	*Angelica*	3 g
Chan Tui	*Cryptotympana*	3 - 6 g
Da Zao	*Ziziphus*	2 - 3 pc

Blood deficiency causing wind which results in an itchy skin.

T pale

P thin, weak

XUE XU SHEN FENG

Blood Deficiency and Calm Wind Decoction

Gou Qi Zi	*Lycium*	6 - 12 g
He Shou Wu	*Polygonum*	6 - 9 g
Fang Feng	*Ledebouriella*	6 - 9 g
Chan Tui	*Cryptotympana*	6 - 9 g
Yu Zhu	*Polygonatum*	6 - 9 g

COLD IN THE LIVER CHANNEL

- testicular pain or pain in the scrotum
- contraction of the testis or shrinking sensation of the vagina
- ilioinguinal hernia

T pale, moist, thin white coat

P deep, slow, maybe wiry

Cold in the lower jiao causing a running piglet disorder. Symptoms include a tingling sensation around the umbilicus, abdomen, and sternum.

T pale, thin white coat

P wiry or tight

☞ Herbs should be cooked with a little sugar, then formed into 6 g pills. Adults take 2 - 3 pills a day with salt water.

BEN TUN WAN

Running Piglet Pill

Wu Zhu Yu	*Evodia*	3 - 6 g
Chuan Lian Zi	*Melia*	15 - 30 g
Ju He	*Citrus*	15 - 45 g
Fu Ling	*Poria*	15 - 45 g
Xiao Hui Xiang	*Foeniculum*	9 - 20 g
Mu Xiang	*Saussurea*	9 - 20 g
Li Zhi He	*Litchi*	15 - 25 g
Rou Gui	*Cinnamomum*	6 - 12 g
Fu Zi	*Aconitum*	6 - 12 g

Blood deficiency with external cold after childbirth. This leads to spasms or hernia pain which are both relieved by pressure.

T pale

P deep, wiry, weak

☞ This formula should be prepared as a stew with eight cups of water. Simmer until it is reduced to three to four cups.

DANG GUI SHENG JIANG YANG ROU TANG

Mutton Stew with Dang Gui and Fresh Ginger Decoction

Dang Gui	*Angelica*	9 - 12 g
Sheng Jiang	*Zingiber*	9 - 15 g
Yang Rou	*Mutton*	40 - 50 g

Liver qi stagnation with cold in the Liver channel causing a hernia.

T pale, light purple

P wiry

DAO QI TANG

Conduct the Qi Decoction

Mu Xiang	*Saussurea*	3 - 9 g
Chuan Lian Zi	*Melia*	9 - 12 g
Wu Zhu Yu	*Evodia*	3 - 6 g
Xiao Hui Xiang	*Foeniculum*	3 - 6 g

Cold damp stagnation in the lower jiao or cold and qi stagnation causing hard masses and nodules, testicular swelling, swelling of the scrotum, hernia, or fibroid tumors.

T pale, thin sticky white coat

P slow, wiry

JU HE WAN

Tangerine Seed Pill

Chuan Lian Zi	*Melia*	9 - 12 g
Ju He	*Citrus*	9 - 12 g
Tao Ren	*Prunus*	9 g
Rou Gui	*Cinnamomum*	3 - 6 g
Mu Tong	*Akebia*	6 g
Hai Dai	*Laminaria*	6 g
Hai Zao	*Sargassum*	6 g
Kun Bu	*Laminaria*	6 g
Mu Xiang	*Saussurea*	3 - 6 g
Yan Hu Suo	*Corydalis*	6 g
Hou Po	*Magnolia*	6 - 12 g
Zhi Shi	*Citrus*	3 - 6 g

Kidney qi/yang deficiency causing qi/cold stagnation in the Liver channel. Symptoms include hernia, nodules in the lower jiao, impotence, or cold uterus with cramps prior to menses.

T pale, purple

P wiry or tight

✪ **Major Formula**

NUAN GAN JIAN

Warm the Liver Decoction

Dang Gui	*Angelica*	6 - 9 g
Gou Qi Zi	*Lycium*	6 - 9 g
Wu Yao	*Lindera*	3 - 6 g
Chen Xiang	*Aquilaria*	3 - 6 g
Fu Ling	*Poria*	6 - 9 g
Rou Gui	*Cinnamomum*	3 - 6 g
Xiao Hui Xiang	*Foeniculum*	3 - 6 g
Sheng Jiang	*Zingiber*	3 - 6 g

Blood and cold stagnation in the lower jiao with mass formation, blood clots, and dysmenorrhea. This formula is also useful for liver cirrhosis.

T pale, purple

P wiry or choppy

✘ Do not use during pregnancy.

SHAO FU ZHU YU TANG

Drive Out Blood Stasis in the Lower Abdomen Decoction

Extract Formula Name: Cnidium and Bulrush Combination

Yan Hu Suo	*Corydalis*	3 - 6 g
Dang Gui	*Angelica*	6 - 9 g
Mo Yao	*Commiphora*	3 - 6 g
Rou Gui	*Cinnamomum*	3 - 6 g
Xiao Hui Xiang	*Foeniculum*	1.5 - 3 g
Gan Jiang	*Zingiber*	3 - 6 g
Pu Huang	*Typha*	6 - 9 g
Chi Shao Yao	*Paeonia*	6 - 9 g
Wu Ling Zhi	*Trogopterus*	6 - 9 g
Chuan Xiong	*Ligusticum*	3 - 9 g

Post-partum retention of lochia due to blood and cold stagnation.

T pale, purple

P choppy

☞ Add yellow wine to the decoction.

SHENG HUA TANG

Generation and Transformation Decoction

Extract Formula Name: Tang-Kuei and Ginger Combination

Dang Gui	*Angelica*	15 - 28 g
Tao Ren	*Prunus*	6 - 9 g
Pao Jiang	*Zingiber*	3 - 6 g
Chuan Xiong	*Ligusticum*	6 - 9 g
Gan Cao	*Glycyrrhiza*	3 - 6 g

External cold causing stagnation in the Liver channel. This leads to testicle pain and swelling in men, or to clear leukorrhea in women.

T pale, purple, thin white coat

P slow, wiry, or tight

☞ Ba Dou - Croton and Chuan Lian Zi - Melia should be dry fried for 5 - 10 minutes. Discard Ba Dou, then decoct as usual. This way the effect of Chuan Lian Zi is to actually warm the Liver channel.

TIAN TAI WU YAO SAN

Top-Quality Lindera Powder

Wu Yao	*Lindera*	6 - 9 g
Xiao Hui Xiang	*Foeniculum*	3 - 6 g
Gao Liang Jiang	*Alpinia*	3 - 6 g
Mu Xiang	*Saussurea*	3 - 6 g
Qing Pi	*Citrus*	3 - 6 g
Chuan Lian Zi	*Melia*	6 - 9 g
Bing Lang	*Areca*	6 - 9 g
Ba Dou	*Croton*	6 - 15 g

Liver

Deficient cold and blood stagnation causing menstrual irregularities, spotting between periods (lou syndrome), clots at the end of the period, coldness in the lower abdomen, or low-grade fever at night only.

T pale, purple, dark purple spots

P deep, slow, or tight

☞ E Jiao - Equus should be added at the end to the strained tea.

WEN JING TANG

Warm the Menses Decoction

Extract Formula Name: Tang-Kuei and Evodia Combination

Gui Zhi	*Cinnamomum*	6 - 9 g
Wu Zhu Yu	*Evodia*	6 - 9 g
Bai Shao Yao	*Paeonia*	6 - 9 g
Mai Men Dong	*Ophiopogon*	6 - 9 g
Mu Dan Pi	*Paeonia*	6 - 9 g
Ban Xia	*Pinellia*	6 - 9 g
Ren Shen	*Panax*	6 - 9 g
Dang Gui	*Angelica*	6 - 9 g
E Jiao	*Equus*	6 - 9 g
Chuan Xiong	*Ligusticum*	6 g
Sheng Jiang	*Zingiber*	3 - 6 g
Gan Cao	*Glycyrrhiza*	3 - 6 g

Spleen qi deficiency with cold which restricts the Liver and Stomach. This results in tight abdominal pain, cold in the middle and lower jiao, vomiting, or acid regurgitation; or cold causes vertex headaches via the Liver channel. This Liver qi stagnation is not due to emotional reasons but is caused by cold.

T pale, purplish, moist white coat

P slow, or wiry, thin

WU ZHU YU TANG

Evodia Decoction

Extract Formula Name: Evodia Combination

Wu Zhu Yu	*Evodia*	3 - 6 g
Ren Shen	*Panax'*	6 - 9 g
Sheng Jiang	*Zingiber*	12 - 20 g
Da Zao	*Ziziphus*	6 - 12 pc

Cold causing severe abdominal distention with absence of bowel movements and urination, or vomiting right after meals. This formula is also for running piglet disorder (tingling sensation in the epigastrium or abdomen) or cold hernias.

T pale

P slow

☞ Herbs should be ground into a powder. Take as a draft in 3 - 9 g doses before meals.

ZHONG MAN FEN XIAO TANG

Separate and Reduce Fullness in the Middle Decoction

Chuan Wu	*Aconitum*	3 - 6 g
Huang Lian	*Coptis*	3 - 6 g
Qing Pi	*Citrus*	3 - 6 g
Ma Huang	*Ephedra*	3 - 6 g
Bi Cheng Qie	*Litsea*	3 - 6 g
Fu Ling	*Poria*	9 - 15 g
Ban Xia	*Pinellia*	9 - 15 g
Sheng Ma	*Cimicifuga*	9 - 15 g
Sheng Jiang	*Zingiber*	3 - 6 g
Gan Jiang	*Zingiber*	3 - 6 g
Wu Zhu Yu	*Evodia*	9 - 15 g
Cao Dou Kou	*Alpinia*	9 - 15 g
Ze Xie	*Alisma*	3 - 6 g
Yi Zhi Ren	*Alpinia*	9 - 15 g
Mu Xiang	*Saussurea*	9 - 15 g
Hou Po	*Magnolia*	9 - 15 g
Huang Bai	*Phellodendron*	9 - 15 g
Huang Qi	*Astragalus*	9 - 15 g
Ren Shen	*Panax*	3 - 6 g
Dang Gui	*Angelica*	3 - 6 g
Chai Hu	*Bupleurum*	3 - 6 g

DAMP HEAT IN THE LIVER AND LOWER JIAO

- fullness or pain in chest and hypochondriac region
- decreased appetite with nausea and vomiting
- vaginal itching or leukorrhea
- herpes lesions

T red, sticky yellow coat

P slippery, wiry, rapid

Herpes zoster around the waist. The cause is damp heat in the lower jiao.

T sticky yellow coat

P slippery

CHU SHI WEI LING TANG

Eliminate Dampness Decoction by Combining Calm the Stomach and Five-Ingredient Powder with Poria

Hou Po	*Magnolia*	6 - 12 g
Cang Zhu	*Atractylodes*	3 - 6 g
Zhu Ling	*Polyporus*	6 - 9 g
Chi Fu Ling	*Poria*	6 - 9 g
Ze Xie	*Alisma*	6 - 9 g
Chen Pi	*Citrus*	3 - 6 g
Bai Zhu	*Atractylodes*	3 - 6 g
Rou Gui	*Cinnamomum*	3 - 6 g
Hua Shi	*Talcum*	6 g
Zhi Zi	*Gardenia*	3 - 6 g
Fang Feng	*Ledebouriella*	6 - 9 g
Mu Tong	*Akebia*	6 - 9 g
Deng Xin Cao	*Juncus*	3 - 6 g
Gan Cao	*Glycyrrhiza*	3 - 6 g

Damp heat in the lower jiao causing low back pain, hot, swollen knees or feet, or odorous leukorrhea.

T sticky yellow coat

P slippery, rapid

ER MIAO SAN

Two-Marvel Powder

Cang Zhu	*Atractylodes*	15 g
Huang Bai	*Phellodendron*	15 g

Yang jaundice from damp heat lodged in the shaoyang level; or damp heat in the Gallbladder causing alternating fever and chills, bitter taste, or malaria.

T red, thick sticky yellow coat

P slippery, wiry, rapid

☞ Bi Yu San - Green Jade Powder consists of: Hua Shi - Talcum, 3 - 6 g; Gan Cao - Glycyrrhiza, 3 - 6 g; and Qing Dai - Indigo, 9 - 12 g. All three ingredients should be cooked separately in a cheesecloth, then decocted with the rest of the herbs.

HAO QIN QING DAN TANG

Artemisia Annua and Scutellaria Decoction to Clear the Gallbladder

Qing Hao	*Artemisia*	6 g
Zhu Ru	*Bambusa*	9 g
Huang Qin	*Scutellaria*	6 g
Zhi Ke	*Citrus*	5 g
Chi Fu Ling	*Poria*	9 g
Ban Xia	*Pinellia*	5 g
Chen Pi	*Citrus*	5 g
Bi Yu San	*Green Jade Powder*	9 g

Damp heat leukorrhea with low back pain, heat sensation along the leg, or eczema.

T red, sticky yellow coat

P wiry, rapid, slippery

JIA WEI ER MIAO SAN

Augmented Two-Marvel Powder

Huang Bai	*Phellodendron*	6 - 12 g
Cang Zhu	*Atractylodes*	9 - 15 g
Dang Gui Wei	*Angelica*	6 - 9 g
Bei Xie	*Dioscorea*	6 - 9 g
Han Fang Ji	*Stephania*	6 - 9 g
Chuan Niu Xi	*Cyathula*	6 - 9 g
Gui Ban	*Chinemys*	6 - 9 g

Damp heat in the lower jiao, or Liver fire. Symptoms include red and itchy eyes, temple headaches, odorous leukorrhea, or pruritus.

T red, sticky yellow coating

P wiry, rapid, slippery

✪ Major Formula

LONG DAN XIE GAN TANG

Gentiana Decoction to Drain the Liver

Extract Formula Name: Gentiana Combination

Long Dan Cao	Gentiana	6 - 9 g
Zhi Zi	Gardenia	3 - 9 g
Mu Tong	Akebia	6 - 9 g
Huang Qin	Scutellaria	6 - 9 g
Ze Xie	Alisma	6 - 9 g
Che Qian Zi	Plantago	6 - 9 g
Dang Gui	Angelica	6 - 9 g
Sheng Di Huang	Rehmannia	6 - 12 g
Chai Hu	Bupleurum	6 - 9 g
Gan Cao	Glycyrrhiza	3 - 6 g

Liver qi stagnation overacting on Spleen. This leads to damp which in turn heats up and then causes red leukorrhea. Or, the Liver fails to store the blood which also manifests as red leukorrhea.

T purple or pale

P wiry, or weak, thin

☞ E Jiao - Equus should be dissolved into the strained tea.

QING GAN ZHI LIN TANG

Clear Liver and Stop Leukorrhea Decoction

Bai Shao Yao	Paeonia	30 g
Dang Gui	Angelica	30 g
Shu Di Huang	Rehmannia	15 g
E Jiao	Equus	9 g
Mu Dan Pi	Paeonia	9 g
Huang Bai	Phellodendron	6 g
Huai Niu Xi	Achyranthes	6 g
Xiang Fu	Cyperus	3 g
Da Zao	Ziziphus	7 - 10 pc
no pinyin name	Small Black beans	30 g

Yellow leukorrhea with dark yellow urination from heat and damp in the lower jiao.

T red, sticky yellowish coat

P slippery, rapid

QING XIN LIAN ZI YIN

Clear the Heart with Lotus Seed Decoction

Extract Formula Name: Lotus Seed Combination

Huang Qin	*Scutellaria*	6 - 9 g
Mai Men Dong	*Ophiopogon*	6 - 9 g
Ren Shen	*Panax*	6 - 9 g
Huang Qi	*Astragalus*	6 - 15g
Di Gu Pi	*Lycium*	6 - 9 g
Che Qian Zi	*Plantago*	6 - 9 g
Lian Zi	*Nelumbo*	3 - 9 g
Chai Hu	*Bupleurum*	6 - 9 g
Fu Ling	*Poria*	6 - 9 g

Damp heat in the lower jiao with atrophy in the lower extremities, weakness and numbness, or swollen feet.

T red, sticky yellow coat

P rapid, slippery

SAN MIAO SAN

Three-Marvel Powder

Extract Formula Name: Phellodendron and Achyranthes Formula

Huai Niu Xi	*Achyranthes*	3 - 9 g
Huang Bai	*Phellodendron*	6 - 9 g
Cang Zhu	*Atractylodes*	6 - 12 g

Trichomonas due to damp. External wash only!

T not important

P not important

☞ Herbs should be ground into a powder, then prepared as a draft.

✘ For external use only.

SHE CHUANG ZI SAN

Cnidium Powder

She Chuang Zi	*Cnidium*	9 - 15 g
Bai Bu	*Stemona*	9 - 15 g
Chuan Jiao	*Zanthoxylum*	9 - 15 g
Ming Fan	*Alumen*	9 - 15 g
Ku Shen	*Sophora*	9 - 15 g

Damp heat in the lower jiao. Odorous leukorrhea, cloudy urine, and painful swollen feet.

T red, sticky yellow coat

P slippery, rapid

Major Formula

SI MIAO SAN

Four-Marvel Powder

Cang Zhu	*Atractylodes*	6 - 9 g
Huang Bai	*Phellodendron*	6 - 9 g
Yi Yi Ren	*Coix*	6 - 12 g
Huai Niu Xi	*Achyranthes*	6 - 12 g

Trichomonas infection: damp heat causing yellow, odorous leukorrhea, and severe itching.

T red, sticky yellow coat

P rapid, slippery

WU MEI YIN CHEN TANG

Mume and Artemisia Yinchenhao Decoction

Wu Mei	*Prunus*	20 - 30 g
Yin Chen Hao	*Artemisia*	9 - 15 g
Hua Jiao	*Zanthoxylum*	6 - 9 g
Jin Yin Hua	*Lonicera*	6 - 12 g
Bian Xu	*Polygonum*	6 - 9 g
Bai Zhu	*Atractylodes*	6 - 9 g
Fu Ling	*Poria*	6 - 15 g
Long Dan Cao	*Gentiana*	6 - 9 g
Huang Bai	*Phellodendron*	6 - 9 g

Whole body yang jaundice due to damp heat in the Liver and Gallbladder.

T Red, thick sticky yellow coat

P slippery, rapid, forceful

✘ Do not use during pregnancy.

YIN CHEN HAO TANG

Artemisia Yinchenhao Decoction

Extract Formula Name: Capillaris Combination

Yin Chen Hao	*Artemisia*	15 - 30 g
Da Huang	*Rheum*	6 - 9 g
Zhi Zi	*Gardenia*	6 - 9 g

Damp heat accumulation in the middle jiao (Liver/Gallbladder) causing yang jaundice, dysurea, or hepatitis with mild fever.

T slightly red, thick sticky coat

P slippery, slightly rapid

YIN CHEN WU LING SAN

Artemisia Yinchenhao and Five-Ingredient Powder with Poria

Extract Formula Name: Capillaris and Hoelen Five Formula

Yin Chen Hao	*Artemisia*	10 - 20 g
Fu Ling	*Poria*	6 - 12 g
Zhu Ling	*Polyporus*	6 - 9 g
Bai Zhu	*Atractylodes*	3 - 9 g
Ze Xie	*Alisma*	6 - 9 g
Gui Zhi	*Cinnamomum*	3 - 9 g

Damp heat accumulation leading to leukorrhea. The discharge is very odorous, yellow, thick, and may be profuse.

T red, thick yellow sticky coat

P slippery, rapid

ZHI DAI TANG

Stop Leukorrhea Decoction

Fu Ling	*Poria*	6 - 9 g
Zhu Ling	*Polyporus*	6 - 9 g
Ze Xie	*Alisma*	6 - 9 g
Che Qian Zi	*Plantago*	3 - 9 g
Yin Chen Hao	*Artemisia*	15 g
Zhi Zi	*Gardenia*	3 - 6 g
Huang Bai	*Phellodendron*	3 - 9 g
Mu Dan Pi	*Paeonia*	6 - 12 g
Chi Shao Yao	*Paeonia*	6 - 9 g
Huai Niu Xi	*Achyranthes*	3 - 6 g

Yang jaundice due to damp heat in the interior. The heat is greater than the damp.

T red, sticky yellow coat

P slippery, rapid

ZHI ZI BAI PI TANG

Gardenia and Phellodendron Decoction

Extract Formula Name: Gardenia and Phellodendron Combination

Zhi Zi	*Gardenia*	9 - 15 g
Huang Bai	*Phellodendron*	6 - 9 g
Zhi Gan Cao	*Glycyrrhiza*	3 - 6 g

Damp heat accumulation in the middle jiao. There is more damp than heat causing fullness in the abdomen, thirst without desire to drink, or immediate fullness upon eating or drinking. This formula is also useful for yang jaundice.

T red, thick sticky coat

P slippery, rapid

ZHONG JIAO XIAN BI TANG

Middle Jiao and Clear Damp Decoction

Xing Ren	*Prunus*	3 - 6 g
Yi Yi Ren	*Coix*	9 - 12 g
Hua Shi	*Talcum*	6 g
Dou Juan	*Glycine*	9 g
Zhi Zi	*Gardenia*	6 - 9 g
Lian Qiao	*Forsythia*	6 g
Ban Xia	*Pinellia*	6 - 9 g
Han Fang Ji	*Stephania*	6 - 9 g
Can Sha	*Bombyx*	3 - 6 g
Shan Zha	*Crataegus*	3 - 9 g
Bian Dou	*Dolichos*	6 - 9 g

Damp heat in the lower jiao causing urinary difficulty and pain.

T red, sticky coat

P slippery

ZHU LING TANG II

Polyporus Decoction from Comprehensive Recordings

Zhu Ling	*Polyporus*	6 - 9 g
Mu Tong	*Akebia*	6 - 9 g
Sang Bai Pi	*Morus*	6 - 9 g
[Deng Xin Cao	*Juncus*	3 g]

Liver

LIVER FIRE

- uncontrolled anger outbursts
- bitter taste
- constipation and dark-yellow urine
- loud tinnitus
- bleeding in the upper parts like epistaxis, hemoptysis

T red, or red sides, yellow coat

P wiry, rapid, forceful

Liver fire causing sores on the head, severe headaches, bad breath, or hearing difficulty.

T red, yellow coat

P rapid, wiry

CHAI HU QING GAN TANG

Bupleurum Decoction to Clear the Liver

Extract Formula Name: Bupleurum and Rehmannia Combination

Chai Hu	*Bupleurum*	6-9 g
Chi Shao Yao	*Paeonia*	6-9 g
Lian Qiao	*Forsythia*	6-9 g
Chuan Xiong	*Ligusticum*	3-6 g
Dang Gui	*Angelica*	6-9 g
Sheng Di Huang	*Rehmannia*	6-9 g
Zhi Zi	*Gardenia*	3-6 g
Tian Hua Fen	*Trichosanthes*	6-9 g
Huang Qin	*Scutellaria*	3-9 g
Niu Bang Zi	*Arctium*	6-9 g
Fang Feng	*Ledebouriella*	3-6 g
Gan Cao	*Glycyrrhiza*	3-6 g

Liver/Spleen disharmony with heat. Symptoms include irregular menstruation, red or bloodshot eyes, or irritability.

T red sides, light purple, thin white coat

P wiry, rapid

DAN ZHI XIAO YAO SAN (JIA WEI XIAO YAO SAN)

Moutan, Gardenia, and Rambling Powder

Extract Formula Name: Bupleurum and Peony Formula

Mu Dan Pi	*Paeonia*	6 - 9 g
Zhi Zi	*Gardenia*	3 - 6 g
Chai Hu	*Bupleurum*	6 - 9 g
Bo He	*Mentha*	3 - 6 g
Dang Gui	*Angelica*	6 - 9 g
Bai Shao Yao	*Paeonia*	6 - 9 g
Bai Zhu	*Atractylodes*	3 - 9 g
Fu Ling	*Poria*	6 - 9 g
Gan Cao	*Glycyrrhiza*	3 - 6 g
[Sheng Jiang	*Zingiber*	3 - 6 g]

Liver/Gallbladder fire with headaches, mania, restlessness, bleeding gums, hypertension, purpura, otitis media, bitter taste, low-pitched tinnitus, melena, and possible coma.

T red, cracks, yellow coat

P rapid, wiry

☞ Herbs should be ground into a powder, then formed into pills with honey.

✘ Do not use during pregnancy.

✪ Major Formula

DANG GUI LONG HUI WAN

Dang Gui, Gentiana, and Aloe Pill

Extract Formula Name: Tang-Kuei, Gentian and Aloe Formula

Dang Gui	*Angelica*	30 g
Long Dan Cao	*Gentiana*	15 g
Lu Hui	*Aloe*	15 g
Zhi Zi	*Gardenia*	30 g
Huang Lian	*Coptis*	30 g
Huang Qin	*Scutellaria*	30 g
Huang Bai	*Phellodendron*	6 - 9 g
Da Huang	*Rheum*	15 g
Mu Xiang	*Saussurea*	3 - 6 g
She Xiang	*Moschus*	1.5 g

Liver fire attacking the Lung yin. This leads to thick blood-tinged phlegm, thirst, or bitter taste.

T red, cracked, sticky yellow coat

P wiry, rapid

KE XUE FANG

Coughing of Blood Formula

Zhi Zi	*Gardenia*	6-9 g
Gua Lou Ren	*Trichosanthes*	6-9 g
Qing Dai	*Indigo*	6-9 g
Fu Hai Shi	*Pumice*	6-9 g
He Zi	*Terminalia*	3-9 g

Liver wind due to Liver fire causing hypertension, twitches, or headaches.

T dark red, raw, dry

P rapid, wiry

☞ Ling Yang Jiao - Saiga should be cooked one hour prior to adding the other herbs.

LING JIAO GOU TENG TANG

Antelope Horn and Uncaria Decoction

Extract Formula Name: Antelope Horn and Uncaria Combination

Ling Yang Jiao	*Saiga*	3-6 g
Sang Ye	*Morus*	6-9 g
Sheng Di Huang	*Rehmannia*	9-15 g
Zhu Ru	*Bambusa*	9-15 g
Bai Shao Yao	*Paeonia*	6-9 g
Gou Teng	*Uncaria*	6-9 g
Chuan Bei Mu	*Fritillaria*	6-12 g
Ju Hua	*Chrysanthemum*	6-9 g
Fu Shen	*Poria*	6-9 g
Gan Cao	*Glycyrrhiza*	3-6 g

Damp heat in the lower jiao, or Liver fire. Symptoms include red and itchy eyes, temple headaches, odorous leukorrhea, or pruritus.

T red, sticky yellow coating

P wiry, rapid, slippery

✪ Major Formula

LONG DAN XIE GAN TANG

Gentiana Decoction to Drain the Liver

Extract Formula Name: Gentiana Combination

Long Dan Cao	*Gentiana*	6 - 9 g
Zhi Zi	*Gardenia*	3 - 9 g
Mu Tong	*Akebia*	6 - 9 g
Huang Qin	*Scutellaria*	6 - 9 g
Ze Xie	*Alisma*	6 - 9 g
Che Qian Zi	*Plantago*	6 - 9 g
Dang Gui	*Angelica*	6 - 9 g
Sheng Di Huang	*Rehmannia*	6 - 12 g
Chai Hu	*Bupleurum*	6 - 9 g
Gan Cao	*Glycyrrhiza*	3 - 6 g

Liver and Stomach fire causing dizziness, bad breath, anger outbursts, oral sores or ulcers, or constipation.

T red, sticky yellow coat

P rapid, wiry, forceful

☞ Niu Huang - Bos should be added at the end of the decoction process. Bing Pian - Dryobalanops and Xiong Huang - Realgar should be powdered prior to the decoction. This prescription is available in prepared form.

✘ Do not use during pregnancy

NIU HUANG JIE DU PIEN

Antiphlogistic Pills with Bos Calculus

Niu Huang	*Bos*	3 - 6 g
Xiong Huang	*Realgar*	3 - 6 g
Da Huang	*Rheum*	6 - 9 g
Jie Geng	*Platycodon*	3 - 6 g
Bing Pian	*Dryobalanops*	3 - 6 g
Shi Gao	*Gypsum*	9 - 15 g
Huang Qin	*Scutellaria*	6 - 9 g
Gan Cao	*Glycyrrhiza*	3 - 6 g

Qi stagnation with fire causing acute pancreatitis. The patient will vomit immediately after food or liquid intake, and experiences epigastric discomfort. Acute pancreatitis can cause shock or sudden death.

T red, thin yellow coat

P rapid, wiry

☞ Mu Xiang - Saussurea and Da Huang - Rheum should be added near the end of decoction process. Mang Xiao - Mirabilitum should be added to the strained tea.

✘ Do not use during pregnancy.

QING YI TANG

Clear the Pancreas Decoction

Chai Hu	*Bupleurum*	6 - 15 g
Bai Shao Yao	*Paeonia*	6 - 15 g
Huang Qin	*Scutellaria*	9 - 12 g
Yan Hu Suo	*Corydalis*	6 - 9 g
Da Huang	*Rheum*	9 - 15 g
Mu Xiang	*Saussurea*	6 - 9 g
Hu Huang Lian	*Picrorhiza*	6 - 9 g
Mang Xiao	*Mirabilitum*	6 - 9 g

Liver fire attacking the Lungs causing hemoptysis and pain in the chest.

T red, sticky yellow coat

P rapid, wiry

SANG DAN XIE BAI TANG

Mulberry Leaf and Paeonia Decoction to Drain the White

Sang Ye	*Morus*	6 - 9 g
Sang Bai Pi	*Morus*	6 - 12 g
Mu Dan Pi	*Paeonia*	3 - 9 g
Di Gu Pi	*Lycium*	6 - 12 g
Chuan Bei Mu	*Fritillaria*	6 - 9 g
Zhu Ru	*Bambusa*	3 - 6 g
Jing Mi	*Oryza*	6 - 9 g
Da Zao	*Ziziphus*	2 - 4 pc
Gan Cao	*Glycyrrhiza*	3 - 6 g

Liver and Stomach fire causing any kind of sudden bleeding disorder. The fire heats up the blood leading to hematemesis, epistaxis, or hemoptysis.

T dark red, yellow coat

P rapid, forceful, wiry

☞ The herbs should be partially charred prior to the decoction process.

✘ Caution during pregnancy.

SHI HUI SAN

Ten Partially-Charred Substance Powder

Xiao Ji	*Cephalanoplos*	9 - 15 g
Da Ji	*Cirsium*	9 - 12 g
Ce Bai Ye	*Biota*	9 - 12 g
Qian Cao Gen	*Rubia*	9 - 12 g
Da Huang	*Rheum*	9 - 12 g
He Ye	*Nelumbo*	9 - 12 g
Zhi Zi	*Gardenia*	6 - 12 g
Bai Mao Gen	*Imperata*	9 - 12 g
Zong Lu Pi	*Trachycarpus*	6 - 9 g
Mu Dan Pi	*Paeonia*	6 - 9 g

Liver heat/fire giving rise to wind causing itchy rash, hypertension, red eyes, high fever, or easily angered.

T red, dry, thin yellow coat

P rapid, wiry, or flooding

XIE QING WAN

Drain the Green Pill

Long Dan Cao	*Gentiana*	6 - 9 g
Zhi Zi	*Gardenia*	6 - 9 g
Chuan Xiong	*Ligusticum*	6 - 9 g
Qiang Huo	*Notopterygium*	6 - 9 g
Fang Feng	*Ledebouriella*	6 - 9 g
Dang Gui	*Angelica*	6 - 9 g
Da Huang	*Rheum*	6 - 9 g

Liver qi stagnation causing Liver fire which burns the Stomach. This leads to vomiting or belching, ulcers due to heat, gas, sour or bitter regurgitation. This is a Liver/Stomach imbalance.

T red, dry, yellow coat

P rapid, wiry

☞ This formula may also be prepared as a powder with ten times the dosage.

ZUO JIN WAN

Left Metal Pill

Extract Formula Name: Coptis and Evodia Formula

Huang Lian	*Coptis*	12 - 18 g
Wu Zhu Yu	*Evodia*	1 - 4 g

LIVER YANG RISING

- temple headaches
- tinnitus
- hearing impairment

T red sides

P wiry

Liver yin deficiency with yang/wind rising causing palpitations, hypertension, or restlessness.

T red, thin yellow coat

P thin, rapid, slightly wiry

✪ Major Formula

JIAN LING TANG

Construct Roof Tiles Decoction

Huai Niu Xi	*Achyranthes*	30 g
Shan Yao	*Dioscorea*	30 g
Long Gu	*Os Draconis*	18 g
Mu Li	*Ostrea*	18 g
Dai Zhi Shi	*Haematitum*	24 g
Sheng Di Huang	*Rehmannia*	18 g
Bai Zi Ren	*Biota*	12 g
Bai Shao Yao	*Paeonia*	12 g

Kidney and Liver yin deficiency with yang rising causing vision disturbances, dry red eyes, or blurry vision.

T red, scanty yellow coat

P thin, rapid

MING MU DI HUANG WAN

Improve Vision Pill with Rehmannia

Shu Di Huang	*Rehmannia*	9 - 20 g
Sheng Di Huang	*Rehmannia*	9 - 15 g
Mu Dan Pi	*Paeonia*	6 - 9 g
Shan Yao	*Dioscorea*	6 - 9 g
Shan Zhu Yu	*Cornus*	6 - 9 g
Ze Xie	*Alisma*	6 - 9 g
Dang Gui	*Angelica*	6 - 9 g
Fu Shen	*Poria*	6 - 9 g
Chai Hu	*Bupleurum*	6 - 9 g
Wu Wei Zi	*Schisandra*	6 - 9 g

Liver wind or yang rising due to yin or blood deficiency. Symptoms include spasms, vertigo, or heat in the palms, soles, and chest.

T dark red, dry, or geographic

P thin, rapid, wiry

☞ E Jiao - Equus should be dissoved at the end into the strained tea.

✘ Caution during pregnancy.

SAN JIA FU MAI TANG

Three-Shell Decoction to Restore the Pulse

Zhi Gan Cao	*Glycyrrhiza*	9 - 15 g
Bai Shao Yao	*Paeonia*	9 - 15 g
Sheng Di Huang	*Rehmannia*	9 - 15 g
E Jiao	*Equus*	6 - 9 g
Bie Jia	*Amyda*	9 - 20 g
Gui Ban	*Chinemys*	15 - 30 g
Huo Ma Ren	*Cannabis*	6 - 9 g
Mu Li	*Ostrea*	9 - 15 g
Mai Men Dong	*Ophiopogon*	9 - 15 g

Kidney/Liver yin deficiency with yang rising causing blurry vision, photophobia, excessive tearing, poor night vision, early stage catarract, or blood-shot eyes.

T red, thin and narrow in size, maybe cracked, scanty coat

P thin, rapid

☞ Xi Jiao - Rhinoceros should be substituted with Shui Niu Jiao - Bubalus.

SHI HU YE GUANG WAN

Dendrobium Pill for Night Vision

Tian Men Dong	*Asparagus*	6- 9 g
Fu Ling	*Poria*	6 - 9 g
Ren Shen	*Panax*	6 - 9 g
Shu Di Huang	*Rehmannia*	12 - 15 g
Mai Men Dong	*Ophiopogon*	6 - 9 g
Tu Si Zi	*Cuscuta*	3 - 9 g
Ju Hua	*Chrysanthemum*	3 - 6 g
Xing Ren	*Prunus*	3 - 6 g
Jue Ming Zi	*Cassia*	6 - 9 g
Gou Qi Zi	*Lycium*	6 - 9 g
Shan Yao	*Dioscorea*	6 - 12 g
Wu Wei Zi	*Schisandra*	6 - 9 g
Huai Niu Xi	*Achyranthes*	6 - 12 g
Bai Ji Li	*Tribulus*	6 - 9 g
Chuan Xiong	*Ligusticum*	3 - 6 g
Rou Cong Rong	*Cistanche*	3 - 6 g
Shi Hu	*Dendrobium*	6 - 12 g
Zhi Ke	*Citrus*	3 - 6 g
Qing Xiang Zi	*Celosia*	3 - 9 g
Xi Jiao	*Rhinoceros*	1 - 3 g
Huang Lian	*Coptis*	3 - 6 g
Fang Feng	*Ledebouriella*	6 - 9 g
Ling Yang Jiao	*Saiga*	1 - 3 g
Gan Cao	*Glycyrrhiza*	3 - 6 g

Liver yin deficiency with yang or wind rising causing headaches, hypertension, tinnitus, or dizziness.

T red

P thin, rapid, wiry

✪ Major Formula

TIAN MA GOU TENG YIN

Gastrodia and Uncaria Decoction

Extract Formula Name: Gastrodia and Uncaria Combination

Tian Ma	*Gastrodia*	9 - 12 g
Gou Teng	*Uncaria*	9 - 15 g
Chuan Niu Xi	*Cyathula*	9 - 12 g
Huang Qin	*Scutellaria*	6 - 9 g
Shi Jue Ming	*Haliotis*	15 - 25 g
Zhi Zi	*Gardenia*	3 - 6 g
Yi Mu Cao	*Leonurus*	6 - 12 g
Ye Jiao Teng	*Polygonum*	9 - 20 g
Du Zhong	*Eucommia*	6 - 12 g
Sang Ji Sheng	*Loranthus*	6 - 20 g
Fu Shen	*Poria*	6 - 12 g

Liver wind due to yang rising with underlying Kidney and Liver yin deficiency: headache, dizziness, restlessness, or belching due to Liver/Stomach disharmony, low-pitched tinnitus, wind stroke, or hypertension.

T red or light purple, trembling, yellow coat

P forceful, wiry

ZHEN GAN XI FENG TANG

Sedate the Liver and Extinguish Wind Decoction

Extract Formula Name: Dragon Bone and Two Shells Combination

Dai Zhe Shi	*Haematitum*	15 - 30 g
Huai Niu Xi	*Achyranthes*	15 - 30 g
Xuan Shen	*Scrophularia*	12 - 15 g
Bai Shao Yao	*Paeonia*	9 - 15 g
Tian Men Dong	*Asparagus*	9 - 15 g
Gui Ban	*Chinemys*	9 - 15 g
Long Gu	*Os Draconis*	9 - 15 g
Mu Li	*Ostrea*	9 - 15 g
Chuan Lian Zi	*Melia*	6 - 9 g
Mai Ya	*Hordeum*	6 - 9 g
Yin Chen Hao	*Artemisia*	6 - 9 g
Gan Cao	*Glycyrrhiza*	3 - 6 g

Kidney and Liver yin/blood deficiency with fire which bothers the Heart. This causes Heart and Liver fire or Liver yang excess leading to excessive dreaming, insomnia, or outbursts of anger.

T red, cracks, thin or thick yellow coat

P rapid, wiry, thin

☞ Ingredients should be powdered, made into 9 - 12 g pills and taken three times a day. Xi Jiao - Rhinoceros should be substituted with Shui Niu Jiao - Bubalus.

ZHEN ZHU MU WAN

Mother-Of-Pearl Pill

Zhen Zhu Mu	*Pteria*	15 - 20 g
Ren Shen	*Panax*	9 - 12 g
Dang Gui	*Angelica*	6 - 12 g
Shu Di Huang	*Rehmannia*	9 - 12 g
Suan Zao Ren	*Ziziphus*	6 - 9 g
Bai Zi Ren	*Biota*	6 - 9 g
Fu Shen	*Poria*	6 - 9 g
Chen Xiang	*Aquilaria*	6 - 9 g
Xi Jiao	*Rhinoceros*	1 - 3 g

LIVER WIND

- tremors, tics, convulsions, high fever
- hemiplegia, deviation of mouth or eye
- aphasia, numbness

T deviated, pale or red

P wiry, choppy

Liver wind due to Liver yin deficiency causing spasms and twitches.

T dark red, scanty yellow coat

P thin, wiry, rapid

☞ E Jiao - Equus should be added to the strained tea. Bie Jia - Amyda, Mu Li - Ostrea, and Gui Ban - Chinemys should all be crushed or powdered, and cooked 45 minutes prior to the other herbs. The egg-yolks are boiled hard, then made into a soft mass and mixed into the tea.

DA DING FENG ZHU

Major Arrest Wind Pearl

Ji Zi Huang	*Egg Yolk*	2
Wu Wei Zi	*Schisandra*	6 - 9 g
E Jiao	*Equus*	6 - 9 g
Bai Shao Yao	*Paeonia*	9 - 15 g
Mai Men Dong	*Ophiopogon*	9 - 15 g
Huo Ma Ren	*Cannabis*	3 - 6 g
Sheng Di Huang	*Rehmannia*	9 - 15 g
Bie Jia	*Amyda*	6 - 12 g
Gui Ban	*Chinemys*	6 - 12 g
Mu Li	*Ostrea*	6 - 12 g
Gan Cao	*Glycyrrhiza*	6 - 12 g

Liver wind and phlegm causing seizures, especially in children or from emotional upset. There may be loss of consciousness.

T quivery, thick sticky white coat

P slippery, wiry

☞ Form 6 g pills out of the powdered herbs with the liquid made from the herbs listed in brackets. Adults take one pill in the morning and one in the evening.

✘ Do not use during pregnancy. Zhu Sha - Cinnabaris is toxic and should only be used short-term.

DING XIAN WAN

Arrest Seizures Pill

Tian Ma	*Gastrodia*	20 - 30 g
Jiang Ban Xia	*Pinellia*	20 - 30 g
Dan Nan Xing	*Arisaema*	12 - 15 g
Chuan Bei Mu	*Fritillaria*	20 - 30 g
Fu Shen	*Poria*	20 - 30 g
Fu Ling	*Poria*	20 - 30 g
Jiang Can	*Bombyx*	12 - 15 g
Shi Chang Pu	*Acorus*	12 - 15 g
Deng Xin Cao	*Juncus*	12 - 15 g
Quan Xie	*Buthus*	12 - 15 g
Dan Shen	*Salvia*	40 - 60 g
Mai Men Dong	*Ophiopogon*	40 - 60 g
Hu Po	*Succinum*	12 - 15 g
Yuan Zhi	*Polygala*	15 - 20 g
Chen Pi	*Citrus*	15 - 20 g
Zhu Sha	*Cinnabaris*	9 g
[Gan Cao	*Glycyrrhiza*	120 g]
[Zhu Li	*Bambusa*	100 ml]
[Sheng Jiang Zhi	*Zingiber juice*	50 ml]

Blood/yin deficiency giving rise to wind. Symptoms include twitches, or rigidity in the extremities.

T red, scanty yellow coat

P thin, rapid

☞ The egg yolks and E Jiao - Equus should be added to the strained tea.

E JIAO JI ZI HUANG TANG

Ass-Hide Gelatin and Egg Yolk Decoction

E Jiao	*Equus*	6 - 9 g
Ji Zi Huang	*Egg Yolks*	2
Gou Teng	*Uncaria*	6 - 9 g
Mu Li	*Ostrea*	9 - 12 g
Shi Jue Ming	*Haliotis*	12 - 15 g
Bai Shao Yao	*Paeonia*	6 - 9 g
Sheng Di Huang	*Rehmannia*	9 - 12 g
Luo Shi Teng	*Trachelospermum*	6 - 9 g
Fu Shen	*Poria*	9 - 12 g
Zhi Gan Cao	*Glycyrrhiza*	3 g

Acute childhood convulsions due to severe heat with underlying qi deficiency causing wind. Symptoms include the eyes turning upward, drooling, fever, or rigidity in the jaw.

T red, yellow coat

P rapid, wiry

☞ Ling Yang Jiao - Saiga powder should be added to the strained tea.

GOU TENG YIN

Uncaria Decoction

Extract Formula Name: Gambir Formula

Gou Teng	*Uncaria*	9 - 12 g
Quan Xie	*Buthus*	.9 g
Ren Shen	*Panax*	3 - 6 g
Ling Yang Jiao	*Saiga*	0.5 g
Tian Ma	*Gastrodia*	6 - 9 g
Gan Cao	*Glycyrrhiza*	1 - 3 g

Liver

Blood deficiency giving rise to internal wind which then leads to tendon or muscle spasms, itchy skin rashes, or blurry vision.

T pale, quivery

P weak, maybe superficial

GUI XIONG SI WU TANG

Altered Four-Substance Decoction

Shu Di Huang	*Rehmannia*	9 - 15 g
Chuan Xiong	*Ligusticum*	3 - 9 g
Bai Shao Yao	*Paeonia*	6 - 9 g
Dang Gui	*Angelica*	6 - 9 g
Fang Feng	*Ledebouriella*	9 - 15 g
Bai Zhu	*Atractylodes*	6 - 9 g
Huai Niu Xi	*Achyranthes*	6 - 12 g
Tian Men Dong	*Asparagus*	9 - 12 g

Liver yin deficiency with yang/wind rising causing palpitations, hypertension, or restlessness.

T red, thin yellow coat

P thin, rapid, slightly wiry

JIAN LING TANG

Construct Roof Tiles Decoction

Huai Niu Xi	*Achyranthes*	30 g
Shan Yao	*Dioscorea*	30 g
Long Gu	*Os Draconis*	18 g
Mu Li	*Ostrea*	18 g
Dai Zhi Shi	*Haematitum*	24 g
Sheng Di Huang	*Rehmannia*	18 g
Bai Zi Ren	*Biota*	12 g
Bai Shao Yao	*Paeonia*	12 g

Liver wind due to Liver fire causing hypertension, twitches, or headaches.

T dark red, raw, dry

P rapid, wiry

☞ Ling Yang Jiao - Saiga should be cooked one hour prior to adding the other herbs.

LING JIAO GOU TENG TANG

Antelope Horn and Uncaria Decoction

Extract Formula Name: Antelope Horn and Uncaria Combination

Ling Yang Jiao	*Saiga*	3 - 6 g
Sang Ye	*Morus*	6 - 9 g
Sheng Di Huang	*Rehmannia*	9 - 15 g
Zhu Ru	*Bambusa*	9 - 15 g
Bai Shao Yao	*Paeonia*	6 - 9 g
Gou Teng	*Uncaria*	6 - 9 g
Chuan Bei Mu	*Fritillaria*	6 - 12 g
Ju Hua	*Chrysanthemum*	6 - 9 g
Fu Shen	*Poria*	6 - 9 g
Gan Cao	*Glycyrrhiza*	3 - 6 g

Liver wind or yang rising due to yin or blood deficiency. Symptoms include spasms, vertigo, or heat in the palms, soles, and chest.

T dark red, dry, or geographic

P thin, rapid, wiry

☞ E Jiao - Equus should be dissoved at the end into the strained tea.

✘ Caution during pregnancy.

SAN JIA FU MAI TANG

Three-Shell Decoction to Restore the Pulse

Zhi Gan Cao	*Glycyrrhiza*	9 - 15 g
Bai Shao Yao	*Paeonia*	9 - 15 g
Sheng Di Huang	*Rehmannia*	9 - 15 g
E Jiao	*Equus*	6 - 9 g
Bie Jia	*Amyda*	9 - 20 g
Gui Ban	*Chinemys*	15 - 30 g
Huo Ma Ren	*Cannabis*	6 - 9 g
Mu Li	*Ostrea*	9 - 15 g
Mai Men Dong	*Ophiopogon*	9 - 15 g

Liver yin deficiency with yang or wind rising causing headaches, hypertension, tinnitus, or dizziness.

T red

P thin, rapid, wiry

TIAN MA GOU TENG YIN

Gastrodia and Uncaria Decoction

Extract Formula Name: Gastrodia and Uncaria Combination

Tian Ma	*Gastrodia*	9 - 12 g
Gou Teng	*Uncaria*	9 - 15 g
Chuan Niu Xi	*Cyathula*	9 - 12 g
Huang Qin	*Scutellaria*	6 - 9 g
Shi Jue Ming	*Haliotis*	15 - 25 g
Zhi Zi	*Gardenia*	3 - 6 g
Yi Mu Cao	*Leonurus*	6 - 12 g
Ye Jiao Teng	*Polygonum*	9 - 20 g
Du Zhong	*Eucommia*	6 - 12 g
Sang Ji Sheng	*Loranthus*	6 - 20 g
Fu Shen	*Poria*	6 - 12 g

Liver wind or external wind with phlegm accumulation in the channels causing stroke, aphasia, cerebral hemorrhage, or numbness; or cold attacking the chest and axillae causing severe localized pain in the flanks.

T sticky white coat

P slippery or wiry

WU YAO SHUN QI SAN

Lindera Powder to Smooth the Flow of Qi

Extract Formula Name: Lindera Formula

Wu Yao	*Lindera*	9 - 15 g
Chen Pi	*Citrus*	9 - 15 g
Ma Huang	*Ephedra*	6 - 9 g
Bai Zhi	*Angelica*	3 - 9 g
Zhi Ke	*Citrus*	3 - 6 g
Jiang Can	*Bombyx*	3 g
Jie Geng	*Platycodon*	3 g
Chuan Xiong	*Ligusticum*	3 - 9 g
Pao Jiang	*Zingiber*	3 - 6 g
Gan Cao	*Glycyrrhiza*	3 - 6 g
[Da Zao	*Ziziphus*	3 - 8 pc]
[Sheng Jiang	*Zingiber*	3 - 6 g]

Liver heat/fire giving rise to wind causing itchy rash, hypertension, red eyes, high fever, or easily angered.

T red, dry, thin yellow coat

P rapid, wiry, or flooding

XIE QING WAN

Drain the Green Pill

Long Dan Cao	*Gentiana*	6-9 g
Zhi Zi	*Gardenia*	6-9 g
Chuan Xiong	*Ligusticum*	6-9 g
Qiang Huo	*Notopterygium*	6-9 g
Fang Feng	*Ledebouriella*	6-9 g
Dang Gui	*Angelica*	6-9 g
Da Huang	*Rheum*	6-9 g

External wind attacks the channels with pre-existing qi/Blood deficiency; or Liver wind with heat causing flaccid hemiplegia, aphasia, or mild fever. There may also be slight mental confusion.

T sticky yellow coat

P wiry, forceful, or rapid, slippery

XU MING TANG

Prolong Life Decoction

Extract Formula Name: Ma-Huang and Ginseng Combination

Gui Zhi	*Cinnamomum*	6-9 g
Ma Huang	*Ephedra*	6-9 g
Chuan Xiong	*Ligusticum*	3-6 g
Xing Ren	*Prunus*	6-9 g
Shi Gao	*Gypsum*	6-9 g
Ren Shen	*Panax*	6-9 g
Dang Gui	*Angelica*	6-9 g
Gan Jiang	*Zingiber*	6-9 g
Gan Cao	*Glycyrrhiza*	3-9 g

Liver wind due to yang rising with underlying Kidney and Liver yin deficiency: headache, dizziness, restlessness, or belching due to Liver/Stomach disharmony, low-pitched tinnitus, wind stroke, or hypertension.

T red or light purple, trembling, yellow coat

P forceful, wiry

✪ Major Formula

ZHEN GAN XI FENG TANG

Sedate the Liver and Extinguish Wind Decoction

Extract Formula Name: Dragon Bone and Two Shells Combination

Dai Zhe Shi	*Haematitum*	15 - 30 g
Huai Niu Xi	*Achyranthes*	15 - 30 g
Xuan Shen	*Scrophularia*	12 - 15 g
Bai Shao Yao-	*Paeonia*	9 - 15 g
Tian Men Dong	*Asparagus*	9 - 15 g
Gui Ban	*Chinemys*	9 - 15 g
Long Gu	*Os Draconis*	9 - 15 g
Mu Li	*Ostrea*	9 - 15 g
Chuan Lian Zi	*Melia*	6 - 9 g
Mai Ya	*Hordeum*	6 - 9 g
Yin Chen Hao	*Artemisia*	6 - 9 g
Gan Cao	*Glycyrrhiza*	3 - 6 g

Liver wind due to fire in the pericardium, or phlegm heat obstructing the orifice causing stroke, high fever, irritability, loss of consciousness, or a raspy voice.

T dark red, sticky yellow grey coat

P rapid, slippery

☞ Herbs should be ground separately, then sifted together. Make into 3 g pills. Adults take one pill 2 - 3 times a day. Xi Jiao - Rhinoceros should be substituted with Shui Niu Jiao - Bubalus or 50 - 60 g of Bai Mao Gen - Imperata.

✘ Do not use during pregnancy. Zhu Sha - Cinnabaris is toxic and should not be used over a prolonged period of time.

ZHI BAO DAN

Greatest Treasure Special Pill

Extract Formula Name: Rhinoceros and Succinum Formula

Xi Jiao	*Rhinoceros*	20 - 30 g
Niu Huang	*Bos*	12 - 15 g
She Xlang	*Moschus*	0.1 - 0.3 g
Dai Mao	*Eretmochelydis*	20 - 30 g
An Xi Xiang	*Styrax*	30 - 45 g
Hu Po	*Succinum*	20 - 30 g
Xiong Huang	*Realgar*	20 - 30 g
Zhu Sha	*Cinnabaris*	20 - 30 g
Bing Pian	*Dryobalanops*	0.1 - 0.3 g

Severe heat causing Liver wind. This causes muscle twitches, convulsions, or spasms.

T red, deviated, yellow coat

P forceful

✘ Do not use during pregnancy. The formula is toxic and should not be taken over a prolonged period of time.

ZHI JING SAN

Stop Spasms Powder

Wu Gong	*Scolopendra*	10 g
Quan Xie	*Buthus*	10 g

GALLBLADDER DISHARMONIES

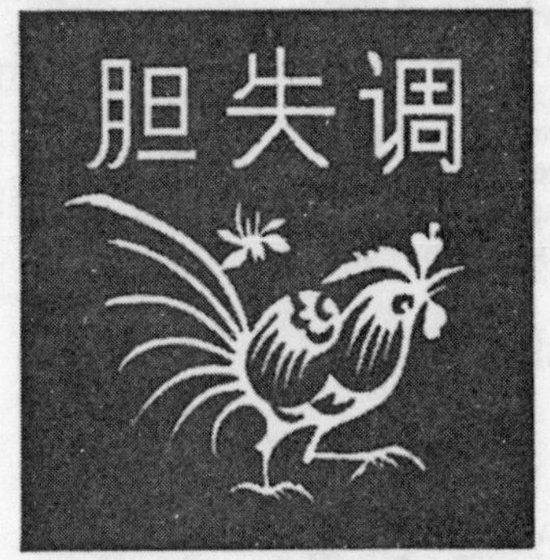

DAMP HEAT IN THE GALLBLADDER

- costal pain and distention
- gallstones
- bitter taste
- nausea and vomiting
- fever and thirst

T thick sticky yellow coat

P wiry, slippery

1. Yangming organ disease (pi man zao shi - glomus, fullness, dryness, excess) causing masses in the abdomen; or yang jaundice with gallstones where the heat is greater than damp. 2. Fire and toxin are severe, so the water escapes causing watery dysentery with odorous stools, bowel incontinence while in a coma; mania, or convulsions with high fever.

T bright red, dry yellow or black coat

P rapid, forceful

☞ Da Huang - Rheum should be added during the last 3 - 5 minutes of the decoction process, and Mang Xiao - Mirabilite should be added into the strained tea.

✘ Do not use during pregnancy. The formula is very cold and can cause diarrhea and vomiting.

DA CHENG QI TANG

Major Order the Qi Decoction

Extract Formula Name: Major Rhubarb Combination

Da Huang	*Rheum*	6 - 12 g
Mang Xiao	*Mirabilitum*	6 - 12 g
Zhi Shi	*Citrus*	6 - 9 g
Hou Po	*Magnolia*	6 - 15 g

Damp heat with qi stagnation and pain causing gallstones.

T red, sticky yellow coat

P slippery, wiry, rapid

DAN DAO PAI SHI TANG

Biliary Lithagogue Decoction

Jin Qian Cao	*Lysimachia*	6 - 9 g
Yu Jin	*Curcuma*	6 - 9 g
Yin Chen Hao	*Artemisia*	6 - 9 g
Mu Xiang	*Saussurea*	3 - 6 g
Zhi Ke	*Citrus*	3 - 6 g
Da Huang	*Rheum*	6 - 9 g

Yang jaundice from damp heat lodged in the shaoyang level; or damp heat in the Gallbladder causing alternating fever and chills, bitter taste, or malaria.

T red, thick sticky yellow coat

P slippery, wiry, rapid

☞ Bi Yu San - Green Jade Powder consists of: Hua Shi - Talcum, 3 - 6 g; Gan Cao - Glycyrrhiza, 3 - 6 g; and Qing Dai - Indigo, 9 - 12 g. All three ingredients should be cooked separately in a cheesecloth, then decocted with the rest of the herbs.

✪ Major Formula

HAO QIN QING DAN TANG

Artemisia Annua and Scutellaria Decoction to Clear the Gallbladder

Qing Hao	*Artemisia*	6 g
Zhu Ru	*Bambusa*	9 g
Huang Qin	*Scutellaria*	6 g
Zhi Ke	*Citrus*	5 g
Chi Fu Ling	*Poria*	9 g
Ban Xia	*Pinellia*	5 g
Chen Pi	*Citrus*	5 g
Bi Yu San	*Green Jade Powder*	9 g

Middle jiao phlegm heat with Gallbladder heat causing severe restlessness or bitter taste.

T red, sticky yellow coat

P rapid, slippery

HUANG LIAN WEN DAN TANG

Coptis Decoction to Warm the Gallbladder

Ban Xia	*Pinellia*	6 - 9 g
Chen Pi	*Citrus*	3 - 6 g
Fu Ling	*Poria*	6 - 9 g
Zhi Ke	*Citrus*	3 - 6 g
Zhu Ru	*Bambusa*	3 - 9 g
Huang Lian	*Coptis*	3 - 6 g
Sheng Jiang	*Zingiber*	3 - 6 g
Da Zao	*Ziziphus*	3 - 4 pc
Gan Cao	*Glycyrrhiza*	3 - 6 g

Wind cold causes facial edema and scanty urination. This formula is also useful for jaundice accompanied by taiyang symptoms.

T thin white coat

P superficial, tight

MA HUANG LIAN QIAO CHI XIAO DOU TANG

Ephedra, Forsythia, and Aduki Bean Decoction

Ma Huang	*Ephedra*	3 - 9 g
Lian Qiao	*Forsythia*	6 - 9 g
Chi Xiao Dou	*Phaseolus*	6 - 9 g
Sang Bai Pi	*Morus*	6 - 9 g
Xing Ren	*Prunus*	6 - 9 g
Sheng Jiang	*Zingiber*	3 - 6 g
Da Zao	*Ziziphus*	3 - 4 pc
Gan Cao	*Glycyrrhiza*	3 - 6 g

Excess fire cholecystitis with Liver qi and damp stagnation causing alternating fever and chills or severe hypochondriac pain.

T deep red, sticky yellow coat

P wiry, slippery, rapid, or flooding

☞ Mang Xiao - Mirabilitum should be dissolved into the strained tea. Da Huang - Rheum should be added within the last 3 - 5 minutes of the decoction process.

✗ Do not use during pregnancy

QING DAN XIE HUO TANG

Clear the Gallbladder and Drain Fire Decoction

Chai Hu	*Bupleurum*	9 - 15 g
Ban Xia	*Pinellia*	6 - 9 g
Yin Chen Hao	*Artemisia*	15 - 25 g
Long Dan Cao	*Gentiana*	6 - 9 g
Yu Jin	*Curcuma*	6 - 9 g
Da Huang	*Rheum*	6 - 9 g
Huang Qin	*Scutellaria*	6 - 15 g
Zhi Zi	*Gardenia*	6 - 9 g
Mang Xiao	*Mirabilitum*	6 - 9 g
Mu Xiang	*Saussurea*	3 - 6 g

Liver and Stomach imbalance with phlegm accumulation and Gallbladder heat. Symptoms include fullness in the chest, bitter taste, thirst without desire to drink, or vomiting. In severe cases, mental confusion or a rattly throat may be seen.

T red, sticky yellow coat

P rapid, slippery and/or wiry

WEN DAN TANG

Warm the Gallbladder Decoction

Extract Formula Name: Hoelen and Bamboo Combination

Ban Xia	*Pinellia*	6 - 9 g
Chen Pi	*Citrus*	9 - 12 g
Fu Ling	*Poria*	6 - 12 g
Zhi Shi	*Citrus*	3 - 6 g
Zhu Ru	*Bambusa*	6 g
Sheng Jiang	*Zingiber*	3 - 6 g
Gan Cao	*Glycyrrhiza*	3 - 6 g
Da Zao	*Ziziphus*	2 pc

Whole body yang jaundice due to damp heat in the Liver and Gallbladder.

T Red, thick sticky yellow coat

P slippery, rapid, forceful

✗ Do not use during pregnancy.

YIN CHEN HAO TANG

Artemisia Yinchenhao Decoction

Extract Formula Name: Capillaris Combination

Yin Chen Hao	*Artemisia*	15 - 30 g
Da Huang	*Rheum*	6 - 9 g
Zhi Zi	*Gardenia*	6 - 9 g

Damp heat accumulation in the middle jiao (Liver/Gallbladder) causing yang jaundice, dysurea, or hepatitis with mild fever.

T slightly red, thick sticky coat

P slippery, slightly rapid

YIN CHEN WU LING SAN

Artemisia Yinchenhao and Five-Ingredient Powder with Poria

Extract Formula Name: Capillaris and Hoelen Five Formula

Yin Chen Hao	*Artemisia*	10 - 20 g
Fu Ling	*Poria*	6 - 12 g
Zhu Ling	*Polyporus*	6 - 9 g
Bai Zhu	*Atractylodes*	3 - 9 g
Ze Xie	*Alisma*	6 - 9 g
Gui Zhi	*Cinnamomum*	3 - 9 g

Yang jaundice due to damp heat in the interior. The heat is greater than the damp.

T red, sticky yellow coat

P slippery, rapid

ZHI ZI BAI PI TANG

Gardenia and Phellodendron Decoction

Extract Formula Name: Gardenia and Phellodendron Combination

Zhi Zi	*Gardenia*	9 - 15 g
Huang Bai	*Phellodendron*	6 - 9 g
Zhi Gan Cao	*Glycyrrhiza*	3 - 6 g

Damp heat accumulation in the middle jiao. There is more damp than heat causing fullness in the abdomen, thirst without desire to drink, or immediate fullness upon eating or drinking. This formula is also useful for yang jaundice.

T red, thick sticky coat

P slippery, rapid

ZHONG JIAO XIAN BI TANG

Middle Jiao and Clear Damp Decoction

Xing Ren	*Prunus*	3 - 6 g
Yi Yi Ren	*Coix*	9 - 12 g
Hua Shi	*Talcum*	6 g
Dou Juan	*Glycine*	9 g
Zhi Zi	*Gardenia*	6 - 9 g
Lian Qiao	*Forsythia*	6 g
Ban Xia	*Pinellia*	6 - 9 g
Han Fang Ji	*Stephania*	6 - 9 g
Can Sha	*Bombyx*	3 - 6 g
Shan Zha	*Crataegus*	3 - 9 g
Bian Dou	*Dolichos*	6 - 9 g

DEFICIENCY IN THE GALLBLADDER

- lack of initiative
- timidity
- startled easily
- sighing

T pale
P weak

This formula treats insomnia due to Heart and Gallbladder qi deficiency. This is commonly seen in children causing them to appear timid and scared of everything, fear ghosts and burglars, or not want to sleep alone. They sweat easily, especially in the hands and soles.

T pale or normal color, slightly swollen

P weak, thready, deep

✪ Major Formula

AN SHEN DING ZHI TANG

Calm Spirit and Stop Fear Decoction

Ren Shen	*Panax*	9 - 12 g
Fu Ling	*Poria*	6 - 9 g
Fu Shen	*Poria*	6 - 9 g
Shi Chang Pu	*Acorus*	3 - 9 g
Long Gu	*Os Draconis*	6 - 9 g
Yuan Zhi	*Polygala*	6 - 9 g

Heart/Gallbladder qi deficiency with edema in the extremities, tight chest, palpitations, anxiety, or timidity.

T pale

P weak

SHI WEI WEN DAN TANG

Ten-Ingredient Decoction to Warm the Gallbladder

Ban Xia	*Pinellia*	6 - 9 g
Chen Pi	*Citrus*	3 - 6 g
Zhi Shi	*Citrus*	6 g
Fu Ling	*Poria*	6 g
Ren Shen	*Panax*	3 - 6 g
Suan Zao Ren	*Ziziphus*	3 - 6 g
Shu Di Huang	*Rehmannia*	3 - 9 g
Wu Wei Zi	*Schisandra*	3 - 6 g
Yuan Zhi	*Polygala*	3 - 6 g
Zhi Gan Cao	*Glycyrrhiza*	3 g
Da Zao	*Ziziphus*	2 pc
Sheng Jiang	*Zingiber*	5 pc

KIDNEY DISHARMONIES

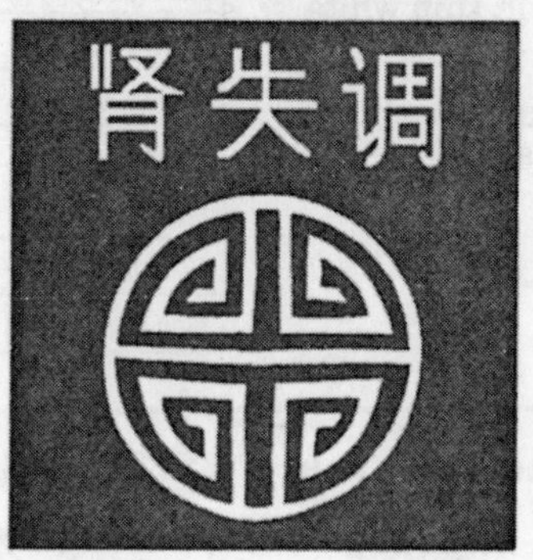

Kidney

KIDNEY QI DEFICIENCY

- sore and weak lower back and knees
- urinary incontinence, frequency, or dribbling
- spermatorrhea, or chronic leukorrhea

T pale, swollen

P deep, weak

Kidney qi/yin deficiency causing menorrhagia. Other symptoms may include low back pain, frequent urination, or weakness in the knees.

T red or normal color, thin white coat

P weak, especially in both chi (third) positions, slightly rapid

BAO YIN JIAN

Augment Yin Decoction

Huang Qin	*Scutellaria*	9 - 12 g
Huang Bai	*Phellodendron*	9 - 12 g
Sheng Di Huang	*Rehmannia*	9 - 15 g
Shu Di Huang	*Rehmannia*	9 - 15 g
Shan Yao	*Dioscorea*	6 - 9 g
Bai Shao Yao	*Paeonia*	6 - 12 g
Xu Duan	*Dipsacus*	6 - 9 g
Gan Cao	*Glycyrrhiza*	3 - 6 g

Kidney qi deficiency with cold and damp leading to frequent, or cloudy, painful urination.

T pale

P weak, or slippery

BEI XIE FEN QIN YIN I

Discorea Hypoglauca Decoction to Separate the Clear

Extract Formula Name: Tokoro Combination

Bei Xie	*Dioscorea*	6 - 12 g
Wu Yao	*Lindera*	6 - 9 g
Shi Chang Pu	*Acorus*	6 - 9 g
Yi Zhi Ren	*Alpinia*	6 - 9 g

Kidney/Lung qi/yin deficiency with wheezing, shortness of breath, or chronic cough. This formula is also known as 'Qi Wu Du Qi Wan'.

T red, slight coat

P thin, rapid

DU QI WAN

Capital Qi Pill

Extract Formula Name: Rehmannia and Schizandra Formula

Shan Zhu Yu	*Cornus*	6 - 9 g
Shan Yao	*Dioscorea*	6 - 9 g
Sheng Di Huang	*Rehmannia*	9 - 12 g
Fu Ling	*Poria*	6 - 9 g
Mu Dan Pi	*Paeonia*	6 - 9 g
Ze Xie	*Alisma*	6 - 9 g
Wu Wei Zi	*Schisandra*	6 - 9 g

Kidney qi and yang deficiency causing edema which manifests mostly in the superficial and muscle layers.

T pale, swollen, sticky white coat

P weak, deep, slippery

FANG JI FU LING TANG

Stephania and Poria Decoction

Extract Formula Name: Stephania and Hoelen Combination

Han Fang Ji	*Stephania*	9 - 12 g
Fu Ling	*Poria*	9 - 18 g
Gui Zhi	*Cinnamomum*	9 - 12 g
Huang Qi	*Astragalus*	9 - 12 g
Gan Cao	*Glycyrrhiza*	3 - 6 g

Turbid leukorrhea due to Kidney qi/yang deficiency. The Kidneys are unable to astringe.

T pale, swollen, slight teeth-marks, wet, thin white coat

P minute or frail

FEN QING YIN

Separate Pure from Impure Powder

Bei Xie	*Dioscorea*	6 - 9 g
Yi Yi Ren	*Coix*	12 - 15 g
Wu Yao	*Lindera*	6 - 9 g
Shi Chang Pu	*Acorus*	6 - 9 g
Fu Ling	*Poria*	6 - 9 g
Chen Pi	*Citrus*	3 - 6 g
Gan Cao	*Glycyrrhiza*	3 - 6 g

Spleen/Kidney qi deficiency resulting in spermatorrhea, no appetite, and weakness.

T pale, thin white coat

P deep, weak

✪ Major Formula

FU TU DAN

Poria and Cuscuta Special Pill

Extract Formula Name: Hoelen and Cuscuta Formula

Tu Si Zi	*Cuscuta*	6 - 9 g
Fu Ling	*Poria*	6 - 9 g
Wu Wei Zi	*Schisandra*	6 - 9 g
Lian Zi	*Nelumbo*	6 - 9 g
Shan Yao	*Dioscorea*	6 - 9 g

Kidney qi/yin deficiency causing irregular periods, leukorrhea, or a bearing-down sensation.

T red, thin white coat

P weak, especially the chi (third) positions

GU YIN JIAN

Stabilize the Yin Decoction

Shu Di Huang	*Rehmannia*	6 - 12 g
Shan Yao	*Dioscorea*	6 - 9 g
Wu Wei Zi	*Schisandra*	6 - 9 g
Shan Zhu Yu	*Cornus*	6 - 9 g
Tu Si Zi	*Cuscuta*	6 - 9 g
Ren Shen	*Panax*	6 - 9 g
Yuan Zhi	*Polygala*	3 g
Zhi Gan Cao	*Glycyrrhiza*	3 - 6 g

Kidney qi deficiency with Kidney/Liver yin deficiency causing amenorrhea, or back and knee pain.

T pale or red, thin white or scanty coat

P weak, maybe thin especially in the left chi (third) position

GUI SHEN TANG

Comeback Kidney Decoction

Shu Di Huang	*Rehmannia*	6 - 15 g
Shan Yao	*Dioscorea*	9 - 15 g
Shan Zhu Yu	*Cornus*	9 - 12 g
Gou Qi Zi	*Lycium*	9 - 15 g
Dang Gui	*Angelica*	9 - 12 g
Du Zhong	*Eucommia*	6 - 12 g
Fu Ling	*Poria*	6 - 12 g
Tu Si Zi	*Cuscuta*	9 - 12 g

Kidney qi and yang deficiency causing low back pain, coldness in the back, urinary difficulties, or pedal edema.

T pale, swollen, thin white coat

P frail

JIN GUI SHEN QI WAN

Kidney Qi Pill from the Golden Cabinet

Extract Formula Name: Rehmannia Eight Formula

Shu Di Huang	*Rehmannia*	24 g
Shan Zhu Yu	*Cornus*	12 g
Shan Yao	*Dioscorea*	12 g
Mu Dan Pi	*Paeonia*	9 g
Ze Xie	*Alisma*	9 g
Fu Ling	*Poria*	9 g
Rou Gui	*Cinnamomum*	3 g
Fu Zi	*Aconitum*	3 g

Kidney qi deficiency causing white leukorrhea.

T thin white coat

P weak

NEI BU WAN

Internal Tonification Pill

Lu Rong	*Cervus*	1 - 3 g
Rou Cong Rong	*Cistanche*	6 - 9 g
Tu Si Zi	*Cuscuta*	6 - 9 g
Huang Qi	*Astralagus*	6 -15 g
Rou Gui	*Cinnamomum*	6 - 9 g
Fu Zi	*Aconitum*	3 - 6 g
Sha Yuan Ji Li	*Astragalus*	6 - 9 g
Zi Wan	*Aster*	6 - 9 g
Sang Piao Xiao	*Paratenodera*	6 - 9 g

Kidney

Liver blood/yin deficiency with Kidney qi deficiency causing early greying, hairloss, poor teeth, and seminal emissions.

T pale

P thin, weak

QI BAO MEI RAN DAN

Seven-Treasure Special Pill for Beautiful Whiskers

He Shou Wu	*Polygonum*	6 - 9 g
Huai Niu Xi	*Achyranthes*	6 - 12 g
Fu Ling	*Poria*	6 - 9 g
Tu Si Zi	*Cuscuta*	6 - 9 g
Gou Qi Zi	*Lycium*	6 - 9 g
Bu Gu Zhi	*Psoralea*	6 - 9 g
Dang Gui	*Angelica*	6 - 9 g

Lung/Kidney qi deficiency causing cough/asthma with wheezing. There are slightly more cold symptoms.

T pale, thin sticky white coat

P weak or frail

REN SHEN HU TAO TANG

Ginseng and Walnut Decoction

Extract Formula Name: Ginseng and Walnut Combination

Ren Shen	*Panax*	6 - 9 g
Hu Tao Ren	*Juglans*	3 - 6 pc
Sheng Jiang	*Zingiber*	3 - 6 pc
Da Zao	*Ziziphus*	3 pc

Heart/Kidney qi/yin deficiency causing incontinence, spermatorrhea, frequent urination, and forgetfulness.

T pale or red

P weak, thin

SANG PIAO XIAO SAN

Mantis Egg-Case Powder

Extract Formula Name: Mantis Formula

Sang Piao Xiao	*Paratenodera*	9 - 12 g
Long Gu	*Os Draconis*	12 - 25 g
Fu Shen	*Poria*	9 - 12 g
Ren Shen	*Panax*	9 - 12 g
Shi Chang Pu	*Acorus*	6 - 9 g
Dang Gui	*Angelica*	6 - 9 g
Gui Ban	*Chinemys*	9 - 15 g
Yuan Zhi	*Polygala*	9 - 15 g

Lung/Kidney qi deficiency causing cough, asthma, and dyspnea.

T pale

P slow, weak

SHEN JIE SAN

Ginseng and Gecko Powder

Ren Shen	*Panax*	9 - 12 g
Ge Jie	*Gekko*	1 pair

Spleen/Kidney qi and yang deficiency causing edema which manifests mostly in the lower body. Other symptoms include cold limbs, poor appetite, decreased urination, or heaviness.

T pale, sticky coat

P deep, slow, maybe thin

SHI PI YIN

Bolster the Spleen Decoction

Extract Formula Name: Magnolia and Atractylodes Combination

Fu Zi	*Aconitum*	6 - 9 g
Bai Zhu	*Atractylodes*	6 - 9 g
Mu Gua	*Chaenomeles*	6 - 9 g
Hou Po	*Magnolia*	6 - 12 g
Gan Jiang	*Zingiber*	6 - 9 g
Mu Xiang	*Saussurea*	6 - 9 g
Fu Ling	*Poria*	6 - 9 g
Da Fu Pi	*Areca*	3 - 6 g
Cao Guo	*Amomum*	3 - 6 g
Zhi Gan Cao	*Glycyrrhiza*	3 - 6 g
[Da Zao	*Ziziphus*	1 - 3 pc]
[Sheng Jiang	*Zingiber*	3 - 6 g]

Kidney qi deficiency causing a restless fetus with spotting, threatened miscarriage, or frequent urination.

T pale

P frail

☞ E Jiao - Equus should be dissolved in water and used to form the other herbs into 6 g pills.

SHOU TAI WAN

Fetus Longevity Pill

Loranthus and Cuscuta Combination

E Jiao	*Equus*	30
Sang Ji Sheng	*Loranthus*	30 g
Tu Si Zi	*Cuscuta*	60 g
Xu Duan	*Dipsacus*	30 g

Lung phlegm damp with underlying Kidney qi deficiency causing wheezing with profuse phlegm.

T sticky white coat

P weak, slippery

SU ZI JIANG QI TANG

Perilla Fruit Decoction for Directing Qi Downward

Extract Formula Name: Perilla Fruit Combination

Zhi Gan Cao	*Glycyrrhiza*	6 g
Ban Xia	*Pinellia*	6 - 9 g
Zi Su Zi	*Perilla*	6 - 12 g
Dang Gui	*Angelica*	6 - 9 g
Hou Po	*Magnolia*	6 - 12 g
Qian Hu	*Peucedanum*	6 - 9 g
Rou Gui	*Cinnamomum*	3 g
[Sheng Jiang	*Zingiber*	1 - 3 g]
[Zi Su Ye	*Perilla*	3 - 6 g]
[Da Zao	*Ziziphus*	3 g]

Kidney qi/yang deficiency with enuresis or frequent, clear urination.

T pale, swollen, teethmarks, white coat

P minute

SUO QUAN WAN

Shut the Sluice Pill

Yi Zhi Ren	*Alpinia*	6 - 15 g
Shan Yao	*Dioscorea*	9 - 15 g
Wu Yao	*Lindera*	6 - 9 g

Chronic lin-syndrome due to Kidney qi deficiency causing urinary frequency with turbidity, incontinence, or enuresis.

T pale or normal color, thin white or yellowish coat

P weak, especially in the chi (third) positions

WU BI SHAN YAO WAN

Dioscorea Pill

Shu Di Huang	*Rehmannia*	12 - 15 g
Shan Yao	*Dioscorea*	12 - 15 g
Shan Zhu Yu	*Cornus*	6 - 9 g
Rou Cong Rong	*Cistanche*	6 - 9 g
Tu Si Zi	*Cuscuta*	6 - 9 g
Wu Wei Zi	*Schisandra*	6 - 12 g
Ze Xie	*Alisma*	6 - 9 g
Ba Ji Tian	*Morinda*	3 - 6 g
Du Zhong	*Eucommia*	9 - 12 g
Huai Niu Xi	*Achyranthes*	12 - 15 g
Fu Shen	*Poria*	9 - 12 g
Chi Shi Zhi	*Halloysitum Rubrum*	12 - 15 g

Kidney qi deficiency causing infertility, urinary frequency, or incontinence.

T pale or normal color, thin white coat

P weak

☞ For infertility and a stronger qi and blood tonifying effect add 'Dang Gui Bu Xue Tang - Dang Gui Decoction to Tonify the Blood' and 'Si Jun Zi Tang - Four-Gentlemen Decoction.'

WU ZI YAN ZONG WAN

Five-Seeds Normalizing Pill

Wu Wei Zi	*Schisandra*	6 - 12 g
Fu Pen Zi	*Rubus*	6 - 9 g
Tu Si Zi	*Cuscuta*	6 - 9 g
Che Qian Zi	*Plantago*	6 - 9 g
Gou Qi Zi	*Lycium*	6 - 12 g

Kidney qi deficiency leading to spermatorrhea, or white leukorrhea in women.

T pale or normal color, thin white coat

P weak

YI YUAN JIAN

Benefit the Source Decoction

Yuan Zhi	*Polygala*	3 g
Shan Yao	*Dioscorea*	6 g
Qian Shi	*Euryale*	6 g
Suan Zao Ren	*Ziziphus*	6 g
Bai Zhu	*Atractylodes*	4.5 g
Fu Ling	*Poria*	4.5 g
Ren Shen	*Panax*	3 - 6 g
Wu Wei Zi	*Schisandra*	14 pc
Jin Ying Zi	*Rosa*	6 g
Gan Cao	*Glycyrrhiza*	3 g

Infertility due to Kidney qi deficiency.

T normal color or pale, thin white coat

P weak, especially in both chi (third) positions

YU LIN WAN

Nourish Cute Animal Pill

Lu Jiao Shuang	*Cervus*	6 - 9 g
Tu Si Zi	*Cuscuta*	6 - 9 g
Du Zhong	*Eucommia*	6 - 12 g
Chuan Jiao	*Zanthoxylum*	3 - 6 g
Zi He Che	*Placenta Hominis*	3 - 9 g
Xiang Fu	*Cyperus*	6 - 9 g

KIDNEY YANG DEFICIENCY

- cold and sore knees and lower back
- frequent, clear and profuse or scanty urination
- infertility, impotence

T pale, swollen, teethmarks, moist

P deep, weak

Cold accumulation or yang deficiency in the abdomen leading to constipation with cramping pain. The qi stagnates and heats up which can cause a mild fever. Other symptoms include cold extremities and chills.

T normal or pale, white coat

P wiry or tight, deep

☞ Fu Zi - Aconitum should be powdered. Da Huang - Rheum should be added during the last 3 - 5 minutes of the decoction process.

✘ Do not use during pregnancy.

DA HUANG FU ZI TANG

Rhubarb and Aconite Decoction

Extract Formula Name: Rhubarb and Aconite Combination

Da Huang	*Rheum*	6 - 9 g
Fu Zi	*Aconitum*	6 g
Xi Xin	*Asarum*	3 - 6 g

Spleen/Kidney yang deficiency causing dawn diarrhea with middle jiao qi stagnation symptoms such as excruciating abdominal pain and severe fullness feelings.

T pale, swollen, teethmarks, light purple, white coat

P deep, weak, or slippery

DAN LIAO SI SHEN WAN

Four-Miracle Pill from the Tranquil Hut

Bu Gu Zhi	*Psoralea*	6 - 12 g
Xiao Hui Xiang	*Foeniculum*	3 - 9 g
Rou Dou Kou	*Myristica*	9 - 12 g
Mu Xiang	*Saussurea*	3 - 6 g

Bone bi-syndrome: wind cold damp with Kidney yang deficiency and yin and blood deficiency. Symptoms include chronic joint pain, cold knees, joint deformities, or stiffness or weakness in the joints.

T pale, thin white coat

P frail

DU HUO JI SHENG TANG

Angelica Pubescens and Sangjisheng Decoction

Extract Formula Name: Tuhuo and Loranthus Combination

Du Huo	*Angelica*	6 - 9 g
Sang Ji Sheng	*Loranthus*	6 - 12 g
Qin Jiao	*Gentiana*	6 - 9 g
Fang Feng	*Ledebouriella*	6 - 9 g
Dang Gui	*Angelica*	6 - 9 g
Rou Gui	*Cinnamomum*	6 g
Ren Shen	*Panax*	6 - 9 g
Huai Niu Xi	*Achyranthes*	6 - 9 g
Du Zhong	*Eucommia*	6 - 9 g
Sheng Di Huang	*Rehmannia*	6 - 9 g
Fu Ling	*Poria*	6 - 9 g
Chuan Xiong	*Ligusticum*	3 - 6 g
Bai Shao Yao	*Paeonia*	6 - 9 g
Xi Xin	*Asarum*	3 - 6 g
Gan Cao	*Glycyrrhiza*	3 - 6 g

Kidney yin and yang deficiency with fire causing menopause, hot flashes, or urinary frequency.

T red

P rapid or normal rate, thin

ER XIAN TANG

Two-Immortal Decoction

Extract Formula Name: Curculigo and Epimedium Combination

Yin Yang Huo	*Epimedium*	9 - 15 g
Xian Mao	*Curculigo*	9 - 15 g
Dang Gui	*Angelica*	6 - 9 g
Huang Bai	*Phellodendron*	6 - 9 g
Zhi Mu	*Anemarrhena*	6 - 9 g
Ba Ji Tian	*Morinda*	6 - 9 g

Kidney qi and yang deficiency causing edema which manifests mostly in the superficial and muscle layers.

T pale, swollen, sticky white coat

P weak, deep, slippery

FANG JI FU LING TANG

Stephania and Poria Decoction

Extract Formula Name: Stephania and Hoelen Combination

Han Fang Ji	*Stephania*	9 - 12 g
Fu Ling	*Poria*	9 - 18 g
Gui Zhi	*Cinnamomum*	9 - 12 g
Huang Qi	*Astragalus*	9 - 12 g
Gan Cao	*Glycyrrhiza*	3 - 6 g

Turbid leukorrhea due to Kidney qi/yang deficiency. The Kidneys are unable to astringe.

T pale, swollen, slight teeth-marks, wet, thin white coat

P minute or frail

FEN QING YIN

Separate Pure from Impure Powder

Bei Xie	*Dioscorea*	6 - 9 g
Yi Yi Ren	*Coix*	12 - 15 g
Wu Yao	*Lindera*	6 - 9 g
Shi Chang Pu	*Acorus*	6 - 9 g
Fu Ling	*Poria*	6 - 9 g
Chen Pi	*Citrus*	3 - 6 g
Gan Cao	*Glycyrrhiza*	3 - 6 g

Severe Kidney yang deficiency where the yang is unable to nourish the limbs leading to edema, and severe body aches with cold and damp symptoms: cold bi-syndrome.

T pale, moist white coat

P deep, minute, or choppy

FU ZI TANG

Prepared Aconite Decoction

Extract Formula Name: Aconite Combination

Fu Zi	*Aconitum*	9 - 15 g
Ren Shen	*Panax*	3 - 6 g
Fu Ling	*Poria*	9 - 12 g
Bai Zhu	*Atractylodes*	3 - 12 g
Bai Shao Yao	*Paeonia*	6 - 9 g

Spleen/Kidney yang deficiency causing watery diarrhea with undigested food, spasms in hands and feet, fatigue, and spontanous severe sweating.

T pale, swollen, teethmarks, wet, white coat

P minute

GU ZHEN TANG

Stabilize the True Decoction

Fu Zi	*Aconitum*	6 - 9 g
Ren Shen	*Panax*	6 - 9 g
Bai Zhu	*Atractylodes*	6 - 9 g
Fu Ling	*Poria*	6 - 9 g
Huang Qi	*Astragalus*	6 - 15 g
Shan Yao	*Dioscorea*	6 - 9 g
Rou Gui	*Cinnamomum*	3 - 9 g
Gan Cao	*Glycyrrhiza*	3 - 6 g
[Sheng Jiang	*Zingiber*	3 - 6 g]
[Da Zao	*Ziziphus*	1 - 2 pc]

Severe cold stagnation with Spleen/Kidney yang deficiency causing coldness in the face, cramping pain in the center, or dawn diarrhea.

T pale, purple, wet coat

P slow, tight

GUI FU LI ZHONG WAN

Cinnamon and Prepared Aconite Decoction to Regulate the Middle

Ren Shen	*Panax*	10 - 15 g
Bai Zhu	*Atractylodes*	6 - 9 g
Gan Jiang	*Zingiber*	6 - 9 g
Gan Cao	*Glycyrrhiza*	3 - 6 g
Fu Zi	*Aconitum*	3 - 6 g
Gui Zhi	*Cinnamomum*	3 - 9 g

Cold phlegm in the Lungs with underlying Kidney yang deficiency. This produces cough with clear watery fluids, or shortness of breath.

T pale, thick sticky white coat

P frail or slippery

GUI LING WU WEI GAN CAO TANG

Cinnamon Twig, Poria, Schisandra, and Licorice Decoction

Gui Zhi	*Cinnamomum*	6 - 12 g
Fu Ling	*Poria*	6 - 12 g
Wu Wei Zi	*Schisandra*	9 - 15 g
Gan Cao	*Glycyrrhiza*	6 - 9 g

Kidney yin and yang deficiency with qi and blood deficiency causing impotence, low back and knee pain, or weight loss. The deficiency is very severe, and the formula is deep-acting.

T pale, thin white coat

P frail, or rapid

☞ Ingredients should be prepared as a syrup. Herbs should be decocted and cane sugar then added to the tea. Doses of about 6 g should be taken with salt water.

GUI LU ER XIAN JIAO

Tortoise Shell and Deer Antler Syrup

Lu Jiao	*Cervus*	500 g
Ren Shen	*Panax*	45 g
Gou Qi Zi	*Lycium*	250 g
Gui Ban	*Chinemys*	150 g

Kidneys and Heart are not harmonizing accompanied with yin and yang deficiency. Symptoms include spermatorrhea, sexual dreams, or poor sleep.

T pale

P slow, hollow, weak

GUI ZHI JIA LONG GU MU LI TANG

Cinnamon Twig Decoction plus Dragon Bone and Oyster Shell

Extract Formula Name: Cinnamon and Dragon Bone Combination

Gui Zhi	*Cinnamomum*	6 - 9 g
Bai Shao Yao	*Paeonia*	6 - 9 g
Sheng Jiang	*Zingiber*	6 - 9 g
Da Zao	*Ziziphus*	4 - 12 pc
Mu Li	*Ostrea*	6 - 9 g
Long Gu	*Os Draconis*	6 - 9 g
Gan Cao	*Glycyrrhiza*	3 - 6 g

Kidney

Phlegm in the Lungs with underlying Kidney yang deficiency. The Kidneys are unable to grasp Lung qi, so qi ascends to the chest causing fullness in chest and epigastrium. This is known as running piglet disorder. Symptoms also include wheezing, spontaneous sweating, and cold hands and feet.

T pale, sticky white coat

P minute

Hei Xi - Plumbum and Liu Huang - Sulphur should both be dry fried. The remaining herbs are ground and made into pills with wine. Adults take 6 - 9 g per day, children take 2-3 g per day.

✘ To prevent lead poisoning, do not take longer than 3 days. Do not use during pregnancy.

HEI XI DAN

Lead Special Pill

Hei Xi	*Plumbum*	60 g
Liu Huang	*Sulphur*	60 g
Fu Zi	*Aconitum*	30 g
Rou Gui	*Cinnamomum*	60 g
Xiao Hui Xiang	*Foeniculum*	30 g
Rou Dou Kou	*Amomun*	30 g
Chen Xiang	*Aquilaria*	30 g
Yang Qi Shi	*Actinolitum*	30 g
Bu Gu Zhi	*Psoralea*	30 g
Mu Xiang	*Saussurea*	30 g
Chuan Lian Zi	*Melia*	30 g
Hu Lu Ba	*Trigonella*	30 g

Kidney and Spleen yang deficiency with cold which has invaded all three yin channels (taiyin, shaoyin, and jueyin). Symptoms include shivering from cold, icy limbs and face, watery diarrhea, or cough with profuse saliva production.

T pale, wet, thin white moist coat

P minute or frail

☞ Remove She Xiang - Moschus, decoct the rest of the formula as usual, then add powdered Moschus to each dosage.

HUI YANG JIU JI TANG

Restore and Revive the Yang Decoction

Fu Zi	*Aconitum*	9 g
Rou Gui	*Cinnamomum*	3 - 6 g
Ren Shen	*Panax*	6 - 9 g
Gan Jiang	*Zingiber*	3 - 6 g
Fu Ling	*Poria*	6 - 9 g
Chen Pi	*Citrus*	3 - 6 g
Bai Zhu	*Atractylodes*	6 - 9 g
Wu Wei Zi	*Schisandra*	3 - 6 g
Ban Xia	*Pinellia*	6 - 9 g
Gan Cao	*Glycyrrhiza*	3 - 6 g
She Xiang	*Moschus*	0.3 g
[Sheng Jiang	*Zingiber*	1 - 3 g]

Kidney qi/yang deficiency resulting in constipation.

T pale, white coat

P weak, deep, or minute

JI CHUAN JIAN

Benefit the River Decoction

Dang Gui	*Angelica*	9 - 15 g
Rou Cong Rong	*Cistanche*	6 - 9 g
Huai Niu Xi	*Achyranthes*	6 g
Zhi Ke	*Citrus*	3 g
Ze Xie	*Alisma*	4.5 g
Sheng Ma	*Cimicifuga*	2 - 3 g

Kidney yang deficiency causing edema, scanty urination, or benign prostate hypertrophy.

T pale, swollen, teethmarks, white sticky coat

P deep, wiry, slippery, thin

JI SHENG SHEN QI WAN

Kidney Qi Pill from Formulas to Aid the Living

Shu Di Huang	*Rehmannia*	6 - 12 g
Shan Yao	*Dioscorea*	6 - 12 g
Shan Zhu Yu	*Cornus*	6 - 9 g
Mu Dan Pi	*Paeonia*	6 - 12 g
Ze Xie	*Alisma*	6 - 9 g
Fu Ling	*Poria*	6 - 9 g
Fu Zi	*Aconitum*	6 - 9 g
Rou Gui	*Cinnamomum*	3 - 9 g
Che Qian Zi	*Plantago*	6 - 9 g
Chuan Niu Xi	*Cyathula*	6 - 9 g

Heart and Kidneys are not communicating. Kidney yang deficiency leads to Heart yang deficiency causing palpitations, cool limbs, or insomnia.

T pale, swollen, thin moist white coat

P deep, weak

JIAO TAI WAN

Grand Communication Pill

Extract Formula Name: Coptis and Cinnamon Formula

Huang Lian	*Coptis*	18 - 20 g
Rou Gui	*Cinnamomum*	3 - 6 g

Kidney qi and yang deficiency causing low back pain, coldness in the back, urinary difficulties, or pedal edema.

T pale, swollen, thin white coat

P frail

✪ Major Formula

JIN GUI SHEN QI WAN

Kidney Qi Pill from the Golden Cabinet

Extract Formula Name: Rehmannia Eight Formula

Shu Di Huang	*Rehmannia*	24 g
Shan Zhu Yu	*Cornus*	12 g
Shan Yao	*Dioscorea*	12 g
Mu Dan Pi	*Paeonia*	9 g
Ze Xie	*Alisma*	9 g
Fu Ling	*Poria*	9 g
Rou Gui	*Cinnamomum*	3 g
Fu Zi	*Aconitum*	3 g

Kidney and Liver yin deficiency, yang deficiency, or jing deficiency causing spermatorrhea, tinnitus, or impotence.

T pale or red, thin white coat

P thin, weak

JIN SUO GU JING WAN

Metal Lock Pill to Stabilize the Essence

Extract Formula Name: Lotus Stamen Formula

Qian Shi	*Euryale*	6 - 12 g
Sha Yuan Ji Li	*Astragalus*	6 - 12 g
Long Gu	*Os Draconis*	6 - 9 g
Mu Li	*Ostrea*	6 - 9 g
Lian Xu	*Nelumbo*	6 - 9 g
Lian Zi	*Nelumbo*	9 - 15 g

Kidney yang deficiency causing pronounced low back pain with severe immobility of the back, and weak legs.

T pale

P deep, weak, thin

☞ Herbs should be made into 3 g pills with honey. Du Zhong - Eucommia should be fried in ginger juice. Bu Gu Zhi - Psoralea should be fried with wine.

QING E WAN

Young Maiden Pill

Du Zhong	*Eucommia*	200 g
Hu Tao Ren	*Juglans*	6 g
Bu Gu Zhi	*Psoralea*	100 g
Da Suan	*Allium*	20 g

Kidney yang deficiency causing pedal edema, dark face, and low back pain, dribbling urination, or chronic deafness.

T pale, swollen, teethmarks, white coat

P frail

SHI BU WAN

Ten-Tonic Pill

Fu Zi	*Aconitum*	6 - 12 g
Rou Gui	*Cinnamomum*	3 - 6 g
Wu Wei Zi	*Schisandra*	6 - 12 g
Shan Yao	*Dioscorea*	6 - 12 g
Lu Rong	*Cervus*	3 - 6 g
Mu Dan Pi	*Paeonia*	3 - 6 g
Shan Zhu Yu	*Cornus*	3 - 6 g
Fu Ling	*Poria*	3 - 6 g
Ze Xie	*Alisma*	3 - 6 g
Shu Di Huang	*Rehmannia*	3 - 6 g

Leukorrhea or cloudy spermatorrhea due to Kidney yang deficiency.

T pale

P frail

SHUI LU ER XIAN DAN

Water and Earth Immortals Special Pill

Qian Shi	*Euryale*	10 g
Jin Ying Zi	*Rosa*	10 g

Kidney/Spleen yang deficiency leading to dawn diarrhea.

T pale, white coat

P deep, weak, slow

SI SHEN WAN

Four-Miracle Pill

Extract Formula Name: Psoralea and Myristica Formula

Bu Gu Zhi	*Psoralea*	12 - 18 g
Rou Dou Kou	*Myristica*	6 - 9 g
Wu Zhu Yu	*Evodia*	3 - 6 g
Wu Wei Zi	*Schisandra*	6 - 9 g
[Sheng Jiang	*Zingiber*	3 - 6 g]
[Da Zao	*Ziziphus*	3 - 5 pc]

Kidney and Spleen yang deficiency which developed after a chronic damp heat dysentery causing damp cold. This obstructs the Large Intestines, manifesting as dark blood in the stools with pus.

T pale

P minute

☞ Ingredients should be ground into a powder.

TAO HUA TANG

Peach Blossom Decoction

Extract Formula Name: Kaolin and Oryza Combination

Chi Shi Zhi	*Halloysitum Rubrum*	20 - 30 g
Jing Mi	*Oryza*	20 - 30 g
Gan Jiang	*Zingiber*	6 - 9 g

Kidney qi and yang deficiency with severe urinary incontinence and frequency or low back pain.

T pale

P frail

TU SI ZI WAN

Cuscuta Seed Pill

Tu Si Zi	*Cuscuta*	6 - 12 g
Rou Cong Rong	*Cistanche*	6 - 12 g
Wu Wei Zi	*Schisandra*	6 - 9 g
Lu Rong	*Cervus*	6 - 9 g
Shan Yao	*Dioscorea*	6 - 9 g
Sang Piao Xiao	*Paratenodera*	6 - 9 g
Wu Yao	*Lindera*	6 - 9 g
Yi Zhi Ren	*Alpinia*	6 - 9 g
Fu Zi	*Aconitum*	6 - 9 g
Mu Li	*Ostrea*	6 - 12 g
Ji Nei Jin	*Gallus*	3 g

Yin jaundice due to Kidney yang deficiency.

T pale, swollen, teethmarks, moist white coat

P deep, weak, thin

YIN CHEN SI NI TANG

Artemisia Yinchenhao Decoction for Frigid Extremities

Yin Chen Hao	*Artemisia*	3 - 9 g
Fu Zi	*Aconitum*	3 - 6 g
Pao Jiang	*Zingiber*	3 - 6 g
Gan Cao	*Glycyrrhiza*	3 - 6 g

Kidney yang and essence deficiency causing amenorrhea, infertility, cold back or knees, pedal edema, or impotence.

T pale, swollen, teethmarks, thin white coat

P minute

YOU GUI WAN

Restore the Right Pill

Extract Formula Name: Eucommia and Rehmannia Formula

Rou Gui	*Cinnamomum*	6 - 9 g
Fu Zi	*Aconitum*	3 - 6 g
Gou Qi Zi	*Lycium*	6 - 9 g
Shan Yao	*Dioscorea*	6 - 9 g
Shu Di Huang	*Rehmannia*	12 - 20 g
Shan Zhu Yu	*Cornus*	6 - 9 g
Du Zhong	*Eucommia*	6 - 9 g
Dang Gui	*Angelica*	6 - 9 g
Tu Si Zi	*Cuscuta*	6 - 9 g
Lu Jiao Jiao	*Cervus*	6 - 9 g

Kidney yang deficiency causing cold extremities, frequent urination, incontinence, decreased sexual function, or cold uterus. If the yang deficiency is chronic there will be heat symptoms: true yang deficiency with false heat symptoms such as redness in the face or thirst.

T pale, swollen, teethmarks, white coat

P frail or minute

YOU GUI YIN

Restore the Right Decoction

Shu Di Huang	*Rehmannia*	9 - 20 g
Gou Qi Zi	*Lycium*	6 - 9 g
Shan Zhu Yu	*Cornus*	6 g
Du Zhong	*Eucommia*	6 - 9 g
Fu Zi	*Aconitum*	6 - 9 g
Shan Yao	*Dioscorea*	6 - 9 g
Rou Gui	*Cinnamomum*	3 - 6 g
Zhi Gan Cao	*Glycyrrhiza*	3 - 6 g

Impotence or infertility due to Kidney yang deficiency with simultaneous qi and blood deficiency. Symptoms include blurry vision, low back pain, and poor memory.

T pale, thin white coat

P frail

ZAN YU DAN

Special Pill to Aid Fertility

Rou Cong Rong	*Cistanche*	6 - 12 g
Fu Zi	*Aconitum*	6 g
Ba Ji Tian	*Morinda*	6 - 12 g
Rou Gui	*Cinnamomum*	6 g
She Chuang Zi	*Cnidium*	6 g
Xian Mao	*Curculigo*	6 - 12 g
Dang Gui	*Angelica*	9 - 15 g
Bai Zhu	*Atractylodes*	12 - 18 g
Gou Qi Zi	*Lycium*	9 - 15 g
Yin Yang Huo	*Epimedium*	6 - 12 g
Shan Zhu Yu	*Cornus*	6 - 12 g
Shu Di Huang	*Rehmannia*	6 - 12 g
Jiu Zi	*Allium*	6 - 12 g
Du Zhong	*Eucommia*	6 - 12 g

Spleen/Kidney qi and yang deficient patient suffers easily from wind cold with internal water accumulation, or experiences urinary difficulty, diarrhea, or edema.

T pale, swollen, teethmarks, moist, thin white coat

P frail or minute

ZHEN WU TANG

True Warrior Decoction

Extract Formula Name: Vitality Combination

Fu Zi	*Aconitum*	6 - 9 g
Bai Zhu	*Atractylodes*	6 - 9 g
Bai Shao Yao	*Paeonia*	6 - 9 g
Fu Ling	*Poria*	6 - 9 g
Sheng Jiang	*Zingiber*	6 - 9 g

KIDNEY JING DEFICIENCY

- weak or brittle bones
- premature greying of hair or hair loss
- decreased sexual desire
- in children: slow bone development, mental slowness or retardation

T red, peeled

P empty

Lung/Kidney yin deficiency or jing deficiency with fire causing sweating, low back pain, slow mental and physical development in children, cough with scanty sticky blood-tinged phlegm, weight loss, or afternoon fever.

T red, slight yellow or no coat

P rapid, thin, or empty

HE CHE DA ZAO WAN

Pills of Human Placenta

Zi He Che	*Placenta Hominis*	9 - 30 g
Tian Men Dong	*Asparagus*	6 - 9 g
Mai Men Dong	*Ophiopogon*	6 - 9 g
Gui Ban	*Chinemys*	6 - 9 g
Shu Di Huang	*Rehmannia*	12 - 15 g
Huang Bai	*Phellodendron*	6 - 9 g
Du Zhong	*Eucommia*	6 - 9 g
Huai Niu Xi	*Achyranthes*	6 - 9 g

Kidney qi/yin deficiency causing slow mental development in children or low energy.

T pale, scanty coat

P thin

JIA WEI LIU WEI DI HUANG WAN

Augmented Six-Ingredient Pill with Rehmannia

Shu Di Huang	*Rehmannia*	6 - 12 g
Shan Yao	*Dioscorea*	6 - 9 g
Shan Zhu Yu	*Cornus*	6 - 9 g
Fu Ling	*Poria*	6 - 9 g
Ze Xie	*Alisma*	6 - 9 g
Mu Dan Pi	*Paeonia*	6 - 9 g
Lu Rong	*Cervus*	3 - 9 g
She Xiang	*Moschus*	1 - 2 g
Wu Jia Pi	*Acanthopanax*	6 - 12 g

Kidney and Liver yin deficiency, yang deficiency, or jing deficiency causing spermatorrhea, tinnitus, or impotence.

T pale or red, thin white coat

P thin, weak

JIN SUO GU JING WAN

Metal Lock Pill to Stabilize the Essence

Extract Formula Name: Lotus Stamen Formula

Qian Shi	*Euryale*	6 - 12 g
Sha Yuan Ji Li	*Astragalus*	6 - 12 g
Long Gu	*Os Draconis*	6 - 9 g
Mu Li	*Ostrea*	6 - 9 g
Lian Xu	*Nelumbo*	6 - 9 g
Lian Zi	*Nelumbo*	9 - 15 g

Liver blood/yin deficiency with Kidney qi deficiency causing early greying, hairloss, poor teeth, and seminal emissions.

T pale

P thin, weak

QI BAO MEI RAN DAN

Seven-Treasure Special Pill for Beautiful Whiskers

He Shou Wu	*Polygonum*	6 - 9 g
Huai Niu Xi	*Achyranthes*	6 - 12 g
Fu Ling	*Poria*	6 - 9 g
Tu Si Zi	*Cuscuta*	6 - 9 g
Gou Qi Zi	*Lycium*	6 - 9 g
Bu Gu Zhi	*Psoralea*	6 - 9 g
Dang Gui	*Angelica*	6 - 9 g

Liver/Kidney yin and jing (essence) deficiency causing slow development in children; or premature aging in adults, in addition to common yin deficiency signs and symptoms. The formula is also for early menopause, spermatorrhea, low sex drive, infertility, or low sperm count.

T red, scanty coat

P thin, rapid

✪ Major Formula

ZUO GUI YIN

Restore the Left [Kidney] Decoction

Shu Di Huang	*Rehmannia*	6 - 15 g
Shan Zhu Yu	*Cornus*	6 - 9 g
Shan Yao	*Dioscorea*	6 - 9 g
Gou Qi Zi	*Lycium*	6 - 9 g
Fu Ling	*Poria*	6 - 9 g
Zhi Gan Cao	*Glycyrrhiza*	3 - 6 g

KIDNEY YIN DEFICIENCY

- nightsweats, or five-palm heat
- thirst and dry mouth, especially at night
- dizziness, tinnitus

T red, peeled, scanty coat, cracks

P thin, rapid, or empty

Kidney/Liver yin deficiency with blood deficiency causing post-partum sweating, or night sweats.

T red, thin yellow coat

P thin, rapid

BA WEI DI HUANG WAN

Eight-Ingredient Pill with Rehmannia

Sheng Di Huang	*Rehmannia*	6 - 12 g
Shan Zhu Yu	*Cornus*	6 - 9 g
Shan Yao	*Dioscorea*	6 - 9 g
Fu Ling	*Poria*	6 - 9 g
Ze Xie	*Alisma*	6 - 9 g
Mu Dan Pi	*Paeonia*	6 - 9 g
Wu Wei Zi	*Schisandra*	6 - 9 g
Huang Qi	*Astragalus*	9 - 15 g

Lung/Kidney yin deficiency with cough and asthma, hemoptysis, tidal fever, or night sweats. This formula is also known as 'Mai Wei Di Huang Wan'.

T red, slight coat

P rapid, thin

BA XIAN CHANG SHOU WAN

Eight-Immortal Pill for Longevity

Shan Zhu Yu	*Cornus*	6 - 9 g
Shan Yao	*Dioscorea*	6 - 9 g
Sheng Di Huang	*Rehmannia*	6 - 12 g
Mu Dan Pi	*Paeonia*	6 - 9 g
Ze Xie	*Alisma*	6 - 9 g
Fu Ling	*Poria*	6 - 9 g
Wu Wei Zi	*Schisandra*	6 - 9 g
Mai Men Dong	*Ophiopogon*	6 - 9 g

Lung/Kidney yin deficiency with bleeding in the upper body due to false heat breaking the blood vessels; or chronic cough due to dryness in the throat.

T red, slight coat

P rapid, thin

BAI HE GU JIN TANG

Lily Bulb Decoction to Preserve the Metal

Extract Formula Name: Lily Combination

Bai He	*Lilium*	3 - 12 g
Mai Men Dong	*Ophiopogon*	6 - 12 g
Sheng Di Huang	*Rehmannia*	6 - 12 g
Shu Di Huang	*Rehmannia*	6 - 12 g
Bei Mu	*Fritillaria*	3 - 6 g
Xuan Shen	*Scrophularia*	6 - 9 g
Dang Gui	*Angelica*	6 - 9 g
Bai Shao Yao	*Paeonia*	6 - 9 g
Jie Geng	*Platycodon*	3 - 6 g
Gan Cao	*Glycyrrhiza*	3 - 6 g

Kidney yin deficiency can't nourish the Heart which leads to Heart blood deficiency. Symptoms include insomnia, dizziness, poor memory, excessive dreaming, or night sweating.

T slightly red, or pale, scanty coat

P thin, rapid

BAI ZI YANG XIN WAN

Biota Seed Pill to Nourish the Heart

Bai Zi Ren	*Biota*	3 - 9 g
Mai Men Dong	*Ophiopogon*	6 - 9 g
Dang Gui	*Angelica*	6 - 12 g
Gou Qi Zi	*Lycium*	6 - 9 g
Xuan Shen	*Scrophularia*	6 - 12 g
Fu Shen	*Poria*	6 - 9 g
Shi Chang Pu	*Acorus*	6 - 9 g
Shu Di Huang	*Rehmannia*	12 - 15 g
Gan Cao	*Glycyrrhiza*	3 - 6 g

Kidney qi/yin deficiency causing menorrhagia. Other symptoms may include low back pain, frequent urination, or weakness in the knees.

T red or normal color, thin white coat

P weak, especially in both chi (third) positions, slightly rapid

BAO YIN JIAN

Augment Yin Decoction

Huang Qin	*Scutellaria*	9 - 12 g
Huang Bai	*Phellodendron*	9 - 12 g
Sheng Di Huang	*Rehmannia*	9 - 15 g
Shu Di Huang	*Rehmannia*	9 - 15 g
Shan Yao	*Dioscorea*	6 - 9 g
Bai Shao Yao	*Paeonia*	6 - 12 g
Xu Duan	*Dipsacus*	6 - 9 g
Gan Cao	*Glycyrrhiza*	3 - 6 g

Purpura due to yin deficiency with heat. Strong false fire due to Kidney and Liver yin deficiency which leads to tidal fever and night sweats.

T red, thin yellow coat or no coat

P rapid, thin, or empty

DA BU YIN WAN

Great Tonify the Yin Pill

Shu Di Huang	*Rehmannia*	6 - 12 g
Gui Ban	*Chinemys*	6 - 12 g
Huang Bai	*Phellodendron*	6 - 9 g
Zhi Mu	*Anemarrhena*	6 - 9 g

Kidney yin and Spleen qi/blood deficiency causing uterine prolapse with low back pain, night urination, or hearing loss and tinnitus.

T red or pale

P frail

DA BU YUAN JIAN

Great Tonify the Basal Decoction

Ren Shen	*Panax*	6 - 12 g
Shu Di Huang	*Rehmannia*	9 - 25 g
Shan Yao	*Dioscorea*	6 - 9 g
Shan Zhu Yu	*Cornus*	3 - 6 g
Gou Qi Zi	*Lycium*	6 - 9 g
Dang Gui	*Angelica*	6 - 9 g
Du Zhong	*Eucommia*	6 - 9 g
Gan Cao	*Glycyrrhiza*	3 - 6 g

Lung/Kidney yin deficiency with bone steaming fever, cough with sticky phlegm, and five-palm heat.

T red, scanty coat

P thin, rapid

DA ZAO WAN

Great Creation Pill

Gui Ban	*Chinemys*	6 - 12 g
Huang Bai	*Phellodendron*	6 - 9 g
Zi He Che	*Placenta Hominis*	1 - 2 g
Huai Niu Xi	*Achyranthes*	6 - 9 g
Ren Shen	*Panax*	6 - 9 g
Du Zhong	*Eucommia*	6 - 9 g
Mai Men Dong	*Ophiopogon*	6 - 9 g
Tian Men Dong	*Asparagus*	6 - 9 g
Sheng Di Huang	*Rehmannia*	6 - 12 g

Kidney and Liver yin deficiency causing irregular menses, scanty menstrual flow, tinnitus, dizziness, or night sweating.

T red, scanty coat

P thin, rapid

DANG GUI DI HUANG YIN

Dang Gui and Rehmannia Decoction

Dang Gui	*Angelica*	6 - 9 g
Shu Di Huang	*Rehmannia*	6 - 12 g
Huai Niu Xi	*Achyranthes*	6 - 9 g
Shan Yao	*Dioscorea*	6 - 9 g
Du Zhong	*Eucommia*	6 - 9 g
Shan Zhu Yu	*Cornus*	6 - 9 g
Zhi Gan Cao	*Glycyrrhiza*	3 - 6 g

Yin deficient patient has very high fever, profuse sweating, thirst, or yellow, scanty urine.

T red, cracked, slight coat

P rapid, thin

DANG GUI LIU HUANG TANG

Dang Gui and Six-Yellow Decoction

Extract Formula Name: Tang-Kuei and Six-Yellows Combination

Dang Gui	*Angelica*	6 - 9 g
Shu Di Huang	*Rehmannia*	6 - 9 g
Sheng Di Huang	*Rehmannia*	6 - 12 g
Huang Qi	*Astralagus*	12 - 15 g
Huang Qin	*Scutellaria*	6 - 12 g
Huang Lian	*Coptis*	3 - 6 g
Huang Bai	*Phellodendron*	6 - 12 g

Kidney/Lung qi/yin deficiency with wheezing, shortness of breath, or chronic cough. This formula is also known as 'Qi Wu Du Qi Wan'.

T red, slight coat

P thin, rapid

DU QI WAN

Capital Qi Pill

Extract Formula Name: Rehmannia and Schizandra Formula

Shan Zhu Yu	*Cornus*	6 - 9 g
Shan Yao	*Dioscorea*	6 - 9 g
Sheng Di Huang	*Rehmannia*	9 - 12 g
Fu Ling	*Poria*	6 - 9 g
Mu Dan Pi	*Paeonia*	6 - 9 g
Ze Xie	*Alisma*	6 - 9 g
Wu Wei Zi	*Schisandra*	6 - 9 g

Kidney yin deficiency with hearing problems, high-pitched tinnitus, dizziness, or hearing loss in the elderly.

T red, scanty yellow coat

P thin, rapid

ER LONG ZUO CI WAN

Pill for Deafness that is Kind to the Left [Kidney]

Shu Di Huang	*Rehmannia*	6 - 12 g
Shan Yao	*Dioscorea*	6 - 9 g
Shan Zhu Yu	*Cornus*	6 - 9 g
Mu Dan Pi	*Paeonia*	6 - 9 g
Fu Ling	*Poria*	6 - 9 g
Ze Xie	*Alisma*	6 - 9 g
Ci Shi	*Magnetitum*	6 - 9 g
Wu Wei Zi	*Schisandra*	6 - 9 g
Shi Chang Pu	*Acorus*	6 - 9 g

Kidney yin and yang deficiency with fire causing menopause, hot flashes, or urinary frequency.

T red

P rapid or normal rate, thin

ER XIAN TANG

Two-Immortal Decoction

Extract Formula Name: Curculigo and Epimedium Combination

Yin Yang Huo	*Epimedium*	9 - 15 g
Xian Mao	*Curculigo*	9 - 15 g
Dang Gui	*Angelica*	6 - 9 g
Huang Bai	*Phellodendron*	6 - 9 g
Zhi Mu	*Anemarrhena*	6 - 9 g
Ba Ji Tian	*Morinda*	6 - 9 g

Liver/Kidney yin deficiency causing weakness in the low back and knees, or atrophy; or Liver cannot store the soul (hun) causing insomnia or bad dreams.

T red, dry, scanty coat

P thin, rapid

☞ Equal amounts of both herbs should be used.

ER ZHI WAN

Two-Ultimate Pill

Han Lian Cao	*Eclipta*	10 g
Nu Zhen Zi	*Ligustrum*	10 g

Kidney qi/yin deficiency causing irregular periods, leukorrhea, or a bearing-down sensation.

T red, thin white coat

P weak, especially the chi (third) positions

GU YIN JIAN

Stabilize the Yin Decoction

Shu Di Huang	*Rehmannia*	6 - 12 g
Shan Yao	*Dioscorea*	6 - 9 g
Wu Wei Zi	*Schisandra*	6 - 9 g
Shan Zhu Yu	*Cornus*	6 - 9 g
Tu Si Zi	*Cuscuta*	6 - 9 g
Ren Shen	*Panax*	6 - 9 g
Yuan Zhi	*Polygala*	3 g
Zhi Gan Cao	*Glycyrrhiza*	3 - 6 g

Kidney yin and yang deficiency with qi and blood deficiency causing impotence, low back and knee pain, or weight loss. The deficiency is very severe, and the formula is deep-acting.

T pale, thin white coat

P frail, or rapid

☞ Ingredients should be prepared as a syrup. Herbs should be decocted and cane sugar then added to the tea. Doses of about 6 g should be taken with salt water.

GUI LU ER XIAN JIAO

Tortoise Shell and Deer Antler Syrup

Lu Jiao	*Cervus*	500 g
Ren Shen	*Panax*	45 g
Gou Qi Zi	*Lycium*	250 g
Gui Ban	*Chinemys*	150 g

Kidney qi deficiency with Kidney/Liver yin deficiency causing amenorrhea, or back and knee pain.

T pale or red, thin white or scanty coat

P weak, maybe thin especially in the left chi (third) position

GUI SHEN TANG

Comeback Kidney Decoction

Shu Di Huang	*Rehmannia*	6 - 15 g
Shan Yao	*Dioscorea*	9 - 15 g
Shan Zhu Yu	*Cornus*	9 - 12 g
Gou Qi Zi	*Lycium*	9 - 15 g
Dang Gui	*Angelica*	9 - 12 g
Du Zhong	*Eucommia*	6 - 12 g
Fu Ling	*Poria*	6 - 12 g
Tu Si Zi	*Cuscuta*	9 - 12 g

Lung/Kidney yin deficiency or jing deficiency with fire causing sweating, low back pain, slow mental and physical development in children, cough with scanty sticky blood-tinged phlegm, weight loss, or afternoon fever.

T red, slight yellow or no coat

P rapid, thin, or empty

HE CHE DA ZAO WAN

Pills of Human Placenta

Zi He Che	*Placenta Hominis*	9 - 30 g
Tian Men Dong	*Asparagus*	6 - 9 g
Mai Men Dong	*Ophiopogon*	6 - 9 g
Gui Ban	*Chinemys*	6 - 9 g
Shu Di Huang	*Rehmannia*	12 - 15 g
Huang Bai	*Phellodendron*	6 - 9 g
Du Zhong	*Eucommia*	6 - 9 g
Huai Niu Xi	*Achyranthes*	6 - 9 g

Kidney and Liver yin deficiency causing bone bi-syndrome or wei syndrome. Deficient yin cannot nourish tendons and false heat burns tendons and muscles. This leads to atrophy, joint swelling, or deformities. The pain tends to be more fixed.

T red, scanty coat

P thin, rapid, weak

☞ All ingredients should be ground up as powder. Take 10 g each time, twice a day.

HU QIAN WAN

Hidden Tiger Pill

Extract Formula Name: Tiger Bone and Tortoise Shell Formula

Gui Ban	*Chinemys*	120 g
Huang Bai	*Phellodendron*	150 g
Shu Di Huang	*Rehmannia*	60 g
Zhi Mu	*Anemarrhena*	60 g
Bai Shao Yao	*Paeonia*	60 g
Suo Yang	*Cynomorium*	45 g
Hu Gu	*Panthera*	30 g
Chen Pi	*Citrus*	60 g
Gan Jiang	*Zingiber*	15 g

Heart/Kidney yin deficiency with fire after febrile disease leading to insomnia, palpitations, or tongue sores: shaoyin deficient heat syndrome.

T red, scanty coat

P rapid, thin

☞ E Jiao - Equus and egg yolks should be dissolved into the strained tea.

HUANG LIAN E JIAO TANG

Coptis and Ass-Hide Gelatin Decoction

Extract Formula Name: Coptis and Gelatin Combination

Huang Lian	*Coptis*	9 - 12 g
E Jiao	*Equus*	6 - 9 g
Huang Qin	*Scutellaria*	6 - 9 g
Bai Shao Yao	*Paeonia*	6 - 9 g
Ji Zi Huang	*Egg yolks*	2

1. Yin/blood deficiency with heat causing arrhythmia of the Heart. 2. High fever causing arrhythmia: yangming disease depleted yin which leads to an irregular Heart beat.

T red, scanty coat

P rapid, irregular

☞ E Jiao - Equus should be dissolved at the end into the strained tea.

JIA JIAN FU MAI TANG

Modified Restore-the-Pulse Decoction

Zhi Gan Cao	*Glycyrrhiza*	12 - 15 g
Bai Shao Yao	*Paeonia*	12 - 15 g
Mai Men Dong	*Ophiopogon*	9 - 12 g
Sheng Di Huang	*Rehmannia*	12 - 15 g
Huo Ma Ren	*Cannabis*	9 - 12 g
E Jiao	*Equus*	6 - 9 g

Kidney qi/yin deficiency causing slow mental development in children or low energy.

T pale, scanty coat

P thin

JIA WEI LIU WEI DI HUANG WAN

Augmented Six-Ingredient Pill with Rehmannia

Shu Di Huang	*Rehmannia*	6 - 12 g
Shan Yao	*Dioscorea*	6 - 9 g
Shan Zhu Yu	*Cornus*	6 - 9 g
Fu Ling	*Poria*	6 - 9 g
Ze Xie	*Alisma*	6 - 9 g
Mu Dan Pi	*Paeonia*	6 - 9 g
Lu Rong	*Cervus*	3 - 9 g
She Xiang	*Moschus*	1 - 2 g
Wu Jia Pi	*Acanthopanax*	6 - 12 g

Kidney/Lung yin deficiency with Lung phlegm causing chronic bronchitis in the elderly, wheezing, or nausea.

T red, slight coat, or geographic

P thin, slightly rapid, slippery

JIN SHUI LIU JUN JIAN

Six-Gentlemen Decoction of Metal and Water

Chen Pi	*Citrus*	3 - 6 g
Ban Xia	*Pinellia*	6 - 9 g
Fu Ling	*Poria*	6 - 9 g
Gan Cao	*Glycyrrhiza*	3 - 6 g
Dang Gui	*Angelica*	6 - 9 g
Sheng Di Huang	*Rehmannia*	6 - 12 g
[Sheng Jiang	*Zingiber*	3 - 6 g]

Kidney and Liver yin deficiency, yang deficiency, or jing deficiency causing spermatorrhea, tinnitus, or impotence.

T pale or red, thin white coat

P thin, weak

JIN SUO GU JING WAN

Metal Lock Pill to Stabilize the Essence

Extract Formula Name: Lotus Stamen Formula

Qian Shi	*Euryale*	6 - 12 g
Sha Yuan Ji Li	*Astragalus*	6 - 12 g
Long Gu	*Os Draconis*	6 - 9 g
Mu Li	*Ostrea*	6 - 9 g
Lian Xu	*Nelumbo*	6 - 9 g
Lian Zi	*Nelumbo*	9 - 15 g

Basic prescription for Kidney/Liver yin deficiency with mild damp. This can cause dry, flaky, pale red rashes, excess sexual activity, or sweating. In women it may lead to irregular menses or night sweating and afternoon heat.

T red, thin yellow coat, or scanty coat

P rapid, thin

✪ **Major Formula**

LIU WEI DI HUANG WAN

Six-Ingredient Pill with Rehmannia

Extract Formula Name: Rehmannia Six Formula

Shan Zhu Yu	*Cornus*	6 - 9 g
Shan Yao	*Dioscorea*	6 - 9 g
Sheng Di Huang	*Rehmannia*	6 - 12 g
Fu Ling	*Poria*	6 - 9 g
Ze Xie	*Alisma*	6 - 9 g
Mu Dan Pi	*Paeonia*	6 - 9 g

Kidney and Liver yin deficiency with yang rising causing vision disturbances, dry red eyes, or blurry vision.

T red, scanty yellow coat

P thin, rapid

MING MU DI HUANG WAN

Improve Vision Pill with Rehmannia

Shu Di Huang	*Rehmannia*	9 - 20 g
Sheng Di Huang	*Rehmannia*	9 - 15 g
Mu Dan Pi	*Paeonia*	6 - 9 g
Shan Yao	*Dioscorea*	6 - 9 g
Shan Zhu Yu	*Cornus*	6 - 9 g
Ze Xie	*Alisma*	6 - 9 g
Dang Gui	*Angelica*	6 - 9 g
Fu Shen	*Poria*	6 - 9 g
Chai Hu	*Bupleurum*	6 - 9 g
Wu Wei Zi	*Schisandra*	6 - 9 g

Liver blood/yin deficiency with Kidney qi deficiency causing early greying, hairloss, poor teeth, and seminal emissions.

T pale

P thin, weak

QI BAO MEI RAN DAN

Seven-Treasure Special Pill for Beautiful Whiskers

He Shou Wu	*Polygonum*	6 - 9 g
Huai Niu Xi	*Achyranthes*	6 - 12 g
Fu Ling	*Poria*	6 - 9 g
Tu Si Zi	*Cuscuta*	6 - 9 g
Gou Qi Zi	*Lycium*	6 - 9 g
Bu Gu Zhi	*Psoralea*	6 - 9 g
Dang Gui	*Angelica*	6 - 9 g

Kidney and Liver yin deficiency with eye disturbances.

T red, scanty yellow coat

P thin, rapid

QI JU DI HUANG WAN

Lycium Fruit, Chrysanthemum, and Rehmannia Pill

Extract Formula Name: Lycium, Chrysanthemum and Rehmannia Formula

Shu Di Huang	*Rehmannia*	6 - 12 g
Shan Yao	*Dioscorea*	6 - 9 g
Shan Zhu Yu	*Cornus*	6 - 9 g
Mu Dan Pi	*Paeonia*	6 - 9 g
Fu Ling	*Poria*	6 - 9 g
Ze Xie	*Alisma*	6 - 9 g
Gou Qi Zi	*Lycium*	6 - 12 g
Ju Hua	*Chrysanthemum*	6 - 9 g

Purpura due to yin deficiency with false heat. This prescription should be used with 'Da Bu Yin Wan' to strengthen the yin tonifying effect.

T red, dry, cracked, thin scanty yellow coat

P thin, rapid

☞ E Jiao - Equus should be dissolved at the end into the strained tea.

QIAN CAO GEN WAN

Rubia Pill

Qian Cao Gen	*Rubia*	6 - 9 g
Huang Qin	*Scutellaria*	6 - 9 g
E Jiao	*Equus*	9 - 15 g
Ce Bai Ye	*Biota*	12 - 20 g
Sheng Di Huang	*Rehmannia*	9 - 15 g
Gan Cao	*Glycyrrhiza*	3 - 6 g

Yin deficiency with severe false heat or tidal/bone steaming fever causing red lips, heat sensation in the bones, five-palm heat, night sweats, or delirium.

T red, slight yellow coat or no coat

P rapid, thin, weak, or empty

P Dissolve Bie Jia - Amyda first for about one hour, then decoct with the remaining herbs.

QING GU SAN

Cool the Bones Powder

Yin Chai Hu	*Stellaria*	6 - 12 g
Hu Huang Lian	*Picrorhiza*	6 - 9 g
Di Gu Pi	*Lycium*	6 - 9 g
Qing Hao	*Artemisia*	6 - 9 g
Bie Jia	*Amyda*	6 - 9 g
Qin Jiao	*Gentiana*	3 - 9 g
Zhi Mu	*Anemarrhena*	6 - 12 g
Gan Cao	*Glycyrrhiza*	3 - 6 g

Febrile disease causing low level chronic fever; or chronic disease damaged yin leading to later stages of febrile disease causing night sweats, AIDS, or tuberculosis.

T red, dry, scanty coat

P thin, rapid

☞ Bie Jia - Amyda should be soaked separately for 30 minutes to one hour, until it starts to dissolve; then soak the rest of the herbs. Qing Hao - Artemisia should be added at the end of the decoction process.

QING HAO BIE JIA TANG

Artemisia Annua and Soft-shelled Turtle Shell Decoction

Bie Jia	*Amyda*	9 - 12 g
Qing Hao	*Artemisia*	6 - 9 g
Mu Dan Pi	*Paeonia*	6 - 9 g
Sheng Di Huang	*Rehmannia*	6 - 12 g
Zhi Mu	*Anemarrhena*	6 - 9 g

Yin deficiency with false heat causing early periods or constipation.

T red, scanty yellowish coat

P thin, rapid

QING JING SAN

Clear the Menses Powder

Shu Di Huang	*Rehmannia*	6 - 12 g
Mu Dan Pi	*Paeonia*	6 - 9 g
Di Gu Pi	*Lycium*	6 - 9 g
Qing Hao	*Artemisia*	3 - 6 g
Bai Shao Yao	*Paeonia*	6 - 9 g
Fu Ling	*Poria*	6 g
Huang Bai	*Phellodendron*	3 g

Heat in the ying level with yin deficiency causing high fever which is worse at night, delirious speech, or mild purpura.

T dark red and dry

P rapid, thin

☞ Xi Jiao - Rhinoceros should be substituted with 9 g of Shui Niu Jiao - Bubalus or 30 g of Bai Mao Gen - Imperata.

QING YING TANG

Clear the Nutritive Level Decoction

Extract Formula Name: Rhinoceros and Scrophularia Combination

Xi Jiao	*Rhinoceros*	3 - 6 g
Sheng Di Huang	*Rehmannia*	9 - 12 g
Mai Men Dong	*Ophiopogon*	6 - 9 g
Huang Lian	*Coptis*	3 - 6 g
Xuan Shen	*Scrophularia*	6 - 9 g
Dan Zhu Ye	*Lophatherum*	6 g
Lian Qiao	*Forsythia*	6 g
Dan Shen	*Salvia*	6 - 9 g
Jin Yin Hua	*Lonicera*	6 - 9 g

Lung and Kidney yin deficiency with dryness in the Lungs causing chronic consumptive disease. Symptoms include thirst, night sweating, or scanty phlegm which is hard to expectorate.

T red, dry, scanty coat

P deep, thin, rapid

QONG YU SAN

Ginseng and Rehmannia Powder

Ren Shen	*Panax*	3 - 6 g
Sheng Di Huang	*Rehmannia*	15 - 30 g
Feng Mi	*Mel*	30 g
Fu Ling	*Poria*	15 - 30 g

Kidney and Liver yin deficiency with blood deficiency and wind damp. This leads to blurry vision, cough, constipation, or bi-syndrome.

T red, scanty yellow coat

P thin

☞ Herbs should be formed into 9 g pills. Adults take one pill two times a day.

SANG MA WAN

Mulberry Leaf and Sesame Seed Pill

Sang Ye	*Morus*	250 - 300 g
Hei Zhi Ma	*Sesamum*	100 - 120 g
Feng Mi	*Mel*	250 - 300 g

Kidney/Liver yin deficiency with yang rising causing blurry vision, photophobia, excessive tearing, poor night vision, early stage catarract, or blood-shot eyes.

T red, thin and narrow in size, maybe cracked, scanty coat

P thin, rapid

☞ Xi Jiao - Rhinoceros should be substituted with Shui Niu Jiao - Bubalus.

SHI HU YE GUANG WAN

Dendrobium Pill for Night Vision

Tian Men Dong	*Asparagus*	6-9 g
Fu Ling	*Poria*	6-9 g
Ren Shen	*Panax*	6-9 g
Shu Di Huang	*Rehmannia*	12-15 g
Mai Men Dong	*Ophiopogon*	6-9 g
Tu Si Zi	*Cuscuta*	3-9 g
Ju Hua	*Chrysanthemum*	3-6 g
Xing Ren	*Prunus*	3-6 g
Jue Ming Zi	*Cassia*	6-9 g
Gou Qi Zi	*Lycium*	6-9 g
Shan Yao	*Dioscorea*	6-12 g
Wu Wei Zi	*Schisandra*	6-9 g
Huai Niu Xi	*Achyranthes*	6-12 g
Bai Ji Li	*Tribulus*	6-9 g
Chuan Xiong	*Ligusticum*	3-6 g
Rou Cong Rong	*Cistanche*	3-6 g
Shi Hu	*Dendrobium*	6-12 g
Zhi Ke	*Citrus*	3-6 g
Qing Xiang Zi	*Celosia*	3-9 g
Xi Jiao	*Rhinoceros*	1-3 g
Huang Lian	*Coptis*	3-6 g
Fang Feng	*Ledebouriella*	6-9 g
Ling Yang Jiao	*Saiga*	1-3 g
Gan Cao	*Glycyrrhiza*	3-6 g

Kidney

Lung/Kidney yin deficiency with severe fire causing nosebleeds, or hemoptysis which occurs during or prior to the menses.

T red, cracks

P rapid, empty

SHUN JING TANG

Smooth the Menses Decoction

Shu Di Huang	*Rehmannia*	9 - 15 g
Mu Dan Pi	*Paeonia*	6 - 9 g
Dang Gui	*Angelica*	6 - 9 g
Bai Shao Yao	*Paeonia*	6 - 9 g
Bei Sha Shen	*Glehnia*	6 - 12 g
Jing Jie	*Schizonepeta*	6 - 9 g
Fu Ling	*Poria*	6 - 9 g

Heart/Kidney yin deficiency, Heart blood deficiency and false heat where Kidneys and Heart don't harmonize. This leads to insomnia, restlessness, palpitations, poor memory, or night sweats.

T red

P rapid, thin

✘ Zhu Sha - Cinnabaris is toxic and should only be used short-term.

TIAN WANG BU XIN DAN

Emperor of Heaven's Special Pill to Tonify the Heart

Extract Formula Name: Ginseng and Zizyphus Formula

Ren Shen	*Panax*	9 - 12 g
Mai Men Dong	*Ophiopogon*	6 - 12 g
Tian Men Dong	*Asparagus*	6 - 9 g
Xuan Shen	*Scrophularia*	6 - 9 g
Dan Shen	*Salvia*	6 - 12 g
Sheng Di Huang	*Rehmannia*	15 - 30 g
Fu Ling	*Poria*	6 - 9 g
Wu Wei Zi	*Schisandra*	6 - 9 g
Jie Geng	*Platycodon*	3 - 6 g
Yuan Zhi	*Polygala*	6 - 9 g
Bai Zi Ren	*Biota*	6 - 9 g
Dang Gui	*Angelica*	6 - 9 g
Suan Zao Ren	*Ziziphus*	6 - 12 g
Zhu Sha	*Cinnabaris*	1 - 3 g

Kidney and Liver yin deficiency causing amenorrhea, cold feeling in the abdomen, retarded growth in puberty, or clear leukorrhea.

T pale or slightly red

P weak, thin

☞ E Jiao - Equus should be added at the end to the strained tea.

TIAO GAN TANG

Regulating the Liver Decoction

Shan Yao	*Dioscorea*	9 - 12 g
E Jiao	*Equus*	6 - 12 g
Ba Ji Tian	*Morinda*	6 - 9 g
Dang Gui	*Angelica*	6 - 9 g
Ze Lan	*Lycopus*	6 - 12 g
Shan Zhu Yu	*Cornus*	6 - 9 g
Bai Shao Yao	*Paeonia*	6 - 9 g
Dan Shen	*Salvia*	6 - 9 g
Gan Cao	*Glycyrrhiza*	3 - 6 g

Lung/Kidney yin deficiency with toxin causing diptheria, laryngitis, coarse breathing, or dry hacking cough.

T red, dry, yellow coat

P thin, rapid, or empty

YANG YIN QING FEI TANG

Nourish the Yin and Clear the Lungs Decoction

Sheng Di Huang	*Rehmannia*	6 - 12 g
Xuan Shen	*Scrophularia*	6 - 9 g
Bai Shao Yao	*Paeonia*	6 - 9 g
Mai Men Dong	*Ophiopogon*	6 - 12 g
Bo He	*Mentha*	3 - 6 g
Chuan Bei Mu	*Fritillaria*	3 - 6 g
Mu Dan Pi	*Paeonia*	6 - 9 g
Gan Cao	*Glycyrrhiza*	3 - 6 g

Liver qi stagnation produces heat which consumes Kidney and Liver yin, or Liver overacts on the Spleen and Stomach causing emotional upset, nausea, belching with sour taste, hiatal hernia, or epigastric or abdominal pain; or Liver yin cannot nourish the tendons and ligaments producing heel or posterior hip pain.

T red, dry

P thin, wiry

YI GUAN JIAN

Linking Decoction

Extract Formula Name: Glehnia and Rehmannia Combination

Sheng Di Huang	*Rehmannia*	15 - 30 g
Gou Qi Zi	*Lycium*	6 - 15 g
Dang Gui	*Angelica*	6 - 12 g
Bei Sha Shen	*Glehnia*	6 - 9 g
Mai Men Dong	*Ophiopogon*	6 - 9 g
Chuan Lian Zi	*Melia*	3 - 6 g

Kidney yin deficiency leading to lower jiao diabetes (xiao ke). Frequent urination is the main symptom.

T red, scanty coat

P thin, slightly rapid

YI YIN TANG

Benefit-Yin Decoction

Shu Di Huang	Rehmannia	15 g
Sheng Di Huang	Rehmannia	15 g
Bai Shao Yao	Paeonia	9 - 15 g
Mai Men Dong	Ophiopogon	9 - 15 g
Huai Niu Xi	Achyranthes	6 - 15 g
Dan Shen	Salvia	12 - 15 g
Gan Cao	Glycyrrhiza	3 - 6 g

Kidney and Liver yin/blood deficiency with fire which bothers the Heart. This causes Heart and Liver fire or Liver yang excess leading to excessive dreaming, insomnia, or outbursts of anger.

T red, cracks, thin or thick yellow coat

P rapid, wiry, thin

☞ Ingredients should be powdered, made into 9 - 12 g pills and taken three times a day. Xi Jiao - Rhinoceros should be substituted with Shui Niu Jiao - Bubalus.

ZHEN ZHU MU WAN

Mother-Of-Pearl Pill

Zhen Zhu Mu	Pteria	15 - 20 g
Ren Shen	Panax	9 - 12 g
Dang Gui	Angelica	6 - 12 g
Shu Di Huang	Rehmannia	9 - 12 g
Suan Zao Ren	Ziziphus	6 - 9 g
Bai Zi Ren	Biota	6 - 9 g
Fu Shen	Poria	6 - 9 g
Chen Xiang	Aquilaria	6 - 9 g
Xi Jiao	Rhinoceros	1 - 3 g

Kidney yin deficiency with heat and mild damp causing afternoon fever, night sweats, spermatorrhea, or malarflush.

T red, scanty coat

P thin, rapid

ZHI BAI DI HUANG WAN

Anemarrhena, Phellodendron, and Rehmannia Pill

Extract Formula Name: Anemarrhena, Phellodendron and Rehmannia Formula

Huang Bai	Phellodendron	3 - 9 g
Zhi Mu	Anemarrhena	6 - 9 g
Sheng Di Huang	Rehmannia	15 - 25 g
Shan Yao	Dioscorea	9 - 12 g
Shan Zhu Yu	Cornus	9 - 12 g
Mu Dan Pi	Paeonia	6 - 9 g
Ze Xie	Alisma	6 - 9 g
Fu Ling	Poria	6 - 9 g

Kidney and Liver yin deficiency with damp stagnation. This causes poor vision, blurry vision, or dry eyes.

T red, sticky yellowish coat

P thin, weak

ZHU JING WAN

Preserve Vistas Pill

Tu Si Zi	Cuscuta	9 - 15 g
Shu Di Huang	Rehmannia	9 - 12 g
Che Qian Zi	Plantago	6 - 9 g

Kidney and Liver yin deficiency with false heat and bone steaming fever, lumbago, involuntary emissions, night sweats, or impotence. Stronger than 'Zuo Gui Yin'.

T red, scanty coat

P thin, rapid, or empty

ZUO GUI WAN

Restore the Left [Kidney] Pill

Extract Formula Name: Achyranthes and Rehmannia Formula

Shu Di Huang	Rehmannia	9 - 25 g
Gou Qi Zi	Lycium	9 - 12 g
Chuan Niu Xi	Cyathula	9 - 12 g
Shan Yao	Dioscorea	9 - 12 g
Shan Zhu Yu	Cornus	9 - 12 g
Lu Jiao Jiao	Cervus	9 - 12 g
Tu Si Zi	Cuscuta	9 - 12 g
Gui Ban	Chinemys	9 - 12 g

Liver/Kidney yin and jing (essence) deficiency causing slow development in children; or premature aging in adults, in addition to common yin deficiency signs and symptoms. The formula is also for early menopause, spermatorrhea, low sex drive, infertility, or low sperm count.

T red, scanty coat

P thin, rapid

ZUO GUI YIN

Restore the Left [Kidney] Decoction

Shu Di Huang	*Rehmannia*	6 - 15 g
Shan Zhu Yu	*Cornus*	6 - 9 g
Shan Yao	*Dioscorea*	6 - 9 g
Gou Qi Zi	*Lycium*	6 - 9 g
Fu Ling	*Poria*	6 - 9 g
Zhi Gan Cao	*Glycyrrhiza*	3 - 6 g

BLADDER DISHARMONIES

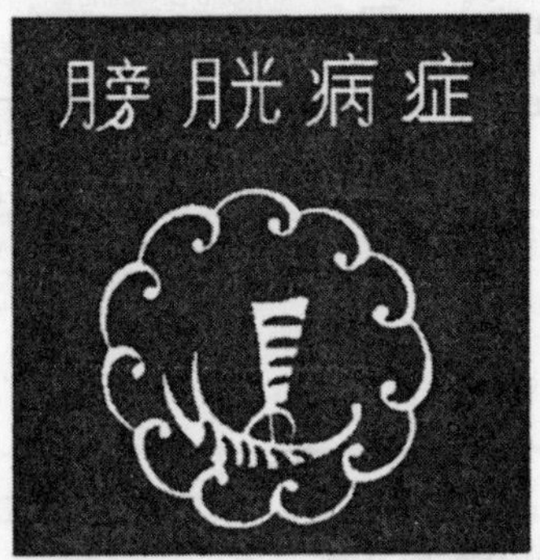

LIN SYNDROME — DISORDERS OF THE BLADDER

- urinary frequency, urgency
- burning or pale turbid urine
- gravel or calculi in urine, or hematurea

T depends on involved syndrome

P depends on involved syndrome

Bladder damp heat: heat lin-syndrome causing burning urination, scanty yellow urine, urgency and frequency.

T red, sticky yellow coat

P wiry, rapid, slippery, forceful

✪ Major Formula

BA ZHENG SAN

Eight-Herb Powder for Rectification

Extract Formula Name: Dianthus Formula

Mu Tong	*Akebia*	6 - 9 g
Qu Mai	*Dianthus*	9 - 12 g
Zhi Zi	*Gardenia*	3 - 6 g
Da Huang	*Rheum*	3 - 9 g
Hua Shi	*Talcum*	9 - 20 g
Bian Xu	*Polygonum*	9 - 12 g
Che Qian Zi	*Plantago*	6 - 12 g
Deng Xin Cao	*Juncus*	6 g
Gan Cao	*Glycyrrhiza*	3 - 6 g

Kidney qi deficiency with cold and damp leading to frequent, or cloudy, painful urination.

T pale

P weak, or slippery

BEI XIE FEN QIN YIN I

Dioscorea Hypoglauca Decoction to Separate the Clear

Extract Formula Name: Tokoro Combination

Bei Xie	*Dioscorea*	6 - 12 g
Wu Yao	*Lindera*	6 - 9 g
Shi Chang Pu	*Acorus*	6 - 9 g
Yi Zhi Ren	*Alpinia*	6 - 9 g

Damp heat in the Bladder causing cloudy and painful urination, urinary retention, or urgency.

T red, sticky yellow coat

P rapid, wiry, slippery

BEI XIE FEN QIN YIN II

Dioscorea Hypoglauca Decoction to Separate the Clear from Medical Revelations

Bei Xie	*Dioscorea*	6 - 9 g
Dan Shen	*Salvia*	3 - 9 g
Huang Bai	*Phellodendron*	6 - 9 g
Che Qian Zi	*Plantago*	3 - 6 g
Shi Chang Pu	*Acorus*	3 - 6 g
Bai Zhu	*Atractylodes*	3 - 9 g
Fu Ling	*Poria*	6 - 9 g
Lian Xin	*Nelumbo*	4 g

Lin-syndrome: urinary distention caused by qi lin-syndrome, which is essentially caused by Liver qi stagnation. Acute type: urinary problems after emotional upset.

T possibly red sides

P wiry

CHEN XIANG SAN

Aquilaria Wood Powder

Chen Xiang	*Aquilaria*	9 - 12 g
Shi Wei	*Pyrrosia*	6 - 9 g
Hua Shi	*Talcum*	3 - 12 g
Bai Shao Yao	*Paeonia*	6 - 9 g
Dang Gui	*Angelica*	6 - 12 g
Dong Kui Zi	*Malva*	6 - 9 g
Wang Bu Liu Xing	*Vaccaria*	3 - 9 g
Gan Cao	*Glycyrrhiza*	3 - 6 g

Heart fire leading to Small Intestine fire, which in turn leads to Bladder damp heat causing hematuria, frequent urination, urinary retention, thirst, or tongue sores.

T bright red, sticky yellow coat

P rapid. wiry

✪ Major Formula

DAO CHI SAN

Guide Out the Red Powder

Extract Formula Name: Rehmannia and Akebia Formula

Sheng Di Huang	*Rehmannia*	9 - 20 g
Dan Zhu Ye	*Lophatherum*	6 - 9 g
Mu Tong	*Akebia*	6 - 9 g
Gan Cao	*Glycyrrhiza*	3 - 6 g

Damp heat in the Bladder causing frequent and burning urination. This may be seen during pregnancy.

T red, sticky yellow coat

P rapid, slippery

JIA WEI WU LIN SAN

Augmented Five-Ingredient Powder for Painful Urinary Dysfunction

Chi Fu Ling	*Poria*	6 - 12 g
Chi Shao Yao	*Paeonia*	6 - 15 g
Dang Gui	*Angelica*	6 - 9 g
Zhi Zi	*Gardenia*	6 - 15 g
Ze Xie	*Alisma*	6 - 9 g
Mu Tong	*Akebia*	6 - 9 g
Che Qian Zi	*Plantago*	6 - 9 g
Hua Shi	*Talcum*	9 - 15 g
Sheng Di Huang	*Rehmannia*	6 - 12 g
Gan Cao	*Glycyrrhiza*	3 - 6 g

Bladder damp heat with calculi.

T red, sticky yellow coat

P slippery, rapid

SAN JIN TANG

Three-Gold Decoction

Jin Qian Cao	*Lysimachia*	6 - 45 g
Jin Sha Teng	*Lygodium*	9 - 25 g
Dong Kui Zi	*Malva*	6 - 9 g
Ji Nei Jin	*Gallus*	6 - 9 g
Shi Wei	*Pyrrosia*	6 - 9 g
Qu Mai	*Dianthus*	9 - 12 g

Bladder damp heat with calculi or gravel. Stone lin syndrome manifesting as severe heat and mild damp.

T sticky coat

P wiry, rapid

SHI WEI SAN

Pyrrosia Leaf Powder

Shi Wei	*Pyrrosia*	6 - 9 g
Dong Kui Zi	*Malva*	3 - 6 g
Mu Tong	*Akebia*	3 - 6 g
Qu Mai	*Dianthus*	6 g
Hua Shi	*Talcum*	6 - 12 g
Che Qian Zi	*Plantago*	6 - 9 g
Gan Cao	*Glycyrrhiza*	3 = 6 g

Kidney qi/yang deficiency with enuresis or frequent, clear urination.

T pale, swollen, teethmarks, white coat

P minute

SUO QUAN WAN

Shut the Sluice Pill

Yi Zhi Ren	*Alpinia*	6 - 15 g
Shan Yao	*Dioscorea*	9 - 15 g
Wu Yao	*Lindera*	6 - 9 g

Chronic lin-syndrome due to Kidney qi deficiency causing urinary frequency with turbidity, incontinence, or enuresis.

T pale or normal color, thin white or yellowish coat

P weak, especially in the chi (third) positions

WU BI SHAN YAO WAN

Dioscorea Pill

Shu Di Huang	*Rehmannia*	12 - 15 g
Shan Yao	*Dioscorea*	12 - 15 g
Shan Zhu Yu	*Cornus*	6 - 9 g
Rou Cong Rong	*Cistanche*	6 - 9 g
Tu Si Zi	*Cuscuta*	6 - 9 g
Wu Wei Zi	*Schisandra*	6 - 12 g
Ze Xie	*Alisma*	6 - 9 g
Ba Ji Tian	*Morinda*	3 - 6 g
Du Zhong	*Eucommia*	9 - 12 g
Huai Niu Xi	*Achyranthes*	12 - 15 g
Fu Shen	*Poria*	9 - 12 g
Chi Shi Zhi	*Halloysitum Rubrum*	12 - 15 g

Bladder damp heat with underlying Kidney qi deficiency causing urgent, painful, or scanty urination.

T red, sticky yellow coat

P rapid, thin, or slippery

WU LIN SAN

Five-Ingredient Powder for Painful Urinary Dysfunction

Extract Formula Name: Gardenia and Hoelen Formula

Zhi Zi	*Gardenia*	6 - 9 g
Chi Fu Ling	*Poria*	6 - 9 g
Dang Gui	*Angelica*	6 - 9 g
Chi Shao Yao	*Paeonia*	6 - 9 g
Gan Cao	*Glycyrrhiza*	3 - 6 g

Heat and water accumulation in the lower jiao (Bladder) with slight taiyang symptoms (wind cold); or Spleen qi deficiency with damp and water causing edema in the skin or muscle layer.

T sticky white or yellow coat

P slippery or superficial

✪ Major Formula

WU LING SAN

Five-Ingredient Powder with Poria

Extract Formula Name: Hoelen Five Herbs Formula

Fu Ling	*Poria*	6 - 9 g
Zhu Ling	*Polyporus*	6 - 9 g
Ze Xie	*Alisma*	6 - 9 g
Gui Zhi	*Cinnamomum*	3 - 9 g
Bai Zhu	*Atractylodes*	6 - 9 g

Liver qi stagnation causing late periods, irritability, premenstrual syndrome, or distention in the urinary tract.

T light purple, thin coat

P wiry

WU YAO TANG

Lindera Decoction

Wu Yao	*Lindera*	3 - 6 g
Dang Gui	*Angelica*	6 - 9 g
Xiang Fu	*Cyperus*	3 - 9 g
Mu Xiang	*Saussurea*	3 - 9 g
Gan Cao	*Zingiber*	3 - 6 g

Blood lin-syndrome causing urinary bleeding with pain, burning urination, frequency, urgency, scanty urination, lower abdominal pain, or Kidney pain.

T red and thin, or red and swollen, yellow coat

P rapid

XIAO JI YIN ZI

Cephalanoplos Decoction

Extract Formula Name: Cephalanoplos Combination

Sheng Di Huang	*Rehmannia*	15 50 g
Dan Zhu Ye	*Lophatherum*	6 - 9 g
Mu Tong	*Akebia*	9 - 15 g
Gan Cao	*Glycyrrhiza*	3 - 6 g
Ou Jie	*Nelumbo*	6 - 9 g
Zhi Zi	*Gardenia*	3 - 6 g
Hua Shi	*Talcum*	9 - 15 g
Pu Huang	*Typha*	3 - 6 g
Dang Gui	*Angelica*	6 - 15 g
Xiao Ji	*Cephalanoplos*	9 - 15 g

Yangming channel syndrome affecting the lower jiao; or wind cold causing heat in the Spleen/Stomach which burns the yin. This leads to water dysfunction and stagnation which heats up leading to Lin-syndrome: Heat Lin or damp heat edema.

T red, sticky yellow coat

P rapid

☞ E Jiao - Equus should be added to the strained tea.

ZHU LING TANG I

Polyporus Decoction

Extract Formula Name: Polyporus Combination

Zhu Ling	*Polyporus*	6 - 9 g
Fu Ling	*Poria*	6 - 9 g
Hua Shi	*Talcum*	6 - 9 g
Ze Xie	*Alisma*	6 - 9 g
E Jiao	*Equus*	6 - 9 g

Damp heat in the lower jiao causing urinary difficulty and pain.

T red, sticky coat

P slippery

ZHU LING TANG II

Polyporus Decoction from Comprehensive Recordings

Zhu Ling	*Polyporus*	6 - 9 g
Mu Tong	*Akebia*	6 - 9 g
Sang Bai Pi	*Morus*	6 - 9 g
[Deng Xin Cao	*Juncus*	3 g]

LARGE INTESTINE DISHARMONIES

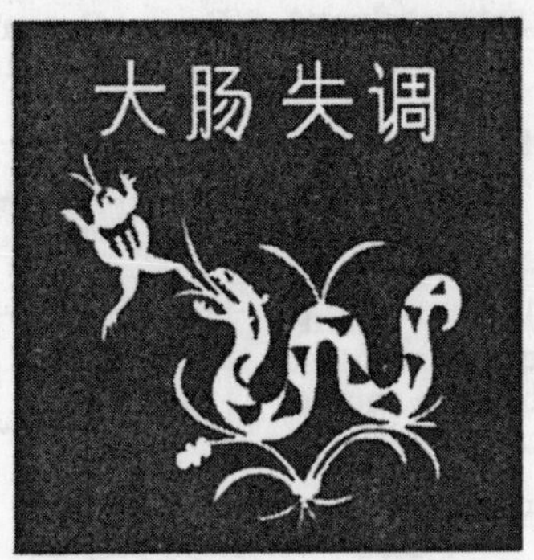

LARGE INTESTINE DISORDERS

- constipation, burning anus
- diarrhea with odorous stools
- abdominal distention or pain

T depends on involved syndrome

P depends on involved syndrome

Toxic heat in the yangming channel causing dysentery, or pus or blood in the stools.

T red, yellow coat

P wiry, rapid, rolling

BAI TOU WENG TANG

Pulsatilla Decoction

Extract Formula Name: Anemone Combination

Bai Tou Weng	*Pulsatilla*	20 - 40 g
Huang Bai	*Phellodendron*	9 - 12 g
Qin Pi	*Fraxinus*	9 - 15 g
Huang Lian	*Coptis*	6 - 9 g

Intestinal abscess or acute appendicitis due to heat and blood stagnation causing mass formation in the lower right quadrant with pain.

T yellow sticky coat

P rapid, slippery

☞ Da Huang - Rheum should be added during the last 3 - 5 minutes of the decoction process. Mang Xiao - Mirabilitum should be added to the strained tea.

✘ Do not use with appendicitis during pregnancy.

DA HUANG MU DAN TANG

Rhubarb and Moutan Decoction

Extract Formula Name: Rhubarb and Moutan Combination

Da Huang	*Rheum*	6 - 12 g
Mang Xiao	*Mirabilitum*	6 - 12 g
Dong Gua Ren	*Benincasa*	12 - 20 g
Tao Ren	*Prunus*	9 - 12 g
Mu Dan Pi	*Paeonia*	6 - 9 g

Water/heat accumulation in the chest and abdomen causing qi obstruction which leads to pancreatitis with edema, intestinal obstruction, or lumps.

T red, sticky coat.

P rapid, slippery

☞ Soak and cook Gan Sui - Euphorbia, add Da Huang - Rheum during the last 3 - 5 minutes, then dissolve Mang Xiao - Mirabilitum into the strained tea.

✘ Gan Sui - Euphorbia is toxic, and should only be taken in small amounts. Do not use during pregnancy.

DA XIAN XIONG TANG

Major Sinking Into the Chest Decoction

Extract Formula Name: Rhubarb and Kansui Combination

Da Huang	*Rheum*	9 - 15 g
Mang Xiao	*Mirabilitum*	9 - 12 g
Gan Sui	*Euphorbia*	0.6 - 1 g

Heat in the yangming channel with pre-existing severe blood stagnation in the lower jiao which affects the uterus and the intestines. Symptoms include jaundice, mania, fever, melena with dry stools which are relatively easy to discharge, dysmenorrhea, amenorrhea, abdominal fullness, or bleeding in the stomach. This formula is stronger than 'Di Dang Wan - Resistance Pill.'

T red, dark purple

P wiry, rapid

✘ Do not use during pregnancy. Use only for a short duration.

DI DANG TANG

Resistance Decoction

Da Huang	*Rheum*	6 - 12 g
Tao Ren	*Prunus*	6 - 9 g
Shui Zhi	*Hirudo*	1 - 3 g
Meng Chong	*Tabanus*	1 - 3 g

Heat in the yangming channel with pre-existing severe blood stagnation in the lower jiao which affects the uterus and the intestines. Symptoms include jaundice, mania, fever, melena with dry stools which are relatively easy to discharge, dysmenorrhea, amenorrhea, abdominal fullness, or bleeding in the stomach. This formula is somewhat milder than 'Di Dang Tang - Resistance Decoction.'

T red, purple

P wiry, rapid

☞ Ingredients should all be ground up, then formed into pills.

✘ Caution during pregnancy.

DI DANG WAN

Resistance Pill

Da Huang	*Rheum*	12 g
Shui Zhi	*Hirudo*	20 - 30 g
Meng Chong	*Tabanus*	20 - 30 g
Tao Ren	*Prunus*	9 - 12 g

Severe damp heat causing bright red blood in stools, bitter taste, or constipation.

T red, sticky yellow coat

P rapid, slippery

DI YU SAN

Sanguisorba Powder

Di Yu	*Sanguisorba*	6 - 9 g
Zhi Zi	*Gardenia*	6 - 9 g
Qian Cao Gen	*Rubia*	6 - 9 g
Huang Lian	*Coptis*	6 - 9 g
Fu Ling	*Poria*	6 - 9 g
Huang Qin	*Scutellaria*	6 - 9 g

Qi and blood stagnation with water accumulation causing intestinal obstruction, lack of gas or bowel movements.

T purple, sticky white or yellow coat

P slippery, rapid

☞ All herbs except Gan Sui - Euphorbia should be decocted. Soak and decoct Gan Sui separately and add at the end.

✘ Gan Sui - Euphorbia is extremely toxic and should be taken with caution. Do not use during pregnancy.

GAN SUI TONG JIE TANG

Euphorbia for Intestinal Obstruction Decoction

Gan Sui	*Euphorbia*	0.5 - 1 g
Tao Ren	*Prunus*	6 - 9 g
Chuan Niu Xi	*Cyathula*	6 - 9 g
Hou Po	*Magnolia*	9 - 30 g
Da Huang	*Rheum*	12 - 25 g
Chi Shao Yao	*Paeonia*	9 - 15 g
Mu Xiang	*Saussurea*	3 - 9 g

Wind heat with internal middle jiao heat and Large Intestine heat and damp causing dysentery: taiyang and yangming disease. Symptoms include fever, thirst, or burning anus.

T red, yellow coat

P rapid, slippery

GE GEN HUANG LIAN HUANG QIN TANG

Kudzu, Coptis, and Scutellaria Decoction

Extract Formula Name: Pueraria, Coptis and Scute Combination

Ge Gen	*Pueraria*	12 - 15 g
Huang Lian	*Coptis*	6 - 9 g
Huang Qin	*Scutellaria*	6 - 9 g
Gan Cao	*Glycyrrhiza*	3 - 6 g

Dry heat accumulation in the Large Intestines with shen (spirit) disturbance causing insomnia, irritability, or constipation.

T red, dry, thin yellow coat

P rapid

☞ Herbs should be ground and formed into 3 g pills.

✘ Do not use during pregnancy. This is a very strong purgative and should only be used once or twice.

GENG YI WAN

Pill Requiring a Change of Clothes

Zhu Sha	*Cinnabaris*	12 - 18 g
Lu Hui	*Aloe*	18 - 25 g

Wind heat enters the Large Intestines; or damp toxin (food) obstructs the intestines. This leads to bleeding which is bright red, lack of pain, or internal hemorrhoids.

T red, yellow coat

P rapid, wiry

HUAI HUA SAN

Sophora Japonica Flower Powder

Extract Formula Name: Sophora Formula

Huai Hua Mi	*Sophora*	12 - 15 g
Jing Jie	*Schizonepeta*	3 - 6 g
Ce Bai Ye	*Biota*	9 - 12 g
Zhi Ke	*Citrus*	3 - 6 g

Bleeding hemorrhoids caused by wind heat, toxic heat, or damp heat in the intestines. This formula is also for prolapse of the rectum.

T red, thin sticky yellow coat

P rapid

☞ All ingredients should be ground into a powder. Take 9 g each time, twice a day.

HUAI JIAO WAN

Sophora Japonica Fruit Pill

Huai Jiao	*Sophora*	500 g
Di Yu	*Sanguisorba*	250 g
Huang Qin	*Scutellaria*	250 g
Fang Feng	*Ledebouriella*	250 g
Zhi Ke	*Citrus*	250 g
Dang Gui	*Angelica*	250 g

Yangming organ heat with qi/blood deficiency causing odorous urgent dysentery with abdominal pain which is worse with pressure, fatigue, or possible hallucinations.

T dry yellow coat

P weak

✘ Do not use during pregnancy.

HUANG LONG TANG

Yellow Dragon Decoction

Da Huang	*Rheum*	12 g
Mang Xiao	*Mirabilitum*	9 g
Hou Po	*Magnolia*	12 g
Zhi Shi	*Citrus*	9 g
Dang Gui	*Angelica*	9 g
Ren Shen	*Panax*	6 g
Jie Geng	*Platycodon*	3 - 6 g
Sheng Jiang	*Zingiber*	3 - 6 g
Da Zao	*Ziziphus*	1 - 3 pc
Gan Cao	*Glycyrrhiza*	3 g

Heat entering the intestines leading to damp heat dysentery. Symptoms include fever, bitter taste, or odorous diarrhea.

T red, yellow coat

P rapid

HUANG QIN TANG

Scutellaria Decoction

Extract Formula Name: Scute and Licorice Combination

Huang Qin	*Scutellaria*	9 g
Bai Shao Yao	*Paeonia*	9 g
Da Zao	*Ziziphus*	4 - 5 pc
Gan Cao	*Glycyrrhiza*	3 g

Externally contracted damp heat dysentery causing explosive, odorous, watery diarrhea, tenesmus, or burning anus.

T sticky yellow coat

P rapid, slippery

JIA WEI BAI TOU WENG TANG

Augmented Pulsatilla Decoction

Bai Tou Weng	*Pulsatilla*	6 - 9 g
Qin Pi	*Fraxinus*	3 - 6 g
Huang Lian	*Coptis*	3 - 6 g
Huang Qin	*Scutellaria*	6 - 9 g
Huang Bai	*Phellodendron*	6 - 9 g
Bai Shao Yao	*Paeonia*	6 - 9 g

Yin/blood deficiency causing constipation with dry stools; or excess heat causing constipation.

T red, dry yellow coat

P rapid, thin, or empty

✘ Do not use during pregnancy.

✪ Major Formula

MA ZI REN WAN

Hemp Seed Pill

Extract Formula Name: Apricot Seed and Linum Formula

Huo Ma Ren	*Cannabis*	6 - 12 g
Da Huang	*Rheum*	6 - 9 g
Xing Ren	*Prunus*	6 - 9 g
Zhi Shi	*Citrus*	3 - 6 g
Bai Shao Yao	*Paeonia*	6 - 9 g
Hou Po	*Magnolia*	6 - 12 g

Constipation due to yin/blood deficiency. This is commonly seen in the elderly, or after giving birth.

T red or pale, dry

P thin

RUN CHANG WAN I

Moisten the Intestines Pill from Master Shen's Book

Huo Ma Ren	*Cannabis*	9 - 15 g
Dang Gui	*Angelica*	9 - 12 g
Sheng Di Huang	*Rehmannia*	6 - 9 g
Tao Ren	*Prunus*	6 - 9 g
Zhi Ke	*Citrus*	6 - 9 g

Large Intestine damp heat with qi and blood stagnation causing hot dysentery with pain and abdominal spasms. This is often associated with food poisoning.

T sticky yellow coat

P rapid

✪ Major Formula

SHAO YAO TANG

Peony Decoction

Extract Formula Name: Peony Combination

Bai Shao Yao	*Paeonia*	9 - 25 g
Bing Lang	*Areca*	3 - 6 g
Da Huang	*Rheum*	6 - 9 g
Huang Qin	*Scutellaria*	6 - 15 g
Huang Lian	*Coptis*	3 - 9 g
Dang Gui	*Angelica*	6 - 9 g
Mu Xiang	*Saussurea*	3 - 6 g
Rou Gui	*Cinnamomum*	1 - 3 g
Gan Cao	*Glycyrrhiza*	3 - 6 g

Water accumulation with heat, damp and qi stagnation; or Stomach deficiency with food stagnation and water. Symptoms include diarrhea, borborygmus, or epigastric distention.

T red, sticky yellow coat

P slippery, rapid

SHENG JIANG XIE XIN TANG

Fresh Ginger Decoction to Drain the Epigastrium

Extract Formula Name: Pinellia and Ginger Combination

Sheng Jiang	*Zingiber*	9 - 12 g
Ban Xia	*Pinellia*	6 - 9 g
Ren Shen	*Panax*	6 - 12 g
Gan Jiang	*Zingiber*	3 - 6 g
Huang Qin	*Scutellaria*	6 - 9 g
Huang Lian	*Coptis*	3 - 6 g
Da Zao	*Ziziphus*	6 - 10 pc
Gan Cao	*Glycyrrhiza*	3 - 6 g

Blood stagnation with fire in the lower jiao causing constipation, sudden abdominal pain, dysmenorrhea, intestinal obstruction, or melena. In severe cases this may lead to restlessness, or even delirium.

T purple

P choppy or forceful

☞ Da Huang - Rheum should be added during the last 3 - 5 minutes of the decoction process. Mang Xiao - Mirabilitum should be added to the strained tea.

✘ Do not use during pregnancy.

TAO HE CHENG QI TANG

Peach Pit Decoction to Order the Qi

Extract Formula Name: Prunus and Rhubarb Combination

Tao Ren	*Prunus*	9 - 15 g
Gui Zhi	*Cinnamomum*	6 - 9 g
Mang Xiao	*Mirabilitum*	3 - 6 g
Da Huang	*Rheum*	9 - 12 g
Gan Cao	*Glycyrrhiza*	3 - 6 g

Kidney and Spleen yang deficiency which developed after a chronic damp heat dysentery causing damp cold. This obstructs the Large Intestines, manifesting as dark blood in the stools with pus.

T pale

P minute

☞ Ingredients should be ground into a powder.

TAO HUA TANG

Peach Blossom Decoction

Extract Formula Name: Kaolin and Oryza Combination

Chi Shi Zhi	*Halloysitum Rubrum*	20 - 30 g
Jing Mi	*Oryza*	20 - 30 g
Gan Jiang	*Zingiber*	6 - 9 g

1. Roundworms have migrated upward due to cold in the Large Intestines to the warmth of the epigastrium/chest. 2. Large Intestine cold and Stomach heat: mixed syndrome - jueyin syndrome.

T pale

P weak

☞ Wu Mei - Prunus should be soaked in vinegar for 12 hours.

WU MEI WAN

Mume Pill

Extract Formula Name: Mume Formula

Wu Mei	*Prunus*	20 - 25 g
Xi Xin	*Asarum*	1 - 3 g
Chuan Jiao	*Zanthoxylum*	1 - 3 g
Gan Jiang	*Zingiber*	12 - 15 g
Fu Zi	*Aconitum*	6 - 9 g
Huang Lian	*Coptis*	9 - 12 g
Huang Bai	*Phellodendron*	6 - 9 g
Gui Zhi	*Cinnamomum*	3 - 9 g
Dang Gui	*Angelica*	6 - 9 g
Ren Shen	*Panax*	6 - 9 g

Blood deficiency causing constipation.

T pale

P weak, thin

WU REN WAN

Five-Seed Pill

Xing Ren	*Prunus*	9 - 20 g
Bai Zi Ren	*Biota*	3 - 6 g
Tao Ren	*Prunus*	9 - 15 g
Yu Li Ren	*Prunus*	3 - 6 g
Sha Ren	*Amomum*	3 - 6 g

Diarrhea due to Spleen qi deficiency with damp and Stomach heat causing dysentery with mucous and possible bleeding.

T sticky yellow coat

P slippery, rapid

XIANG LIAN WAN

Aucklandia and Coptis Pill

Extract Formula Name: Saussurea and Coptis Formula

Mu Xiang	*Saussurea*	6 - 9 g
Huang Lian	*Coptis*	3 - 6 g
Wu Zhu Yu	*Evodia*	3 - 12 g

Damp and blood stagnation causing intestinal abscess, colicky pain in the abdomen with urinary disturbances, or severe pain after menstruation or childbirth.

T purple, sticky coat

P wiry or choppy

YI YI REN TANG

Coix Decoction from the Standards

Yi Yi Ren	*Coix*	9 - 15 g
Mu Dan Pi	*Paeonia*	6 - 9 g
Gua Lou Ren	*Trichosanthes*	9 - 12 g
Tao Ren	*Prunus*	6 - 9 g

Chronic diarrhea has depleted Spleen and Kidney yang causing prolapse of the rectum or bowel incontinence.

T pale, white coat

P deep, slow

ZHEN REN YANG ZANG TANG

True Man's Decoction to Nourish the Organs

Ren Shen	*Panax*	6 - 9 g
Rou Gui	*Cinnamomum*	3 g
Bai Zhu	*Atractylodes*	6 - 12 g
He Zi	*Terminalia*	6 - 9 g
Rou Dou Kou	*Myristica*	9 - 12 g
Ying Su Ke	*Papaver*	6 - 15 g
Mu Xiang	*Saussurea*	3 - 9 g
Dang Gui	*Angelica*	6 - 15 g
Bai Shao Yao	*Paeonia*	9 - 12 g
Zhi Gan Cao	*Glycyrrhiza*	3- 6 g

Food stagnation in the middle jiao with damp and heat accumulation: cold and heat in the middle jiao with Spleen deficiency. Symptoms include fullness with pain, odorous diarrhea, mucus, tenesmus, gas, or constipation.

T red, red sides, rough, thick sticky yellow coat

P slippery, rapid, forceful

✘ Caution during pregnancy.

ZHI SHI DAO ZHI WAN

Immature Bitter Orange Pill to Guide Out Stagnation

Extract Formula Name: Chih-shih and Rhubarb Formula

Zhi Shi	*Citrus*	9 - 15 g
Shen Qu	*Massa Fermentata*	9 - 15 g
Da Huang	*Rheum*	15 - 25 g
Huang Qin	*Scutellaria*	6 - 9 g
Huang Lian	*Coptis*	6 - 9 g
Fu Ling	*Poria*	6 - 9 g
Ze Xie	*Alisma*	6 - 9 g
Bai Zhu	*Atractylodes*	6 - 9 g

JIN YE (BODY FLUID) DISHARMONIES

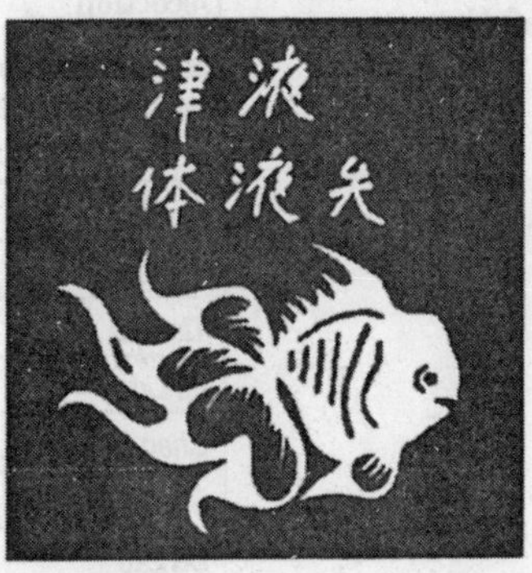

ACCUMULATION OF TAN YIN (DAMP AND PHLEGM)

- fullness in epigastrium or abdomen
- dizziness
- edema
- masses, lumps, or nodules

T thin or thick sticky white or yellowish coat

P slippery

Spleen/Stomach deficiency with damp causing vomiting or diarrhea.

T pale, sticky white coat

P weak, slippery

BAI ZHU SAN

Atractylodes Powder

Extract Formula Name: Atractylodes and Pueraria Formula

Ren Shen	*Panax*	6 - 9 g
Bai Zhu	*Atractylodes*	9 - 15 g
Ge Gen	*Pueraria*	9 - 15 g
Huo Xiang	*Agastache*	9 - 15 g
Fu Ling	*Poria*	9 - 15 g
Mu Xiang	*Saussurea*	3 - 6 g
Gan Cao	*Glycyrrhiza*	3 - 6 g

Liver wind and phlegm rises to the head leading to hypertension, dizziness, nausea, vomiting, or deviation of the eye or mouth.

T sticky white coat

P slippery

BAN XIA BAI ZHU TIAN MA TANG

Pinellia, Atractylodes, and Gastrodia Decoction

Extract Formula Name: Pinellia and Gastrodia Combination

Ban Xia	*Pinellia*	6 - 9 g
Bai Zhu	*Atractylodes*	6 - 15 g
Tian Ma	*Gastrodia*	6 - 9 g
Fu Ling	*Poria*	6 - 9 g
Chen Pi	*Citrus*	3 - 6 g
Sheng Jiang	*Zingiber*	3 - 6 g
Da Zao	*Ziziphus*	1 - 3 pc
Gan Cao	*Glycyrrhiza*	3 g

Phlegm and Liver qi stagnation causing hysteria, plumpit qi, or depression.

T light purple, sticky white or yellowish coat

P slippery or wiry

BAN XIA HOU PO TANG

Pinellia and Magnolia Bark Decoction

Extract Formula Name: Pinellia and Magnolia Combination

Ban Xia	*Pinellia*	6 - 9 g
Hou Po	*Magnolia*	6 - 15 g
Zi Su Ye	*Perilla*	3 - 6 g
Fu Ling	*Poria*	6 - 9 g
Sheng Jiang	*Zingiber*	9 - 12 g

Disharmony between Stomach and Intestines which leads to failure to descend qi which, subsequently, leads to food, damp, or water accumulation (or heat and cold accumulation in the Stomach). This is known as glomus and fullness (pi man). Symptoms include epigastric fullness, gurgling, reflux or loose stools.

T yellow sticky coat

P wiry, rapid

BAN XIA XIE XIN TANG

Pinellia Decoction to Drain the Epigastrium

Extract Formula Name: Pinellia Combination

Ban Xia	*Pinellia*	6 - 12 g
Huang Qin	*Scutellaria*	6 - 9 g
Huang Lian	*Coptis*	3 - 6 g
Gan Jiang	*Zingiber*	3 - 6 g
Ren Shen	*Panax*	6 - 9 g
Da Zao	*Ziziphus*	3 - 5 pc
Gan Cao	*Glycyrrhiza*	3 - 6 g

External wind cold entering the Stomach causing severe damp accumulation which then leads to fever and chills, diarrhea, vomiting, fullness, or abdominal bloating.

T sticky white coat

P slippery, superficial

BU HUAN JING ZHENG QI SAN

Rectify the Qi Powder Worth More Than Gold

Extract Formula Name: Pinellia, Atractylodes, and Agastache Formula

Hou Po	*Magnolia*	9 - 12 g
Cang Zhu	*Atractylodes*	3 - 9 g
Huo Xiang	*Agastache*	6 - 9 g
Ban Xia	*Pinellia*	6 - 9 g
Chen Pi	*Citrus*	3 - 6 g
Gan Cao	*Glycyrrhiza*	3 - 6 g
[Sheng Jiang	*Zingiber*	3 - 6 g]
[Da Zao	*Ziziphus*	3 - 5 pc]

Severe phlegm damp accumulation causing dizziness, headache, sticky phlegm expectoration, or amenorrhea due to phlegm obstruction.

T thick sticky white or slightly yellowish coat

P slippery

CANG FU DAO TAN TANG

Atractylodes, Cyperus, and Guide Out Phlegm Decoction

Ban Xia	*Pinellia*	6 - 9 g
Chen Pi	*Citrus*	3 - 6 g
Fu Ling	*Poria*	6 - 9 g
Tian Nan Xing	*Arisaema*	1 - 3 g
Zhi Shi	*Citrus*	3 - 9 g
Gan Cao	*Glycyrrhiza*	3 - 6 g
Cang Zhu	*Atractylodes*	3 - 9 g
Xiang Fu	*Cyperus*	3 - 9 g
Sheng Jiang	*Zingiber*	6 - 9 g

Spleen qi deficiency causing tan yin: damp or water accumulation. Symptoms include borborygmus, and loose, watery stools.

T pale, swollen, teethmarks, wet

P slippery

DA BAN XIA TANG

Major Pinellia Decoction

Ban Xia	*Pinellia*	6 - 9 g
Fu Ling	*Poria*	6 - 9 g
Bai Feng Mi	*Mel*	9 - 15 g

(Lung) phlegm damp with cough or coma causing wind phlegm, dizziness, or hypertension.

T thick sticky coat

P slippery

✘ Tian Nan Xing - Arisaema is slightly toxic.

DAO TAN TANG

Guide Out Phlegm Decoction

Ban Xia	*Pinellia*	6 - 9 g
Chen Pi	*Citrus*	3 - 6 g
Fu Ling	*Poria*	6 - 9 g
Gan Cao	*Glycyrrhiza*	3 - 6 g
Zhi Shi	*Citrus*	3 - 6 g
Tian Nan Xing	*Arisaema*	1 - 3 g
Sheng Jiang	*Zingiber*	3 g

Wind and phlegm accumulation causing hypertension, vertigo, and aphasia.

T rigid, sticky white or yellowish coat

P slippery

DI TAN TANG

Scour Phlegm Decoction

Extract Formula Name: Arisaema and Acorus Combination

Ban Xia	*Pinellia*	6 - 9 g
Fu Ling	*Poria*	6 - 9 g
Zhi Shi	*Citrus*	3 - 6 g
Chen Pi	*Citrus*	3 - 6 g
Zhu Ru	*Bambusa*	1 - 3 g
Dan Nan Xing	*Arisaema*	1 - 3 g
Ren Shen	*Panax*	3 - 6 g
Shi Chang Pu	*Acorus*	6 g
Gan Cao	*Glycyrrhiza*	3 - 6 g
[Sheng Jiang	*Zingiber*	3 - 6 g]
[Da Zao	*Ziziphus*	1 - 3 pc]

Basic formula for phlegm and damp accumulation from Stomach and Spleen qi deficiency. Symptoms include nausea and vomiting, or epigastric distention.

T sticky coat

P slippery

✪ **Major Formula**

ER CHEN TANG

Two-Cured Decoction

Extract Formula Name: Citrus and Pinellia Combination

Ban Xia	*Pinellia*	6 - 9 g
Chen Pi	*Citrus*	3 - 6 g
Fu Ling	*Poria*	6 - 9 g
Gan Cao	*Glycyrrhiza*	3 - 6 g
[Sheng Jiang	*Zingiber*	3 - 6 g]
[Da Zao	*Ziziphus*	3 pc]

Damp heat in the lower jiao causing low back pain, hot, swollen knees or feet, or odorous leukorrhea.

T sticky yellow coat

P slippery, rapid

ER MIAO SAN

Two-Marvel Powder

Cang Zhu	*Atractylodes*	15 g
Huang Bai	*Phellodendron*	15 g

Wind heat with internal middle jiao heat and Large Intestine heat and damp causing dysentery: taiyang and yangming disease. Symptoms include fever, thirst, or burning anus.

T red, yellow coat

P rapid, slippery

GE GEN HUANG LIAN HUANG QIN TANG

Kudzu, Coptis, and Scutellaria Decoction

Extract Formula Name: Pueraria, Coptis and Scute Combination

Ge Gen	*Pueraria*	12 - 15 g
Huang Lian	*Coptis*	9 g
Huang Qin	*Scutellaria*	6 - 9 g
Gan Cao	*Glycyrrhiza*	3 - 6 g

Blood and phlegm stagnation in the uterus leading to masses or lumps, amenorrhea, dysmenorrhea, or restless fetus.

T purple, sticky coat

P wiry, slippery, choppy

GUI ZHI FU LING WAN

Cinnamon Twig and Poria Pill

Extract Formula Name: Cinnamon and Hoelen Formula

Gui Zhi	*Cinnamomum*	6 - 12 g
Fu Ling	*Poria*	6 - 12 g
Mu Dan Pi	*Paeonia*	6 - 12 g
Tao Ren	*Prunus*	6 - 12 g
Chi Shao Yao	*Paeonia*	9 - 12 g

Phlegm accumulation causing hardenings; or Liver qi stagnation leading to goiter or cancer.

T sticky coat

P slippery, wiry

HAI ZAO YU HU TANG

Sargassum Decoction for the Jade Flask

Hai Zao	*Sargassum*	3 - 6 g
Kun Bu	*Laminaria*	3 - 6 g
Hai Dai	*Laminaria*	1.5 g
Du Huo	*Angelica*	3 - 6 g
Lian Qiao	*Forsythia*	3 - 6 g
Zhe Bei Mu	*Fritillaria*	3 - 6 g
Chuan Xiong	*Ligusticum*	3 - 6 g
Ban Xia	*Pinellia*	3 - 6 g
Dang Gui	*Angelica*	3 - 6 g
Chen Pi	*Citrus*	3 - 6 g
Qing Pi	*Citrus*	3 - 6 g
Gan Cao	*Glycyrrhiza*	3 - 6 g

Cold in the Spleen/Stomach after ingestion of cold food with damp and qi stagnation in the center. Symptoms include lack of appetite, loose stools, or nausea and vomiting.

T pale, sticky white coat

P weak, deep, or tight

HOU PO WEN ZHONG TANG

Magnolia Bark Decoction for Warming the Middle

Extract Formula Name: Magnolia and Saussurea Combination

Hou Po	*Magnolia*	30 g
Gan Jiang	*Zingiber*	2 g
Mu Xiang	*Saussurea*	15 g
Chen Pi	*Citrus*	30 g
Fu Ling	*Poria*	15 g
Cao Dou Kou	*Alpinia*	15 g
Zhi Gan Cao	*Glycyrrhiza*	15 g
[Sheng Jiang —	*Zingiber*	3 g]

Wind damp heat invasion affecting the middle jiao causing recurring fevers and slight thirst.

T sticky yellowish coat, moist

P moderate

HUANG QIN HUA SHI TANG

Scutellaria and Talcum Decoction

Huang Qin	*Scutellaria*	6 - 9g
Hua Shi	*Talcum*	6 - 12 g
Bai Dou Kou	*Amomum*	1 - 3 g
Da Fu Pi	*Areca*	3 - 6 g
Fu Ling Pi	*Poria*	6 - 9 g
Zhu Ling	*Polyporus*	6 - 9 g
Tong Cao	*Tetrapanax*	3 - 6 g

Wind damp heat invasion with internal pre-existing damp accumulation and qi/yang deficiency.

T thin sticky white coat

P slippery, soggy, slightly slow

HUO PO XIA LING TANG

Agastache, Magnolia Bark, Pinellia, and Poria Decoction

Huo Xiang	*Agastache*	6 g
Hou Po	*Magnolia*	3 g
Ban Xia	*Pinellia*	4.5 g
Chi Fu Ling	*Poria*	9 g
Zhu Ling	*Polyporus*	4.5 g
Dan Dou Chi	*Glycine*	9 g
Ze Xie	*Alisma*	4.5 g
Bai Dou Kou	*Amomum*	2 g
Yi Yi Ren	*Coix*	12 g
Xing Ren	*Prunus*	9 g

Wind cold and damp accumulation, with qi stagnation in the middle jiao causing diarrhea, nausea, vomiting, headache, or fever and chills.

T white sticky coat

P soggy or slippery

☞ All ingredients should be ground into a powder. Take 6 g two to three times a day.

HUO XIANG ZHENG QI SAN

Agastache Powder to Rectify the Qi

Extract Formula Name: Agastache Formula

Huo Xiang	*Agastache*	9 g
Hou Po	*Magnolia*	6 - 9 g
Bai Zhi	*Angelica*	3 - 6 g
Zi Su Ye	*Perilla*	3 - 6 g
Chen Pi	*Citrus*	6 g
Bai Zhu	*Atractylodes*	6 g
Fu Ling	*Poria*	3 - 6 g
Ban Xia	*Pinellia*	6 g
Da Fu Pi	*Areca*	3 - 6 g
Jie Geng	*Platycodon*	6 g
Gan Cao	*Glycyrrhiza*	6 - 9 g
[Da Zao	*Ziziphus*	1 - 3 g]
[Sheng Jiang	*Zingiber*	3 - 6 g]

Heated water/phlegm in the Stomach and Large Intestines with qi stagnation causing edema with dyspnea, or a dry mouth.

T red, sticky yellow coat

P rapid, slippery

✘ Do not use during pregnancy.

JI JIAO LI HUANG WAN

Stephania, Zanthoxylum, Lepidium, and Rhubarb Pill

Extract Formula Name: Stephania and Lepidium Formula

Han Fang Ji	*Stephania*	3 g
Chuan Jiao	*Zanthoxylum*	3 g
Da Huang	*Rheum*	3 g
Ting Li Zi	*Lepidium*	3 g

Watery fluids in the Lungs and Spleen yang deficiency causing cough, wheezing, and a stuffy sensation in the chest.

T pale, sticky or slippery white coat

P slippery, wiry

LING GAN WU WEI JIANG XIN TANG

Poria, Licorice, Schisandra, Ginger, and Asarum Decoction

Fu Ling	*Poria*	6 - 12 g
Gan Cao	*Glycyrrhiza*	3 - 9 g
Wu Wei Zi	*Schisandra*	6 - 9 g
Gan Jiang	*Zingiber*	3 - 9 g
Xi Xin	*Asarum*	6 - 9 g

Spleen/Stomach yang deficiency causing phlegm accumulation which affects the Lungs; or taiyang disease was mistreated and guided into the Spleen leading to water accumulation. Symptoms include dyspnea, clear phlegm expectoration, and fullness in the chest and flanks.

T pale, slippery white coat

P slippery, weak, deep

LING GUI ZHU GAN TANG

Poria, Cinnamon Twig, Atractylodes, and Licorice Decoction

Extract Formula Name: Hoelen and Atractylodes Combination

Fu Ling	*Poria*	6 - 12 g
Gui Zhi	*Cinnamomum*	3 - 9 g
Bai Zhu	*Atractylodes*	6 - 9 g
Gan Cao	*Glycyrrhiza*	3 - 6 g

Spleen/Stomach qi deficiency with mild damp symptoms including decreased appetite, middle jiao distention, or nausea and vomiting.

T pale, thin sticky coat

P weak, slightly slippery

LIU JUN ZI TANG

Six-Gentlemen Decoction

Extract Formula Name: Six Major Herbs Combination

Ren Shen	*Panax*	6 - 9 g
Bai Zhu	*Atractylodes*	6 - 9 g
Fu Ling	*Poria*	6 - 9 g
Chen Pi	*Citrus*	3 - 6 g
Ban Xia	*Pinellia*	6 - 9 g
Gan Cao	*Glycyrrhiza*	3 - 6 g

Spleen deficiency with damp which is turning to heat in the middle jiao; or Stomach/Spleen deficiency causing a lack of fluids which leads to deficiency type heat.

T pale or red, sticky coat

P slippery, weak, thin

LIU SHEN SAN

Six-Miracle Powder from Standards of Patterns and Treatments

Ren Shen	*Panax*	6 - 9 g
Bai Zhu	*Atractylodes*	3 - 9 g
Fu Ling	*Poria*	6 - 9 g
Bian Dou	*Dolichos*	6 - 9 g
Huang Qi	*Astragalus*	6 - 12 g
Gan Cao	*Glycyrrhiza*	3 - 6 g
[Sheng Jiang	*Zingiber*	1 - 2 pc]
[Da Zao	*Ziziphus*	1 - 2 pc]

Damp heat in the lower jiao, or Liver fire. Symptoms include red and itchy eyes, temple headaches, odorous leukorrhea, or pruritus.

T red, sticky yellow coating

P wiry, rapid, slippery

LONG DAN XIE GAN TANG

Gentiana Decoction to Drain the Liver

Extract Formula Name: Gentiana Combination

Long Dan Cao	*Gentiana*	6 - 9 g
Zhi Zi	*Gardenia*	3 - 9 g
Mu Tong	*Akebia*	6 - 9 g
Huang Qin	*Scutellaria*	6 - 9 g
Ze Xie	*Alisma*	6 - 9 g
Che Qian Zi	*Plantago*	6 - 9 g
Dang Gui	*Angelica*	6 - 9 g
Sheng Di Huang	*Rehmannia*	6 - 12 g
Chai Hu	*Bupleurum*	6 - 9 g
Gan Cao	*Glycyrrhiza*	3 - 6 g

Stomach/Spleen deficiency with cold damp and middle jiao qi stagnation causing fullness and distention.

T thick sticky white coat

P slippery

PING WEI SAN

Calm the Stomach Powder

Extract Formula Name: Magnolia and Ginger Formula

Hou Po	*Magnolia*	6 - 12 g
Cang Zhu	*Atractylodes*	9 - 15 g
Chen Pi	*Citrus*	6 - 12 g
Gan Cao	*Glycyrrhiza*	3 - 6 g
[Da Zao	*Ziziphus*	3 - 6 pc]
[Sheng Jiang	*Zingiber*	3 - 6 g]

Phlegm damp leading to infertility or leukorrhea.

T thick sticky white coat

P slippery or soggy

QI GONG WAN

Open Uterus Pill

Ban Xia	*Pinellia*	6 - 9 g
Fu Ling	*Poria*	6 - 9 g
Cang Zhu	*Atractylodes*	6 - 9 g
Shen Qu	*Massa Fermentata*	6 - 12 g
Chen Pi	*Citrus*	3 - 6 g
Xiang Fu	*Cyperus*	6 - 9 g
Chuan Xiong	*Ligusticum*	3 - 6 g

Wind phlegm attacking the channels, especially the head and face with pre-existing qi and yang deficiency. This leads to paralysis, facial twitches, stiff muscles, spasms, or loose stools.

T pale, swollen, teethmarks, thick sticky coat

P slippery, deep, frail

✘ The formula is toxic and should not be taken over a long period of time. Do not use during pregnancy.

QIAN ZHENG SAN

Lead to Symmetry Powder

Jiang Can	*Bombyx*	6 g
Bai Fu Zi	*Typhonium*	6 g
Quan Xie	*Buthus*	6 g

Spleen qi deficiency with damp leading to diarrhea and irregular periods. Other symptoms include weight loss, fatigue, poor appetite, or pale face.

T pale, white coat

P weak or thin

SHEN LING BAI ZHU SAN

Ginseng, Poria, and Atractylodes Powder

Extract Formula Name: Ginseng and Atractylodes Formula

Ren Shen	*Panax*	9 - 15 g
Fu Ling	*Poria*	9 - 12 g
Bai Zhu	*Atractylodes*	3 - 9 g
Gan Cao	*Glycyrrhiza*	6 - 9 g
Lian Zi	*Nelumbo*	3 - 9 g
Yi Yi Ren	*Coix*	6 - 15 g
Shan Yao	*Dioscorea*	9 - 15 g
Bian Dou	*Dolichos*	6 - 9 g
Jie Geng	*Platycodon*	3 - 6 g
Sha Ren	*Amomum*	3 g

Damp heat in the lower jiao. Odorous leukorrhea, cloudy urine, and painful swollen feet.

T red, sticky yellow coat

P slippery, rapid

SI MIAO SAN

Four-Marvel Powder

Cang Zhu	*Atractylodes*	6 - 9 g
Huang Bai	*Phellodendron*	6 - 9 g
Yi Yi Ren	*Coix*	6 - 12 g
Huai Niu Xi	*Achyranthes*	6 - 12 g

Spleen qi deficiency with damp and watery leukorrhea, edema, or cramping pain. Other symptoms include loose stools, and urinary retention.

T sticky white coat

P weak, slippery

WEI LING TANG

Calm the Stomach and Poria Decoction

Extract Formula Name: Magnolia and Hoelen Combination

Ze Xie	*Alisma*	6 - 12 g
Zhu Ling	*Polyporus*	6 - 9 g
Fu Ling	*Poria*	6 - 9 g
Bai Zhu	*Atractylodes*	3 - 9 g
Gui Zhi	*Cinnamomum*	3 - 9 g
Hou Po	*Magnolia*	6 - 12 g
Cang Zhu	*Atractylodes*	3 - 9 g
Chen Pi	*Citrus*	3 - 6 g
Sheng Jiang	*Zingiber*	3 - 6 g
Da Zao	*Ziziphus*	3 - 6 pc
Gan Cao	*Glycyrrhiza*	3 - 6 g

Wind cold with internal damp causing a common cold without sweating. Stomach flu, heaviness in the head, cold intolerance, or nausea and vomiting may also be present.

T white sticky coat

P superficial

XIANG RU SAN

Elsholtzia Powder

Extract Formula Name: Elsholtzia Combination

Xiang Ru	*Elsholtzia*	9 - 12 g
Hou Po	*Magnolia*	9 - 12 g
Bian Dou	*Dolichos*	6 - 9 g

Spleen/Stomach qi deficiency with qi stagnation and cold damp in the middle jiao causing abdominal fullness or morning sickness.

T pale, light purple, swollen, sticky white coat

P slippery, weak

XIANG SHA LIU JUN ZI TANG

Six-Gentlemen Decoction with Aucklandia and Amomum

Extract Formula Name: Saussurea and Cardamon Combination

Ren Shen	*Panax*	6 - 9 g
Fu Ling	*Poria*	6 - 9 g
Bai Zhu	*Atractylodes*	3 - 9 g
Chen Pi	*Citrus*	3 - 6 g
Ban Xia	*Pinellia*	6 - 9 g
Sha Ren	*Amomum*	3 g
Mu Xiang	*Saussurea*	3 - 6 g
Zhi Gan Cao	*Glycyrrhiza*	3 - 6 g

Spleen and Stomach qi deficiency with damp accumulation. Symptoms include fullness, nausea and vomiting, loose stools, poor appetite, or morning sickness.

T pale, thin sticky white coat

P slippery, weak

XIANG SHA YANG WEI TANG

Nourish the Stomach Decoction with Aucklandia and Amomum

Extract Formula Name: Cyperus and Cluster Combination

Xiang Fu	*Cyperus*	6 - 9 g
Bai Dou Kou	*Amomum*	3 - 6 g
Sha Ren	*Amomum*	3 - 6 g
Mu Xiang	*Saussurea*	3 - 6 g
Bai Zhu	*Atractylodes*	6 - 9 g
Fu Ling	*Poria*	6 - 9 g
Chen Pi	*Citrus*	3 - 6 g
Dang Shen	*Codonopsis*	9 - 12 g
Hou Po	*Magnolia*	6 - 12 g
Cang Zhu	*Atractylodes*	3 - 9 g
Sheng Jiang	*Zingiber*	3 - 6 g
Da Zao	*Ziziphus*	3 - 6 pc
Zhi Gan Cao	*Glycyrrhiza*	3 - 6 g

Spleen qi and yang deficiency with damp and water accumulation causing loose stools with undigested food.

T pale, swollen, teethmarks, white sticky coat

P weak, deep, or frail

XIAO BAN XIA TANG

Minor Pinellia Decoction

Ban Xia	*Pinellia*	6 - 9 g
Sheng Jiang	*Zingiber*	3 - 6 g

Goiter, scrofula, and lumps due to yin deficieny with false heat. The false heat dries the fluids and causes phlegm accumulation.

T red, coat

P rapid, slippery, or wiry

XIAO LUO WAN

Reduce Scrofula Pill

Chuan Bei Mu	*Fritillaria*	6 - 12 g
Mu Li	*Ostrea*	6 - 12 g
Xuan Shen	*Scrophularia*	6 - 12 g

Phlegm heat in the chest (Heart), or epigastrium (Stomach) leading to bronchitis, constipation, distending pain or pressure in the chest, numbness, or bitter taste.

T red, sticky yellow coat

P rapid, slippery

XIAO XIAN XIONG TANG

Minor Sinking Into the Chest Decoction

Extract Formula Name: Minor Trichosanthes Combination

Gua Lou	*Trichosanthes*	20 g
Huang Lian	*Coptis*	3 g
Ban Xia	*Pinellia*	6 - 9 g

Phlegm accumulation with Stomach qi deficiency causing hiccups, fullness, or nausea and vomiting.

T pale, white sticky coat

P frail, slippery, or wiry

☞ Xuan Fu Hua - Inula should be wrapped in a cheese cloth for decoction.

XUAN FU DAI ZHE TANG

Inula and Hematite Decoction

Extract Formula Name: Inula and Hematite Combination

Xuan Fu Hua	*Inula*	6 - 9 g
Dai Zhe Shi	*Haematitum*	6 - 12 g
Ren Shen	*Panax*	6 - 9 g
Ban Xia	*Pinellia*	6 - 9 g
Da Zao	*Ziziphus*	3 - 6 pc
Sheng Jiang	*Zingiber*	6 - 9 g
Zhi Gan Cao	*Glycyrrhiza*	3 - 6 g

Qi/blood/yang deficient patient gets a cold which leads to damp and phlegm accumulation in the channels, muscles, organs, or under the skin, causing swollen joints with atrophy, scrofula, or multiple abscesses.

T pale, thick sticky white coat

P weak, thin, deep

YANG HE TANG

Yang-Heartening Decoction

Shu Di Huang	*Rehmannia*	20 - 30 g
Rou Gui	*Cinnamomum*	6 - 9 g
Bai Jie Zi	*Brassica*	3 - 6 g
Lu Jiao Jiao	*Cervus*	9 - 12 g
Pao Jiang	*Zingiber*	1 - 3 g
Ma Huang	*Ephedra*	1 - 3 g
Gan Cao	*Glycyrrhiza*	3 - 6 g

Damp accumulation draining downward leading to clear white leukorrhea.

T swollen, thick white coat

P slippery

YI ZHI TANG

Boosting Wisdom Decoction

Bai Zhu	*Atractylodes*	9 g
Fu Ling	*Poria*	9 g
Chen Pi	*Citrus*	6 g
Cang Zhu	*Atractylodes*	6 g
Yi Yi Ren	*Coix*	6 g
Chai Hu	*Bupleurum*	6 g
Sheng Ma	*Cimicifuga*	2 g
Zhi Gan Cao	*Glycyrrhiza*	3 g

Damp heat accumulation in the middle jiao (Liver/Gallbladder) causing yang jaundice, dysurea, or hepatitis with mild fever.

T slightly red, thick sticky coat

P slippery, slightly rapid

YIN CHEN WU LING SAN

Artemisia Yinchenhao and Five-Ingredient Powder with Poria

Extract Formula Name: Capillaris and Hoelen Five Formula

Yin Chen Hao	*Artemisia*	10 - 20 g
Fu Ling	*Poria*	6 - 12 g
Zhu Ling	*Polyporus*	6 - 9 g
Bai Zhu	*Atractylodes*	3 - 9 g
Ze Xie	*Alisma*	6 - 9 g
Gui Zhi	*Cinnamomum*	3 - 9 g

Cold damp has entered the Spleen leading to water accumulation and Spleen yang deficiency. This causes damp in the middle jiao which bothers the Gallbladder so the bile cannot circulate properly. This manifests as yin-type jaundice.

T pale, white coat

P weak, deep

YIN CHEN ZHU FU TANG

Artemisia Yinchenhao, Atractylodes and Prepared Aconite Decoction

Extract Formula Name: Capillaris, Atractylodes and Aconite Combination

Yin Chen Hao	*Artemisia*	3-6 g
Gan Jiang	*Zingiber*	3-6 g
Bai Zhu	*Atractylodes*	6-9 g
Rou Gui	*Cinnamomum*	1-3 g
Fu Zi	*Aconitum*	1-3 g
Zhi Gan Cao	*Glycyrrhiza*	3-6 g

Stagnations of all kinds (qi, blood, food, damp, etc.). Symptoms include epigastric or chest fullness, nausea and vomiting, or poor appetite.

T depends on particular syndrome involved

P depends on particular syndrome involved

YUE JU WAN

Escape Restraint Pill

Chuan Xiong	*Ligusticum*	3-9 g
Cang Zhu	*Atractylodes*	3-9 g
Zhi Zi	*Gardenia*	3-9 g
Xiang Fu	*Cyperus*	3-9 g
Shen Qu	*Massa Fermentata*	3-9 g

Phlegm accumulation in the middle jiao restricts the Spleen. This leads to more damp and water accumulation which then overflows under the skin leading to edema.

T thick white sticky coat

P deep, slippery

ZHI MI FU LING TANG

Small Finger Poria Decoction

Ban Xia	*Pinellia*	6-15 g
Fu Ling	*Poria*	6-15 g
Zhi Ke	*Citrus*	3-9 g
Mang Xiao	*Mirabilitum*	1-3 g
[Sheng Jiang	*Zingiber*	3-6 g]

Food stagnation in the middle jiao with damp and heat accumulation: cold and heat in the middle jiao with Spleen deficiency. Symptoms include fullness with pain, odorous diarrhea, mucus, tenesmus, gas, or constipation.

T red, red sides, rough, thick sticky yellow coat

P slippery, rapid, forceful

✘ Caution during pregnancy.

ZHI SHI DAO ZHI WAN

Immature Bitter Orange Pill to Guide Out Stagnation

Extract Formula Name: Chih-shih and Rhubarb Formula

Zhi Shi	*Citrus*	9 - 15 g
Shen Qu	*Massa Fermentata*	9 - 15 g
Da Huang	*Rheum*	15 - 25 g
Huang Qin	*Scutellaria*	6 - 9 g
Huang Lian	*Coptis*	6 - 9 g
Fu Ling	*Poria*	6 - 9 g
Ze Xie	*Alisma*	6 - 9 g
Bai Zhu	*Atractylodes*	6 - 9 g

Damp heat accumulation in the middle jiao. There is more damp than heat causing fullness in the abdomen, thirst without desire to drink, or immediate fullness upon eating or drinking. This formula is also useful for yang jaundice.

T red, thick sticky coat

P slippery, rapid

ZHONG JIAO XIAN BI TANG

Middle Jiao and Clear Damp Decoction

Xing Ren	*Prunus*	3 - 6 g
Yi Yi Ren	*Coix*	9 - 12 g
Hua Shi	*Talcum*	6 g
Dou Juan	*Glycine*	9 g
Zhi Zi	*Gardenia*	6 - 9 g
Lian Qiao	*Forsythia*	6 g
Ban Xia	*Pinellia*	6 - 9 g
Han Fang Ji	*Stephania*	6 - 9 g
Can Sha	*Bombyx*	3 - 6 g
Shan Zha	*Crataegus*	3 - 9 g
Bian Dou	*Dolichos*	6 - 9 g

ACCUMULATION OF YING (WATER)

- borborygmus
- fullness sensation in the epigastrium or abdomen
- edema

T wet, or white sticky coat

P slippery

Disharmony between Stomach and Intestines which leads to failure to descend qi which, subsequently, leads to food, damp, or water accumulation (or heat and cold accumulation in the Stomach). This is known as glomus and fullness (pi man). Symptoms include epigastric fullness, gurgling, reflux or loose stools.

T yellow sticky coat

P wiry, rapid

BAN XIA XIE XIN TANG

Pinellia Decoction to Drain the Epigastrium

Extract Formula Name: Pinellia Combination

Ban Xia	*Pinellia*	6 - 12 g
Huang Qin	*Scutellaria*	6 - 9 g
Huang Lian	*Coptis*	3 - 6 g
Gan Jiang	*Zingiber*	3 - 6 g
Ren Shen	*Panax*	6 - 9 g
Da Zao	*Ziziphus*	3 - 5 pc
Gan Cao	*Glycyrrhiza*	3 - 6 g

Shaoyang disease with water and damp accumulation causing fullness in the hypochondriac area, malaria symptoms, and more chills than fever.

T thin white coat

P wiry

CHAI HU GUI ZHI GAN JIANG TANG

Bupleurum, Cinnamon Twig, and Ginger Decoction

Extract Formula Name: Bupleurum, Cinnamon and Ginger Combination

Chai Hu	*Bupleurum*	6 - 12 g
Gui Zhi	*Cinnamomum*	6 - 9 g
Gan Jiang	*Zingiber*	6 - 9 g
Huang Qin	*Scutellaria*	6 - 9 g
Mu Li	*Ostrea*	6 - 9 g
Tian Hua Fen	*Trichosanthes*	9 - 12 g
Gan Cao	*Glycyrrhiza*	3 - 6 g

Wind cold invasion which has turned to heat and entered the shaoyang level leading to water accumulation in the hypochondriac region.

T red tip, thin yellow coat

P superficial or wiry

CHAI ZHI BAN XIA TANG

Bupleurum, Bitter Orange and Pinellia Decoction

Chai Hu	*Bupleurum*	9 - 15 g
Zhi Ke	*Citrus*	3 - 9 g
Ban Xia	*Pinellia*	6 - 12 g
Huang Qin	*Scutellaria*	6 - 15 g
Jie Geng	*Platycodon*	3 - 6 g
Xing Ren	*Prunus*	6 - 9 g
Qing Pi	*Citrus*	3 - 9 g
Gan Cao	*Glycyrrhiza*	3 - 6 g

Kidney qi and yang deficiency causing edema which manifests mostly in the superficial and muscle layers.

T pale, swollen, sticky white coat

P weak, deep, slippery

FANG JI FU LING TANG

Stephania and Poria Decoction

Extract Formula Name: Stephania and Hoelen Combination

Han Fang Ji	*Stephania*	9 - 12 g
Fu Ling	*Poria*	9 - 18 g
Gui Zhi	*Cinnamomum*	9 - 12 g
Huang Qi	*Astragalus*	9 - 12 g
Gan Cao	*Glycyrrhiza*	3 - 6 g

Wind edema or wind damp with Spleen and wei qi deficiency causing sweating, urinary difficulty, or edema in the superficial layer.

T pale, thin white coat

P superficial

FANG JI HUANG QI TANG

Stephania and Astragalus Decoction

Extract Formula Name: Stephania and Astragalus Combination

Han Fang Ji	*Stephania*	9 - 12 g
Huang Qi	*Astragalus*	9 - 15 g
Bai Zhu	*Atractylodes*	6 - 9 g
Sheng Jiang	*Zingiber*	3 - 6 g
Da Zao	*Ziziphus*	3 - 4 pc
Gan Cao	*Glycyrrhiza*	3 - 6 g

Damp/water accumulation in the middle jiao causing abdominal fullness, ascites, or scanty urination.

T sticky white coat

P slippery

FEN XIAO TANG

Separate and Reduce Decoction

Extract Formula Name: Hoelen and Alisma Combination

Cang Zhu	*Atractylodes*	3 - 6 g
Bai Zhu	*Atractylodes*	3 - 6 g
Hou Po	*Magnolia*	6 - 9 g
Fu Ling	*Poria*	6 - 9 g
Chen Pi	*Citrus*	3 - 6 g
Zhu Ling	*Polyporus*	3 - 6 g
Deng Xin Cao	*Juncus*	1 pc
Ze Xie	*Alisma*	3 - 6 g
Xiang Fu	*Cyperus*	3 - 6 g
Mu Xiang	*Saussurea*	3 - 6 g
Zhi Shi	*Citrus*	3 - 6 g
Sha Ren	*Amomum*	1 - 3 g
Da Fu Pi	*Areca*	3 - 6 g
Sheng Jiang	*Zingiber*	3 - 6 g

Water accumulation in the middle jiao which restricts the Spleen function causing abdominal or epigastric fullness, borborygmus, fatigue, loose stools, or decreased appetite.

T pink or pale, wet

P slippery

FU LING GAN CAO TANG

Poria and Licorice Decoction

Extract Formula Name: Licorice and Hoelen Combination

Fu Ling	*Poria*	6 g
Gui Zhi	*Cinnamomum*	6 g
Sheng Jiang	*Zingiber*	9 g
Gan Cao	*Glycyrrhiza*	3 g

Heated water/phlegm in the Stomach and Large Intestines with qi stagnation causing edema with dyspnea, or a dry mouth.

T red, sticky yellow coat

P rapid, slippery

✘ Do not use during pregnancy.

JI JIAO LI HUANG WAN

Stephania, Zanthoxylum, Lepidium, and Rhubarb Pill

Extract Formula Name: Stephania and Lepidium Formula

Han Fang Ji	Stephania	3 g
Chuan Jiao	Zanthoxylum	3 g
Da Huang	Rheum	3 g
Ting Li Zi	Lepidium	3 g

Kidney yang deficiency causing edema, scanty urination, or benign prostate hypertrophy.

T pale, swollen, teethmarks, white sticky coat

P deep, wiry, slippery, thin

JI SHENG SHEN QI WAN

Kidney Qi Pill from Formulas to Aid the Living

Shu Di Huang	Rehmannia	6 - 12 g
Shan Yao	Dioscorea	6 - 12 g
Shan Zhu Yu	Cornus	6 - 9 g
Mu Dan Pi	Paeonia	6 - 12 g
Ze Xie	Alisma	6 - 9 g
Fu Ling	Poria	6 - 9 g
Fu Zi	Aconitum	6 - 9 g
Rou Gui	Cinnamomum	3 - 9 g
Che Qian Zi	Plantago	6 - 9 g
Chuan Niu Xi	Cyathula	6 - 9 g

Watery fluids in the Lungs and Spleen yang deficiency causing cough, wheezing, and a stuffy sensation in the chest.

T pale, sticky or slippery white coat

P slippery, wiry

LING GAN WU WEI JIANG XIN TANG

Poria, Licorice, Schisandra, Ginger, and Asarum Decoction

Fu Ling	Poria	6 - 12 g
Gan Cao	Glycyrrhiza	3 - 9 g
Wu Wei Zi	Schisandra	6 - 9 g
Gan Jiang	Zingiber	3 - 9 g
Xi Xin	Asarum	6 - 9 g

Heart yang is not warmed by the Kidneys leading to water accumulation which rises upwards causing abdominal pain, angina, Stomach cramping, tingling sensation in the abdomen, (ben ten qi - running piglet sensation), or scanty urine.

T pale, wet, sticky white coat

P deep, weak, slightly slow

LING GUI ZAO GAN TANG

Poria, Cinnamon Twig, Jujube, and Licorice Decoction

Fu Ling	*Poria*	9 - 12 g
Gui Zhi	*Cinnamomum*	3 - 9 g
Da Zao	*Ziziphus*	3 - 4 pc
Gan Cao	*Glycyrrhiza*	3 - 6 g

Spleen/Stomach yang deficiency causing phlegm accumulation which affects the Lungs; or taiyang disease was mistreated and guided into the Spleen leading to water accumulation. Symptoms include dyspnea, clear phlegm expectoration, and fullness in the chest and flanks.

T pale, slippery white coat

P slippery, weak, deep

✪ Major Formula

LING GUI ZHU GAN TANG

Poria, Cinnamon Twig, Atractylodes, and Licorice Decoction

Extract Formula Name: Hoelen and Atractylodes Combination

Fu Ling	*Poria*	6 - 12 g
Gui Zhi	*Cinnamomum*	3 - 9 g
Bai Zhu	*Atractylodes*	6 - 9 g
Gan Cao	*Glycyrrhiza*	3 - 6 g

Wind cold with pre-existing damp causing wind cold edema, and a headache which feels as if there is a belt around the head.

T white coat

P superficial, maybe slippery

MA HUANG JIA ZHU TANG

Ephedra Decoction plus Atractylodes

Ma Huang	*Ephedra*	6 - 9 g
Xing Ren	*Prunus*	6 - 9 g
Gui Zhi	*Cinnamomum*	3 - 6 g
Gan Cao	*Glycyrrhiza*	3 - 6 g
Bai Zhu	*Atractylodes*	6 - 9 g

Wind cold causes facial edema and scanty urination. This formula is also useful for jaundice accompanied by taiyang symptoms.

T thin white coat

P superficial, tight

MA HUANG LIAN QIAO CHI XIAO DOU TANG

Ephedra, Forsythia, and Aduki Bean Decoction

Ma Huang	*Ephedra*	3 - 9 g
Lian Qiao	*Forsythia*	6 - 9 g
Chi Xiao Dou	*Phaseolus*	6 - 9 g
Sang Bai Pi	*Morus*	6 - 9 g
Xing Ren	*Prunus*	6 - 9 g
Sheng Jiang	*Zingiber*	3 - 6 g
Da Zao	*Ziziphus*	3 - 4 pc
Gan Cao	*Glycyrrhiza*	3 - 6 g

Skin edema due to Spleen-deficiency with abdominal fullness.

T pale, swollen, teethmarks, white coat

P weak

QI PI YIN

Seven-Peel Decoction

Fu Ling Pi	*Poria*	9 g
Chen Pi	*Citrus*	3 - 9 g
Da Fu Pi	*Areca*	3 - 9 g
Di Gu Pi	*Lycium*	9 g
Sheng Jiang Pi	*Zingiber*	3 - 9 g
Qing Pi	*Citrus*	3 - 9 g
Gan Cao Pi	*Glycyrrhiza*	3 - 6 g

Cold packs were used on a patient who had a common cold but also an underlying Spleen yang deficiency. Now the cold has moved into deeper layers and caused severe cold stagnation with water accumulation under the Heart. Symptoms include shortness of breath, watery sputum, angina, or stuffiness in the chest.

T pale, wet

P slow, slightly slippery

✘ Ba Dou - Croton is extremely toxic and should be used with extreme caution. Do not use during pregnancy.

SAN WU BAI SAN

Three-White Herbs Powder

Jie Geng	*Platycodon*	3 - 6 g
Bei Mu	*Fritillaria*	6 - 12 g
Ba Dou	*Croton*	1 - 3 g

Water accumulation with heat, damp and qi stagnation; or Stomach deficiency with food stagnation and water. Symptoms include diarrhea, borborygmus, or epigastric distention.

T red, sticky yellow coat

P slippery, rapid

SHENG JIANG XIE XIN TANG

Fresh Ginger Decoction to Drain the Epigastrium

Extract Formula Name: Pinellia and Ginger Combination

Sheng Jiang	*Zingiber*	9 - 12 g
Ban Xia	*Pinellia*	6 - 9 g
Ren Shen	*Panax*	6 - 12 g
Gan Jiang	*Zingiber*	3 - 6 g
Huang Qin	*Scutellaria*	6 - 9 g
Huang Lian	*Coptis*	3 - 6 g
Da Zao	*Ziziphus*	6 - 10 pc
Gan Cao	*Glycyrrhiza*	3 - 6 g

Spleen/Kidney qi and yang deficiency causing edema which manifests mostly in the lower body. Other symptoms include cold limbs, poor appetite, decreased urination, or heaviness.

T pale, sticky coat

P deep, slow, maybe thin

SHI PI YIN

Bolster the Spleen Decoction

Extract Brion Name: Magnolia and Atractylodes Combination

Fu Zi	*Aconitum*	6 - 9 g
Bai Zhu	*Atractylodes*	6 - 9 g
Mu Gua	*Chaenomeles*	6 - 9 g
Hou Po	*Magnolia*	6 - 12 g
Gan Jiang	*Zingiber*	6 - 9 g
Mu Xiang	*Saussurea*	6 - 9 g
Fu Ling	*Poria*	6 - 9 g
Da Fu Pi	*Areca*	3 - 6 g
Cao Guo	*Amomum*	3 - 6 g
Zhi Gan Cao	*Glycyrrhiza*	3 - 6 g
[Da Zao	*Ziziphus*	1 - 3 pc]
[Sheng Jiang	*Zingiber*	3 - 6 g]

Heart/Gallbladder qi deficiency with edema in the extremities, tight chest, palpitations, anxiety, or timidity.

T pale

P weak

SHI WEI WEN DAN TANG

Ten-Ingredient Decoction to Warm the Gallbladder

Ban Xia	*Pinellia*	6 - 9 g
Chen Pi	*Citrus*	3 - 6 g
Zhi Shi	*Citrus*	6 g
Fu Ling	*Poria*	6 g
Ren Shen	*Panax*	3 - 6 g
Suan Zao Ren	*Ziziphus*	3 - 6 g
Shu Di Huang	*Rehmannia*	3 - 9 g
Wu Wei Zi	*Schisandra*	3 - 6 g
Yuan Zhi	*Polygala*	3 - 6 g
Zhi Gan Cao	*Glycyrrhiza*	3 g
Da Zao	*Ziziphus*	2 pc
Sheng Jiang	*Zingiber*	5 pc

Chronic water accumulation in the chest and hypochondrium causing cough and shortness of breath.

T white sticky coat

P deep, wiry

☞ Grind ingredients into a powder and take in 0.7 g doses in the morning with a warm tea made from ten pieces of Da Zao - Ziziphus. Between five and six bowel movements are expected after each dose.

✘ Do not use during pregnancy or in weak patients. Gan Sui - Euphorbia is toxic.

SHI ZAO TANG

Ten-Jujube Decoction

Extract Formula Name: Jujube Combination

Gan Sui	*Euphorbia*	6 g
Yuan Hua	*Daphne*	6 g
Jing Da Ji	*Euphorbia*	6 g

Damp heat accumulation causing edema.

T Swollen, white or sticky coat

P rapid, slippery

✘ This formula is slightly toxic due to the ingredient Shang Lu - Phytolacca. This prescription should not be taken during pregnancy.

SHU ZUO YIN ZI

Decoction for Diuresis

Extract Formula Name: Alisma and Areca Combination

Qiang Huo	*Notopterygium*	6 - 9 g
Qin Jiao	*Gentiana*	9 - 12 g
Da Fu Pi	*Areca*	6 - 9 g
Fu Ling Pi	*Poria*	20 - 40 g
Shang Lu	*Phytolacca*	3 - 6 g
Mu Tong	*Akebia*	9 - 12 g
Ze Xie	*Alisma*	9 - 15 g
Chi Xiao Dou	*Phaseolus*	15 - 30 g
Chuan Jiao	*Zanthoxylum*	6 - 9 g
Sheng Jiang	*Zingiber*	3 - 6 g

Spleen/Stomach deficiency with mild damp causing loose stools or urinary retention.

T pale, sticky white coat

P slippery, weak

SI LING SAN

Four-Ingredient Powder with Poria

Zhu Ling	*Polyporus*	6 - 9 g
Fu Ling	*Poria*	6 - 9 g
Ze Xie	*Alisma*	6 - 9 g
Bai Zhu	*Atractylodes*	3 - 9 g

Lung phlegm fluid causing eye/facial edema, cough or asthma, or Lung abscess with phlegm.

T sticky white coat

P slippery

TING LI DA ZAO XIE FEI TANG

Lepidium and Jujube Decoction to Drain the Lungs

Extract Formula Name: Lepidium and Jujube Combination

Ting Li Zi	*Lepidium*	6 - 9 g
Da Zao	*Ziziphus*	6 - 12 pc

Spleen qi deficiency with damp and watery leukorrhea, edema, or cramping pain. Other symptoms include loose stools, and urinary retention.

T sticky white coat

P weak, slippery

WEI LING TANG

Calm the Stomach and Poria Decoction

Extract Formula Name: Magnolia and Hoelen Combination

Ze Xie	*Alisma*	6 - 12 g
Zhu Ling	*Polyporus*	6 - 9 g
Fu Ling	*Poria*	6 - 9 g
Bai Zhu	*Atractylodes*	3 - 9 g
Gui Zhi	*Cinnamomum*	3 - 9 g
Hou Po	*Magnolia*	6 - 12 g
Cang Zhu	*Atractylodes*	3 - 9 g
Chen Pi	*Citrus*	3 - 6 g
Sheng Jiang	*Zingiber*	3 - 6 g
Da Zao	*Ziziphus*	3 - 6 pc
Gan Cao	*Glycyrrhiza*	3 - 6 g

Heat and water accumulation in the lower jiao (Bladder) with slight taiyang symptoms (wind cold); or Spleen qi deficiency with damp and water causing edema in the skin or muscle layer.

T sticky white or yellow coat

P slippery or superficial

WU LING SAN

Five-Ingredient Powder with Poria

Extract Formula Name: Hoelen Five Herbs Formula

Fu Ling	*Poria*	6 - 9 g
Zhu Ling	*Polyporus*	6 - 9 g
Ze Xie	*Alisma*	6 - 9 g
Gui Zhi	*Cinnamomum*	3 - 9 g
Bai Zhu	*Atractylodes*	6 - 9 g

Spleen qi deficiency with water/damp and qi stagnation causing edema, dyspnea, or urinary retention.

T pale, swollen, teethmarks, sticky white coat

P slippery

WU PI SAN

Five-Peel Powder

Extract Formula Name: Hoelen and Areca Combination

Sang Bai Pi	*Morus*	6 - 15 g
Sheng Jiang Pi	*Zingiber*	6 - 9 g
Chen Pi	*Citrus*	3 - 9 g
Da Fu Pi	*Areca*	6 - 12 g
Fu Ling Pi	*Poria*	6 - 15 g

Qi and blood stagnation causing chest pain with water/damp accumulation: Liver affects the Lungs. Symptoms include hypochondriac pain, possible coughing, or raspy voice.

T purple, thick sticky coat

P wiry

☞ Xuan Fu Hua - Inula should be wrapped in a cheesecloth.

XIANG FU XUAN FU HUA TANG

Cyperus and Inula Decoction

Xiang Fu	*Cyperus*	6 - 9 g
Xuan Fu Hua	*Inula*	6 - 9 g
Yi Yi Ren	*Coix*	9 - 15 g
Chen Pi	*Citrus*	3 - 6 g
Zi Su Zi	*Perilla*	6 - 9 g
Ban Xia	*Pinellia*	6 - 9 g
Fu Ling	*Poria*	6 - 9 g

Wind cold with internal water accumulation causing profuse phlegm expectoration, bodyaches, or superficial edema.

T moist white coat

P superficial, tight

XIAO QING LONG TANG

Minor Blue Dragon Decoction

Extract Formula Name: Minor Blue Dragon Combination

Ma Huang	*Ephedra*	6 - 9 g
Gui Zhi	*Cinnamomum*	6 - 9 g
Xi Xin	*Asarum*	3 g
Wu Wei Zi	*Schisandra*	6 - 9 g
Gan Jiang	*Zingiber*	3 g
Bai Shao Yao	*Paeonia*	6 - 9 g
Ban Xia	*Pinellia*	6 - 9 g
Gan Cao	*Glycyrrhiza*	3 - 6 g

Cold damp has entered the Spleen leading to water accumulation and Spleen yang deficiency. This causes damp in the middle jiao which bothers the Gallbladder so the bile cannot circulate properly. This manifests as yin-type jaundice.

T pale, white coat

P weak, deep

YIN CHEN ZHU FU TANG

Artemisia Yinchenhao, Atractylodes and Prepared Aconite Decoction

Extract Formula Name: Capillaris, Atractylodes and Aconite Combination

Yin Chen Hao	*Artemisia*	3 - 6 g
Gan Jiang	*Zingiber*	3 - 6 g
Bai Zhu	*Atractylodes*	6 - 9 g
Rou Gui	*Cinnamomum*	1 - 3 g
Fu Zi	*Aconitum*	1 - 3 g
Zhi Gan Cao	*Glycyrrhiza*	3 - 6 g

Wind edema with fever and chills, or decreased urination.

T thin white coat

P superficial, slippery, or deep

YUE BI JIA ZHU TANG

Maidservant from Yue Decoction plus Atractylodes

Extract Formula Name: Atractylodes Combination

Ma Huang	*Ephedra*	6 - 9 g
Shi Gao	*Gypsum*	9 - 20 g
Bai Zhu	*Atractylodes*	6 - 9 g
Sheng Jiang	*Zingiber*	3 - 9 g
Da Zao	*Ziziphus*	3 - 7 pc
Gan Cao	*Glycyrrhiza*	3 - 6 g

Whole body edema due to wind causing wind intolerance, scanty urination, possible sweating, possible fever, or thirst.

T thin white coat

P superficial

YUE BI TANG

Maidservant from Yue Decoction

Extract Formula Name: Ma-Huang and Gypsum Combination

Ma Huang	*Ephedra*	6 - 15 g
Sheng Jiang	*Zingiber*	3 - 9 g
Shi Gao	*Gypsum*	15 - 30 g
Da Zao	*Ziziphus*	6 - 12 pc
Gan Cao	*Glycyrrhiza*	3 - 6 g

Spleen/Kidney qi and yang deficient patient suffers easily from wind cold with internal water accumulation, or experiences urinary difficulty, diarrhea, or edema.

T pale, swollen, teethmarks, moist, thin white coat

P frail or minute

ZHEN WU TANG

True Warrior Decoction

Extract Formula Name: Vitality Combination

Fu Zi	*Aconitum*	6 - 9 g
Bai Zhu	*Atractylodes*	6 - 9 g
Bai Shao Yao	*Paeonia*	6 - 9 g
Fu Ling	*Poria*	6 - 9 g
Sheng Jiang	*Zingiber*	6 - 9 g

Phlegm accumulation in the middle jiao restricts the Spleen. This leads to more damp and water accumulation which then overflows under the skin leading to edema.

T thick white sticky coat

P deep, slippery

ZHI MI FU LING TANG

Small Finger Poria Decoction

Ban Xia	Pinellia	6 - 15 g
Fu Ling	Poria	6 - 15 g
Zhi Ke	Citrus	3 - 9 g
Mang Xiao	Mirabilitum	1 - 3 g
[Sheng Jiang	Zingiber	3 - 6 g]

Severe edema (ascites), water and heat stagnation. This formula is a strong water purgative.

T red, sticky coat

P rapid, deep, forceful

☞ Grind herbs into a powder and take as a 3 - 6 g dose of pills in the morning. Only strong patients may take this dosage more than once.

✘ Do not use during pregnancy or in very weak patients. The formula is highly toxic, and should only be used for a limited time. Do not use with Gan Cao - Glycyrrhiza.

ZHOU CHE WAN

Vessel and Vehicle Pill

Gan Sui	Euphorbia	15 g
Yuan Hua	Daphne	15 g
Qian Niu Zi	Pharbitis	60 g
Jing Da Ji	Euphorbia	15 g
Qing Pi	Citrus	7.5 g
Chen Pi	Citrus	7.5 g
Da Huang	Rheum	30 g
Mu Xiang	Saussurea	7.5 g
Bing Lang	Areca	7.5 g
Qing Fen	Calomelas	1.5 g

SIX DIVISIONS

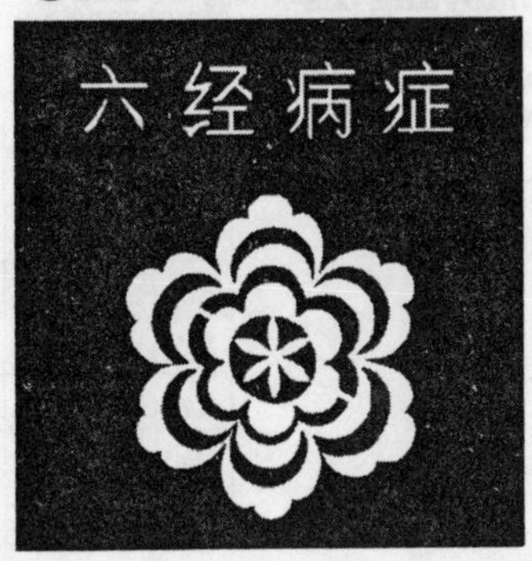

DISEASES IN THE TAIYANG STAGE

Please see WIND INVASIONS

DISEASES IN THE SHAOYANG STAGE

- bitter taste
- alternating chills and fever
- costal pain
- irritability

T white coat

P wiry

Shaoyang and yangming channel disease causing mild chills with severe fever, and thirst.

T red, thin yellow coat

P rapid, maybe flooding

CHAI HU BAI HU TANG

Bupleurum White Tiger Decoction

Chai Hu	*Bupleurum*	3 - 6 g
Huang Qin	*Scutellaria*	3 - 6 g
Shi Gao	*Gypsum*	12 - 20 g
Zhi Mu	*Anemarrhena*	6 - 12 g
Tian Hua Fen	*Trichosanthes*	6 - 9 g
Jing Mi	*Oryza*	6 - 9 g
Gan Cao	*Glycyrrhiza*	3 - 6 g

Phlegm damp obstruction in the chest and epigastrium with a complication of shaoyang disease. Symptoms include alternating fever and chills, bitter taste, or cough with sticky phlegm.

T thick sticky white or yellow coat

P slippery, wiry

CHAI HU DA YUAN YIN

Bupleurum Decoction to Reach the Membrane Source

Zhi Ke	*Citrus*	5 g
Chai Hu	*Bupleurum*	6 - 9 g
Qing Pi	*Citrus*	3 - 6 g
Hou Po	*Magnolia*	6 - 12 g
Huang Qin	*Scutellaria*	6 - 9 g
Cao Guo	*Amomum*	3 - 6 g
He Ye	*Nelumbo*	6 - 15 g
Bing Lang	*Areca*	6 - 9 g
Jie Geng	*Platycodon*	3 - 6 g
Gan Cao	*Glycyrrhiza*	3 - 6 g

Shaoyang disease with water and damp accumulation causing fullness in the hypochondriac area, malaria symptoms, and more chills than fever.

T thin white coat

P wiry

CHAI HU GUI ZHI GAN JIANG TANG

Bupleurum, Cinnamon Twig, and Ginger Decoction

Extract Formula Name: Bupleurum, Cinnamon and Ginger Combination

Chai Hu	*Bupleurum*	6 - 12 g
Gui Zhi	*Cinnamomum*	6 - 9 g
Gan Jiang	*Zingiber*	6 - 9 g
Huang Qin	*Scutellaria*	6 - 9 g
Mu Li	*Ostrea*	6 - 9 g
Tian Hua Fen	*Trichosanthes*	9 - 12 g
Gan Cao	*Glycyrrhiza*	3 - 6 g

Taiyang and shaoyang disease with joint congestion and intolerance to wind, or alternating fever and chills. Also useful for Liver overacting on Spleen.

T thin white coat

P possibly superficial

CHAI HU GUI ZHI TANG

Bupleurum and Cinnamon Twig Decoction

Extract Formula Name: Bupleurum and Cinnamon Combination

Gui Zhi	*Cinnamomum*	3 - 6 g
Chai Hu	*Bupleurum*	6 - 12 g
Ren Shen	*Panax*	3 - 6 g
Ban Xia	*Pinellia*	3 - 6 g
Huang Qin	*Scutellaria*	3 - 9 g
Bai Shao Yao	*Paeonia*	3 - 6 g
Sheng Jiang	*Zingiber*	3 - 6 g
Da Zao	*Ziziphus*	4 - 6 pc
Gan Cao	*Glycyrrhiza*	3 - 6 g

Qi deficient patient gets evil qi invading taiyang, shaoyang, and yangming channels. This causes irritability, constipation, full chest, or heaviness.

T red, sticky coat

P rapid, wiry

☞ Da Huang - Rheum should be added during the last 3 minutes of the decoction process.

✘ Qian Dan - Minium is toxic and should be substituted with Dai Zhe Shi - Haematitum or Sheng Tie Luo - Frusta Ferri. Caution during pregnancy.

CHAI HU JIA LONG GU MU LI TANG

Bupleurum plus Dragon Bone and Oyster Shell Decoction

Extract Formula Name: Bupleurum and D.B. Combination

Chai Hu	*Bupleurum*	9 - 12 g
Huang Qin	*Scutellaria*	6 g
Ren Shen	*Panax*	6 g
Gui Zhi	*Cinnamomum*	3 - 6 g
Ban Xia	*Pinellia*	6 g
Fu Ling	*Poria*	6 g
Da Huang	*Rheum*	6 g
Long Gu	*Os Draconis*	3 - 6 g
Mu Li	*Ostrea*	3 - 6 g
Sheng Jiang	*Zingiber*	3 - 6 g
Da Zao	*Ziziphus*	3 - 6 pc
Qian Dan	*Minium*	1 - 4 g

Shaoyang disorder with constipation, discomfort in the chest or flanks, or vomiting.

T thin yellow coat

P wiry

CHAI HU JIA MANG XIAO TANG

Bupleurum Decoction plus Mirabilite

Chai Hu	*Bupleurum*	6 - 9 g
Ren Shen	*Panax*	3 - 6 g
Ban Xia	*Pinellia*	3 - 6 g
Mang Xiao	*Mirabilitum*	3 - 6 g
Huang Qin	*Scutellaria*	3 - 9 g
Da Zao	*Ziziphus*	3 - 5 pc
Sheng Jiang	*Zingiber*	3 - 6 g
Gan Cao	*Glycyrrhiza*	3 - 6 g

Shaoyang disease with residual heat and injury to the yin. Symptoms include alternating fever and chills, malarflush, or night heat.

T red, scanty yellow coat, dry

P wiry, rapid, thin

CHAI HU QING ZAO TANG

Bupleurum Decoction to Clear Dryness

Chai Hu	*Bupleurum*	9 - 12 g
Huang Qin	*Scutellaria*	3 - 9 g
Tian Hua Fen	*Trichosanthes*	6 - 12 g
Zhi Mu	*Anemarrhena*	6 - 12 g
Chen Pi	*Citrus*	3 - 9 g
Sheng Jiang	*Zingiber*	3 - 6 g
Da Zao	*Ziziphus*	3 - 5 pc
Gan Cao	*Glycyrrhiza*	3 - 6 g

External invasion which has entered the jueyin level but shaoyang symptoms are present as well as blood deficiency and blood stagnation complaints. The main symptoms are alternating fever and chills with chest and back pain.

T pale, purple, or purple spots

P thin, wiry

CHAI HU SI WU TANG

Bupleurum and Four-Substance Decoction

Chai Hu	*Bupleurum*	6 - 12 g
Huang Qin	*Scutellaria*	6 - 9 g
Ren Shen	*Panax*	3 - 6 g
Ban Xia	*Pinellia*	6 g
Chuan Xiong	*Ligusticum*	6 - 15 g
Bai Shao Yao	*Paeonia*	6 - 15 g
Shu Di Huang	*Rehmannia*	6 - 15 g
Dang Gui	*Angelica*	6 - 15 g
Gan Cao	*Glycyrrhiza*	3 - 6 g

Shaoyang disease with accumulation of phlegm causing fullness and distention in the chest and diaphragm.

T thick sticky yellow coat

P wiry, rapid

CHAI HU XIAN XIONG TANG

Bupleurum Decoction for Sinking into the Chest

Chai Hu	*Bupleurum*	6 - 9 g
Huang Qin	*Scutellaria*	3 - 9 g
Huang Lian	*Coptis*	3 g
Ban Xia	*Pinellia*	6 - 12 g
Gua Lou Ren	*Trichosanthes*	9 - 18 g
Jie Geng	*Platycodon*	3 g
Zhi Ke	*Citrus*	3 - 6 g
Sheng Jiang	*Zingiber*	3 - 6 g

Shaoyang disorder with qi stagnation in the chest and diaphragm. Symptoms include fullness in the chest, dizziness, lack of hearing, headache, and alternating fever and chills.

T sticky white coat

P slippery, wiry

CHAI HU ZHI JIE TANG

Bupleurum, Bitter Orange, and Platycodon Decoction

Chai Hu	*Bupleurum*	6 - 9 g
Ban Xia	*Pinellia*	6 - 9 g
Huang Qin	*Scutellaria*	3 - 6 g
Zhi Ke	*Citrus*	3 - 6 g
Jie Geng	*Platycodon*	3 - 6 g
Chen Pi	*Citrus*	3 - 6 g
Sheng Jiang	*Zingiber*	3 - 6 g

Shaoyang disease with damp accumulation causing malaria with severe chills and mild fever.

T sticky white coat

P soggy

CHAI PING TANG

Bupleurum and Calm the Stomach Decoction

Chai Hu	*Bupleurum*	6 - 9 g
Huang Qin	*Scutellaria*	3 - 6 g
Ren Shen	*Panax*	3 - 6 g
Cang Zhu	*Atractylodes*	3 - 6 g
Chen Pi	*Citrus*	3 - 6 g
Hou Po	*Magnolia*	3 - 9 g
Ban Xia	*Pinellia*	3 - 6 g
Gan Cao	*Glycyrrhiza*	3 - 6 g

Wind cold invasion which has turned to heat and entered the shaoyang level leading to water accumulation in the hypochondriac region.

T red tip, thin yellow coat

P superficial or wiry

CHAI ZHI BAN XIA TANG

Bupleurum, Bitter Orange and Pinellia Decoction

Chai Hu	*Bupleurum*	9 - 15 g
Zhi Ke	*Citrus*	3 - 9 g
Ban Xia	*Pinellia*	6 - 12 g
Huang Qin	*Scutellaria*	6 - 15 g
Jie Geng	*Platycodon*	3 - 6 g
Xing Ren	*Prunus*	6 - 9 g
Qing Pi	*Citrus*	3 - 9 g
Gan Cao	*Glycyrrhiza*	3 - 6 g

Shaoyang disease with internal yangming channel heat. The formula purges internal heat stagnation. Symptoms include constipation, severe fever alternating with mild chills, bitter taste, thirst, or hypochondriac discomfort.

T red, yellow coat

P rapid, wiry, forceful

✘ Caution during pregnancy.

DA CHAI HU TANG

Major Bupleurum Decoction

Extract Formula Name: Major Bupleurum Combination

Chai Hu	*Bupleurum*	9 - 15 g
Da Huang	*Rheum*	6 - 9 g
Ban Xia	*Pinellia*	6 - 9 g
Huang Qin	*Scutellaria*	6 - 9 g
Bai Shao Yao	*Paeonia*	6 - 9 g
Zhi Shi	*Citrus*	6 - 9 g
Sheng Jiang	*Zingiber*	3 - 9 g
Da Zao	*Ziziphus*	3 - 6 pc

Shaoyang disease and damp accumulation leading to malaria, fullness in the chest, or nausea and vomiting.

T thick, sticky coat

P wiry, slippery

DA YUAN YIN

Reach the Membrane Source Decoction

Hou Po	*Magnolia*	6 - 9 g
Bing Lang	*Areca*	6 - 12 g
Zhi Mu	*Anemarrhena*	6 - 9 g
Bai Shao Yao	*Paeonia*	6 - 9 g
Cao Guo	*Amomum*	3 g
Huang Qin	*Scutellaria*	6 - 9 g
Gan Cao	*Glycyrrhiza*	3 - 6 g

Yang jaundice from damp heat lodged in the shaoyang level; or damp heat in the Gallbladder causing alternating fever and chills, bitter taste, or malaria.

T red, thick sticky yellow coat

P slippery, wiry, rapid

☞ Bi Yu San - Green Jade Powder consists of: Hua Shi - Talcum, 3 - 6 g; Gan Cao - Glycyrrhiza, 3 - 6 g; and Qing Dai - Indigo, 9 - 12 g. All three ingredients should be cooked separately in a cheesecloth, then decocted with the rest of the herbs.

HAO QIN QING DAN TANG

Artemisia Annua and Scutellaria Decoction to Clear the Gallbladder

Qing Hao	*Artemisia*	6 g
Zhu Ru	*Bambusa*	9 g
Huang Qin	*Scutellaria*	6 g
Zhi Ke	*Citrus*	5 g
Chi Fu Ling	*Poria*	9 g
Ban Xia	*Pinellia*	5 g
Chen Pi	*Citrus*	5 g
Bi Yu San	*Green Jade Powder*	9 g

Chronic malaria has depleted Liver blood and Spleen qi and blood. The patient experiences alternating fever and chills which are aggravated with only mild stress.

T pale

P empty

HE REN YIN

Polygonum Multiflorum Root and Ginseng Decoction

He Shou Wu	*Polygonum*	9 - 20 g
Ren Shen	*Panax*	9 - 12 g
Chen Pi	*Citrus*	3 - 9 g
Dang Gui	*Angelica*	3 - 9 g
Wei Jiang	*Zingiber*	3 - 12 g

Pre-existing phlegm or damp accumulation with shaoyang disease leading to malaria. There is a slight possibility that this formula can cause vomiting.

T thick sticky white coat

P superficial, slippery, wiry

✘ Note that Chang Shan - Dichroa is an emetic. The formula may cause vomiting.

JIE NUE QI BAO YIN

Seven-Treasure Decoction to Check Malarial Conditions

Chang Shan	*Dichroa*	3 - 5 g
Bing Lang	*Areca*	3 g
Chen Pi	*Citrus*	3 g
Hou Po	*Magnolia*	3 g
Cao Guo	*Amomum*	3 g
Qing Pi	*Citrus*	3 g
Gan Cao	*Glycyrrhiza*	3 g

Excess fire cholecystitis with Liver qi and damp stagnation causing alternating fever and chills or severe hypochondriac pain.

T deep red, sticky yellow coat

P wiry, slippery, rapid, or flooding

☞ Mang Xiao - Mirabilitum should be dissolved into the strained tea. Da Huang - Rheum should be added within the last 3 - 5 minutes of the decoction process.

✘ Do not use during pregnancy

QING DAN XIE HUO TANG

Clear the Gallbladder and Drain Fire Decoction

Chai Hu	*Bupleurum*	9 - 15 g
Ban Xia	*Pinellia*	6 - 9 g
Yin Chen Hao	*Artemisia*	15 - 25 g
Long Dan Cao	*Gentiana*	6 - 9 g
Yu Jin	*Curcuma*	6 - 9 g
Da Huang	*Rheum*	6 - 9 g
Huang Qin	*Scutellaria*	6 - 15 g
Zhi Zi	*Gardenia*	6 - 9 g
Mang Xiao	*Mirabilitum*	6 - 9 g
Mu Xiang	*Saussurea*	3 - 6 g

Shaoyang disorder with severe fever and mild chills.

T red, dry

P wiry, rapid

QING PI TANG

Clear the Spleen Decoction

Qing Pi	*Citrus*	3 - 6 g
Chai Hu	*Bupleurum*	6 - 12 g
Ban Xia	*Pinellia*	6 - 12 g
Hou Po	*Magnolia*	6 - 12 g
Cao Guo	*Amomum*	3 - 9 g
Fu Ling	*Poria*	6 - 12 g
Huang Qin	*Scutellaria*	6 - 12 g
Bai Zhu	*Atractylodes*	6 - 12 g
Gan Cao	*Glycyrrhiza*	3 - 6 g
[Sheng Jiang	*Zingiber*	3 - 6 g]

Shaoyang level disease: symptoms include bitter taste, fullness in the abdomen and hypochondrium, intermittent fever and chills, dizziness, or belching.

T red, dry, yellow or white coat

P wiry, rapid

✪ **Major Formula**

XIAO CHAI HU TANG

Minor Bupleurum Decoction

Extract Formula Name: Minor Bupleurum Combination

Chai Hu	*Bupleurum*	9 - 15 g
Huang Qin	*Scutellaria*	6 - 9 g
Ban Xia	*Pinellia*	6 - 12 g
Ren Shen	*Panax*	9 - 12 g
Sheng Jiang	*Zingiber*	3 - 6 g
Da Zao	*Ziziphus*	3 - 4 pc
Gan Cao	*Glycyrrhiza*	3 - 6 g

DISEASES IN THE YANGMING STAGE

DISEASES IN THE YANGMING FU (ORGAN) STAGE

- severe constipation (pi man zao shi - glomus, fullness, dryness, excess)
- abdominal bloating and pain
- profuse sweating, high fever
- severe thirst
- delirium

T red, yellow or dry black coat

P rapid, forceful

1. Yangming organ disease (pi man zao shi - glomus, fullness, dryness, excess) causing masses in the abdomen; or yang jaundice with gallstones where the heat is greater than damp. 2. Fire and toxin are severe, so the water escapes causing watery dysentery with odorous stools, bowel incontinence while in a coma; mania, or convulsions with high fever.

T bright red, dry yellow or black coat

P rapid, forceful

☞ Da Huang - Rheum should be added during the last 3 - 5 minutes of the decoction process, and Mang Xiao - Mirabilitum should be added into the strained tea.

✘ Do not use during pregnancy. The formula is very cold and can cause diarrhea and vomiting.

✪ Major Formula

DA CHENG QI TANG

Major Order the Qi Decoction

Extract Formula Name: Major Rhubarb Combination

Da Huang	*Rheum*	6 - 12 g
Mang Xiao	*Mirabilitum*	6 - 12 g
Zhi Shi	*Citrus*	6 - 9 g
Hou Po	*Magnolia*	6 - 15 g

Intestinal abscess or acute appendicitis due to heat and blood stagnation causing mass formation in the lower right quadrant with pain.

T yellow sticky coat

P rapid, slippery

☞ Da Huang - Rheum should be added during the last 3 - 5 minutes of the decoction process. Mang Xiao - Mirabilitum should be added to the strained tea..

✘ Do not use with appendicitis during pregnancy.

DA HUANG MU DAN TANG

Rhubarb and Moutan Decoction

Extract Formula Name: Rhubarb and Moutan Combination

Da Huang	*Rheum*	6 - 12 g
Mang Xiao	*Mirabilitum*	6 - 12 g
Dong Gua Ren	*Benincasa*	12 - 20 g
Tao Ren	*Prunus*	9 - 12 g
Mu Dan Pi	*Paeonia*	6 - 9 g

Heat in the middle and upper jiao with fullness as the main symptom (pi-syndrome from pi man zhao shi - firmness, fullness, dryness, excess). Symptoms include nausea and vomiting, possible hematemesis, red face, palpitations, diarrhea, or bleeding in the upper body.

T red, yellow coat

P rapid

✘ Do not use during pregnancy.

DA HUANG XIE XIN TANG

Rhubarb to Drain the Epigastrium Decoction

Da Huang	*Rheum*	6 - 12 g
Huang Lian	*Coptis*	3 - 9 g

Water/heat accumulation in the chest and abdomen causing qi obstruction which leads to pancreatitis with edema, intestinal obstruction, or lumps.

T red, dry coat

P rapid, slippery

☞ Soak and cook Gan Sui - Euphorbia, add Da Huang - Rheum during the last 3 - 5 minutes, then dissolve Mang Xiao - Mirabilitum into the strained tea.

✘ Gan Sui - Euphorbia is toxic, and should only be taken in small amounts. Do not use during pregnancy.

DA XIAN XIONG TANG

Major Sinking Into the Chest Decoction

Extract Formula Name: Rhubarb and Kansui Combination

Da Huang	*Rheum*	9 - 15 g
Mang Xiao	*Mirabilitum*	9 - 12 g
Gan Sui	*Euphorbia*	0.6 - 1 g

Wind heat with internal heat: taiyang and yangming organ disease. The heat is severe. Symptoms include dark yellow urine, constipation, severe fever and chills, heat sensations in the body, sores and carbuncles, skin disorders, and a bitter taste.

T bright or dark red, dry, yellow coat

P flooding, rapid, wiry

☞ Ingredients should be ground into powder, then made into a pill with water. Take 6 g each time, twice a day.

✘ Do not use during pregnancy.

FANG FENG TONG SHENG SAN

Ledebouriella Powder that Sagely Unblocks

Extract Formula Name: Siler and Platycodon Formula

Fang Feng	*Ledebouriella*	9 - 15 g
Ma Huang	*Ephedra*	9 - 15 g
Da Huang	*Rheum*	9 - 15 g
Mang Xiao	*Mirabilitum*	9 - 15 g
Jing Jie	*Schizonepeta*	9 - 15 g
Bo He	*Mentha*	9 - 15 g
Zhi Zi	*Gardenia*	9 - 15 g
Hua Shi	*Talcum*	60 - 90 g
Shi Gao	*Gypsum*	15 - 30 g
Huang Qin	*Scutellaria*	15 - 30 g
Lian Qiao	*Forsythia*	9 - 15 g
Jie Geng	*Platycodon*	15 - 30 g
Dang Gui	*Angelica*	9 - 15 g
Bai Shao Yao	*Paeonia*	9 - 15 g
Chuan Xiong	*Ligusticum*	9 - 15 g
Bai Zhu	*Atractylodes*	9 - 15 g
Gan Cao	*Glycyrrhiza*	30 - 60 g

Blockage in the intestines with yangming organ disease and qi stagnation. Symptoms include no bowel movements or severe abdominal pain.

T red, yellow coat

P rapid, wiry, forceful

☞ Give one dose via nasogastric tube, and the next dose by enema a couple of hours later. Da Huang - Rheum is added during the last 3 minutes of the decoction process. Mang Xiao - Mirabilitum is added to the strained tea.

✘ Do not use during pregnancy.

FU FANG DA CHENG QI TANG

Revised Major Order the Qi Decoction

Lai Fu Zi	*Raphanus*	12 - 20 g
Hou Po	*Magnolia*	12 - 20 g
Da Huang	*Rheum*	9 - 12 g
Tao Ren	*Prunus*	6 g
Mang Xiao	*Mirabilitum*	9 - 12 g
Zhi Shi	*Citrus*	9 - 12 g
Chi Shao Yao	*Paeonia*	9 - 12 g

Yangming organ heat with qi/blood deficiency causing odorous urgent dysentery with abdominal pain which is worse with pressure, fatigue, or possible hallucinations.

T dry yellow coat

P weak

✘ Do not use during pregnancy.

HUANG LONG TANG

Yellow Dragon Decoction

Da Huang	*Rheum*	12 g
Mang Xiao	*Mirabilitum*	9 g
Hou Po	*Magnolia*	12 g
Zhi Shi	*Citrus*	9 g
Dang Gui	*Angelica*	9 g
Ren Shen	*Panax*	6 g
Jie Geng	*Platycodon*	3 - 6 g
Sheng Jiang	*Zingiber*	3 - 6 g
Da Zao	*Ziziphus*	1 - 3 pc
Gan Cao	*Glycyrrhiza*	3 g

Yangming organ syndrome in the abdomen (pi man zao shi - glomus, fullness, dryness, excess) with blood stasis causing acute yang jaundice, Gallbladder infection, intestinal obstruction, possible palpable mass, or nausea and vomiting.

T very red, maybe purplish, dry, rough surface, yellow/brown coat

P flooding, rapid

☞ Da Huang - Rheum should be added during the last 3 - 5 minutes of the decoction process. Mang Xiao - Mirabilitum should be dissolved into the strained tea.

✘ Do not use during pregnancy.

JIA JIAN CHENG QI TANG

Modified Order the Qi Decoction

Da Huang	*Rheum*	9 - 12 g
Mang Xiao	*Mirabilitum*	6 - 9 g
Hou Po	*Magnolia*	9 - 12 g
Zhi Shi	*Citrus*	6 g
Tao Ren	*Prunus*	9 - 15 g
Bai Shao Yao	*Paeonia*	9 - 15 g
Lai Fu Zi	*Raphanus*	6 - 12 g

Fire in the upper/middle jiao (chest/diaphragm) causing thirst, red lips, epistaxis, redness in the face, dark yellow urine, constipation, or delirium.

T red, dry yellow coat

P rapid

✘ Do not use during pregnancy.

LIANG GE SAN

Cool the Diaphragm Powder

Extract Formula Name: Forsythia and Rhubarb Formula

Da Huang	*Rheum*	6 - 9 g
Mang Xiao	*Mirabilitum*	6 - 9 g
Zhi Zi	*Gardenia*	3 - 6 g
Huang Qin	*Scutellaria*	6 - 9 g
Bo He	*Mentha*	3 - 6 g
Lian Qiao	*Forsythia*	9 - 12 g
Gan Cao	*Glycyrrhiza*	3 - 6 g
[Dan Zhu Ye	*Lophatherum*	3 - 6 g]

Yin/blood deficiency causing constipation with dry stools; or excess heat causing constipation.

T red, dry yellow coat

P rapid, thin, or empty

✘ Do not use during pregnancy.

MA ZI REN WAN

Hemp Seed Pill

Extract Formula Name: Apricot Seed and Linum Formula

Huo Ma Ren	*Cannabis*	6 - 12 g
Da Huang	*Rheum*	6 - 9 g
Xing Ren	*Prunus*	6 - 9 g
Zhi Shi	*Citrus*	3 - 6 g
Bai Shao Yao	*Paeonia*	6 - 9 g
Hou Po	*Magnolia*	6 - 12 g

Yangming heat with irritability and Spleen qi deficiency causing constipation with very dry feces, yellow urine, possible fever, or bleeding disorders.

T red, yellow coat

P deep, forceful, rapid

☞ Mang Xiao - Mirabilitum should be added to the strained tea.

✘ Do not use during pregnancy.

TIAO WEI CHENG QI TANG

Regulate the Stomach and Order the Qi Decoction

Extract Formula Name: Rhubarb and Mirabilitum Combination

Da Huang	*Rheum*	9 - 15 g
Mang Xiao	*Mirabilitum*	9 - 12 g
Zhi Gan Cao	*Glycyrrhiza*	3 - 9 g

Excess fire with qi stagnation causing fullness, possible palpable mass, or constipation. This is a mild yangming organ disease.

T red, thin sticky yellow coat

P rapid, slightly forceful

✘ Do not use during pregnancy.

XIAO CHENG QI TANG

Minor Order the Qi Decoction

Extract Formula Name: Minor Rhubarb Combination

Da Huang	*Rheum*	9 - 12 g
Zhi Shi	*Citrus*	6 g
Hou Po	*Magnolia*	6 - 12 g

Yin deficiency with dryness and heat in the yangming leading to constipation.

T red, dry yellow coat

P rapid, thin, wiry

☞ Da Huang - Rheum should be added during the last 3 minutes of the cooking process. Mang Xiao - Mirabilitum should be added to the strained tea.

✘ Do not use during pregnancy.

ZENG YE CHENG QI TANG

Increase the Fluids and Order the Qi Decoction

Xuan Shen	*Scrophularia*	15 - 25 g
Sheng Di Huang	*Rehmannia*	15 - 20 g
Mai Men Dong	*Ophiopogón*	15 - 20 g
Mang Xiao	*Mirabilitum*	3 - 6 g
Da Huang	*Rheum*	6 - 9 g

Yangming fire causing jaundice, restlessness, fever, or constipation.

T red, yellow coat

P rapid, forceful

✘ Do not use during pregnancy.

ZHI ZI DA HUANG TANG

Gardenia and Rhubarb Decoction

Zhi Zi	*Gardenia*	6 - 12 g
Da Huang	*Rheum*	3 - 6 g
Zhi Shi	*Citrus*	3 - 9 g
Dan Dou Chi	*Glycine*	6 - 12 g

DISEASES IN THE YANGMING JING (CHANNEL) STAGE

- high fever
- thirst
- profuse sweating
- irritability due to heat

T red, yellow coat

P flooding

Heat in the yangming channel with slight external cold and damp causing obstruction in the channels which leads to joint pain.

T red, yellow coat

P rapid, wiry

☞ Decoct the first four herbs, then add the rice at the end. It will absorb the water to make a thick liquid.

BAI HU JIA GUI ZHI TANG

White Tiger plus Cinnamon Twig Decoction

Shi Gao	*Gypsum*	20 - 30 g
Zhi Mu	*Anemarrhena*	9 - 12 g
Gan Cao	*Glycyrrhiza*	3 - 9 g
Gui Zhi	*Cinnamomum*	3 - 9 g
Jing Mi	*Oryza*	15 - 30 g

Upper jiao diabetes with heat: yangming channel syndrome with qi and yin deficiency causing severe sweating, fever, and thirst.

T red, dry yellow coat

P rapid, flooding, weak

☞ Decoct the first four herbs, then add the rice at the end. It will absorb the water to make a thick liquid.

BAI HU JIA REN SHEN TANG

White Tiger plus Ginseng Decoction

Extract Formula Name: Ginseng and Gypsum Combination

Shi Gao	*Gypsum*	15 - 20 g
Zhi Mu	*Anemarrhena*	9 - 12 g
Gan Cao	*Glycyrrhiza*	3 - 6 g
Ren Shen	*Panax*	3 - 9 g
Jing Mi	*Oryza*	9 - 12 g

Heat in the qi level/yangming channel syndrome causing severe fever, epidemic febrile disease, acute inflammation, encephalitis, or meningitis.

T red, dry yellow coat

P flooding, rapid

☞ Decoct the first five herbs, then add the rice at the end. It will absorb the water to make a thick liquid.

BAI HU JIA YIN QIAO TANG

White Tiger plus Lonicera and Forsythia Decoction

Shi Gao	*Gypsum*	20 - 30 g
Zhi Mu	*Anemarrhena*	9 - 12 g
Gan Cao	*Glycyrrhiza*	3 - 6 g
Jin Yin Hua	*Lonicera*	6 - 9 g
Lian Qiao	*Forsythia*	6 - 9 g
Jing Mi	*Oryza*	15 - 30 g

Summerheat with damp and yangming channel heat/qi level heat. This causes severe sweating, nausea, vomiting, thirst, or fever.

T red, sticky yellow coat

P slippery, rapid

☞ Decoct the first four herbs, then add the rice at the end. It will absorb the water to make a thick liquid.

BAI HU JIA ZHU TANG

White Tiger with White Atractylodes Decoction

Shi Gao	*Gypsum*	20 - 30 g
Zhi Mu	*Anemarrhena*	9 - 12 g
Gan Cao	*Glycyrrhiza*	3 - 6 g
Bai Zhu	*Atractylodes*	3 - 9 g
Jing Mi	*Oryza*	15 - 30 g

Heat in the qi level/yangming channel disease causing high fever, sweating, flooding pulse, or thirst.

T red, yellow coat

P flooding, rapid

☞ Decoct the first three herbs, then add the rice at the end. It will absorb the water to make a thick liquid.

✪ Major Formula

BAI HU TANG

White Tiger Decoction

Extract Formula Name: Gypsum Combination

Shi Gao	*Gypsum*	20 - 30 g
Zhi Mu	*Anemarrhena*	9 - 12 g
Gan Cao	*Glycyrrhiza*	3 - 6 g
Jing Mi	*Oryza*	15 - 30 g

Toxic heat in the yangming channel causing dysentery, or pus or blood in the stools.

T red, yellow coat

P wiry, rapid, rolling

BAI TOU WENG TANG

Pulsatilla Decoction

Extract Formula Name: Anemone Combination

Bai Tou Weng	*Pulsatilla*	20 - 40 g
Huang Bai	*Phellodendron*	9 - 12 g
Qin Pi	*Fraxinus*	9 - 15 g
Huang Lian	*Coptis*	6 - 9 g

Exterior wind cold or heat with internal heat which starts to go from the wei to the qi level into the yangming channel. Only mild exterior symptoms are present. Thirst, constipation, full and painful eye orbits, severe bodyaches, or restlessness are the main symptoms.

T red, dry, thin yellow coat

P superficial, slightly flooding, rapid

CHAI GE JIE JI TANG

Bupleurum and Kudzu Decoction to Release the Muscle Layer

Extract Formula Name: Bupleurum and Pueraria Combination

Chai Hu	*Bupleurum*	3 - 9 g
Ge Gen	*Pueraria*	9 - 12 g
Bai Zhi	*Angelica*	3 - 9 g
Shi Gao	*Gypsum*	6 - 15 g
Bai Shao Yao	*Paeonia*	6 - 9 g
Qiang Huo	*Notopterygium*	3 - 6 g
Huang Qin	*Scutellaria*	6 - 9 g
Jie Geng	*Platycodon*	3 - 6 g
Da Zao	*Ziziphus*	3 - 4 pc
Sheng Jiang	*Zingiber*	3 - 6 g
Gan Cao	*Glycyrrhiza*	3 - 6 g

Shaoyang and yangming channel disease causing mild chills with severe fever, and thirst.

T red, thin yellow coat

P rapid, maybe flooding

CHAI HU BAI HU TANG

Bupleurum White Tiger Decoction

Chai Hu	Bupleurum	3 - 6 g
Huang Qin	Scutellaria	3 - 6 g
Shi Gao	Gypsum	12 - 20 g
Zhi Mu	Anemarrhena	6 - 12 g
Tian Hua Fen	Trichosanthes	6 - 9 g
Jing Mi	Oryza	6 - 9 g
Gan Cao	Glycyrrhiza	3 - 6 g

Qi deficient patient gets evil qi invading taiyang, shaoyang, and yangming channels. This causes irritability, constipation, full chest, or heaviness.

T red, sticky coat

P rapid, wiry

☞ Da Huang - Rheum should be added during the last 3 minutes of the decoction process.

✘ Qian Dan - Minium is toxic and should be substituted with Dai Zhe Shi - Haematitum or Sheng Tie Luo - Frusta Ferri. Caution during pregnancy.

CHAI HU JIA LONG GU MU LI TANG

Bupleurum plus Dragon Bone and Oyster Shell Decoction

Extract Formula Name: Bupleurum and D.B. Combination

Chai Hu	Bupleurum	9 - 12 g
Huang Qin	Scutellaria	6 g
Ren Shen	Panax	6 g
Gui Zhi	Cinnamomum	3 - 6 g
Ban Xia	Pinellia	6 g
Fu Ling	Poria	6 g
Da Huang	Rheum	6 g
Long Gu	Os Draconis	3 - 6 g
Mu Li	Ostrea	3 - 6 g
Sheng Jiang	Zingiber	3 - 6 g
Da Zao	Ziziphus	3 - 6 pc
Qian Dan	Minium	1 - 4 g

Shaoyang disease with internal yangming channel heat. The formula purges internal heat stagnation. Symptoms include constipation, severe fever alternating with mild chills, bitter taste, thirst, or hypochondriac discomfort.

T red, yellow coat

P rapid, wiry, forceful

✘ Caution during pregnancy.

DA CHAI HU TANG

Major Bupleurum Decoction

Extract Formula Name: Major Bupleurum Combination

Chai Hu	*Bupleurum*	9 - 15 g
Da Huang	*Rheum*	6 - 9 g
Ban Xia	*Pinellia*	6 - 9 g
Huang Qin	*Scutellaria*	6 - 9 g
Bai Shao Yao	*Paeonia*	6 - 9 g
Zhi Shi	*Citrus*	6 - 9 g
Sheng Jiang	*Zingiber*	3 - 9 g
Da Zao	*Ziziphus*	3 - 6 pc

Heat in the yangming channel with pre-existing severe blood stagnation in the lower jiao which affects the uterus and the intestines. Symptoms include jaundice, mania, fever, melena with dry stools which are relatively easy to discharge, dysmenorrhea, amenorrhea, abdominal fullness, or bleeding in the stomach. This formula is stronger than 'Di Dang Wan - Resistance Pill.'

T red, dark purple

P wiry, rapid

✘ Do not use during pregnancy. Use only for a short duration.

DI DANG TANG

Resistance Decoction

Da Huang	*Rheum*	6 - 12 g
Tao Ren	*Prunus*	6 - 9 g
Shui Zhi	*Hirudo*	1 - 3 g
Meng Chong	*Tabanus*	1 - 3 g

Heat in the yangming channel with pre-existing severe blood stagnation in the lower jiao which affects the uterus and the intestines. Symptoms include jaundice, mania, fever, melena with dry stools which are relatively easy to discharge, dysmenorrhea, amenorrhea, abdominal fullness, or bleeding in the stomach. This formula is somewhat milder than 'Di Dang Tang - Resistance Decoction.'

T red, purple

P wiry, rapid

☞ Ingredients should all be ground up, then formed into pills.

✘ Caution during pregnancy.

DI DANG WAN

Resistance Pill

Da Huang	*Rheum*	12 g
Shui Zhi	*Hirudo*	20 - 30 g
Meng Chong	*Tabanus*	20 - 30 g
Tao Ren	*Prunus*	9 - 12 g

Yangming channel disease, damp stagnation and yin deficiency leading to mouth sores, swollen, red gums with pus, bad breath, sore throat, or eye disorders.

T thick sticky yellow coat

P rapid, slippery, thin

GAN LU YIN

Sweet Dew Decoction

Extract Formula Name: Sweet Combination

Shu Di Huang	*Rehmannia*	6 - 9 g
Sheng Di Huang	*Rehmannia*	6 - 9 g
Huang Qin	*Scutellaria*	6 - 9 g
Zhi Ke	*Citrus*	3 - 6 g
Mai Men Dong	*Ophiopogon*	6 - 9 g
Tian Men Dong	*Asparagus*	6 - 9 g
Pi Pa Ye	*Eriobotrya*	12 - 18 g
Yin Chen Hao	*Artemisia*	6 - 9 g
Shi Hu	*Dendrobium*	6 - 9 g
Gan Cao	*Glycyrrhiza*	3 - 6 g

Wind cold (deficiency type) with internal fire: taiyang and yangming disorder. This causes sweating, chills, nasal congestion, and constipation with abdominal fullness.

T red, thin white or yellow coat

P superficial, rapid

✘ Caution during pregnancy.

HOU PO QI WU TANG

Seven-Substance Decoction with Magnolia Bark

Extract Formula Name: Magnolia 7 Combination

Hou Po	*Magnolia*	15 g
Da Huang	*Rheum*	9 g
Gui Zhi	*Cinnamomum*	6 g
Zhi Shi	*Citrus*	9 g
Sheng Jiang	*Zingiber*	12 g
Da Zao	*Ziziphus*	12 pc
Gan Cao	*Glycyrrhiza*	6 g

Yangming channel disease/Stomach fire causing bleeding gums, toothache, soreness in the tongue, headaches, or red eyes.

T red, dry

P rapid, flooding

QING WEI SAN

Clear the Stomach Powder

Extract Formula Name: Coptis and Rehmannia Formula

Huang Lian	*Coptis*	3 - 6 g
Sheng Di Huang	*Rehmannia*	9 - 12 g
Mu Dan Pi	*Paeonia*	9 - 12 g
Dang Gui Shen	*Angelica*	9 - 12 g
Sheng Ma	*Cimicifuga*	9 - 15 g

Heat in the chest and Lungs due to taiyang disease; or lingering qi level heat manifesting in the yangming channel layer. In some patients this formula will induce vomiting, after which the symptoms will disappear.

T red, especially the tip, yellow coat

P rapid, forceful, superficial

✘ This prescription can cause vomiting.

ZHI ZI DOU CHI TANG

Gardenia and Prepared Soybean Decoction

Zhi Zi	*Gardenia*	6 - 9 g
Dan Dou Chi	*Glycine*	6 - 9 g

Yangming channel syndrome affecting the lower jiao; or wind cold causing heat in the Spleen/Stomach which burns the yin. This leads to water dysfunction and stagnation which heats up leading to Lin-syndrome: Heat Lin or damp heat edema.

T red, sticky yellow coat

P rapid

☞ E Jiao - Equus should be added to the strained tea.

ZHU LING TANG I

Polyporus Decoction

Extract Formula Name: Polyporus Combination

Zhu Ling	*Polyporus*	6 - 9 g
Fu Ling	*Poria*	6 - 9 g
Hua Shi	*Talcum*	6 - 9 g
Ze Xie	*Alisma*	6 - 9 g
E Jiao	*Equus*	6 - 9 g

DISEASES IN THE TAIYIN STAGE

- no appetite, no thirst
- vomiting
- abdominal fullness
- diarrhea

T pale

P deep, slow

Severe taiyin/taiyang disease with abdominal cramps as the main symptom.

T thin white coat

P superficial

GUI ZHI JIA SHAO YAO TANG

Cinnamon Twig Decoction plus Peony

Extract Formula Name: Cinnamon and Peony Combination

Gui Zhi	*Cinnamomum*	6 - 9 g
Bai Shao Yao	*Paeonia*	15 - 18 g
Sheng Jiang	*Zingiber*	3 - 6 g
Da Zao	*Ziziphus*	3 - 4 pc
Gan Cao	*Glycyrrhiza*	3 - 6 g

Mild taiyin with taiyang syndrome: wind cold with mild Spleen qi deficiency. The chills are predominant, and the patient experiences diarrhea with epigastric fullness.

T pale, thin white coat

P weak, maybe superficial

GUI ZHI REN SHEN TANG

Cinnamon Twig and Ginseng Decoction

Extract Formula Name: Cinnamon and Ginseng Combination

Gui Zhi	*Cinnamomum*	9 - 12 g
Ren Shen	*Panax*	9 - 12 g
Gan Jiang	*Zingiber*	9 g
Bai Zhu	*Atractylodes*	9 g
Zhi Gan Cao	*Glycyrrhiza*	9 - 12 g

Kidney and Spleen yang deficiency with cold which has invaded all three yin channels (taiyin, shaoyin, and jueyin). Symptoms include shivering from cold, icy limbs and face, watery diarrhea, or cough with profuse saliva production.

T pale, wet, thin white moist coat

P minute or frail

☞ Remove She Xiang - Moschus, decoct the rest of the formula as usual, then add powdered Moschus to each dosage.

HUI YANG JIU JI TANG

Restore and Revive the Yang Decoction

Fu Zi	*Aconitum*	9 g
Rou Gui	*Cinnamomum*	3 - 6 g
Ren Shen	*Panax*	6 - 9 g
Gan Jiang	*Zingiber*	3 - 6 g
Fu Ling	*Poria*	6 - 9 g
Chen Pi	*Citrus*	3 - 6 g
Bai Zhu	*Atractylodes*	6 - 9 g
Wu Wei Zi	*Schisandra*	3 - 6 g
Ban Xia	*Pinellia*	6 - 9 g
Gan Cao	*Glycyrrhiza*	3 - 6 g
She Xiang	*Moschus*	0.3 g
[Sheng Jiang	*Zingiber*	1 - 3 g]

Blood level heat and taiyin level disease with lingering summerheat causing thirst and severe sweating.

T red or dark red

P rapid

JIA JIAN SHENG MAI SAN

Modified Generate the Pulse Powder

Mai Men Dong	*Ophiopogon*	6 - 12 g
Wu Wei Zi	*Schisandra*	6 - 12 g
Bei Sha Shen	*Glehnia*	6 - 12 g
Mu Dan Pi	*Paeonia*	6 - 12 g
Sheng Di Huang	*Rehmannia*	6 - 12 g

Middle jiao qi/yang deficiency resulting in loss of appetite, absence of thirst, watery diarrhea with undigested food, or cold or painful limbs.

T pale, swollen, teethmarks, white coat

P deep, weak

✪ Major Formula

LI ZHONG WAN

Regulate the Middle Pill

Extract Formula Name: Ginseng and Ginger Combination

Ren Shen	*Panax*	6 - 9 g
Gan Jiang	*Zingiber*	6 - 9 g
Bai Zhu	*Atractylodes*	6 - 9 g
Gan Cao	*Glycyrrhiza*	3 - 6 g

Exterior cold has gone internally. qi and yang are very weak and Kidney/Spleen yang have been damaged. Symptoms include low blood pressure, cold limbs, shock, or sweating.

T pale, or purple, moist white coat

P minute

☞ The raw type of Aconite is used here since it is much warmer than the prepared kind. 6 - 12 g of honey are often added for detoxification. Fu Zi - Aconitum is soaked in 8 - 10 cups of boiling water for 30 minutes to one hour. The remaining herbs should be added during the last 25 minutes and decocted as usual.

✘ Fu Zi - Aconitum in its raw form is toxic and is intended for short-term use only.

SI NI TANG

Frigid Extremities Decoction

Extract Formula Name: Aconite, Ginger and Licorice Combination

Fu Zi	*Aconitum*	9 - 15 g
Gan Jiang	*Zingiber*	6 - 12 g
Zhi Gan Cao	*Glycyrrhiza*	3 - 6 g

Cold damp has entered the Spleen leading to water accumulation and Spleen yang deficiency. This causes damp in the middle jiao which bothers the Gallbladder so the bile cannot circulate properly. This manifests as yin-type jaundice.

T pale, white coat

P weak, deep

YIN CHEN ZHU FU TANG

Artemisia Yinchenhao, Atractylodes and Prepared Aconite Decoction

Extract Formula Name: Capillaris, Atractylodes and Aconite Combination

Yin Chen Hao	*Artemisia*	3 - 6 g
Gan Jiang	*Zingiber*	3 - 6 g
Bai Zhu	*Atractylodes*	6 - 9 g
Rou Gui	*Cinnamomum*	1 - 3 g
Fu Zi	*Aconitum*	1 - 3 g
Zhi Gan Cao	*Glycyrrhiza*	3 - 6 g

DISEASES IN THE SHAOYIN STAGE

- 1. **Cold type**: cold limps with an aversion to cold and chills
- no appetite, diarrhea
- 2. **Heat type**: fever, irritability
- dry mouth

T pale, or red

P minute, or rapid

Severe yang deficiency and cold causes the yang to be pushed superficially leading to superficial false yang symptoms. The patient gives the appearance that he/she will get better but in reality may die soon. Symptoms include diarrhea, low fever, or red face. Internal cold with superficial false heat: shaoyin syndrome.

T pale, red tip

P deep, faint

BAI TONG TANG

White Penetrating Decoction

Gan Jiang	*Zingiber*	3 - 6 g
Fu Zi	*Aconitum*	3 - 9 g
Cong Bai	*Allium*	3 - 6 g

Stomach/Spleen yang deficiency causing watery diarrhea and epigastric pain. Severe cold symptoms such as cold limbs and vomiting of clear fluids.

T pale, swollen, teethmarks, white coat

P minute

✪ Major Formula

FU ZI LI ZHONG WAN

Prepared Aconite Pill to Regulate the Middle

Extract Formula Name: Aconite, Ginseng, and Ginger Combination

Fu Zi	*Aconitum*	6 - 9 g
Ren Shen	*Panax*	3 - 9 g
Bai Zhu	*Atractylodes*	3 - 9 g
Gan Jiang	*Zingiber*	3 - 9 g
Zhi Gan Cao	*Glycyrrhiza*	3 - 6 g

Severe Kidney yang deficiency where the yang is unable to nourish the limbs leading to edema, and severe body aches with cold and damp symptoms: cold bi-syndrome.

T pale, moist white coat

P deep, minute, or choppy

FU ZI TANG

Prepared Aconite Decoction

Extract Formula Name: Aconite Combination

Fu Zi	*Aconitum*	9 - 15 g
Ren Shen	*Panax*	3 - 6 g
Fu Ling	*Poria*	9 - 12 g
Bai Zhu	*Atractylodes*	3 - 12 g
Bai Shao Yao	*Paeonia*	6 - 9 g

Heart/Kidney yin deficiency with fire after febrile disease leading to insomnia, palpitations, or tongue sores: shaoyin deficient heat syndrome.

T red, scanty coat

P rapid, thin

☞ E Jiao - Equus and egg yolks should be dissolved into the strained tea.

✪ Major Formula

HUANG LIAN E JIAO TANG

Coptis and Ass-Hide Gelatin Decoction

Extract Formula Name: Coptis and Gelatin Combination

Huang Lian	*Coptis*	9 - 12 g
E Jiao	*Equus*	6 - 9 g
Huang Qin	*Scutellaria*	6 - 9 g
Bai Shao Yao	*Paeonia*	6 - 9 g
Ji Zi Huang	*Egg yolks*	2

Kidney and Spleen yang deficiency with cold which has invaded all three yin channels (taiyin, shaoyin, and jueyin). Symptoms include shivering from cold, icy limbs and face, watery diarrhea, or cough with profuse saliva production.

T pale, wet, thin white moist coat

P minute or frail

☞ Remove She Xiang - Moschus, decoct the rest of the formula as usual, then add powdered Moschus to each dosage.

HUI YANG JIU JI TANG

Restore and Revive the Yang Decoction

Fu Zi	*Aconitum*	9 g
Rou Gui	*Cinnamomum*	3 - 6 g
Ren Shen	*Panax*	6 - 9 g
Gan Jiang	*Zingiber*	3 - 6 g
Fu Ling	*Poria*	6 - 9 g
Chen Pi	*Citrus*	3 - 6 g
Bai Zhu	*Atractylodes*	6 - 9 g
Wu Wei Zi	*Schisandra*	3 - 6 g
Ban Xia	*Pinellia*	6 - 9 g
Gan Cao	*Glycyrrhiza*	3 - 6 g
She Xiang	*Moschus*	0.3 g
[Sheng Jiang	*Zingiber*	1 - 3 g]

Mild yang deficiency with external wind cold without sweating. (shaoyin and taiyang disease). Symptoms include extreme chilliness with mild fever and severe fatigue.

T pale, white coat

P minute

MA HUANG FU ZI XI XIN TANG

Ephedra, Prepared Aconite, and Asarum Decoction

Extract Formula Name: Ma-Huang and Asarum Combination

Ma Huang	*Ephedra*	6 - 9 g
Fu Zi	*Aconitum*	3 - 6 g
Xi Xin	*Asarum*	3 - 6 g

Shaoyin disease: severe yang deficiency with cold accumulation which causes false yang to be pushed to the exterior. The yang cannot stay in the interior causing icy limbs upon touch but no cold intolerance, flushed face, thirst without desire to drink, or a dry throat.

T pale, light purple, teethmarks, thin white coat

P slow, minute

TONG MAI SI NI TANG

Unblock the Pulse Decoction for Frigid Extremities

Extract Formula Name: Licorice, Aconite and Ginger Pulse Combination

Fu Zi	*Aconitum*	12 - 15 g
Gan Jiang	*Zingiber*	9 - 12 g
Gan Cao	*Glycyrrhiza*	3 - 6 g

Spleen/Kidney qi and yang deficient patient suffers easily from wind cold with internal water accumulation, or experiences urinary difficulty, diarrhea, or edema.

T pale, swollen, teethmarks, moist, thin white coat

P frail or minute

ZHEN WU TANG

True Warrior Decoction

Extract Formula Name: Vitality Combination

Fu Zi	*Aconitum*	6 - 9 g
Bai Zhu	*Atractylodes*	6 - 9 g
Bai Shao Yao	*Paeonia*	6 - 9 g
Fu Ling	*Poria*	6 - 9 g
Sheng Jiang	*Zingiber*	6 - 9 g

DISEASES IN THE JUEYIN STAGE

- heat sensation and pain in the chest
- hunger without desire to eat
- diarrhea, vomiting
- thirst

T red

P rapid, weak

Kidney and Spleen yang deficiency with cold which has invaded all three yin channels (taiyin, shaoyin, and jueyin). Symptoms include shivering from cold, icy limbs and face, watery diarrhea, or cough with profuse saliva production.

T pale, wet, thin white moist coat

P minute or frail

☞ Remove She Xiang - Moschus, decoct the rest of the formula as usual, then add powdered Moschus to each dosage.

HUI YANG JIU JI TANG

Restore and Revive the Yang Decoction

Fu Zi	*Aconitum*	9 g
Rou Gui	*Cinnamomum*	3 - 6 g
Ren Shen	*Panax*	6 - 9 g
Gan Jiang	*Zingiber*	3 - 6 g
Fu Ling	*Poria*	6 - 9 g
Chen Pi	*Citrus*	3 - 6 g
Bai Zhu	*Atractylodes*	6 - 9 g
Wu Wei Zi	*Schisandra*	3 - 6 g
Ban Xia	*Pinellia*	6 - 9 g
Gan Cao	*Glycyrrhiza*	3 - 6 g
She Xiang	*Moschus*	0.3 g
[Sheng Jiang	*Zingiber*	1 - 3 g]

1. Roundworms have migrated upward due to cold in the Large Intestines to the warmth of the epigastrium/chest. 2. Large Intestine cold and Stomach heat: mixed syndrome - jueyin syndrome.

T pale

P weak

☞ Wu Mei - Prunus should be soaked in vinegar for 12 hours.

✪ Major Formula

WU MEI WAN

Mume Pill

Extract Formula Name: Mume Formula

Wu Mei	*Prunus*	20 - 25 g
Xi Xin	*Asarum*	1 - 3 g
Chuan Jiao	*Zanthoxylum*	1 - 3 g
Gan Jiang	*Zingiber*	12 - 15 g
Fu Zi	*Aconitum*	6 - 9 g
Huang Lian	*Coptis*	9 - 12 g
Huang Bai	*Phellodendron*	6 - 9 g
Gui Zhi	*Cinnamomum*	3 - 9 g
Dang Gui	*Angelica*	6 - 9 g
Ren Shen	*Panax*	6 - 9 g

FOUR STAGES

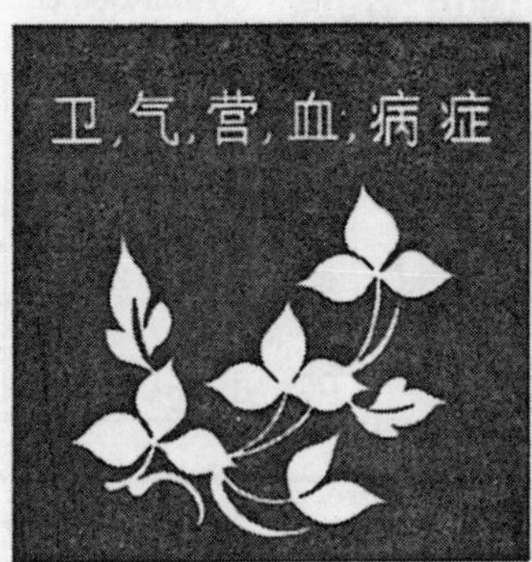

HEAT IN THE WEI (DEFENSIVE) LEVEL

Please see WIND INVASIONS

HEAT IN THE QI LEVEL

- high fever
- thirst
- profuse sweating
- cough or asthma with yellow expectoration

T red, dry, thick yellow coat

P flooding, rapid

Damp heat febrile disease or damp bi-syndrome with heat causing severe sweating and joint pain with swelling and redness. Joints feel hot to the touch.

T red, sticky yellow coat

P slippery, rapid, or flooding

☞ Decoct the first four herbs, then add the rice at the end. It will absorb the water to make a thick liquid.

BAI HU JIA CANG ZHU TANG

White Tiger plus Atractylodes Decoction

Shi Gao	*Gypsum*	20 - 30 g
Zhi Mu	*Anemarrhena*	9 - 12 g
Gan Cao	*Glycyrrhiza*	3 - 6 g
Cang Zhu	*Atractylodes*	3 - 9 g
Jing Mi	*Oryza*	15 - 30 g

Heat in the qi level/yangming channel syndrome causing severe fever, epidemic febrile disease, acute inflammation, encephalitis, or meningitis.

T red, dry yellow coat

P flooding, rapid

☞ Decoct the first five herbs, then add the rice at the end. It will absorb the water to make a thick liquid.

BAI HU JIA YIN QIAO TANG

White Tiger plus Lonicera and Forsythia Decoction

Shi Gao	Gypsum	20 - 30 g
Zhi Mu	Anemarrhena	9 - 12 g
Gan Cao	Glycyrrhiza	3 - 6 g
Jin Yin Hua	Lonicera	6 - 9 g
Lian Qiao	Forsythia	6 - 9 g
Jing Mi	Oryza	15 - 30 g

Summerheat with damp and yangming channel heat/qi level heat. This causes severe sweating, nausea, vomiting, thirst, or fever.

T red, sticky yellow coat

P slippery, rapid

☞ Decoct the first four herbs, then add the rice at the end. It will absorb the water to make a thick liquid.

BAI HU JIA ZHU TANG

White Tiger with White Atractylodes Decoction

Shi Gao	Gypsum	20 - 30 g
Zhi Mu	Anemarrhena	9 - 12 g
Gan Cao	Glycyrrhiza	3 - 6 g
Bai Zhu	Atractylodes	3 - 9 g
Jing Mi	Oryza	15 - 30 g

Heat in the qi level/yangming channel disease causing high fever, sweating, flooding pulse, or thirst.

T red, yellow coat

P flooding, rapid

☞ Decoct the first three herbs, then add the rice at the end. It will absorb the water to make a thick liquid.

✪ Major Formula

BAI HU TANG

White Tiger Decoction

Extract Formula Name: Gypsum Combination

Shi Gao	Gypsum	20 - 30 g
Zhi Mu	Anemarrhena	9 - 12 g
Gan Cao	Glycyrrhiza	3 - 6 g
Jing Mi	Oryza	15 - 30 g

Shaoyang and yangming channel disease causing mild chills with severe fever, and thirst.

T red, thin yellow coat

P rapid, maybe flooding

CHAI HU BAI HU TANG

Bupleurum White Tiger Decoction

Chai Hu	*Bupleurum*	3 - 6 g
Huang Qin	*Scutellaria*	3 - 6 g
Shi Gao	*Gypsum*	12 - 20 g
Zhi Mu	*Anemarrhena*	6 - 12 g
Tian Hua Fen	*Trichosanthes*	6 - 9 g
Jing Mi	*Oryza*	6 - 9 g
Gan Cao	*Glycyrrhiza*	3 - 6 g

Shaoyang disease with internal yangming channel heat. The formula purges internal heat stagnation. Symptoms include constipation, severe fever alternating with mild chills, bitter taste, thirst, or hypochondriac discomfort.

T red, yellow coat

P rapid, wiry, forceful

✘ Caution during pregnancy.

DA CHAI HU TANG

Major Bupleurum Decoction

Extract Formula Name: Major Bupleurum Combination

Chai Hu	*Bupleurum*	9 - 15 g
Da Huang	*Rheum*	6 - 9 g
Ban Xia	*Pinellia*	6 - 9 g
Huang Qin	*Scutellaria*	6 - 9 g
Bai Shao Yao	*Paeonia*	6 - 9 g
Zhi Shi	*Citrus*	6 - 9 g
Sheng Jiang	*Zingiber*	3 - 9 g
Da Zao	*Ziziphus*	3 - 6 pc

Damp accumulation with heat toxin in the qi level causing gastritis, hepatitis, fever, bodyaches, diarrhea, or vomiting.

T sticky yellow coat

P rapid, soggy

☞ All ingredients should be dried in sunlight and ground into powder. Take 9 g each time, twice a day.

GAN LU XIAO DU DAN

Sweet Dew Special Pill to Eliminate Toxin

Extract Formula Name: Talc and Scute Formula

She Gan	*Belamcanda*	120 g
Lian Qiao	*Forsythia*	120 g
Hua Shi	*Talcum*	450 g
Chuan Bei Mu	*Fritillaria*	150 g
Bo He	*Mentha*	120 g
Huang Qin	*Scutellaria*	300 g
Bai Dou Kou	*Amomum*	120 g
Yin Chen Hao	*Artemisia*	330 g
Shi Chang Pu	*Acorus*	180 g
Huo Xiang	*Agastache*	120 g
Mu Tong	*Akebia*	150 g

Heat in the qi and blood levels resulting in purpura.

T red, thin yellow coat

P flooding, rapid

☞ Shi Gao - Gypsum should be decocted first for 20 minutes. Xi Jiao - Rhinoceros is powdered and added to the strained decoction. Shui Niu Jiao - Bubalus should be substituted for Xi Jiao.

HUA BAN TANG

Transform Blotches Decoction

Shi Gao	*Gypsum*	30 g
Zhi Mu	*Anemarrhena*	12 g
Xuan Shen	*Scrophularia*	10 g
Xi Jiao	*Rhinoceros*	2 - 6 g
Jing Mi	*Oryza*	9 g
Gan Cao	*Glycyrrhiza*	10 g

Wind heat with fever, possible sweating, thirst, dyspnea, or asthma: heat in the qi level.

T red tip or border, yellow coat

P rapid, flooding

MA XING SHI GAN TANG

Ephedra, Apricot Kernel, Gypsum, and Licorice Decoction

Extract Formula Name: Ma-Huang and Apricot Seed Combination

Ma Huang	*Ephedra*	6 - 15 g
Xing Ren	*Prunus*	6 - 9 g
Shi Gao	*Gypsum*	6 - 20 g
Gan Cao	*Glycyrrhiza*	3 - 6 g

Mild summer heat invading the qi level with residual pathogens lingering causing mild superficial and damp symptoms. The patient feels thirst but can only sip fluids, and experiences diarrhea, gas, vomiting, or cold limbs.

T red, thin white coat

P rapid, maybe superficial

☞ The prepared form of Xi Gua - Citrullus is used.

☞ The outer skin of Si Gua Luo - Luffa is used.

QING LUO YIN

Clear the Collaterals Decoction

Bian Dou Hua	*Dolichos*	6 - 9 g
Xi Gua Shuang	*Citrullus*	6 - 9 g
Si Gua Pi	*Luffa*	6 - 9 g
Jin Yin Hua	*Lonicera*	6 - 9 g
He Ye	*Nelumbo*	6 g
Dan Zhu Ye	*Lophatherum*	6 - 9 g

Qi and blood level heat: qi level heat causing high fever, thirst, sweating; and blood level heat causing bleeding conditions, coma, or restlessness. This formula also treats toxic heat.

T dark red, dry, yellow coat

P flooding, rapid

☞ Shi Gao - Gypsum should be decocted first for 20 minutes. Xi Jiao - Rhinoceros should be powdered and added to the strained decoction. It should be substituted with 6 - 9 g of Shui Niu Jiao - Bubalus, or 30 g of Bai Mao Gen - Imperata.

QING WEN BAI DU YIN

Clear Epidemics and Overcome Toxin Decoction

Shi Gao	*Gypsum*	40 - 100 g
Zhi Mu	*Anemarrhena*	9 - 12 g
Xuan Shen	*Scrophularia*	6 - 9 g
Dan Zhu Ye	*Lophatherum*	3 - 6 g
Xi Jiao	*Rhinoceros*	1 - 3 g
Chi Shao Yao	*Paeonia*	6 - 9 g
Huang Qin	*Scutellaria*	6 - 9 g
Huang Lian	*Coptis*	3 - 6 g
Mu Dan Pi	*Paeonia*	6 - 9 g
Sheng Di Huang	*Rehmannia*	6 - 12 g
Zhi Zi	*Gardenia*	3 - 6 g
Jie Geng	*Platycodon*	3 - 6 g
Lian Qiao	*Forsythia*	6 - 9 g
Gan Cao	*Glycyrrhiza*	3 - 6 g

Qi level heat with toxin in the upper body causing throat swelling, fever, sweating, and thirst for cold fluids.

T red, yellow coat

P flooding, rapid

QING XIN LIANG GE SAN

Clear the Heart and Cool the Diaphragm Powder

Lian Qiao	*Forsythia*	6 - 15 g
Huang Qin	*Scutellaria*	6 - 9 g
Zhi Zi	*Gardenia*	3 - 6 g
Bo He	*Mentha*	3 - 6 g
Jie Geng	*Platycodon*	3 - 6 g
Shi Gao	*Gypsum*	12 - 15 g
Gan Cao	*Glycyrrhiza*	3 - 6 g

Heat or damp heat has entered the Stomach leading to fever, thirst, nausea and vomiting, and distention in the middle jiao.

T red

P rapid

ZHEN NI BAI HU TANG

White Tiger Decoction to Suppress Rebellion

Shi Gao	Gypsum	20 - 35 g
Zhi Mu	Anemarrhena	12 - 18 g
Zhu Ru	Bambusa	6 - 9 g
Ban Xia	Pinellia	6 - 12 g

Heat in the chest and Lungs due to taiyang disease; or lingering qi level heat manifesting in the yangming channel layer. In some patients this formula will induce vomiting, after which the symptoms will disappear.

T red, especially the tip, yellow coat

P rapid, forceful, superficial

✘ This prescription can cause vomiting.

ZHI ZI DOU CHI TANG

Gardenia and Prepared Soybean Decoction

Zhi Zi	Gardenia	6 - 9 g
Dan Dou Chi	Glycine	6 - 9 g

Qi level heat damaged the qi and yin. Now there is residual heat and a mild fever, dry mouth, and irritability.

T red

P rapid, weak, thin

ZHU YE SHI GAO TANG

Lophatherum and Gypsum Decoction

Extract Formula Name: Bamboo Leaves and Gypsum Combination

Dan Zhu Ye	Lophatherum	6 - 15 g
Shi Gao	Gypsum	20 - 30 g
Ban Xia	Pinellia	6 - 9 g
Ren Shen	Panax	3 - 6 g
Zhi Gan Cao	Glycyrrhiza	3 - 6 g
Jing Mi	Oryza	9 - 15 g
Mai Men Dong	Ophiopogon	12 - 15 g

HEAT IN THE YING (NUTRITIVE) LEVEL

- mental restlessness
- dry mouth without desire to drink
- night fevers
- skin eruptions

T deep red, no coat

P thin, rapid

Heat in the ying level with yin deficiency causing high fever which is worse at night, delirious speech, or mild purpura.

T dark red and dry

P rapid, thin

☞ Xi Jiao - Rhinoceros should be substituted with 9 g of Shui Niu Jiao - Bubalus or 30 g of Bai Mao Gen - Imperata.

QING YING TANG

Clear the Nutritive Level Decoction

Extract Formula Name: Rhinoceros and Scrophularia Combination

Xi Jiao	*Rhinoceros*	3 - 6 g
Sheng Di Huang	*Rehmannia*	9 - 12 g
Mai Men Dong	*Ophiopogon*	6 - 9 g
Huang Lian	*Coptis*	3 - 6 g
Xuan Shen	*Scrophularia*	6 - 9 g
Dan Zhu Ye	*Lophatherum*	6 g
Lian Qiao	*Forsythia*	6 g
Dan Shen	*Salvia*	6 - 9 g
Jin Yin Hua	*Lonicera*	6 - 9 g

HEAT IN THE XUE (BLOOD) LEVEL

- skin eruptions, purpura
- hematemesis, melena
- high fever
- mania

T dark red
P rapid, wiry

Heat in the qi and blood levels resulting in purpura.

T red, thin yellow coat

P flooding, rapid

☞ Shi Gao - Gypsum should be decocted first for 20 minutes. Xi Jiao - Rhinoceros is powdered and added to the strained decoction. Shui Niu Jiao - Bubalus should be substituted for Xi Jiao.

HUA BAN TANG

Transform Blotches Decoction

Shi Gao	*Gypsum*	30 g
Zhi Mu	*Anemarrhena*	12 g
Xuan Shen	*Scrophularia*	10 g
Xi Jiao	*Rhinoceros*	2 - 6 g
Jing Mi	*Oryza*	9 g
Gan Cao	*Glycyrrhiza*	10 g

Blood level heat and taiyin level disease with lingering summer-heat causing thirst and severe sweating.

T red or dark red

P rapid

JIA JIAN SHENG MAI SAN

Modified Generate the Pulse Powder

Mai Men Dong	*Ophiopogon*	6 - 12 g
Wu Wei Zi	*Schisandra*	6 - 12 g
Bei Sha Shen	*Glehnia*	6 - 12 g
Mu Dan Pi	*Paeonia*	6 - 12 g
Sheng Di Huang	*Rehmannia*	6 - 12 g

Heat in the blood level causing menorrhagia where the yin has already been damaged. Symptoms include thirst, dry mouth, and restlessness.

T red, yellow coat

P rapid, thin, forceful

☞ Ce Bai Ye Tan - Biota is charred to strenghten the stop bleeding effect.

QING RE ZHI BENG TANG

Clear Heat and Stop Excessive Uterine Bleeding Decoction

Huang Qin	*Scutellaria*	9 - 15 g
Huang Bai	*Phellodendron*	9 - 12 g
Zhi Zi	*Gardenia*	6 - 9 g
Mu Dan Pi	*Paeonia*	6 - 9 g
Chun Gen Bai Pi	*Ailanthus*	9 - 25 g
Sheng Di Huang	*Rehmannia*	9 - 18 g
Bai Shao Yao	*Paeonia*	9 - 25 g
Ce Bai Ye Tan	*Biota*	9 - 25 g
Gui Ban	*Chinemys*	9 - 15 g
Di Yu	*Sanguisorba*	9 - 18 g

Qi and blood level heat: qi level heat causing high fever, thirst, sweating; and blood level heat causing bleeding conditions, coma, or restlessness. This formula also treats toxic heat.

T dark red, dry, yellow coat

P flooding, rapid

☞ Shi Gao - Gypsum should be decocted first for 20 minutes. Xi Jiao - Rhinoceros should be powdered and added to the strained decoction. It should be substituted with 6 - 9 g of Shui Niu Jiao - Bubalus, or 30 g of Bai Mao Gen - Imperata.

QING WEN BAI DU YIN

Clear Epidemics and Overcome Toxin Decoction

Shi Gao	*Gypsum*	40 - 100 g
Zhi Mu	*Anemarrhena*	9 - 12 g
Xuan Shen	*Scrophularia*	6 - 9 g
Dan Zhu Ye	*Lophatherum*	3 - 6 g
Xi Jiao	*Rhinoceros*	1 - 3 g
Chi Shao Yao	*Paeonia*	6 - 9 g
Huang Qin	*Scutellaria*	6 - 9 g
Huang Lian	*Coptis*	3 - 6 g
Mu Dan Pi	*Paeonia*	6 - 9 g
Sheng Di Huang	*Rehmannia*	6 - 12 g
Zhi Zi	*Gardenia*	3 - 6 g
Jie Geng	*Platycodon*	3 - 6 g
Lian Qiao	*Forsythia*	6 - 9 g
Gan Cao	*Glycyrrhiza*	3 - 6 g

Severe toxin, epidemic summer heat, and blood heat causing delirious speech, purpura, or red eyes. This formula opens the orifice.

T scarlet

P rapid or flooding

☞ Herbs should be made into pills. Xi Jiao - Rhinoceros should be substituted with Shui Niu Jiao - Bubalus.

SHEN XI DAN

Magical Rhinoceros Special Pill

Xi Jiao	*Rhinoceros*	60 - 90 g
Jin Yin Hua	*Lonicera*	200 - 225 g
Ban Lan Gen	*Isatis*	100 - 135 g
Huang Qin	*Scutellaria*	60 - 90 g
Sheng Di Huang	*Rehmannia*	200 - 225 g
Lian Qiao	*Forsythia*	125 - 150 g
Xuan Shen	*Scrophularia*	90 - 105 g
Dan Dou Chi	*Glycine*	100 - 120 g
Shi Chang Pu	*Acorus*	60 - 90 g
Tian Hua Fen	*Trichosanthes*	40 - 60 g
Zi Cao	*Lithospermum*	40 - 60 g

Heat in the blood resulting in various types of upper jiao bleeding such as hemoptysis or epistaxis.

T red or dark red

P wiry, forceful, rapid

SI SHENG WAN

Four-Fresh Pill

Ce Bai Ye	*Biota*	9 - 12 g
Sheng Di Huang	*Rehmannia*	15 - 20 g
He Ye	*Nelumbo*	9 - 12 g
Ai Ye	*Artemisia*	6 - 9 g

Four Stages

Blood level heat with blood stagnation causing various bleeding disorders such as melena, hematurea, hematemesis, purpura, or thirst but no desire to drink.

T dark red, or purple, dry, yellow coat

P rapid, thin

☞ Xi Jiao - Rhinoceros should be powdered and then added into the strained decoction. It should be substituted with 60 g Shui Niu Jiao - Bubalus. Powder and cook separately for 20 minutes before including the other herbs. Xi Jiao may also be substituted with 30 - 60 g of Bai Mao Gen - Imperata.

✪ **Major Formula**

XI JIAO DI HUANG TANG

Rhinoceros Horn and Rehmannia Decoction

Extract Formula Name: Rhinoceros and Rehmannia Combination

Xi Jiao	*Rhinoceros*	3 - 9 g
Sheng Di Huang	*Rehmannia*	15 - 30 g
Mu Dan Pi	*Paeonia*	9 - 15 g
Chi Shao Yao	*Paeonia*	9 - 15 g

INTERNAL MEDICINE DISHARMONIES AND MISCELLANEOUS SYNDROMES

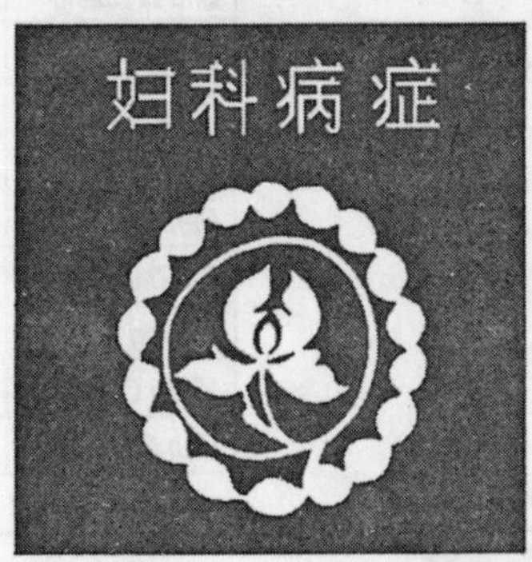

OB-GYN/MENSTRUAL DISORDERS

- irregular menstruation
- dysmenorrhea, amenorrhea
- uterine bleeding

T depends on involved syndrome

P depends on involved syndrome

Late periods due to yang deficiency or cold in the uterus. This formula is also useful during pregnancy to warm the uterus.

T pale, white coat

P frail

☞ Herbs should be ground into a powder and made into 6 g pills with rice vinegar.

AI FU NUAN GONG WAN

Mugwort and Cyperus Pill for Warming the Womb

Ai Ye	*Artemisia*	60 - 90 g
Xiang Fu	*Cyperus*	150 - 180 g
Wu Zhu Yu	*Evodia*	40 - 60 g
Bai Shao Yao	*Paeonia*	40 - 60 g
Huang Qi	*Astragalus*	40 - 60 g
Dang Gui	*Angelica*	60 - 90 g
Xu Duan	*Dipsacus*	30 - 45 g
Shu Di Huang	*Rehmannia*	15 - 30 g
Chuan Xiong	*Ligusticum*	40 - 60 g
Rou Gui	*Cinnamomum*	9 - 15 g

Qi and blood deficiency with blood stagnation. This formula is for a restless fetus, infertility, irregular periods, poor appetite, weakness, or fatigue.

T pale, thin white coat

P weak, maybe wiry

BA ZHEN YI MU WAN

Eight-Treasure Pill to Benefit Mothers

Shu Di Huang	Rehmannia	6 - 15 g
Chuan Xiong	Ligusticum	3 - 9 g
Dang Gui	Angelica	6 - 9 g
Bai Shao Yao	Paeonia	6 - 12 g
Ren Shen	Panax	6 - 12 g
Bai Zhu	Atractylodes	3 - 9 g
Fu Ling	Poria	6 - 9 g
Yi Mu Cao	Leonurus	6 - 18 g
Gan Cao	Glycyrrhiza	3 - 6 g

Kidney qi/yin deficiency causing menorrhagia. Other symptoms may include low back pain, frequent urination, or weakness in the knees.

T red or normal color, thin white coat

P weak, especially in both chi (third) positions, slightly rapid

BAO YIN JIAN

Augment Yin Decoction

Huang Qin	Scutellaria	9 - 12 g
Huang Bai	Phellodendron	9 - 12 g
Sheng Di Huang	Rehmannia	9 - 15 g
Shu Di Huang	Rehmannia	9 - 15 g
Shan Yao	Dioscorea	6 - 9 g
Bai Shao Yao	Paeonia	6 - 12 g
Xu Duan	Dipsacus	6 - 9 g
Gan Cao	Glycyrrhiza	3 - 6 g

Spleen/Stomach qi deficiency where the Spleen qi is sinking, or the Spleen is not governing the blood. qi deficiency can lead to (morning) fever, early periods, weakness, diarrhea, or pallor.

T pale, swollen, teethmarks, thin white coat

P weak

BU ZHONG YI QI TANG

Tonify the Middle and Augment the Qi Decoction

Extract Formula Name: Ginseng and Astragalus Combination

Ren Shen	*Panax*	6 - 12 g
Huang Qi	*Astragalus*	9 - 15 g
Dang Gui	*Angelica*	6 - 9 g
Chen Pi	*Citrus*	3 - 6 g
Sheng Ma	*Cimicifuga*	3 - 6 g
Chai Hu	*Bupleurum*	3 - 9 g
Bai Zhu	*Atractylodes*	3 - 9 g
Zhi Gan Cao	*Glycyrrhiza*	3 - 6 g

Severe phlegm damp accumulation causing dizziness, headache, sticky phlegm expectoration, or amenorrhea due to phlegm obstruction.

T thick sticky white or slightly yellowish coat

P slippery

CANG FU DAO TAN TANG

Atractylodes, Cyperus, and Guide Out Phlegm Decoction

Ban Xia	*Pinellia*	6 - 9 g
Chen Pi	*Citrus*	3 - 6 g
Fu Ling	*Poria*	6 - 9 g
Tian Nan Xing	*Arisaema*	1 - 3 g
Zhi Shi	*Citrus*	3 - 9 g
Gan Cao	*Glycyrrhiza*	3 - 6 g
Cang Zhu	*Atractylodes*	3 - 9 g
Xiang Fu	*Cyperus*	3 - 9 g
Sheng Jiang	*Zingiber*	6 - 9 g

Yin and blood deficiency with blood stagnation causing emaciation, no appetite, amenorrhea, tidal fever, or abdominal distention.

T red, pale, purple or purple spots

P thin, choppy

✘ Do not use during pregnancy.

DA HUANG ZHE CHONG WAN

Rhubarb and Eupolyphaga Pill

Da Huang	*Rheum*	12 - 18 g
Tu Bie Chong	*Eupolyphaga*	3 g
Xing Ren	*Prunus*	3 - 6 g
Gan Qi	*Sinica*	3 g
Sheng Di Huang	*Rehmannia*	12 - 18 g
Bai Shao Yao	*Paeonia*	6 - 12 g
Meng Chong	*Tabanus*	3 - 6 g
Qi Cao	*Holotrichia*	3 - 6 g
Tao Ren	*Prunus*	6 - 9 g
Shui Zhi	*Hirudo*	3 - 6 g
Huang Qin	*Scutellaria*	6 g
Gan Cao	*Glycyrrhiza*	3 - 6 g

Liver/Spleen disharmony with heat. Symptoms include irregular menstruation, red or bloodshot eyes, or irritability.

T red sides, light purple, thin white coat

P wiry, rapid

DAN ZHI XIAO YAO SAN (JIA WEI XIAO YAO SAN)

Moutan, Gardenia, and Rambling Powder

Extract Formula Name: Bupleurum and Peony Formula

Mu Dan Pi	*Paeonia*	6 - 9 g
Zhi Zi	*Gardenia*	3 - 6 g
Chai Hu	*Bupleurum*	6 - 9 g
Bo He	*Mentha*	3 - 6 g
Dang Gui	*Angelica*	6 - 9 g
Bai Shao Yao	*Paeonia*	6 - 9 g
Bai Zhu	*Atractylodes*	3 - 9 g
Fu Ling	*Poria*	6 - 9 g
Gan Cao	*Glycyrrhiza*	3 - 6 g
[Sheng Jiang	*Zingiber*	3 - 6 g]

Qi/blood deficiency with bleeding, fever, heat feelings in the muscles, thirst with a desire for warm liquids, or irregular periods.

T pale, thin coat

P empty

DANG GUI BU XUE TANG

Dang Gui Decoction to Tonify the Blood

Extract Formula Name: Tang-Kuei and Astragalus Combination

Huang Qi	*Astragalus*	30 g
Dang Gui	*Angelica*	6 g

Kidney and Liver yin deficiency causing irregular menses, scanty menstrual flow, tinnitus, dizziness, or night sweating.

T red, scanty coat

P thin, rapid

DANG GUI DI HUANG YIN

Dang Gui and Rehmannia Decoction

Dang Gui	*Angelica*	6 - 9 g
Shu Di Huang	*Rehmannia*	6 - 12 g
Huai Niu Xi	*Achyranthes*	6 - 9 g
Shan Yao	*Dioscorea*	6 - 9 g
Du Zhong	*Eucommia*	6 - 9 g
Shan Zhu Yu	*Cornus*	6 - 9 g
Zhi Gan Cao	*Glycyrrhiza*	3 - 6 g

Heat in the yangming channel with pre-existing severe blood stagnation in the lower jiao which affects the uterus and the intestines. Symptoms include jaundice, mania, fever, melena with dry stools which are relatively easy to discharge, dysmenorrhea, amenorrhea, abdominal fullness, or bleeding in the stomach. This formula is stronger than 'Di Dang Wan - Resistance Pill.'

T red, dark purple

P wiry, rapid

✘ Do not use during pregnancy. Use only for a short duration.

DI DANG TANG

Resistance Decoction

Da Huang	*Rheum*	6 - 12 g
Tao Ren	*Prunus*	6 - 9 g
Shui Zhi	*Hirudo*	1 - 3 g
Meng Chong	*Tabanus*	1 - 3 g

Chronic uterine bleeding due to blood deficiency and cold. This formula is also useful for spotting or clear leukorrhea.

T pale, white coat

P weak, thin

☞ E Jiao - Equus should be dissolved into the strained tea.

DING XIANG JIAO AI TANG

Clove, Ass-Hide Gelatin, and Mugwort Decoction

Ding Xiang	*Eugenia*	3 - 6 g
E Jiao	*Equus*	3 - 9 g
Ai Ye	*Artemisia*	6 g
Shu Di Huang	*Rehmannia*	6 - 9 g
Dang Gui	*Angelica*	6 - 9 g
Bai Shao Yao	*Paeonia*	6 - 9 g
Chuan Xiong	*Ligusticum*	3 - 9 g

Kidney yin and yang deficiency with fire causing menopause, hot flashes, or urinary frequency.

T red

P rapid or normal rate, thin

ER XIAN TANG

Two-Immortal Decoction

Extract Formula Name: Curculigo and Epimedium Combination

Yin Yang Huo	*Epimedium*	9 - 15 g
Xian Mao	*Curculigo*	9 - 15 g
Dang Gui	*Angelica*	6 - 9 g
Huang Bai	*Phellodendron*	6 - 9 g
Zhi Mu	*Anemarrhena*	6 - 9 g
Ba Ji Tian	*Morinda*	6 - 9 g

Qi/blood stagnation under the diaphragm and epigastrium, or masses in the abdomen or epigastrium.

T purple

P wiry or choppy

✘ Do not use during pregnancy.

GE XIA ZHU YU TANG

Drive Out Blood Stasis Below the Diaphragm Decoction

Extract Formula Name: Persica and Carthamus Combination

Dang Gui	*Angelica*	6 - 9 g
Chuan Xiong	*Ligusticum*	6 - 9 g
Tao Ren	*Prunus*	6 - 9 g
Hong Hua	*Carthamus*	3 - 6 g
Mu Dan Pi	*Paeonia*	6 - 9 g
Chi Shao Yao	*Paeonia*	6 - 9 g
Yan Hu Suo	*Corydalis*	3 - 6 g
Xiang Fu	*Cyperus*	3 - 9 g
Zhi Ke	*Citrus*	3 - 6 g
Wu Ling Zhi	*Trogopterus*	6 - 9 g
Wu Yao	*Lindera*	3 - 6 g
Gan Cao	*Glycyrrhiza*	6 - 9 g

Spleen qi deficiency leading to uncontrolled menstrual bleeding which is pale and watery (ben lou syndrome).

T pale, swollen, teethmarks, thin coat

P hollow or thin, deep, weak

GU BEN ZHI BENG TANG

Stabilize the Root and Stop Excessive Uterine Bleeding Decoction

Shu Di Huang	*Rehmannia*	6 - 20 g
Bai Zhu	*Atractylodes*	6 - 15 g
Huang Qi	*Astragalus*	6 - 15 g
Dang Gui	*Angelica*	6 - 9 g
Ren Shen	*Panax*	6 - 9 g
Pao Jiang	*Zingiber*	3 - 6 g

Spleen qi deficiency causing ben lou syndrome - excessive uterine bleeding or spotting.

T pale, swollen, slight teeth-marks, thin white coat

P weak, thin

GU BEN ZHI LOU TANG

Stabilize the Root and Stop Spotting Decoction

Ren Shen	*Panax*	9 - 15 g
Bai Zhu	*Atractylodes*	6 - 12 g
Gan Jiang	*Zingiber*	3 - 6 g
Shu Di Huang	*Rehmannia*	9 - 12 g
Dang Gui	*Angelica*	9 - 12 g
Sheng Ma	*Cimicifuga*	6 - 9 g
Shan Yao	*Dioscorea*	6 - 12 g
Da Zao	*Ziziphus*	3 - 4 pc

Menorrhagia or spotting due to Kidney and Liver yin deficiency, false heat, blood stagnation, or Spleen qi deficiency.

T pale, thin coat

P weak, thin

☞ Zong Lu Pi Tan - Trachycarpus should be charred to maximize the stop bleeding function.

GU CHONG TANG

Stabilize Gushing Decoction

Bai Zhu	*Atractylodes*	9 - 30 g
Shan Zhu Yu	*Cornus*	9 - 24 g
Long Gu	*Os Draconis*	12 - 24 g
Mu Li	*Ostrea*	12 - 24 g
Zong Lu Pi Tan	*Trachycarpus*	3 - 6 g
Huang Qi	*Astragalus*	9 - 18 g
Bai Shao Yao	*Paeonia*	9 - 12 g
Qian Cao Gen	*Rubia*	6 - 9 g
Hai Piao Xiao	*Sepia*	9 - 12 g
Wu Bei Zi	*Rhus/Melaphis*	1 - 2 g

Liver qi stagnation with heat causing uterine bleeding which depletes yin (ben lou syndrome).

T red, no coat

P thin, rapid

GU JING WAN

Stabilize the Menses Pill

Extract Formula Name: Tortoise Shell and Scute Combination

Gui Ban	Chinemys	15 - 30 g
Chun Pi	Ailanthus	6 - 12 g
Bai Shao Yao	Paeonia	15 - 30 g
Huang Bai	Phellodendron	6 - 9 g
Huang Qin	Scutellaria	15 - 30 g
Xiang Fu	Cyperus	3 - 6 g

Kidney qi/yin deficiency causing irregular periods, leukorrhea, or a bearing-down sensation.

T red, thin white coat

P weak, especially the chi (third) positions

GU YIN JIAN

Stabilize the Yin Decoction

Shu Di Huang	Rehmannia	6 - 12 g
Shan Yao	Dioscorea	6 - 9 g
Wu Wei Zi	Schisandra	6 - 9 g
Shan Zhu Yu	Cornus	6 - 9 g
Tu Si Zi	Cuscuta	6 - 9 g
Ren Shen	Panax	6 - 9 g
Yuan Zhi	Polygala	3 g
Zhi Gan Cao	Glycyrrhiza	3 - 6 g

Blood deficiency with yang deficiency and cold causing coldness in the uterus with dysmenorrhea. The blood is scanty, pale, and watery. The patient experiences severe cramping upon menstrual onset.

T pale, light purple, some cracks, thin white coat

P slow, thin, weak

GUI FU SI WU TANG

Cinnamon Bark, Aconite, and Four-Substance Decoction

Sheng Di Huang	Rehmannia	6 - 12 g
Dang Gui	Angelica	6 - 9 g
Chuan Xiong	Ligusticum	3 - 9 g
Bai Shao Yao	Paeonia	6 - 9 g
Rou Gui	Cinnamomum	3 - 9 g
Fu Zi	Aconitum	1 - 6 g

Kidney qi deficiency with Kidney/Liver yin deficiency causing amenorrhea, or back and knee pain.

T pale or red, thin white or scanty coat

P weak, maybe thin especially in the left chi (third) position

GUI SHEN TANG

Comeback Kidney Decoction

Shu Di Huang	*Rehmannia*	6 - 15 g
Shan Yao	*Dioscorea*	9 - 15 g
Shan Zhu Yu	*Cornus*	9 - 12 g
Gou Qi Zi	*Lycium*	9 - 15 g
Dang Gui	*Angelica*	9 - 12 g
Du Zhong	*Eucommia*	6 - 12 g
Fu Ling	*Poria*	6 - 12 g
Tu Si Zi	*Cuscuta*	9 - 12 g

Blood and phlegm stagnation in the uterus leading to masses or lumps, amenorrhea, dysmenorrhea, or restless fetus.

T purple, sticky coat

P wiry, slippery, choppy

GUI ZHI FU LING WAN

Cinnamon Twig and Poria Pill

Extract Formula Name: Cinnamon and Hoelen Formula

Gui Zhi	*Cinnamomum*	6 - 12 g
Fu Ling	*Poria*	6 - 12 g
Mu Dan Pi	*Paeonia*	6 - 12 g
Tao Ren	*Prunus*	6 - 12 g
Chi Shao Yao	*Paeonia*	9 - 12 g

Liver qi stagnation with blood deficiency causing delayed periods with clots.

T pale, purple

P choppy, wiry

GUO QI YIN

Delayed Menstruation Decoction

Shu Di Huang	*Rehmannia*	6 - 9 g
Dang Gui	*Angelica*	6 - 9 g
Bai Shao Yao	*Paeonia*	6 - 9 g
Chuan Xiong	*Ligusticum*	3 - 6 g
Hong Hua	*Carthamus*	3 - 6 g
Tao Ren	*Prunus*	3 - 6 g
Xiang Fu	*Cyperus*	3 - 6 g
Mu Tong	*Akebia*	3 - 6 g
E Zhu	*Curcuma*	3 - 6 g
Rou Gui	*Cinnamomum*	1 - 3 g
Gan Cao	*Glycyrrhiza*	3 - 6 g

Epistaxis or hematemesis during menses due to Stomach deficiency and rebellious qi.

T pale

P weak, thin

JIA WEI MAI MEN DONG TANG

Augmented Ophiopogon Decoction

Mai Men Dong	*Ophiopogon*	9 - 15 g
Shan Yao	*Dioscorea*	9 - 12 g
Ren Shen	*Panax*	9 - 12 g
Dan Shen	*Salvia*	9 - 12 g
Ban Xia	*Pinellia*	6 - 9 g
Bai Shao Yao	*Paeonia*	6 - 9 g
Tao Ren	*Prunus*	3 - 6 g
Da Zao	*Ziziphus*	3 - 5 pc
Gan Cao	*Glycyrrhiza*	3 - 6 g

Cold uterus with underlying blood deficiency causing excessive uterine bleed with pale, watery blood.

T pale

P slow, thin, weak

JIAO AI SI WU TANG

Gelatin and Artemisia and Four-Substance Decoction

Extract Formula Name: Gelatin and Artemisia Combination

Shu Di Huang	*Rehmannia*	6 - 12 g
Bai Shao Yao	*Paeonia*	6 - 9 g
Chuan Xiong	*Ligusticum*	3 - 6 g
Dang Gui	*Angelica*	6 - 9 g
E Jiao	*Equus*	3 - 9 g
Ai Ye	*Artemisia*	6 - 9 g
Gan Cao	*Glycyrrhiza*	3 - 6 g

Chong and Ren imbalance with blood deficiency causing restless fetus, pale post-partum bleeding, abdominal pain, a weak low back, or a cold uterus.

T pale

P frail, slow

☞ E Jiao - Equus should be dissolved at the end into the strained tea.

JIAO AI TANG

Ass-Hide Equus and Mugwort Decoction

Extract Formula Name: Tang-kuei and Equus Combination

E Jiao	*Equus*	6 - 9 g
Ai Ye	*Artemisia*	6 - 9 g
Dang Gui	*Angelica*	6 - 9 g
Sheng Di Huang	*Rehmannia*	18 g
Bai Shao Yao	*Paeonia*	12 g
Chuan Xiong	*Ligusticum*	6 g
Gan Cao	*Glycyrrhiza*	3 - 6 g

Spleen qi deficiency causing severe uterine bleeding which is pale in color, or early or irregular periods. The Spleen qi is sinking causing a restless fetus.

T pale, swollen, teethmarks, thin white coat

P weak

JU YUAN JIAN

Lift the Source Decoction

Ren Shen	*Panax*	6 - 9 g
Huang Qi	*Astragalus*	9 - 12 g
Sheng Ma	*Cimicifuga*	3 - 6 g
Bai Zhu	*Atractylodes*	3 - 6 g
Gan Cao	*Glycyrrhiza*	3 - 6 g

Liver qi stagnation with cold in the Stomach causing abdominal pain which is relieved by warmth. The Formula is also useful for dysmenorrhea.

T pale, white coat

P weak, slow, or wiry

LIANG FU WAN

Galanga and Cyperus Pill

Extract Formula Name: Galanga and Cyperus Formula

Gao Liang Jiang	*Alpinia*	6 - 9 g
Xiang Fu	*Cyperus*	6 - 9 g

Blood deficiency with deficient or excess heat causing purple menstrual blood, early periods, or thick leukorrhea with tidal fever.

T pale

P rapid, thin, weak

QIN LIAN SI WU TANG

Four-Substance Decoction with Scutellaria and Coptis

Huang Qin	*Scutellaria*	6 - 9 g
Huang Lian	*Coptis*	3 - 6 g
Chuan Xiong	*Ligusticum*	3 - 6 g
Bai Shao Yao	*Paeonia*	6 - 9 g
Dang Gui	*Angelica*	6 - 9 g
Mai Men Dong	*Ophiopogon*	6 - 9 g
Sheng Di Huang	*Rehmannia*	9 - 12 g

Yin deficiency with false heat causing early periods or constipation.

T red, scanty yellowish coat

P thin, rapid

QING JING SAN

Clear the Menses Powder

Shu Di Huang	*Rehmannia*	6 - 12 g
Mu Dan Pi	*Paeonia*	6 - 9 g
Di Gu Pi	*Lycium*	6 - 9 g
Qing Hao	*Artemisia*	3 - 6 g
Bai Shao Yao	*Paeonia*	6 - 9 g
Fu Ling	*Poria*	6 g
Huang Bai	*Phellodendron*	3 g

Excess heat or heat in the blood leading to gushing uterine bleeding.

T red, yellow coat

P forceful, rapid, slippery

☞ Zong Lu Pi Tan - Trachycarpus is charred to maximize the stop bleeding function.

QING JING ZHI XUE TANG

Cool the Menses and Stop Bleeding Decoction

Sheng Di Huang	*Rehmannia*	6 - 25 g
Huang Bai	*Phellodendron*	6 - 12 g
Huang Qin	*Scutellaria*	9 - 15 g
Di Yu	*Sanguisorba*	9 - 25 g
Yi Mu Cao	*Leonurus*	9 - 15 g
Bai Mao Gen	*Imperata*	12 - 25 g
Mu Dan Pi	*Paeonia*	6 - 9 g
Pu Huang	*Typha*	9 - 15 g
Zong Lu Pi Tan	*Trachycarpus*	9 - 18 g

Blood heat causing severe uterine bleeding, heavy periods, and the blood is bright red and gushing (ben syndrome).

T red

P rapid, forceful

☞ Zong Lu Pi Tan - Trachycarpus and Di Yu Tan - Sanguisorba are charred to strengthen the stop bleeding effect. E Jiao - Equus should be dissolved into the strained tea.

QING RE GU JING TANG I

Clear Heat and Stabilize Menses Decoction I

Di Gu Pi	*Lycium*	6 - 9 g
Huang Qin	*Scutellaria*	6 - 9 g
Zhi Zi	*Gardenia*	6 - 9 g
Bai Mao Gen	*Imperata*	6 - 9 g
Mu Dan Pi	*Paeonia*	6 - 12 g
Sheng Di Huang	*Rehmannia*	6 - 12 g
Zong Lu Pi Tan	*Trachycarpus*	6 - 9 g
Di Yu Tan	*Sanguisorba*	6 - 9 g
Gan Cao	*Glycyrrhiza*	6 - 9 g
Ou Jie	*Nelumbo*	6 - 9 g
Gui Ban	*Chinemys*	12 g
Mu Li	*Ostrea*	12 g
E Jiao	*Equus*	12 g

Damp heat obstruction causing dysmenorrhea, pain prior to onset of the menstruation, cramps, or leukorrhea.

T light purple or red, thick sticky yellow coat

P slippery, slightly rapid, or wiry

QING RE GU JING TANG II

Clear Heat and Stabilize Menses Decoction II

Huang Bai	*Phellodendron*	6 - 9 g
Huang Lian	*Coptis*	3 - 9 g
Mu Dan Pi	*Paeonia*	6 - 12 g
Sheng Di Huang	*Rehmannia*	6 - 12 g
Dang Gui	*Angelica*	6 - 9 g
Chi Shao Yao	*Paeonia*	6 - 9 g
Chuan Xiong	*Ligusticum*	3 - 9 g
Yan Hu Suo	*Corydalis*	6 - 9 g

Heat in the blood level causing menorrhagia where the yin has already been damaged. Symptoms include thirst, dry mouth, and restlessness.

T red, yellow coat

P rapid, thin, forceful

☞ Ce Bai Ye Tan - Biota is charred to strenghten the stop bleeding effect.

QING RE ZHI BENG TANG

Clear Heat and Stop Excessive Uterine Bleeding Decoction

Huang Qin	*Scutellaria*	9 - 15 g
Huang Bai	*Phellodendron*	9 - 12 g
Zhi Zi	*Gardenia*	6 - 9 g
Mu Dan Pi	*Paeonia*	6 - 9 g
Chun Gen Bai Pi	*Ailanthus*	9 - 25 g
Sheng Di Huang	*Rehmannia*	9 - 18 g
Bai Shao Yao	*Paeonia*	9 - 25 g
Ce Bai Ye Tan	*Biota*	9 - 25 g
Gui Ban	*Chinemys*	9 - 15 g
Di Yu	*Sanguisorba*	9 - 18 g

Spleen/Lung qi and blood deficiency with Heart yang deficiency, or ying level deficiency. The patient is easily startled, experiences shortness of breath, lack of taste sensation, insomnia, or palpitations. This formula is also useful for irregular periods or uterine bleeding.

T pale, swollen

P weak

REN SHEN YANG YING TANG

Ginseng Decoction to Nourish the Nutritive Qi

Extract Formula Name: Ginseng Combination

Bai Shao Yao	*Paeonia*	9 - 15 g
Chen Pi	*Citrus*	3 - 6 g
Dang Gui	*Angelica*	3 - 9 g
Ren Shen	*Panax*	6 - 9 g
Huang Qi	*Astragalus*	6 - 12 g
Bai Zhu	*Atractylodes*	6 - 9 g
Shu Di Huang	*Rehmannia*	3 - 6 g
Wu Wei Zi	*Schisandra*	3 - 6 g
Fu Ling	*Poria*	3 - 6 g
Yuan Zhi	*Polygala*	2 - 6 g
Rou Gui	*Cinnamomum*	6 - 9 g
Gan Cao	*Glycyrrhiza*	3 - 6 g
[Da Zao	*Ziziphus*	2 pc]
[Gan Jiang	*Zingiber*	3 pc]

Heart fire and excess heat leading to nose bleeding or premenstrual vomiting.

T red, yellow coat

P rapid, or empty

✘ Caution during pregnancy.

SAN HUANG SI WU TANG

Three-Yellow and Four-Substance Decoction

Shu Di Huang	*Rehmannia*	6 - 15 g
Bai Shao Yao	*Paeonia*	6 - 9 g
Chuan Xiong	*Ligusticum*	3 - 9 g
Dang Gui	*Angelica*	6 - 9 g
Huang Lian	*Coptis*	3 - 9 g
Da Huang	*Rheum*	6 - 12 g
Huang Qin	*Scutellaria*	6 - 9 g

Severe qi deficiency with yang and blood deficiency and cold symptoms. Irregular menstruation with a pale and watery flow, dizziness, pale or sallow face, cold limbs, or chills.

T pale, wet, thin white coat

P deep, weak, thready

SHAN HE YIN

Mountain and River Decoction

Shu Di Huang	*Rehmannia*	15 - 25 g
Dang Gui	*Angelica*	6 - 9 g
Bai Shao Yao	*Paeonia*	6 - 9 g
Chuan Xiong	*Ligusticum*	3 - 9 g
Rou Gui	*Cinnamomum*	3 - 9 g
Huang Qi	*Astragalus*	6 - 15 g

Blood and cold stagnation in the lower jiao with mass formation, blood clots, and dysmenorrhea. This formula is also useful for liver cirrhosis.

T pale, purple

P wiry or choppy

✘ Do not use during pregnancy.

SHAO FU ZHU YU TANG

Drive Out Blood Stasis in the Lower Abdomen Decoction

Extract Formula Name: Cnidium and Bulrush Combination

Yan Hu Suo	*Corydalis*	3 - 6 g
Dang Gui	*Angelica*	6 - 9 g
Mo Yao	*Commiphora*	3 - 6 g
Rou Gui	*Cinnamomum*	3 - 6 g
Xiao Hui Xiang	*Foeniculum*	1.5 - 3 g
Gan Jiang	*Zingiber*	3 - 6 g
Pu Huang	*Typha*	6 - 9 g
Chi Shao Yao	*Paeonia*	6 - 9 g
Wu Ling Zhi	*Trogopterus*	6 - 9 g
Chuan Xiong	*Ligusticum*	3 - 9 g

Spleen qi deficiency with damp leading to diarrhea and irregular periods. Other symptoms include weight loss, fatigue, poor appetite, or pale face.

T pale, white coat

P weak or thin, slow

SHEN LING BAI ZHU SAN

Ginseng, Poria, and Atractylodes Powder

Extract Formula Name: Ginseng and Atractylodes Formula

Ren Shen	*Panax*	9 - 15 g
Fu Ling	*Poria*	9 - 12 g
Bai Zhu	*Atractylodes*	3 - 9 g
Gan Cao	*Glycyrrhiza*	6 - 9 g
Lian Zi	*Nelumbo*	3 - 9 g
Yi Yi Ren	*Coix*	6 - 15 g
Shan Yao	*Dioscorea*	9 - 15 g
Bian Dou	*Dolichos*	6 - 9 g
Jie Geng	*Platycodon*	3 - 6 g
Sha Ren	*Amomum*	3 g

Post-partum retention of lochia due to blood and cold stagnation.

T pale, purple

P choppy

☞ Add yellow wine to the decoction.

SHENG HUA TANG

Generation and Transformation Decoction

Extract Formula Name: Tang-Kuei and Ginger Combination

Dang Gui	*Angelica*	15 - 28 g
Tao Ren	*Prunus*	6 - 9 g
Pao Jiang	*Zingiber*	3 - 6 g
Chuan Xiong	*Ligusticum*	6 - 9 g
Gan Cao	*Glycyrrhiza*	3 - 6 g

Spleen qi/blood deficiency causing slow blood circulation with deficiency type abdominal pain during menstruation, or bleeding sores.

T pale, light purple, thin white coat

P thin, weak

SHENG YU TANG

Sage-like Healing Decoction

Shu Di Huang	*Rehmannia*	15 - 25 g
Ren Shen	*Panax*	12 - 15 g
Dang Gui	*Angelica*	12 - 15 g
Huang Qi	*Astragalus*	15 - 20 g
Chuan Xiong	*Ligusticum*	6 - 9 g
Bai Shao Yao	*Paeonia*	15 - 20 g

Qi/yang/blood deficiency. Symptoms include poor appetite, general malaise, mild cold symptoms, severe deficiency, rashes, dysmenorrhea, uterine bleeding, or post-partum deficiency.

T pale, thin white coat

P weak, thin, deep

SHI QUAN DA BU TANG

All-Inclusive Great Tonifying Decoction

Extract Formula Name: Ginseng and Tang-Kuei Ten Combination

Ren Shen	*Panax*	6 - 9 g
Fu Ling	*Poria*	9 - 12 g
Bai Zhu	*Atractylodes*	9 - 12 g
Gan Cao	*Glycyrrhiza*	3 - 6 g
Dang Gui	*Angelica*	12 - 15 g
Shu Di Huang	*Rehmannia*	15 - 20 g
Bai Shao Yao	*Paeonia*	12 - 15 g
Chuan Xiong	*Ligusticum*	3 - 9 g
Rou Gui	*Cinnamomum*	6 - 9 g
Huang Qi	*Astragalus*	15 - 20 g
[Da Zao	*Ziziphus*	1 - 3 g]
[Sheng Jiang	*Zingiber*	3 - 6 g]

Post-partum blood (lochia) retention with dark clots and severe abdominal pain. The stagnation is in the Chong and Ren channels.

T purple

P wiry

✘ Do not use during pregnancy.

SHI XIAO SAN

Sudden Smile Powder

Extract Formula Name: Pteropus and Bulrush Formula

Pu Huang	*Typha*	6 - 12 g
Wu Ling Zhi	*Trogopterus*	6 - 9 g

Spleen qi deficiency causing gushing uterine bleeding (ben syndrome).

T pale

P weak

SHOU PI JIAN

Consolidate Spleen Decoction

Cang Zhu	*Atractylodes*	3 - 6 g
Lian Zi	*Nelumbo*	3 - 9 g
Ren Shen	*Panax*	6 - 9 g
Suan Zao Ren	*Ziziphus*	6 - 12 g
Dang Gui	*Angelica*	3 - 9 g
Shan Yao	*Dioscorea*	6 - 9 g
Yuan Zhi	*Polygala*	3 - 6 g
Sheng Jiang	*Zingiber*	3 - 6 g
Zhi Gan Cao	*Glycyrrhiza*	3 - 6 g

Lung/Kidney yin deficiency with severe fire causing nosebleeds, or hemoptysis which occurs during or prior to the menses.

T red, cracks

P rapid, empty

SHUN JING TANG

Smooth the Menses Decoction

Shu Di Huang	*Rehmannia*	9 - 15 g
Mu Dan Pi	*Paeonia*	6 - 9 g
Dang Gui	*Angelica*	6 - 9 g
Bai Shao Yao	*Paeonia*	6 - 9 g
Bei Sha Shen	*Glehnia*	6 - 12 g
Jing Jie	*Schizonepeta*	6 - 9 g
Fu Ling	*Poria*	6 - 9 g

Blood stagnation with fire in the lower jiao causing constipation, sudden abdominal pain, dysmenorrhea, intestinal obstruction, or melena. In severe cases this may lead to restlessness, or even delirium.

T purple

P choppy or forceful

☞ Da Huang - Rheum should be added during the last 3 - 5 minutes of the decoction process. Mang Xiao - Mirabilitum should be added to the strained tea.

✘ Do not use during pregnancy.

TAO HE CHENG QI TANG

Peach Pit Decoction to Order the Qi

Extract Formula Name: Prunus and Rhubarb Combination

Tao Ren	*Prunus*	9 - 15 g
Gui Zhi	*Cinnamomum*	6 - 9 g
Mang Xiao	*Mirabilitum*	3 - 6 g
Da Huang	*Rheum*	9 - 12 g
Gan Cao	*Glycyrrhiza*	3 - 6 g

Mild blood deficiency with severe blood stagnation causing early periods or dysmenorrhea.

T pale or purple

P choppy or wiry

✘ Do not use during pregnancy.

TAO HONG SI WU TANG

Four-Substance Decoction with Safflower and Peach Pit

Shu Di Huang	*Rehmannia*	6 - 12 g
Bai Shao Yao	*Paeonia*	6 - 9 g
Chuan Xiong	*Ligusticum*	3 - 6 g
Dang Gui	*Angelica*	6 - 9 g
Tao Ren	*Prunus*	3 - 9 g
Hong Hua	*Carthamus*	3 - 6 g

Kidney and Liver yin deficiency causing amenorrhea, cold feeling in the abdomen, retarded growth in puberty, or clear leukorrhea.

T pale or slightly red

P weak, thin

☞ E Jiao - Equus should be added at the end to the strained tea.

TIAO GAN TANG

Regulating the Liver Decoction

Shan Yao	*Dioscorea*	9 - 12 g
E Jiao	*Equus*	6 - 12 g
Ba Ji Tian	*Morinda*	6 - 9 g
Dang Gui	*Angelica*	6 - 9 g
Ze Lan	*Lycopus*	6 - 12 g
Shan Zhu Yu	*Cornus*	6 - 9 g
Bai Shao Yao	*Paeonia*	6 - 9 g
Dan Shen	*Salvia*	6 - 9 g
Gan Cao	*Glycyrrhiza*	3 - 6 g

Deficient cold and blood stagnation causing menstrual irregularities, spotting between periods (lou syndrome), clots at the end of the period, coldness in the lower abdomen, or low-grade fever at night only.

T pale, purple, dark purple spots

P deep, slow, or tight

☞ E Jiao - Equus should be added at the end to the strained tea.

WEN JING TANG

Warm the Menses Decoction

Extract Formula Name: Tang-Kuei and Evodia Combination

Gui Zhi	*Cinnamomum*	6 - 9 g
Wu Zhu Yu	*Evodia*	6 - 9 g
Bai Shao Yao	*Paeonia*	6 - 9 g
Mai Men Dong	*Ophiopogon*	6 - 9 g
Mu Dan Pi	*Paeonia*	6 - 9 g
Ban Xia	*Pinellia*	6 - 9 g
Ren Shen	*Panax*	6 - 9 g
Dang Gui	*Angelica*	6 - 9 g
E Jiao	*Equus*	6 - 9 g
Chuan Xiong	*Ligusticum*	6 g
Sheng Jiang	*Zingiber*	3 - 6 g
Gan Cao	*Glycyrrhiza*	3 - 6 g

Liver qi stagnation causing late periods, irritability, premenstrual syndrome, or distention in the urinary tract.

T light purple, thin coat

P wiry

WU YAO TANG

Lindera Decoction

Wu Yao	*Lindera*	3 - 6 g
Dang Gui	*Angelica*	6 - 9 g
Xiang Fu	*Cyperus*	3 - 9 g
Mu Xiang	*Saussurea*	3 - 9 g
Gan Cao	*Zingiber*	3 - 6 g

Excess heat causing early periods, heavy periods with clots, flushed face, thirst, dry mouth, or irritability.

T red, cracks, rough, yellow coat

P rapid, forceful

☞ E Jiao - Equus should be dissolved into the strained tea.

XIANG QI TANG

Earlier-Time Decoction

Dang-Gui	*Angelica*	6 - 9 g
Chuan Xiong	*Ligusticum*	3 - 9 g
Bai Shao Yao	*Paeonia*	6 - 9 g
Ai Ye	*Artemisia*	6 - 9 g
E Jiao	*Equus*	3 - 6 g
Huang Bai	*Phellodendron*	6 - 9 g
Huang Qin	*Scutellaria*	6 - 9 g
Huang Lian	*Coptis*	3 - 6 g
Zhi Mu	*Anemarrhena*	6 - 12g
Xiang Fu	*Cyperus*	6 - 9 g
Gan Cao	*Glycyrrhiza*	3 - 6 g

Liver qi stagnation manifesting mostly as irregular periods. Menstruation is sometimes early or sometimes late, and the patient experiences severe premenstrual syndrome, cramping prior to the onset of bleeding, or breast distention.

T light purple, thin coat

P wiry

XIANG WU SAN

Cyperus and Lindera Powder

Xiang Fu	*Cyperus*	6 - 12 g
Wu Yao	*Lindera*	3 - 9 g
Chai Hu	*Bupleurum*	6 - 9 g
Bai Zhu	*Atractylodes*	3 - 9 g
Bai Shao Yao	*Paeonia*	6 - 9 g
Dang Gui	*Angelica*	6 - 9 g
Fu Ling	*Poria*	6 - 9 g

Blood deficiency causing delayed periods, a pale watery flow, scanty period, dizziness, poor memory, blurry vision.

T pale

P weak, thin

XIAO YIN JIAN

Minor Yin Decoction

Dang Gui	*Angelica*	6 - 9 g
Sheng Di Huang	*Rehmannia*	12 - 25 g
Bai Shao Yao	*Paeonia*	6 - 12 g
Gou Qi Zi	*Lycium*	6 - 12 g
Shan Yao	*Dioscorea*	6 - 9 g
Gan Cao	*Glycyrrhiza*	3 - 6 g

Blood stagnation in head, chest, and diaphragm causing angina, palpitations, insomnia, nightmares, or dysmenorrhea.

T purple or purple spots

P wiry

✘ Do not use during pregnancy.

XUE FU ZHU YU TANG

Drive out Stasis in the Mansion of Blood Decoction

Extract Formula Name: Persica and Achyranthes Combination

Dang Gui	Angelica	6 - 9 g
Chuan Xiong	Ligusticum	3 - 9 g
Sheng Di Huang	Rehmannia	6 - 9 g
Chi Shao Yao	Paeonia	6 - 9 g
Tao Ren	Prunus	6 - 12 g
Hong Hua	Carthamus	6 - 9 g
Chuan Niu Xi	Cyathula	9 - 12 g
Jie Geng	Platycodon	3 - 6 g
Zhi Ke	Citrus	3 - 6 g
Chai Hu	Bupleurum	3 - 9 g
Gan Cao	Glycyrrhiza	3 - 6 g

Blood stagnation with abdominal pain, severe spasms, and irregular periods.

T purple, or purple spots

P choppy, wiry

✘ Do not use during pregnancy.

YAN HU SUO TANG

Corydalis Decoction

Yan Hu Suo	Corydalis	30 - 45 g
Chi Shao Yao	Paeonia	9 - 15 g
Rou Gui	Cinnamomum	9 - 15 g
Ru Xiang	Boswellia	60 - 90 g
Mo Yao	Commiphora	60 - 90 g
Jiang Huang	Curcuma	60 - 90 g
Dang Gui	Angelica	9 - 15 g
Mu Xiang	Saussurea	60 - 90 g
Pu Huang	Typha	9 - 15 g
Gan Cao	Glycyrrhiza	6 - 9 g
[Sheng Jiang	Zingiber	3 - 6 g]

Spleen qi deficiency causing damp which heats up. This leads to heat type leukorrhea with a fishy smell or delayed periods from qi and blood deficiency.

T pale, thin sticky yellow or white coat

P slippery, weak

YI HUANG TANG

Change Yellow (Discharge) Decoction

Shan Yao	*Dioscorea*	9 - 30 g
Huang Bai	*Phellodendron*	6 - 9 g
Qian Shi	*Euryale*	9 - 30 g
Bai Guo	*Gingko*	6 - 10 pc
Che Qian Zi	*Plantago*	3 - 6 g

Kidney yang and essence deficiency causing amenorrhea, infertility, cold back or knees, pedal edema, or impotence.

T pale, swollen, teethmarks, thin white coat

P minute

YOU GUI WAN

Restore the Right Pill

Extract Formula Name: Eucommia and Rehmannia Formula

Rou Gui	*Cinnamomum*	6 - 9 g
Fu Zi	*Aconitum*	3 - 6 g
Gou Qi Zi	*Lycium*	6 - 9 g
Shan Yao	*Dioscorea*	6 - 9 g
Shu Di Huang	*Rehmannia*	12 - 20 g
Shan Zhu Yu	*Cornus*	6 - 9 g
Du Zhong	*Eucommia*	6 - 9 g
Dang Gui	*Angelica*	6 - 9 g
Tu Si Zi	*Cuscuta*	6 - 9 g
Lu Jiao Jiao	*Cervus*	6 - 9 g

Blood deficiency with interior excess heat causing constipation; or blood stagnation with excess heat resulting in amenorrhea.

T red or purple, yellow coat

P rapid

✘ Do not use during pregnancy.

YU ZHU SAN

Jade Candle Powder

Chuan Xiong	*Ligusticum*	3 - 9 g
Shu Di Huang	*Rehmannia*	6 - 12 g
Dang Gui	*Angelica*	6 - 9 g
Bai Shao Yao	*Paeonia*	6 - 9 g
Da Huang	*Rheum*	6 - 9 g
Mang Xiao	*Mirabilitum*	3 - 6 g
Gan Cao	*Glycyrrhiza*	3 - 6 g

Deficient cold with blood stagnation causing uterine bleeding with pain which is better with the passage of clots.

T pale, dark purple

P choppy or wiry

☞ The first seven ingredients (which may be calcined) should be ground and made into 9 - 12 g pills with glutinous rice and water. The pills should be coated with Zhu Sha - Cinnabaris. One pill per day with wine is the recommeded dosage.

✘ Do not use during pregnancy. Zhu Sha - Cinnabaris is toxic and should therefore not be taken long-term.

ZHEN LING DAN

Rouse the Spirits Special Pill

Zi Shi Ying	*Fluoritum*	60 g
Yu Liang Shi	*Limonite*	60 g
Dai Zhe Shi	*Haematitum*	60 g
Wu Ling Zhi	*Trogoptérus*	30 g
Ru Xiang	*Boswellia*	30 g
Chi Shi Zhi	*Halloysitum Rubrum*	60 g
Mo Yao	*Commiphora*	30 g
Zhu Sha	*Cinnabaris*	15 g

Liver/Kidney yin and jing (essence) deficiency causing slow development in children; or premature aging in adults, in addition to common yin deficiency signs and symptoms. The formula is also for early menopause, spermatorrhea, low sex drive, infertility, or low sperm count.

T red, scanty coat

P thin, rapid

ZUO GUI YIN

Restore the Left [Kidney] Decoction

Shu Di Huang	*Rehmannia*	6 - 15 g
Shan Zhu Yu	*Cornus*	6 - 9 g
Shan Yao	*Dioscorea*	6 - 9 g
Gou Qi Zi	*Lycium*	6 - 9 g
Fu Ling	*Poria*	6 - 9 g
Zhi Gan Cao	*Glycyrrhiza*	3 - 6 g

OB-GYN/LEUKORRHEA

- vaginal discharge

T usually sticky coat

P usually slippery

Chronic uterine bleeding due to blood deficiency and cold. This formula is also useful for spotting or clear leukorrhea.

T pale, white coat

P weak, thin

☞ E Jiao - Equus should be dissolved into the strained tea.

DING XIANG JIAO AI TANG

Clove, Ass-Hide Gelatin, and Mugwort Decoction

Ding Xiang	*Eugenia*	3 - 6 g
E Jiao	*Equus*	3 - 9 g
Ai Ye	*Artemisia*	6 g
Shu Di Huang	*Rehmannia*	6 - 9 g
Dang Gui	*Angelica*	6 - 9 g
Bai Shao Yao	*Paeonia*	6 - 9 g
Chuan Xiong	*Ligusticum*	3 - 9 g

Damp heat in the lower jiao causing low back pain, hot, swollen knees or feet, or odorous leukorrhea.

T sticky yellow coat

P slippery, rapid

ER MIAO SAN

Two-Marvel Powder

Cang Zhu	*Atractylodes*	15 g
Huang Bai	*Phellodendron*	15 g

Turbid leukorrhea due to Kidney qi/yang deficiency. The Kidneys are unable to astringe.

T pale, swollen, slight teethmarks, wet, thin white coat

P minute or frail

FEN QING YIN

Separate Pure from Impure Powder

Bei Xie	*Dioscorea*	6 - 9 g
Yi Yi Ren	*Coix*	12 - 15 g
Wu Yao	*Lindera*	6 - 9 g
Shi Chang Pu	*Acorus*	6 - 9 g
Fu Ling	*Poria*	6 - 9 g
Chen Pi	*Citrus*	3 - 6 g
Gan Cao	*Glycyrrhiza*	3 - 6 g

Kidney qi/yin deficiency causing irregular periods, leukorrhea, or a bearing-down sensation.

T red, thin white coat

P weak, especially the chi (third) positions

GU YIN JIAN

Stabilize the Yin Decoction

Shu Di Huang	*Rehmannia*	6 - 12 g
Shan Yao	*Dioscorea*	6 - 9 g
Wu Wei Zi	*Schisandra*	6 - 9 g
Shan Zhu Yu	*Cornus*	6 - 9 g
Tu Si Zi	*Cuscuta*	6 - 9 g
Ren Shen	*Panax*	6 - 9 g
Yuan Zhi	*Polygala*	3 g
Zhi Gan Cao	*Glycyrrhiza*	3 - 6 g

Damp heat leukorrhea with low back pain, heat sensation along the leg, or eczema.

T red, sticky yellow coat

P wiry, rapid, slippery

JIA WEI ER MIAO SAN

Augmented Two-Marvel Powder

Huang Bai	*Phellodendron*	6 - 12 g
Cang Zhu	*Atractylodes*	9 - 15 g
Dang Gui Wei	*Angelica*	6 - 9 g
Bei Xie	*Dioscorea*	6 - 9 g
Han Fang Ji	*Stephania*	6 - 9 g
Chuan Niu Xi	*Cyathula*	6 - 9 g
Gui Ban	*Chinemys*	6 - 9 g

White turbid leukorrhea due to cold and deficiency in the lower jiao. This formula is also useful for spermatorrhea.

T pale

P weak

☞ This formula should be decocted twice. Stew tea into a thick paste. It should be taken on an empty stomach with three tablespoons of boiling water.

JIN YING GAO

Rosa Paste

Jin Ying Zi	*Rosa*	60 g
Ren Shen	*Panax*	60 g
Sang Piao Xiao	*Paratenodera*	60 g
Shan Yao	*Dioscorea*	60 g
Du Zhong	*Eucommia*	60 g
Yi Zhi Ren	*Alpinia*	30 g
Yi Yi Ren	*Coix*	30 g
Wu Zhu Yu	*Evodia*	30 g
Qian Shi	*Euryale*	30 g
Gou Qi Zi	*Lycium*	120 g
no pinyin name	*Sodium Chloride*	9 g

Black colored leukorrhea due to severe heat with abdominal pain, dysurea, genital swelling, thirst, increased appetite; purgative.

T very red, dry, sticky yellow coat

P rapid

✘ Caution during pregnancy

LI HUO TANG

Move Fire Decoction

Da Huang	*Rheum*	9 g
Bai Zhu	*Atractylodes*	15 g
Fu Ling	*Poria*	9 g
Che Qian Zi	*Plantago*	9 g
Huang Lian	*Coptis*	3 g
Zhi Zi	*Gardenia*	9 g
Bei Mu	*Fritillaria*	6 g
Wang Bu Liu Xing	*Vaccaria*	9 g

Damp heat in the lower jiao, or Liver fire. Symptoms include red and itchy eyes, temple headaches, odorous leukorrhea, or pruritus.

T red, sticky yellow coating

P wiry, rapid, slippery

LONG DAN XIE GAN TANG

Gentiana Decoction to Drain the Liver

Extract Formula Name: Gentiana Combination

Long Dan Cao	*Gentiana*	6 - 9 g
Zhi Zi	*Gardenia*	3 - 9 g
Mu Tong	*Akebia*	6 - 9 g
Huang Qin	*Scutellaria*	6 - 9 g
Ze Xie	*Alisma*	6 - 9 g
Che Qian Zi	*Plantago*	6 - 9 g
Dang Gui	*Angelica*	6 - 9 g
Sheng Di Huang	*Rehmannia*	6 - 12 g
Chai Hu	*Bupleurum*	6 - 9 g
Gan Cao	*Glycyrrhiza*	3 - 6 g

Kidney qi deficiency causing white leukorrhea.

T thin white coat

P weak

NEI BU WAN

Internal Tonification Pill

Lu Rong	*Cervus*	1 - 3 g
Rou Cong Rong	*Cistanche*	6 - 9 g
Tu Si Zi	*Cuscuta*	6 - 9 g
Huang Qi	*Astralagus*	6 - 15 g
Rou Gui	*Cinnamomum*	6 - 9 g
Fu Zi	*Aconitum*	3 - 6 g
Sha Yuan Ji Li	*Astragalus*	6 - 9 g
Zi Wan	*Aster*	6 - 9 g
Sang Piao Xiao	*Paratenodera*	6 - 9 g

Phlegm damp leading to infertility or leukorrhea.

T thick sticky white coat

P slippery or soggy

QI GONG WAN

Open Uterus Pill

Ban Xia	*Pinellia*	6 - 9 g
Fu Ling	*Poria*	6 - 9 g
Cang Zhu	*Atractylodes*	6 - 9 g
Shen Qu	*Massa Fermentata*	6 - 12 g
Chen Pi	*Citrus*	3 - 6 g
Xiang Fu	*Cyperus*	6 - 9 g
Chuan Xiong	*Ligusticum*	3 - 6 g

Blood deficiency with deficient or excess heat causing purple menstrual blood, early periods, or thick leukorrhea with tidal fever.

T pale

P rapid, thin, weak

QIN LIAN SI WU TANG

Four-Substance Decoction with Scutellaria and Coptis

Huang Qin	*Scutellaria*	6 - 9 g
Huang Lian	*Coptis*	3 - 6 g
Chuan Xiong	*Ligusticum*	3 - 6 g
Bai Shao Yao	*Paeonia*	6 - 9 g
Dang Gui	*Angelica*	6 - 9 g
Mai Men Dong	*Ophiopogon*	6 - 9 g
Sheng Di Huang	*Rehmannia*	9 - 12 g

Spleen qi deficiency causing thin, clear or reddish leukorrhea, with low back pain.

T pale, thin white coat

P deep, thin, slippery

QING DAI TANG

Clear Discharge Decoction

Shan Yao	*Dioscorea*	9 - 30 g
Mu Li	*Ostrea*	9 - 15 g
Long Gu	*Os Draconis*	9 - 15 g
Qian Cao Gen	*Rubia*	6 - 9 g
Hai Piao Xiao	*Sepia*	9 - 12 g

Liver qi stagnation overacting on Spleen. This leads to damp which in turn heats up and then causes red leukorrhea. Or, the Liver fails to store the blood which also manifests as red leukorrhea.

T purple or pale

P wiry, or weak, thin

☞ E Jiao - Equus should be dissolved into the strained tea.

QING GAN ZHI LIN TANG

Clear Liver and Stop Leukorrhea Decoction

Bai Shao Yao	*Paeonia*	30 g
Dang Gui	*Angelica*	30 g
Shu Di Huang	*Rehmannia*	15 g
E Jiao	*Equus*	9 g
Mu Dan Pi	*Paeonia*	9 g
Huang Bai	*Phellodendron*	6 g
Huai Niu Xi	*Achyranthes*	6 g
Xiang Fu	*Cyperus*	3 g
Da Zao	*Ziziphus*	7 - 10 pc
no pinyin name	*Small Black beans*	30 g

Damp heat obstruction causing dysmenorrhea, pain prior to onset of the menstruation, cramps, or leukorrhea.

T light purple or red, thick sticky yellow coat

P slippery, slightly rapid, or wiry

QING RE GU JING TANG II

Clear Heat and Stabilize Menses Decoction II

Huang Bai	*Phellodendron*	6 - 9 g
Huang Lian	*Coptis*	3 - 9 g
Mu Dan Pi	*Paeonia*	6 - 12 g
Sheng Di Huang	*Rehmannia*	6 - 12 g
Dang Gui	*Angelica*	6 - 9 g
Chi Shao Yao	*Paeonia*	6 - 9 g
Chuan Xiong	*Ligusticum*	3 - 9 g
Yan Hu Suo	*Corydalis*	6 - 9 g

Yellow leukorrhea with dark yellow urination from heat and damp in the lower jiao.

T red, sticky yellowish coat

P slippery, rapid

QING XIN LIAN ZI YIN

Clear the Heart with Lotus Seed Decoction

Extract Formula Name: Lotus Seed Combination

Huang Qin	Scutellaria	6 - 9 g
Mai Men Dong	Ophiopogon	6 - 9 g
Ren Shen	Panax	6 - 9 g
Huang Qi	Astragalus	6 - 15g
Di Gu Pi	Lycium	6 - 9 g
Che Qian Zi	Plantago	6 - 9 g
Lian Zi	Nelumbo	3 - 9 g
Chai Hu	Bupleurum	6 - 9 g
Fu Ling	Poria	6 - 9 g

Trichomonas due to damp. External wash only!

T not important

P not important

☞ Herbs should be ground into a powder, then prepared as a draft.

✘ For external use only.

SHE CHUANG ZI SAN

Cnidium Powder

She Chuang Zi	Cnidium	9 - 15 g
Bai Bu	Stemona	9 - 15 g
Chuan Jiao	Zanthoxylum	9 - 15 g
Ming Fan	Alumen	9 - 15 g
Ku Shen	Sophora	9 - 15 g

Leukorrhea or cloudy spermatorrhea due to Kidney yang deficiency.

T pale

P frail

SHUI LU ER XIAN DAN

Water and Earth Immortals Special Pill

Qian Shi	Euryale	10 g
Jin Ying Zi	Rosa	10 g

External cold causing stagnation in the Liver channel. This leads to testicle pain and swelling in men, or to clear leukorrhea in women.

T pale, purple, thin white coat

P slow, wiry, or tight

☞ Ba Dou - Croton and Chuan Lian Zi - Melia should be dry fried for 5 - 10 minutes. Discard Ba Dou, then decoct as usual. This way the effect of Chuan Lian Zi is to actually warm the Liver channel.

TIAN TAI WU YAO SAN

Top-Quality Lindera Powder

Wu Yao	*Lindera*	6 - 9 g
Xiao Hui Xiang	*Foeniculum*	3 - 6 g
Gao Liang Jiang	*Alpinia*	3 - 6 g
Mu Xiang	*Saussurea*	3 - 6 g
Qing Pi	*Citrus*	3 - 6 g
Chuan Lian Zi	*Melia*	6 - 9 g
Bing Lang	*Areca*	6 - 9 g
Ba Dou	*Croton*	6 - 15 g

Spleen qi deficiency with Liver qi stagnation causing leukorrhea. The discharge is thin, watery, or white. Other symptoms include loose stools, poor appetite, and possible irritability.

T pale, light purple, swollen, sticky white coat

P slippery, slow

WAN DAI TANG

End Discharge Decoction

Bai Zhu	*Atractylodes*	20 - 30 g
Cang Zhu	*Atractylodes*	3 - 6 g
Shan Yao	*Dioscorea*	20 - 30 g
Chen Pi	*Citrus*	3 - 6 g
Bai Shao Yao	*Paeonia*	6 - 12 g
Chai Hu	*Bupleurum*	3 - 6 g
Jing Jie	*Schizonepeta*	6 - 9 g
Che Qian Zi	*Plantago*	6 - 9 g
Ren Shen	*Panax*	6 - 9 g
Gan Cao	*Glycyrrhiza*	3 - 6 g

Spleen qi deficiency with damp and watery leukorrhea, edema, or cramping pain. Other symptoms include loose stools, and urinary retention.

T sticky white coat

P weak, slippery

WEI LING TANG

Calm the Stomach and Poria Decoction

Extract Formula Name: Magnolia and Hoelen Combination

Ze Xie	*Alisma*	6 - 12 g
Zhu Ling	*Polyporus*	6 - 9 g
Fu Ling	*Poria*	6 - 9 g
Bai Zhu	*Atractylodes*	3 - 9 g
Gui Zhi	*Cinnamomum*	3 - 9 g
Hou Po	*Magnolia*	6 - 12 g
Cang Zhu	*Atractylodes*	3 - 9 g
Chen Pi	*Citrus*	3 - 6 g
Sheng Jiang	*Zingiber*	3 - 6 g
Da Zao	*Ziziphus*	3 - 6 pc
Gan Cao	*Glycyrrhiza*	3 - 6 g

Trichomonas infection: damp heat causing yellow, odorous leukorrhea, and severe itching.

T red, sticky yellow coat

P rapid, slippery

WU MEI YIN CHEN TANG

Mume and Artemisia Yinchenhao Decoction

Wu Mei	*Prunus*	20 - 30 g
Yin Chen Hao	*Artemisia*	9 - 15 g
Chuan Jiao	*Zanthoxylum*	6 - 9 g
Jin Yin Hua	*Lonicera*	6 - 12 g
Bian Xu	*Polygonum*	6 - 9 g
Bai Zhu	*Atractylodes*	6 - 9 g
Fu Ling	*Poria*	6 - 15 g
Long Dan Cao	*Gentiana*	6 - 9 g
Huang Bai	*Phellodendron*	6 - 9 g

Internal Medicine & Misc. Syndromes

Spleen qi deficiency causing damp which heats up. This leads to heat type leukorrhea with a fishy smell, or delayed periods from qi and blood deficiency.

T pale, thin sticky yellow or white coat

P slippery, weak

YI HUANG TANG

Change Yellow (Discharge) Decoction

Shan Yao	*Dioscorea*	9 - 30 g
Huang Bai	*Phellodendron*	6 - 9 g
Qian Shi	*Euryale*	9 - 30 g
Bai Guo	*Gingko*	6 - 10 pc
Che Qian Zi	*Plantago*	3 - 6 g

Kidney qi deficiency leading to spermatorrhea, or white leukorrhea in women.

T pale or normal color, thin white coat

P weak

YI YUAN JIAN

Benefit the Source Decoction

Yuan Zhi	*Polygala*	3 g
Shan Yao	*Dioscorea*	6 g
Qian Shi	*Euryale*	6 g
Suan Zao Ren	*Ziziphus*	6 g
Bai Zhu	*Atractylodes*	4.5 g
Fu Ling	*Poria*	4.5 g
Ren Shen	*Panax*	3 - 6 g
Wu Wei Zi	*Schisandra*	14 pc
Jin Ying Zi	*Rosa*	6 g
Gan Cao	*Glycyrrhiza*	3 g

Damp accumulation draining downward leading to clear white leukorrhea.

T swollen, thick white coat

P slippery

YI ZHI TANG

Boosting Wisdom Decoction

Bai Zhu	*Atractylodes*	9 g
Fu Ling	*Poria*	9 g
Chen Pi	*Citrus*	6 g
Cang Zhu	*Atractylodes*	6 g
Yi Yi Ren	*Coix*	6 g
Chai Hu	*Bupleurum*	6 g
Sheng Ma	*Cimicifuga*	2 g
Zhi Gan Cao	*Glycyrrhiza*	3 g

Damp heat accumulation causing leukorrhea which smells fishy and is thick, yellow, or reddish.

T red, sticky yellow coat

P rapid, slippery

☞ Herbs should be ground and made into pills of 3 g with glutenous rice. Take 2 - 3 pills once or twice daily. Huang Bai - Phellodendron and Gao Liang Jiang - Alpinia should both be charred.

YU DAI WAN

Cure Discharge Pill

Bai Shao Yao	*Paeonia*	20 - 30 g
Chun Pi	*Ailanthus*	60 - 90 g
Huang Bai	*Phellodendron*	9 - 12 g
Gao Liang Jiang	*Alpinia*	9 - 18 g

Damp heat accumulation leading to leukorrhea. The discharge is very odorous, yellow, thick, and may be profuse.

T red, thick yellow sticky coat

P slippery, rapid

ZHI DAI TANG

Stop Leukorrhea Decoction

Fu Ling	*Poria*	6 - 9 g
Zhu Ling	*Polyporus*	6 - 9 g
Ze Xie	*Alisma*	6 - 9 g
Che Qian Zi	*Plantago*	3 - 9 g
Yin Chen Hao	*Artemisia*	15 g
Zhi Zi	*Gardenia*	3 - 6 g
Huang Bai	*Phellodendron*	3 - 9 g
Mu Dan Pi	*Paeonia*	6 - 12 g
Chi Shao Yao	*Paeonia*	6 - 9 g
Huai Niu Xi	*Achyranthes*	3 - 6 g

OB-GYN/PREGNANCY DISORDERS AND INFERTILITY

- spotting during pregnancy
- threatened miscarriage
- infertility

T depends on involved syndrome

P depends on involved syndrome

Late periods due to yang deficiency or cold in the uterus. This formula is also useful during pregnancy to warm the uterus.

T pale, white coat

P frail

☞ Herbs should be ground into a powder and made into 6 g pills with rice vinegar.

AI FU NUAN GONG WAN

Mugwort and Cyperus Pill for Warming the Womb

Ai Ye	*Artemisia*	60 - 90 g
Xiang Fu	*Cyperus*	150 - 180 g
Wu Zhu Yu	*Evodia*	40 - 60 g
Bai Shao Yao	*Paeonia*	40 - 60 g
Huang Qi	*Astragalus*	40 - 60 g
Dang Gui	*Angelica*	60 - 90 g
Xu Duan	*Dipsacus*	30 - 45 g
Shu Di Huang	*Rehmannia*	15 - 30 g
Chuan Xiong	*Ligusticum*	40 - 60 g
Rou Gui	*Cinnamomum*	9 - 15 g

Kidney/Liver yin deficiency with blood deficiency causing post-partum sweating, or night sweats.

T red, thin yellow coat

P thin, rapid

BA WEI DI HUANG WAN

Eight-Ingredient Pill with Rehmannia

Sheng Di Huang	*Rehmannia*	6 - 12 g
Shan Zhu Yu	*Cornus*	6 - 9 g
Shan Yao	*Dioscorea*	6 - 9 g
Fu Ling	*Poria*	6 - 9 g
Ze Xie	*Alisma*	6 - 9 g
Mu Dan Pi	*Paeonia*	6 - 9 g
Wu Wei Zi	*Schisandra*	6 - 9 g
Huang Qi	*Astragalus*	9 - 15 g

Qi and blood deficiency with blood stagnation. This formula is for a restless fetus, infertility, irregular periods, poor appetite, weakness, or fatigue.

T pale, thin white coat

P weak, maybe wiry

BA ZHEN YI MU WAN

Eight-Treasure Pill to Benefit Mothers

Shu Di Huang	*Rehmannia*	6 - 15 g
Chuan Xiong	*Ligusticum*	3 - 9 g
Dang Gui	*Angelica*	6 - 9 g
Bai Shao Yao	*Paeonia*	6 - 12 g
Ren Shen	*Panax*	6 - 12 g
Bai Zhu	*Atractylodes*	3 - 9 g
Fu Ling	*Poria*	6 - 9 g
Yi Mu Cao	*Leonurus*	6 - 18 g
Gan Cao	*Glycyrrhiza*	3 - 6 g

Spleen qi deficiency causing morning sickness, a restless fetus, loose stools, or poor appetite.

T pale, swollen, white coat

P weak

BAO TAI ZI SHENG WAN

Protect the Fetus and Aid Life Pill

Ren Shen	*Panax*	6 - 9 g
Fu Ling	*Poria*	6 - 9 g
Bai Zhu	*Atractylodes*	6 - 9 g
Gan Cao	*Glycyrrhiza*	3 - 6 g
Lian Zi	*Nelumbo*	6 - 9 g
Bian Dou	*Dolichos*	6 - 9 g
Huo Xiang	*Agastache*	6 - 9 g
Bai Dou Kou	*Amomum*	3 - 6 g
Chen Pi	*Citrus*	3 - 6 g
Jie Geng	*Platycodon*	3 - 6 g
Shan Yao	*Dioscorea*	6 - 9 g
Yi Yi Ren	*Coix*	6 - 12 g
Ze Xie	*Alisma*	6 - 9 g
Mai Ya	*Hordeum*	12 - 20 g
Qian Shi	*Euryale*	6 - 9 g
Shan Zha	*Crataegus*	6 - 12 g
Huang Lian	*Coptis*	3 g

Post-partum abdominal pain of the deficiency type after qi and blood loss from giving birth.

T pale

P frail

☞ E Jiao - Equus should be added to the strained tea.

CHANG NING TANG

Intestinal Serenity Decoction

Shu Di Huang	*Rehmannia*	6 - 12 g
Dang Gui	*Angelica*	6 - 12 g
Mai Men Dong	*Ophiopogon*	6 - 9 g
Ren Shen	*Panax*	6 - 9 g
Xu Duan	*Dipsacus*	6 - 9 g
Rou Gui	*Cinnamomum*	3 g
E Jiao	*Equus*	6 - 9 g
Shan Yao	*Dioscorea*	6 - 9 g
Gan Cao	*Glycyrrhiza*	3 - 6 g

Kidney yin and Spleen qi/blood deficiency causing uterine prolapse with low back pain, night urination, or hearing loss and tinnitus.

T red or pale

P frail

DA BU YUAN JIAN

Great Tonify the Basal Decoction

Ren Shen	*Panax*	6 - 12 g
Shu Di Huang	*Rehmannia*	9 - 25 g
Shan Yao	*Dioscorea*	6 - 9 g
Shan Zhu Yu	*Cornus*	3 - 6 g
Gou Qi Zi	*Lycium*	6 - 9 g
Dang Gui	*Angelica*	6 - 9 g
Du Zhong	*Eucommia*	6 - 9 g
Gan Cao	*Glycyrrhiza*	3 - 6 g

Spleen qi and blood deficiency with slight cold leading to spasm pain or post-partum emaciation.

T pale, white coat

P weak

☞ Yi Tang - Saccharum Granorum is added to the strained tea.

DANG GUI JIAN ZHONG TANG

Dang Gui Decoction to Construct the Middle

Extract Formula Name: Tang-Kuei, Cinnamon and Peony Combination

Yi Tang	*Saccharum Granorum*	6 - 20 g
Gui Zhi	*Cinnamomum*	3 - 9 g
Bai Shao Yao	*Paeonia*	6 - 9 g
Sheng Jiang	*Zingiber*	3 - 6 g
Da Zao	*Ziziphus*	3 - 6 pc
Gan Cao	*Glycyrrhiza*	3 - 6 g
Dang Gui	*Angelica*	6 - 9 g

Spleen qi and blood deficiency with yin deficiency and restless fetus. This prescription can be taken as a preventative during pregnancy.

T pale or red

P thin, weak

DANG GUI SAN

Dang Gui Powder

Extract Formula Name: Tang-Kuei Formula

Dang Gui	*Angelica*	6 - 12 g
Huang Qin	*Scutellaria*	6 - 12 g
Chuan Xiong	*Ligusticum*	3 g
Bai Zhu	*Atractylodes*	3 - 9 g
Bai Shao Yao	*Paeonia*	6 - 9 g

Liver overacting on Spleen causing mild cramping in the abdomen with Liver blood deficiency and some damp accumulation. Symptoms include urinary retention and lower body edema. This is often seen during pregnancy.

T pale, orange color on the sides

P weak, thin, or slightly wiry

DANG GUI SHAO YAO SAN

Dang Gui and Peony Powder

Extract Formula Name: Tang-Kuei and Peony Formula

Dang Gui	*Angelica*	6 - 9 g
Bai Shao Yao	*Paeonia*	3 - 9 g
Bai Zhu	*Atractylodes*	3 - 9 g
Fu Ling	*Poria*	6 - 9 g
Chuan Xiong	*Ligusticum*	3 - 6 g
Ze Xie	*Alisma*	6 - 9 g

Blood deficiency with external cold after childbirth. This leads to spasms or hernia pain which are both relieved by pressure.

T pale

P deep, wiry, weak

☞ This formula should be prepared as a stew with eight cups of water. Simmer until it is reduced to three to four cups.

DANG GUI SHENG JIANG YANG ROU TANG

Mutton Stew with Dang Gui and Fresh Ginger Decoction

Dang Gui	*Angelica*	9 - 12 g
Sheng Jiang	*Zingiber*	9 - 15 g
Yang Rou	*Mutton*	40 - 50 g

Spleen/Stomach qi deficiency and cold causing vomiting during pregnancy.

T pale, thin white coat

P weak

GAN JIANG REN SHEN BAN XIA WAN

Ginger, Ginseng, and Pinellia Pill

Extract Formula Name: G.P. and Ginseng Formula

Gan Jiang	*Zingiber*	3 g
Ren Shen	*Panax*	3 g
Ban Xia	*Pinellia*	6 g
[Sheng Jiang	*Zingiber*	1 - 3 g]

Spleen qi deficiency during pregnancy with lethargy, spotting, or low back pain.

T pale, swollen, teethmarks, thin white coat

P weak, thin

☞ E Jiao - Equus should be added at the end to the strained tea.

JIA JIAN BU ZHONG YI QI TANG

Modified Tonify the Middle and Augment the Qi Decoction

Ren Shen	*Panax*	6 - 9 g
Huang Qi	*Astragalus*	6 - 12 g
Chen Pi	*Citrus*	3 - 6 g
Bai Zhu	*Atractylodes*	3 - 9 g
Sheng Ma	*Cimicifuga*	3 - 6 g
Chai Hu	*Bupleurum*	3 - 9 g
E Jiao	*Equus*	3 - 9 g
Ai Ye	*Artemisia*	3 - 9 g
Gan Cao	*Glycyrrhiza*	3 - 6 g

Chong and Ren imbalance with blood deficiency causing restless fetus, pale post-partum bleeding, abdominal pain, a weak low back, or a cold uterus.

T pale

P frail, slow

☞ E Jiao - Equus should be dissolved at the end into the strained tea.

JIAO AI TANG

Ass-Hide Equus and Mugwort Decoction

Extract Formula Name: Tang-kuei and Equus Combination

E Jiao	*Equus*	6 - 9 g
Ai Ye	*Artemisia*	6 - 9 g
Dang Gui	*Angelica*	6 - 9 g
Sheng Di Huang	*Rehmannia*	18 g
Bai Shao Yao	*Paeonia*	12 g
Chuan Xiong	*Ligusticum*	6 g
Gan Cao	*Glycyrrhiza*	3 - 6 g

Spleen qi deficiency causing severe uterine bleeding which is pale in color, or early or irregular periods. The Spleen qi is sinking causing a restless fetus.

T pale, swollen, teethmarks, thin white coat

P weak

JU YUAN JIAN

Lift the Source Decoction

Ren Shen	Panax	6 - 9 g
Huang Qi	Astragalus	9 - 12 g
Sheng Ma	Cimicifuga	3 - 6 g
Bai Zhu	Atractylodes	3 - 6 g
Gan Cao	Glycyrrhiza	3 - 6 g

Phlegm damp leading to infertility or leukorrhea.

T thick sticky white coat

P slippery or soggy

QI GONG WAN

Open Uterus Pill

Ban Xia	*Pinellia*	6 - 9 g
Fu Ling	*Poria*	6 - 9 g
Cang Zhu	*Atractylodes*	6 - 9 g
Shen Qu	*Massa Fermentata*	6 - 12 g
Chen Pi	*Citrus*	3 - 6 g
Xiang Fu	*Cyperus*	6 - 9 g
Chuan Xiong	*Ligusticum*	3 - 6 g

Post-partum retention of lochia due to blood and cold stagnation.

T pale, purple

P choppy

☞ Add yellow wine to the decoction.

SHENG HUA TANG

Generation and Transformation Decoction

Extract Formula Name: Tang-Kuei and Ginger Combination

Dang Gui	*Angelica*	15 - 28 g
Tao Ren	*Prunus*	6 - 9 g
Pao Jiang	*Zingiber*	3 - 6 g
Chuan Xiong	*Ligusticum*	6 - 9 g
Gan Cao	*Glycyrrhiza*	3 - 6 g

Kidney qi deficiency causing a restless fetus with spotting, threatened miscarriage, or frequent urination.

T pale

P frail

☞ E Jiao - Equus should be dissolved in water and used to form the other herbs into 6 g pills.

SHOU TAI WAN

Fetus Longevity Pill

Loranthus and Cuscuta Combination

E Jiao	*Equus*	30
Sang Ji Sheng	*Loranthus*	30 g
Tu Si Zi	*Cuscuta*	60 g
Xu Duan	*Dipsacus*	30 g

Spleen qi/blood deficiency during pregnancy causing restless fetus, or use formula if the woman has a history of miscarriage or infertility.

T pale, thin white coat

P weak, thin, slippery

TAI SHAN PAN SHI SAN

Powder that Gives the Stability of Mount Tai

Ren Shen	*Panax*	6 - 9 g
Huang Qi	*Astragalus*	12 - 15 g
Shu Di Huang	*Rehmannia*	9 - 12 g
Chuan Xiong	*Ligusticum*	3 - 6 g
Bai Zhu	*Atractylodes*	9 - 12 g
Sha Ren	*Amomum*	1 - 3 g
Huang Qin	*Scutellaria*	6 - 9 g
Xu Duan	*Dipsacus*	3 - 6 g
Bai Shao Yao	*Paeonia*	6 - 9 g
Zhi Gan Cao	*Glycyrrhiza*	3 - 6 g
Nuo Mi	*Glutinous Oryza*	3 - 6 g

Kidney qi deficiency causing infertility, urinary frequency, or incontinence.

T pale or normal color, thin white coat

P weak

☞ For infertility and a stronger qi and blood tonifying effect add 'Dang Gui Bu Xue Tang - Dang Gui Decoction to Tonify the Blood' and 'Si Jun Zi Tang - Four-Gentlemen Decoction.'

WU ZI YAN ZONG WAN

Five-Seeds Normalizing Pill

Wu Wei Zi	*Schisandra*	6 - 12 g
Fu Pen Zi	*Rubus*	6 - 9 g
Tu Si Zi	*Cuscuta*	6 - 9 g
Che Qian Zi	*Plantago*	6 - 9 g
Gou Qi Zi	*Lycium*	6 - 12 g

Spleen/Stomach qi deficiency with qi stagnation and cold damp in the middle jiao causing abdominal fullness or morning sickness.

T pale, light purple, swollen, sticky white coat

P slippery, weak

XIANG SHA LIU JUN ZI TANG

Six-Gentlemen Decoction with Aucklandia and Amomum

Extract Formula Name: Saussurea and Cardamon Combination

Ren Shen	*Panax*	6 - 9 g
Fu Ling	*Poria*	6 - 9 g
Bai Zhu	*Atractylodes*	3 - 9 g
Chen Pi	*Citrus*	3 - 6 g
Ban Xia	*Pinellia*	6 - 9 g
Sha Ren	*Amomum*	3 g
Mu Xiang	*Saussurea*	3 - 6 g
Zhi Gan Cao	*Glycyrrhiza*	3 - 6 g

Pronounced wind cold with mild qi stagnation, or wind cold invasion during pregnancy.

T thin white coat

P superficial, tight

XIANG SU CONG CHI TANG

Cyperus, Perilla Leaf, Scallion, and Prepared Soybean Decoction

Zi Su Ye	*Perilla*	6 - 9 g
Xiang Fu	*Cyperus*	6 - 9 g
Cong Bai	*Allium*	2 - 4 pc
Dan Dou Chi	*Glycine*	9 - 12 g
Chen Pi	*Citrus*	3 - 6 g
Zhi Gan Cao	*Glycyrrhiza*	3 - 6 g

Kidney yang and essence deficiency causing amenorrhea, infertility, cold back or knees, pedal edema, or impotence.

T pale, swollen, teethmarks, thin white coat

P minute

YOU GUI WAN

Restore the Right Pill

Extract Formula Name: Eucommia and Rehmannia Formula

Rou Gui	*Cinnamomum*	6 - 9 g
Fu Zi	*Aconitum*	3 - 6 g
Gou Qi Zi	*Lycium*	6 - 9 g
Shan Yao	*Dioscorea*	6 - 9 g
Shu Di Huang	*Rehmannia*	12 - 20 g
Shan Zhu Yu	*Cornus*	6 - 9 g
Du Zhong	*Eucommia*	6 - 9 g
Dang Gui	*Angelica*	6 - 9 g
Tu Si Zi	*Cuscuta*	6 - 9 g
Lu Jiao Jiao	*Cervus*	6 - 9 g

Infertility due to Kidney qi deficiency.

T normal color or pale, thin white coat

P weak, especially in both chi (third) positions

YU LIN WAN

Nourish Cute Animal Pill

Lu Jiao Shuang	*Cervus*	6 - 9 g
Tu Si Zi	*Cuscuta*	6 - 9 g
Du Zhong	*Eucommia*	6 - 12 g
Chuan Jiao	*Zanthoxylum*	3 - 6 g
Zi He Che	*Placenta Hominis*	3 - 9 g
Xiang Fu	*Cyperus*	6 - 9 g

Impotence or infertility due to Kidney yang deficiency with simultaneous qi and blood deficiency. Symptoms include blurry vision, low back pain, and poor memory.

T pale, thin white coat

P frail

ZAN YU DAN

Special Pill to Aid Fertility

Rou Cong Rong	*Cistanche*	6 - 12 g
Fu Zi	*Aconitum*	6 g
Ba Ji Tian	*Morinda*	6 - 12 g
Rou Gui	*Cinnamomum*	6 g
She Chuang Zi	*Cnidium*	6 g
Xian Mao	*Curculigo*	6 - 12 g
Dang Gui	*Angelica*	9 - 15 g
Bai Zhu	*Atractylodes*	12 - 18 g
Gou Qi Zi	*Lycium*	9 - 15 g
Yin Yang Huo	*Epimedium*	6 - 12 g
Shan Zhu Yu	*Cornus*	6 - 12 g
Shu Di Huang	*Rehmannia*	6 - 12 g
Jiu Zi	*Allium*	6 - 12 g
Du Zhong	*Eucommia*	6 - 12 g

Liver/Kidney yin and jing (essence) deficiency causing slow development in children; or premature aging in adults, in addition to common yin deficiency signs and symptoms. The formula is also for early menopause, spermatorrhea, low sex drive, infertility, or low sperm count.

T red, scanty coat

P thin, rapid

ZUO GUI YIN

Restore the Left [Kidney] Decoction

Shu Di Huang	*Rehmannia*	6 - 15 g
Shan Zhu Yu	*Cornus*	6 - 9 g
Shan Yao	*Dioscorea*	6 - 9 g
Gou Qi Zi	*Lycium*	6 - 9 g
Fu Ling	*Poria*	6 - 9 g
Zhi Gan Cao	*Glycyrrhiza*	3 - 6 g

WIND DAMP BI - SYNDROME

- joint pain
- joint deformities
- heaviness
- numbness or paralysis in the extremities

T sticky coat

P slippery

Damp heat febrile disease or damp bi-syndrome with heat causing severe sweating and joint pain with swelling and redness. Joints feel hot to the touch.

T red, sticky yellow coat

P slippery, rapid, or flooding

☞ Decoct the first four herbs, then add the rice at the end. It will absorb the water to make a thick liquid.

BAI HU JIA CANG ZHU TANG

White Tiger plus Atractylodes Decoction

Shi Gao	*Gypsum*	20 - 30 g
Zhi Mu	*Anemarrhena*	9 - 12 g
Gan Cao	*Glycyrrhiza*	3 - 6 g
Cang Zhu	*Atractylodes*	3 - 9 g
Jing Mi	*Oryza*	15 - 30 g

Heat in the yangming channel with slight external cold and damp causing obstruction in the channels which leads to joint pain.

T red, yellow coat

P rapid, wiry

☞ Decoct the first four herbs, then add the rice at the end. It will absorb the water to make a thick liquid.

BAI HU JIA GUI ZHI TANG

White Tiger plus Cinnamon Twig Decoction

Shi Gao	*Gypsum*	20 - 30 g
Zhi Mu	*Anemarrhena*	9 - 12 g
Gan Cao	*Glycyrrhiza*	3 - 9 g
Gui Zhi	*Cinnamomum*	3 - 9 g
Jing Mi	*Oryza*	15 - 30 g

Dysentery weakens the legs severely causing difficulty walking; or wind invades the knees causing atrophy in the legs with severe swelling and pain in one or both knees.

T pale, sticky coat

P slippery

DA FANG FENG TANG

Major Ledebouriella Decoction

Extract Formula Name: Major Siler Combination

Fu Zi	*Aconitum*	6 - 9 g
Chuan Xiong	*Ligusticum*	6 - 9 g
Fang Feng	*Ledebouriella*	6 - 12 g
Shu Di Huang	*Rehmannia*	6 - 12 g
Qiang Huo	*Notopterygium*	6 - 12 g
Bai Shao Yao	*Paeonia*	6 - 12 g
Dang Gui	*Angelica*	6 - 12 g
Bai Zhu	*Atractylodes*	3 - 9 g
Huang Qi	*Astragalus*	6 - 12 g
Ren Shen	*Panax*	3 - 9 g
Du Zhong	*Eucommia*	6 - 12 g
Huai Niu Xi	*Achyranthes*	3 - 9 g
Gan Jiang	*Zingiber*	3 g
Da Zao	*Ziziphus*	1 - 3 pc
Zhi Gan Cao	*Glycyrrhiza*	3 - 6 g

Internal Medicine & Misc. Syndromes

External wind attacks the channels where there is an underlying qi and blood deficiency. Wind cold changes to heat causing chronic hemiplegia, spasms, numbness and pain, or slurred speech.

T red, yellow coat, deviated

P wiry, rapid

DA QIN JIAO TANG

Major Gentiana Qinjiao Decoction

Qin Jiao	*Gentiana*	9 - 12 g
Chuan Xiong	*Ligusticum*	6 - 9 g
Dang Gui	*Angelica*	6 - 9 g
Bai Shao Yao	*Paeonia*	6 - 9 g
Shu Di Huang	*Rehmannia*	9 - 15 g
Sheng Di Huang	*Rehmannia*	9 - 15 g
Fu Ling	*Poria*	6 - 9 g
Bai Zhu	*Atractylodes*	6 - 9 g
Qiang Huo	*Notopterygium*	6 - 9 g
Du Huo	*Angelica*	6 - 9 g
Fang Feng	*Ledebouriella*	6 - 9 g
Bai Zhi	*Angelica*	3 - 6 g
Xi Xin	*Asarum*	3 - 6 g
Huang Qin	*Scutellaria*	6 - 12 g
Shi Gao	*Gypsum*	6 - 9 g
Gan Cao	*Glycyrrhiza*	3 - 6 g

Heat bi-syndrome: wind damp heat causing redness and heat in the joints, stabbing or severe fullness pain, or restlessness. The symptoms are better with cold weather. This formula is also useful for damp heat skin disorders.

T normal color or red, dry, rough texture, yellow coat

P rapid, superficial, slightly slippery

DANG GUI LIAN TONG TANG

Dang Gui and Anemarrhena Decoction

Extract Formula Name: Tang-Kuei and Anemarrhena Combination

Ren Shen	*Panax*	6 - 9 g
Huang Qin	*Scutellaria*	9 - 12 g
Bai Zhu	*Atractylodes*	6 - 9 g
Cang Zhu	*Atractylodes*	3 - 9 g
Dang Gui	*Angelica*	6 - 9 g
Ze Xie	*Alisma*	6 - 9 g
Zhu Ling	*Polyporus*	6 - 9 g
Yin Chen Hao	*Artemisia*	6 - 12 g
Ge Gen	*Pueraria*	6 - 12 g
Zhi Mu	*Anemarrhena*	9 - 12 g
Sheng Ma	*Cimicifuga*	6 - 9 g
Qiang Huo	*Notopterygium*	6 - 12 g
Fang Feng	*Ledebouriella*	6 - 12 g
Ku Shen	*Sophora*	6 - 9 g
Gan Cao	*Glycyrrhiza*	3 - 6 g

Blood and yin deficient patient with cold evil qi which leads to obstruction of the channels which causes pain. The patient feels cold subjectively and may feel cold to the touch. Raynaud's disease.

T pale, white coat

P deep, thin, or minute

DANG GUI SI NI TANG

Dang Gui Decoction for Frigid Extremities

Extract Formula Name: Tang-Kuei and Jujube Combination

Dang Gui	*Angelica*	6 - 12 g
Gui Zhi	*Cinnamomum*	3 - 9 g
Bai Shao Yao	*Paeonia*	6 - 9 g
Mu Tong	*Akebia*	6 - 9 g
Xi Xin	*Asarum*	3 - 6 g
Da Zao	*Ziziphus*	3 - 5 pc
Gan Cao	*Glycyrrhiza*	3 - 6 g

Bone bi-syndrome: wind cold damp with Kidney yang deficiency and yin and blood deficiency. Symptoms include chronic joint pain, cold knees, joint deformities, or stiffness or weakness in the joints.

T pale, thin white coat

P frail

✪ Major Formula

DU HUO JI SHENG TANG

Angelica Pubescens and Sangjisheng Decoction

Extract Formula Name: Tuhuo and Loranthus Combination

Du Huo	*Angelica*	6 - 9 g
Sang Ji Sheng	*Loranthus*	6 - 12 g
Qin Jiao	*Gentiana*	6 - 9 g
Fang Feng	*Ledebouriella*	6 - 9 g
Dang Gui	*Angelica*	6 - 9 g
Rou Gui	*Cinnamomum*	6 g
Ren Shen	*Panax*	6 - 9 g
Huai Niu Xi	*Achyranthes*	6 - 9 g
Du Zhong	*Eucommia*	6 - 9 g
Sheng Di Huang	*Rehmannia*	6 - 9 g
Fu Ling	*Poria*	6 - 9 g
Chuan Xiong	*Ligusticum*	3 - 6 g
Bai Shao Yao	*Paeonia*	6 - 9 g
Xi Xin	*Asarum*	3 - 6 g
Gan Cao	*Glycyrrhiza*	3 - 6 g

Wind bi-syndrome: wind cold damp causing migrating joint pain.

T pale, sticky white coat, wet

P maybe superficial, slow, slippery

FANG FENG TANG

Ledebouriella Decoction

Fang Feng	*Ledebouriella*	12 g
Qin Jiao	*Gentiana*	9-12 g
Dang Gui	*Angelica*	6-9 g
Fu Ling	*Poria*	6-9 g
Xing Ren	*Prunus*	6-9 g
Qiang Huo	*Notopterygium*	3-6 g
Gui Zhi	*Cinnamoum*	3-6 g
Ge Gen	*Pueraria*	9-12 g
Sheng Jiang	*Zingiber*	3-6 g
Da Zao	*Ziziphus*	3-4 pc
Gan Cao	*Glycyrrhiza*	3-6 g
For the lower limbs add:		
Du Huo	*Angelica*	6-9 g
Huai Niu Xi	*Achyranthes*	6-12 g
Bei Xie	*Dioscorea*	6-9 g
For the upper limbs:		
Bai Zhi	*Angelica*	6-9 g
Wei Ling Xian	*Clematis*	6-9 g
Chuan Xiong	*Ligusticum*	3-9 g
Jiang Huang	*Curcuma*	6-9 g
For the low back add:		
Du Zhong	*Eucommia*	6-12 g
Sang Ji Sheng	*Loranthus*	6-12 g
Xu Duan	*Dipsacus*	6-9 g
Ba Ji Tian	*Morinda*	6-9 g

Severe Kidney yang deficiency where the yang is unable to nourish the limbs leading to edema, and severe body aches with cold and damp symptoms: cold bi-syndrome.

T pale, moist white coat

P deep, minute, or choppy

FU ZI TANG

Prepared Aconite Decoction

Extract Formula Name: Aconite Combination

Fu Zi	*Aconitum*	9 - 15 g
Ren Shen	*Panax*	3 - 6 g
Fu Ling	*Poria*	9 - 12 g
Bai Zhu	*Atractylodes*	3 - 12 g
Bai Shao Yao	*Paeonia*	6 - 9 g

Chronic wind cold damp causing heat which is worse at night, or joints which are swollen, hot, and painful.

T sticky white coat

P slippery, wiry

GUI ZHI SHAO YAO ZHI MU TANG

Cinnamon Twig, Peony, and Anemarrhena Decoction

Extract Formula Name: Cinnamon and Anemarrhena Combination

Gui Zhi	*Cinnamomum*	9 - 12 g
Bai Shao Yao	*Paeonia*	9 - 12 g
Zhi Mu	*Anemarrhena*	9 - 12 g
Ma Huang	*Ephedra*	3 - 6 g
Bai Zhu	*Atractylodes*	12 - 15 g
Fu Zi	*Aconitum*	3 - 6 g
Fang Feng	*Ledebouriella*	9 - 12 g
Sheng Jiang	*Zingiber*	12 - 15 g
Gan Cao	*Glycyrrhiza*	3 - 6 g

Kidney and Liver yin deficiency causing bone bi-syndrome or wei syndrome. Deficient yin cannot nourish tendons and false heat burns tendons and muscles. This leads to atrophy, joint swelling, or deformities. The pain tends to be more fixed.

T red, scanty coat

P thin, rapid, weak

☞ All ingredients should be ground up as powder. Take 10 g each time, twice a day.

✪ Major Formula

HU QIAN WAN

Hidden Tiger Pill

Extract Formula Name: Tiger Bone and Tortoise Shell Formula

Gui Ban	*Chinemys*	120 g
Huang Bai	*Phellodendron*	150 g
Shu Di Huang	*Rehmannia*	60 g
Zhi Mu	*Anemarrhena*	60 g
Bai Shao Yao	*Paeonia*	60 g
Suo Yang	*Cynomorium*	45 g
Hu Gu	*Panthera*	30 g
Chen Pi	*Citrus*	60 g
Gan Jiang	*Zingiber*	15 g

Blood stagnation in the channels with a mild wind invasion. This leads to a superficial numbness sensation without pain.

T purple or pale

P choppy or tight

HUANG QI GUI ZHI WU WU TANG

Astragalus and Cinnamon Twig Five-Substance Decoction

Extract Formula Name: Astragalus and Cinnamon Five Herb Combination

Huang Qi	*Astragalus*	9 g
Gui Zhi	*Cinnamomum*	9 g
Bai Shao Yao	*Paeonia*	9 g
Sheng Jiang	*Zingiber*	18 g
Da Zao	*Ziziphus*	9 - 12 pc

Cold damp stagnation in the channels of the legs causing weakness in the legs, difficulty walking, spasms, numbness, polio, or cold intolerance.

T sticky white coat

P rolling, slow

JI MING SAN

Powder to Take at Cock's Crow

Extract Formula Name: Areca Seed and Chaenomeles Formula

Bing Lang	*Areca*	15 g
Wu Zhu Yu	*Evodia*	1 - 3 g
Mu Gua	*Chaenomeles*	9 g
Chen Pi	*Citrus*	9 g
Zi Su Ye	*Perilla*	3 g
Jie Geng	*Platycodon*	5 g
Sheng Jiang	*Zingiber*	5 g

Weakness in the extremities with difficulty walking and muscle atrophy due to blood deficiency and damp stagnation.

T pale, sticky coat

P thin, slippery

JIA WEI SI WU TANG

Augmented Four-Substance Decoction

Dang Gui	*Angelica*	6 - 9 g
Huang Bai	*Phellodendron*	6 - 9 g
Mai Men Dong	*Ophiopogon*	6 - 9 g
Shu Di Huang	*Rehmannia*	9 - 12 g
Cang Zhu	*Atractylodes*	3 - 9 g
Du Zhong	*Eucommia*	3 - 6 g
Bai Shao Yao	*Paeonia*	3 - 9 g
Ren Shen	*Panax*	3 g
Wu Wei Zi	*Schisandra*	3 - 6 g
Zhi Mu	*Anemarrhena*	6 - 9 g
Huai Niu Xi	*Achyranthes*	3 - 9 g
Huang Lian	*Coptis*	3 g
Chuan Xiong	*Ligusticum*	3 - 6 g

Wind damp cold bi-syndrome with qi deficiency leading to numbness, heavy sensation, cold and wind intolerance, slight joint swelling, or acute rheumatic fever.

T pale, thin white coat

P superficial, slightly slow

JUAN BI TANG I

Remove Painful Obstruction Decoction from Selected Formulas

Extract Formula Name: Chianghuo and Turmeric Combination

Qiang Huo	*Notopterygium*	6 - 15 g
Huang Qi	*Astragalus*	6 - 15
Dang Gui	*Angelica*	6 - 12 g
Chi Shao Yao	*Paeonia*	6 - 12 g
Fang Feng	*Ledebouriella*	6 - 9 g
Jiang Huang	*Curcuma*	6 - 9 g
Sheng Jiang	*Zingiber*	3 - 6 g
Da Zao	*Ziziphus*	3 - 6 pc
Gan Cao	*Glycyrrhiza*	3 - 6 g

Wind damp cold bi-syndrome with numbness, heavy sensation, migrating joint pain, or cold and wind intolerance.

T sticky white coat

P slippery, slow

JUAN BI TANG II

Remove Painful Obstruction from Medical Revelations

Qiang Huo	*Notopterygium*	6 - 12 g
Du Huo	*Angelica*	6 - 12 g
Sang Zhi	*Morus*	9 - 18 g
Dang Gui	*Angelica*	6 - 12 g
Mu Xiang	*Saussurea*	3 - 9 g
Hai Feng Teng	*Piper*	9 - 18 g
Gui Zhi	*Cinnamomum*	6 - 9 g
Qin Jiao	*Gentiana*	6 - 12 g
Chuan Xiong	*Ligusticum*	3 - 9 g
Ru Xiang	*Boswellia*	3 - 6 g
Gan Cao	*Glycyrrhiza*	3 - 6 g

Wind cold damp with pre-existing internal damp causing muscle aches; or external wind damp cold and internal heat causing intolerance to wind and cold, joint- or bodyaches, lack of sweating, or thirst.

T normal color, or red, thin yellowish coat

P superficial, rapid, maybe slippery

JIU WEI QIANG HUO TANG

Nine-Ingredient Decoction with Notopterygium

Extract Formula Name: Chianghuo Combination

Qiang Huo	*Notopterygium*	3 - 6 g
Cang Zhu	*Atractylodes*	3 - 6 g
Xi Xin	*Asarum*	1 - 3 g
Fang Feng	*Ledebouriella*	3 - 6 g
Chuan Xiong	*Ligusticum*	3 - 6 g
Huang Qin	*Scutellaria*	3 - 9 g
Bai Zhi	*Angelica*	3 - 6 g
Sheng Di Huang	*Rehmannia*	3 - 9 g
Gan Cao	*Glycyrrhiza*	3 - 6 g

Acute wind damp cold lodged in the channels causing acute bi-syndrome. Symptoms include heaviness and pain in the body, belt-type headache, or lack of sweating.

T normal color, thin white coat

P superficial

✪ Major Formula

QIANG HUO SHENG SHI TANG

Notopterygium Decoction to Overcome Dampness

Extract Formula Name: Chianghuo and Vitex Combination

Qiang Huo	*Notopterygium*	3 - 6 g
Gao Ben	*Ligusticum*	3 - 6 g
Fang Feng	*Ledebouriella*	6 - 9 g
Du Huo	*Angelica*	6 - 9 g
Chuan Xiong	*Ligusticum*	3 - 9 g
Man Jing Zi	*Vitex*	3 - 9 g
Gan Cao	*Glycyrrhiza*	3 - 6 g

Qi and blood stasis with underlying Kidney and Liver yin deficiency and qi/blood deficiency manifesting as wind damp bi-syndrome. Symptoms include tremors and weakness in the extremities.

T pale

P wiry, weak, thin

SAN BI TANG

Three-Painful Obstruction Decoction

Xu Duan	*Dipsacus*	6 - 9 g
Fang Feng	*Ledebouriella*	6 - 9 g
Rou Gui	*Cinnamomum*	6 - 9 g
Dang Gui	*Angelica*	6 - 9 g
Xi Xin	*Asarum*	3 g
Fu Ling	*Poria*	6 - 9 g
Qin Jiao	*Gentiana*	6 - 9 g
Du Zhong	*Eucommia*	6 - 9 g
Ren Shen	*Panax*	3 - 6 g
Huai Niu Xi	*Achyranthes*	6 - 9 g
Bai Shao Yao	*Paeonia*	6 - 9 g
Huang Qi	*Astragalus*	6 - 9 g
Du Huo	*Angelica*	6 - 9 g
Chuan Xiong	*Ligusticum*	3 - 9 g
Sheng Di Huang	*Rehmannia*	6 - 9 g
Gan Cao	*Glycyrrhiza*	3 - 6 g
Gan Jiang	*Zingiber*	3 - 6 g

Kidney and Liver yin deficiency with blood deficiency and wind damp. This leads to blurry vision, cough, constipation, or bi-syndrome.

T red, scanty yellow coat

P thin

☞ Herbs should be formed into 9 g pills. Adults take one pill two times a day.

SANG MA WAN

Mulberry Leaf and Sesame Seed Pill

Sang Ye	*Morus*	250 - 300 g
Hei Zhi Ma	*Sesamum*	100 - 120 g
Feng Mi	*Mel*	250 - 300 g

Qi and blood stagnation in the channels causing pain in the extremities or muscles.

T purple

P wiry

SHEN TONG ZHU YU TANG

Drive Out Blood Stasis from a Painful Body Decoction

Chuan Xiong	*Ligusticum*	3 - 9 g
Tao Ren	*Prunus*	6 - 9 g
Hong Hua	*Carthamus*	6 - 9 g
Qin Jiao	*Gentiana*	6 - 9 g
Qiang Huo	*Notopterygium*	3 - 6 g
Dang Gui	*Angelica*	6 - 9 g
Chuan Niu Xi	*Cyathula*	6 - 12 g
Mo Yao	*Commiphora*	6 - 9 g
Wu Ling Zhi	*Trogopterus*	6 - 9 g
Di Long	*Pheretima*	6 - 9 g
Xiang Fu	*Cyperus*	3 - 6 g
Gan Cao	*Glycyrrhiza*	3 - 6 g

Wind damp bi-syndrome with phlegm and blood stagnation causing sharp piercing pain in all joints.

T purple, sticky coat

P wiry, slippery

SHU FENG HUO XUE TANG

Disperse Wind and Invigorate the Blood Decoction

Extract Formula Name: Stephania and Carthamus Combination

Dang Gui	*Angelica*	6 - 9 g
Han Fang Ji	*Stephania*	6 - 9 g
Chuan Xiong	*Ligusticum*	3 - 9 g
Bai Zhi	*Angelica*	6 - 9 g
Wei Ling Xian	*Clematis*	3 - 9 g
Cang Zhu	*Atractylodes*	3 - 9 g
Hong Hua	*Carthamus*	3 - 9 g
Dan Nan Xing	*Arisaema*	3 g
Huang Bai	*Phellodendron*	6 - 9 g
Gui Zhi	*Cinnamomum*	3 - 9 g
Qiang Huo	*Notopterygium*	6 - 9 g
Gan Jiang	*Zingiber*	3 - 6 g

Lower body wind cold damp bi-syndrome with blood stagnation causing low back pain, muscle aches, sciatica, or hemiplegia.

T purple

P wiry, slippery

✘ Do not use during pregnancy.

SHU JING HUO XUE TANG

Relax the Channels and Invigorate the Blood Decoction

Extract Formula Name: Clematis and Stephania Combination

Bai Shao Yao	*Paeonia*	6 - 9 g
Chuan Xiong	*Ligusticum*	3 - 9 g
Sheng Di Huang	*Rehmannia*	6 - 9 g
Dang Gui	*Angelica*	6 - 9 g
Cang Zhu	*Atractylodes*	3 - 6 g
Fu Ling	*Poria*	6 - 9 g
Long Dan Cao	*Gentiana*	6 - 9 g
Tao Ren	*Prunus*	3 - 6 g
Wei Ling Xian	*Clematis*	3 - 6 g
Huai Niu Xi	*Achyranthes*	6 - 9 g
Qiang Huo	*Notopterygium*	3 - 6 g
Chen Pi	*Citrus*	3 - 6 g
Fang Feng	*Ledebouriella*	6 - 9 g
Han Fang Ji	*Stephania*	6 - 9 g
Bai Zhi	*Angelica*	3 - 6 g
Sheng Jiang	*Zingiber*	3 - 6 g
Gan Cao	*Glycyrrhiza*	3 - 6 g

Internal Medicine & Misc. Syndromes

Blood stagnation in the head, face, and neck area leading to migraines or cyanotic lips.

T purple or purple spots

P wiry or choppy

☞ Decoct all herbs except She Xiang - Moschus for 15 minutes. Add 230 cc of rice wine and let cook for another 5 - 10 minutes, then add powdered She Xiang - Moschus and dissolve into the tea.

✗ Do not use during pregnancy.

TONG QIAO HUO XUE TANG

Unblock the Orifices and Invigorate the Blood Decoction

Extract Formula Name: Persica and Cnidium Combination

Hong Hua	*Carthamus*	6 - 9 g
Tao Ren	*Prunus*	6 - 9 g
Chuan Xiong	*Ligusticum*	3 - 9 g
Chi Shao Yao	*Paeonia*	6 - 9 g
Cong Bai	*Allium*	3 - 6 g
She Xiang	*Moschus*	0.1 - 0.3 g
Da Zao	*Ziziphus*	3 - 6 pc
Sheng Jiang	*Zingiber*	3 - 6 g

Severe joint pain due to wind damp cold bi-syndrome with significant pain in the hands and feet.

T moist, white coat

P slow, slippery

☞ Decoct Chuan Wu - Aconitum one hour prior to adding the other herbs. The prepared type of Aconite should be used.

✗ This formula can be somewhat toxic. Caution during pregnancy.

WU TOU TANG

Aconite Decoction

Zhi Chuan Wu	*Aconitum*	6 - 15 g
Huang Qi	*Astragalus*	9 - 12 g
Ma Huang	*Ephedra*	6 - 9 g
Bai Shao Yao	*Paeonia*	6 - 9 g
Gan Cao	*Glycyrrhiza*	3 - 6 g

Wind stroke leading to paralysis and numbness; or wind cold damp in the channels resulting in wandering or fixed pain in the joints and muscles. The patient has difficulty controlling the muscles due to weakness and spasms.

T moist, white coat

P slow, slippery

☞ The formula should be taken as a powder. The prepared types of Aconite are used here.

✘ Do not use during pregnancy. It is a very strong prescription. Use only for a short period of time.

XIAO HUO LUO DAN

Minor Invigorate the Collaterals Special Pill

Cao Wu	*Aconitum*	60 g
Chuan Wu	*Aconitum*	60 g
Tian Nan Xing	*Arisaema*	60 g
Di Long	*Pheretima*	60 g
Ru Xiang	*Boswellia*	30 g
Mo Yao	*Commiphora*	30 g

Damp heat obstruction in the channels causing joint pain with fever and shivering.

T red, sticky coat

P slippery, rapid

XUAN BI TANG

Disband Painful Obstruction Decoction

Guang Fang Ji	*Aristolochia*	9 - 15 g
Lian Qiao	*Forsythia*	6 - 9 g
Xing Ren	*Prunus*	9 - 15 g
Yi Yi Ren	*Coix*	9 - 15 g
Zhi Zi	*Gardenia*	6 - 9 g
Hua Shi	*Talcum*	9 - 15 g
Ban Xia	*Pinellia*	6 - 9 g
Can Sha	*Bombyx*	6 - 9 g
Chi Xiao Dou	*Phaseolus*	6 - 9 g

Wind damp heat causing joint pain with swelling and pain in hands and feet, and fever.

T red, sticky coat

P rapid, slippery

YI YI REN TANG II

Coix Decoction from the Enlightened Physicians

Extract Formula Name: Coix Combination

Yi Yi Ren	*Coix*	9 - 20 g
Dang Gui	*Angelica*	6 - 9 g
Ma Huang	*Ephedra*	6 - 9 g
Cang Zhu	*Atractylodes*	6 - 9 g
Bai Shao Yao	*Paeonia*	6 - 9 g
Gui Zhi	*Cinnamomum*	6 - 9 g
Zhi Gan Cao	*Glycyrrhiza*	3 - 6 g

BLOOD STAGNATION DUE TO TRAUMA

- pain caused by a traumatic injury
- swelling and/or hematoma

T purple or unremarkable

P tends to be wiry

Trauma causing qi and blood stagnation which leads to bruising and swelling.

T purple

P wiry

☞ Herbs should be made into 3 g pills with honey. Adults take one or two pills two times a day.

✘ Do not use during pregnancy.

✪ Major Formula

DIE DA WAN

Trauma Pill

Chuan Xiong	*Ligusticum*	20 - 30 g
Dang Gui	*Angelica*	20 - 30 g
Mo Yao	*Commiphora*	20 - 30 g
Tu Bie Chong	*Eupolyphaga*	20 - 30 g
Ma Huang	*Ephedra*	50 - 60 g
Ru Xiang	*Boswellia*	20 - 30 g
Xue Jie	*Dracaena*	20 - 30 g
Zi Ran Tong	*Pyritum*	20 - 30 g

Blood stagnation due to trauma. The pain is mostly in the chest and flanks. Symptoms include large bruises or stabbing pain.

T purple

P wiry, slippery

☞ A few drops of wine should be added at the end.

✘ Do not use during pregnancy.

FU YUAN HUO XUE TANG

Revive Health by Invigorating the Blood Decoction

Extract Formula Name: Tang-Kuei and Persica Combination

Tao Ren	*Prunus*	6 - 9 g
Hong Hua	*Carthamus*	6 - 9 g
Da Huang	*Rheum*	9 - 30 g
Chai Hu	*Bupleurum*	6 - 15 g
Tian Hua Fen	*Trichosanthes*	9 - 12 g
Dang Gui	*Angelica*	6 - 9 g
Chuan Shan Jia	*Manis*	6 - 9 g
Gan Cao	*Glycyrrhiza*	3 - 6 g

Qi and blood stagnation in the channels causing pain, ulcerations, or swellings.

T purple

P wiry, choppy

✘ Do not use during pregnancy.

HUO LUO XIAO LING DAN

Fantastically Effective Pill to Invigorate the Collaterals

Dan Shen	*Salvia*	15 g
Dang Gui	*Angelica*	15 g
Mo Yao	*Commiphora*	15 g
Ru Xiang	*Boswellia*	15 g

Qi/blood stagnation from external or internal injury of all kinds causing pain and bleeding.

T purple

P wiry or choppy

☞ Powder herbs and take in a 0.2 - 1.5 g dosage internally. For external use mix herbs with wine.

✘ Do not use during pregnancy. Zhu Sha - Cinnabaris is toxic, and should only be used short-term.

✪ Major Formula

QI LI SAN

Seven-Thousandths of a Tael Powder

Extract Formula Name: Musk and Catechu Formula

Xue Jie	*Dracaena*	30 g
Ru Xiang	*Boswellia*	3 - 6 g
Hong Hua	*Carthamus*	3 - 6 g
Mo Yao	*Commiphora*	3 - 6 g
Er Cha	*Acacia*	6 - 9 g
Zhu Sha	*Cinnabaris*	3 - 5 g
She Xiang	*Moschus*	0.5 g
Bing Pian	*Dryobalanops*	0.5 g

TOXIC HEAT

- fever
- bleeding disorders
- sore, swollen throat or diptheria
- boils, carbuncles

T red, yellow coat

P rapid, forceful

Heart/Pericardium fire with toxic heat and fever which congeals into phlegm. This leads to delirium, coma, aphasia, or convulsions in children.

T dark red, sticky yellow coat

P rapid, forceful, wiry

☞ Herbs should be ground and made into 3 g pills. The adult dosage is one pill two to three times a day. Xi Jiao - Rhinoceros should be substituted with Shui Niu Jiao - Bubalus.

✘ Do not use during pregnancy. Do not take over a prolonged period of time. Note that Zhu Sha - Cinnabaris is toxic.

AN GONG NIU HUANG WAN

Calm the Palace Pill with Cattle Gallstone

Extract Formula Name: Bos and Curcuma Formula

Niu Huang	*Bos*	25 - 30 g
Xi Jiao	*Rhinoceros*	25 - 30 g
She Xiang	*Moschus*	7.5 g
Huang Lian	*Coptis*	25 - 30 g
Zhi Zi	*Gardenia*	25 - 30 g
Huang Qin	*Scutellaria*	25 - 30 g
Bing Pian	*Dryobalanops*	7.5 g
Zhen Zhu Mu	*Pteria*	12 - 15 g
Yu Jin	*Curcuma*	25 - 30 g
Xiong Huang	*Realgar*	25 - 30 g
Zhu Sha	*Cinnabaris*	25 - 30 g

Heat in the qi level/yangming channel syndrome causing severe fever, epidemic febrile disease, acute inflammation, encephalitis, or meningitis.

T red, dry yellow coat

P flooding, rapid

☞ Decoct the first five herbs, then add the rice at the end. It will absorb the water to make a thick liquid.

BAI HU JIA YIN QIAO TANG

White Tiger plus Lonicera and Forsythia Decoction

Shi Gao	*Gypsum*	20 - 30 g
Zhi Mu	*Anemarrhena*	9 - 12 g
Gan Cao	*Glycyrrhiza*	3 - 6 g
Jin Yin Hua	*Lonicera*	6 - 9 g
Lian Qiao	*Forsythia*	6 - 9 g
Jing Mi	*Oryza*	15 - 30 g

Toxic heat in the yangming channel causing dysentery, or pus or blood in the stools.

T red, yellow coat

P wiry, rapid, rolling

BAI TOU WENG TANG

Pulsatilla Decoction

Extract Formula Name: Anemone Combination

Bai Tou Weng	*Pulsatilla*	20 - 40 g
Huang Bai	*Phellodendron*	9 - 12 g
Qin Pi	*Fraxinus*	9 - 15 g
Huang Lian	*Coptis*	6 - 9 g

Damp accumulation with heat toxin in the qi level causing gastritis, hepatitis, fever, bodyaches, diarrhea, or vomiting.

T sticky yellow coat

P rapid, soggy

☞ All ingredients should be dried in sunlight and ground into powder. Take 9 g each time, twice a day.

GAN LU XIAO DU DAN

Sweet Dew Special Pill to Eliminate Toxin

Extract Formula Name: Talc and Scute Formula

She Gan	*Belamcanda*	120 g
Lian Qiao	*Forsythia*	120 g
Hua Shi	*Talcum*	450 g
Chuan Bei Mu	*Fritillaria*	150 g
Bo He	*Mentha*	120 g
Huang Qin	*Scutellaria*	300 g
Bai Dou Kou	*Amomum*	120 g
Yin Chen Hao	*Artemisia*	330 g
Shi Chang Pu	*Acorus*	180 g
Huo Xiang	*Agastache*	120 g
Mu Tong	*Akebia*	150 g

Heat is creating fire, then toxin which affects the three jiaos. The heat may be internal or external. Symptoms include high fever, mania, delirium, or bleeding in the upper parts.

T red, dry, rough

P rapid, forceful

✪ **Major Formula**

HUANG LIAN JIE DU TANG

Coptis Decoction to Relieve Toxicity

Extract Formula Name: Coptis and Scute Combination

Huang Lian	*Coptis*	3 - 9 g
Huang Bai	*Phellodendron*	6 g
Huang Qin	*Scutellaria*	6 g
Zhi Zi	*Gardenia*	9 g

Toxic heat with underlying Kidney and Lung yin deficiency causing diphtheria, laryngitis, or tonsillitis. The patient experiences sore, swollen throat, dry nose and lips, cough, or wheezing.

T red, scanty yellow coat

P rapid

KANG BAI HOU HE JI

Treat Diphtheria Decoction

Sheng Di Huang	*Rehmannia*	12 - 30 g
Huang Qin	*Scutellaria*	6 - 18 g
Lian Qiao	*Forsythia*	6 - 18 g
Mai Men Dong	*Ophiopogon*	6 - 9 g
Xuan Shen	*Scrophularia*	6 - 9 g

Toxic heat and phlegm from chronic heat in the middle jiao complicated by wind heat affects the throat leading to tonsillitis with pus and difficulty swallowing.

T red, sticky yellow coat

P rapid, forceful

☞ Herbs should be powdered and mixed with wine. Adults should take 3 - 8 small pills each time.

✘ Do not use during pregnancy.

LIU SHEN WAN

Six-Miracle Pill

Niu Huang	*Bos*	3 - 6 g
Xiong Huang	*Realgar*	2 - 3 g
Chan Su	*Bufo*	2 - 3 g
Bing Pian	*Dryobalanops*	2 - 3 g
She Xiang	*Moschus*	3 - 6 g
Zhen Zhu	*Pteria*	3 - 6 g

Toxic heat causing swelling and abscess, fever, thirst, or scanty urination.

T red or dark red, yellow coat

P rapid, forceful

✘ Formula is very cold. Use caution during pregnancy.

NEI SHU HUANG LIAN TANG

Internal Dispersing Decoction with Coptis

Huang Lian	*Coptis*	3 - 9 g
Zhi Zi	*Gardenia*	3 - 9 g
Huang Qin	*Scutellaria*	6 - 9 g
Da Huang	*Rheum*	3 - 6 g
Lian Qiao	*Forsythia*	3 - 9 g
Dang Gui	*Angelica*	6 - 9 g
Bing Lang	*Areca*	3 - 6 g
Bo He	*Mentha*	6 - 9 g
Bai Shao Yao	*Paeonia*	3 - 9 g
Mu Xiang	*Saussurea*	3 - 6 g
Jie Geng	*Platycodon*	3 - 6 g
Gan Cao	*Glycyrrhiza*	3 - 6 g

Wind heat with toxic fire causing throat and gum swelling or oral ulcers.

T red or dark red, cracked

P rapid, forceful

✘ Do not use during pregnancy.

NIU HUANG SHANG QING WAN

Cattle Gallstone Pill to Ascend and Clear

Huang Lian	*Coptis*	3 - 9 g
Huang Bai	*Phellodendron*	6 - 9 g
Zhi Zi	*Gardenia*	3 - 6 g
Huang Qin	*Scutellaria*	6 - 9 g
Da Huang	*Rheum*	9 - 20 g
Fang Feng	*Ledebouriella*	6 - 9 g
Jing Jie	*Schizonepeta*	6 - 9 g
Chuan Xiong	*Ligusticum*	3 - 6 g
Niu Huang	*Bos*	2 - 3 g
Shi Gao	*Gypsum*	9 - 20 g
Bing Pian	*Dryobalanops*	3 - 9 g
Bai Zhi	*Angelica*	3 - 6 g
Bo He	*Mentha*	3 - 6 g
Dang Gui	*Angelica*	6 - 9 g
Chi Shao Yao	*Paeonia*	6 - 12 g
Lian Xin	*Nelumbo*	9 - 15 g
Lian Qiao	*Forsythia*	6 - 9 g
Xiong Huang	*Realgar*	3 - 6 g
Ju Hua	*Chrysanthemum*	6 - 9 g
Jie Geng	*Platycodon*	3 g
Gan Cao	*Glycyrrhiza*	3 g

Toxic heat with wind heat, sore, swollen throat, and facial swelling.

T red, dry yellow coat

P forceful, rapid

PU JI XIAO DU YIN

Universal Benefit Decoction to Eliminate Toxin

Extract Formula Name: Scute and Cimicifuga Combination

Huang Qin	*Scutellaria*	6 - 18 g
Huang Lian	*Coptis*	6 - 18 g
Ban Lan Gen	*Isatis*	3 - 6 g
Lian Qiao	*Forsythia*	3 - 6 g
Niu Bang Zi	*Arctium*	3 - 6 g
Chen Pi	*Citrus*	3 - 6 g
Sheng Ma	*Cimicifuga*	1 - 3 g
Jiang Can	*Bombyx*	1 - 3 g
Bo He	*Mentha*	3 - 6 g
Ma Bo	*Lasiosphaera*	3 - 6 g
Chai Hu	*Bupleurum*	3 - 6 g
Xuan Shen	*Scrophularia*	3 - 6 g
Jie Geng	*Platycodon*	3 - 6 g
Gan Cao	*Glycyrrhiza*	3 - 6 g

Wind heat with toxin affecting the neck and head with swollen sore throat or glands, tonsillitis, or pharyngitis.

T red

P rapid

QIANG LAN TANG

Notopterygium and Isatis Root Decoction

Qiang Huo	*Notopterygium*	9 - 12 g
Ban Lan Gen	*Isatis*	12 - 20 g

Qi and blood level heat: qi level heat causing high fever, thirst, sweating; and blood level heat causing bleeding conditions, coma, or restlessness. This formula also treats toxic heat.

T dark red, dry, yellow coat

P flooding, rapid

☞ Shi Gao - Gypsum should be decocted first for 20 minutes. Xi Jiao - Rhinoceros should be powdered and added to the strained decoction. It should be substituted with 6 - 9 g of Shui Niu Jiao - Bubalus, or 30 g of Bai Mao Gen - Imperata.

QING WEN BAI DU YIN

Clear Epidemics and Overcome Toxin Decoction

Shi Gao	*Gypsum*	40 - 100 g
Zhi Mu	*Anemarrhena*	9 - 12 g
Xuan Shen	*Scrophularia*	6 - 9 g
Dan Zhu Ye	*Lophatherum*	3 - 6 g
Xi Jiao	*Rhinoceros*	1 - 3 g
Chi Shao Yao	*Paeonia*	6 - 9 g
Huang Qin	*Scutellaria*	6 - 9 g
Huang Lian	*Coptis*	3 - 6 g
Mu Dan Pi	*Paeonia*	6 - 9 g
Sheng Di Huang	*Rehmannia*	6 - 12 g
Zhi Zi	*Gardenia*	3 - 6 g
Jie Geng	*Platycodon*	3 - 6 g
Lian Qiao	*Forsythia*	6 - 9 g
Gan Cao	*Glycyrrhiza*	3 - 6 g

Qi level heat with toxin in the upper body causing throat swelling, fever, sweating, and thirst for cold fluids.

T red, yellow coat

P flooding, rapid

QING XIN LIANG GE SAN

Clear the Heart and Cool the Diaphragm Powder

Lian Qiao	*Forsythia*	6 - 15 g
Huang Qin	*Scutellaria*	6 - 9 g
Zhi Zi	*Gardenia*	3 - 6 g
Bo He	*Mentha*	3 - 6 g
Jie Geng	*Platycodon*	3 - 6 g
Shi Gao	*Gypsum*	12 - 15 g
Gan Cao	*Glycyrrhiza*	3 - 6 g

Qi and blood deficiency with toxic abscess causing mastitis, intestinal abscess, or fever and chills.

T pale or red, yellow coat

P rapid

SHEN XIAO TUO LI SAN

Miraculous Powder for Supporting the Interior

Ren Dong Cao	*Lonicera*	15 g
Dang Gui	*Angelica*	9 g
Huang Qi	*Astragalus*	15 g
Gan Cao	*Glycyrrhiza*	15 - 20 g

Toxic heat with blood stagnation causing gangrene or ulcers in the extremities.

T red or purple spots

P rapid, wiry

SI MIAO YONG AN TANG

Four-Valiant Decoction for Well-Being

Jin Yin Hua	*Lonicera*	60 - 90 g
Dang Gui	*Angelica*	35 g
Xuan Shen	*Scrophularia*	60 - 90 g
Gan Cao	*Glycyrrhiza*	20 g

Phlegm heat toxin and blood stagnation with pus causing Lung abscess, measles, whooping cough, cough with blood-streaked sputum, chest congestion, or low-grade fever.

T red, sticky yellow coat

P rapid, slippery

WEI JING TANG

Reed Decoction

Phragmites Combination

Lu Gen	*Phragmitis*	40 - 60 g
Dong Gua Ren	*Benincasa*	15 - 25 g
Yi Yi Ren	*Coix*	15 - 20 g
Tao Ren	*Prunus*	6 - 9 g

Damp heat with toxin causing abscess, skin rash in the lower limbs, or erysipelas.

T red, sticky coat

P rapid, slippery

WU SHEN TANG

Five-Miracle Decoction

Jin Yin Hua	*Lonicera*	30 - 60 g
Zi Hua Di Ding	*Viola*	15 - 20 g
Fu Ling	*Poria*	9 - 12 g
Huai Niu Xi	*Achyranthes*	3 - 6 g
Che Qian Zi	*Plantago*	6 - 9 g

Any organ heat or toxin causing boils or sores. They are painful, hot, swollen, and may be hard to the touch.

T red or dark red, yellow dry coat

P rapid

WU WEI XIAO DU YIN

Five-Ingredient Decoction to Eliminate Toxin

Jin Yin Hua	*Lonicera*	12 - 15 g
Zi Hua Di Ding	*Viola*	9 - 15 g
Pu Gong Ying	*Taraxacum*	9 - 15 g
Zi Bei Tian Kuei	*Begonia*	9 - 15 g
Ye Ju Hua	*Chrysanthemum*	9 - 15 g

Phlegm fire or toxic fire causing qi and blood stagnation. This manifests as carbuncles and boils with redness, mild chills, and severe fever.

T red, thin yellow coat

P rapid, forceful

☞ The formula should be decocted with 50 % wine and 50 % water. It may also be applied topically.

✘ Zao Jiao Ci - Gleditsia is slightly toxic and should not be used during pregnancy.

XIAN FANG HUO MING YIN

Sublime Formula for Sustaining Life

Extract Formula Name: Angelica and Mastic Combination

Jin Yin Hua	*Lonicera*	6 - 9 g
Zhe Bei Mu	*Fritillaria*	3 - 6 g
Dang Gui Wei	*Angelica*	9 - 12 g
Tian Hua Fen	*Trichosanthes*	3 - 6 g
Ru Xiang	*Boswellia*	2 - 3 g
Zao Jiao Ci	*Gleditsia*	2 - 3 g
Fang Feng	*Ledebouriella*	3 - 6 g
Chi Shao Yao	*Paeonia*	6 g
Mo Yao	*Commiphora*	3 - 6 g
Bai Zhi	*Angelica*	3 g
Chuan Shan Jia	*Manis*	3 - 6 g
Chen Pi	*Citrus*	3 - 6 g
Gan Cao	*Glycyrrhiza*	3 - 6 g

External invasion with toxic heat causing carbuncles, mastitis, or red rashes.

T red, thin yellow coat

P superficial, rapid

XIAO YAN JIE DU WAN

Reduce Inflammation and Relieve Toxicity Pill

Jin Yin Hua	*Lonicera*	9 - 20 g
Pu Gong Ying	*Taraxacum*	9 - 20 g
Fang Feng	*Ledebouriella*	6 - 9 g
Lian Qiao	*Forsythia*	9 - 15 g
Gan Cao	*Glycyrrhiza*	3 - 6 g

Wind heat and toxin causing measles, lack of sweating, cough, dark urine, or severe sore throat.

T red tip

P superficial, rapid

XUAN DU FA BIAO TANG

Dissipate Toxin and Release the Exterior Decoction

Sheng Ma	*Cimicifuga*	6 - 9 g
Ge Gen	*Pueraria*	6 - 9 g
Xing Ren	*Prunus*	6 - 9 g
Qian Hu	*Peucedanum*	6 - 9 g
Jie Geng	*Platycodon*	3 - 6 g
Bo He	*Mentha*	3 - 6 g
Fang Feng	*Ledebouriella*	3 - 6 g
Jing Jie	*Schizonepeta*	3 - 6 g
Lian Qiao	*Forsythia*	3 - 9 g
Niu Bang Zi	*Arctium*	3 - 6 g
Dan Zhu Ye	*Lophatherum*	3 - 6 g
Zhi Ke	*Citrus*	3 - 6 g
Mu Tong	*Akebia*	6 - 9 g
Gan Cao	*Glycyrrhiza*	3 - 6 g

Lung/Kidney yin deficiency with toxin causing diptheria, laryngitis, coarse breathing, or dry hacking cough.

T red, dry, yellow coat

P thin, rapid, or empty

YANG YIN QING FEI TANG

Nourish the Yin and Clear the Lungs Decoction

Sheng Di Huang	*Rehmannia*	6 - 12 g
Xuan Shen	*Scrophularia*	6 - 9 g
Bai Shao Yao	*Paeonia*	6 - 9 g
Mai Men Dong	*Ophiopogon*	6 - 12 g
Bo He	*Mentha*	3 - 6 g
Chuan Bei Mu	*Fritillaria*	3 - 6 g
Mu Dan Pi	*Paeonia*	6 - 9 g
Gan Cao	*Glycyrrhiza*	3 - 6 g

Fire toxin from wind damp heat causing skin lesions with pus and redness.

T red

P rapid, slippery

☞ Xi Jiao - Rhinoceros should be substituted with 6 - 9 g of Shui Niu Jiao - Bubalus or 30 g of Bai Mao Gen - Imperata.

YIN HUA JIE DU TANG

Honeysuckle Decoction to Relieve Toxicity

Jin Yin Hua	*Lonicera*	9 - 20 g
Zi Hua Di Ding	*Viola*	9 - 20 g
Lian Qiao	*Forsythia*	6 - 18 g
Huang Lian	*Coptis*	6 g
Xia Ku Cao	*Prunella*	6 - 18 g
Xi Jiao	*Rhinoceros*	2 - 3 g
Mu Dan Pi	*Paeonia*	6 - 9 g
Chi Fu Ling	*Poria*	6 - 9 g

Wind/toxic heat with damp and qi deficiency causing red, swollen sores or carbuncles.

T thin sticky white coat

P superficial

YIN QIAO BAI DU SAN

Honeysuckle and Forsythia Powder to Overcome Pathogenic Influences

Qiang Huo	Notopterygium	6 - 9 g
Chuan Xiong	Ligusticum	3 - 6 g
Du Huo	Angelica	3 - 6 g
Chai Hu	Bupleurum	6 - 9 g
Qian Hu	Peucedanum	6 - 9 g
Ren Shen	Panax	6 - 9 g
Jie Geng	Platycodon	3 - 6 g
Zhi Ke	Citrus	3 - 6 g
Fu Ling	Poria	3 - 6 g
Gan Cao	Glycyrrhiza	3 - 6 g
Jin Yin Hua	Lonicera	6 - 9 g
Lian Qiao	Forsythia	6 - 9 g

Damp heat in the Lungs causing toxin in the throat with obstruction and soreness.

T red, sticky yellow coat

P rapid, slippery

YIN QIAO MA BO SAN

Honeysuckle, Forsythia, and Puffball Powder

Lian Qiao	Forsythia	15 - 25 g
Jin Yin Hua	Lonicera	9 - 12 g
Niu Bang Zi	Arctium	12 - 15 g
Ma Bo	Lasiosphaera	6 - 9 g
She Gan	Belamcanda	6 - 9 g
[Lu Gen	Phragmites	12 - 20 g]

SUMMERHEAT INVASION

- fever and chills after exposure to the sun
- nausea and vomiting
- thirst
- sweating

T red tip, yellow coat

P superficial, rapid

Summerheat with damp and yangming channel heat/qi level heat. This causes severe sweating, nausea, vomiting, thirst, or fever.

T red, sticky yellow coat

P slippery, rapid

☞ Decoct the first four herbs, then add the rice at the end. It will absorb the water to make a thick liquid.

BAI HU JIA ZHU TANG

White Tiger with White Atractylodes Decoction

Shi Gao	*Gypsum*	20 - 30 g
Zhi Mu	*Anemarrhena*	9 - 12 g
Gan Cao	*Glycyrrhiza*	3 - 6 g
Bai Zhu	*Atractylodes*	3 - 9 g
Jing Mi	*Oryza*	15 - 30 g

Longstanding summer damp heat with urinary problems and fever.

T red, thin yellow coat

P rapid

CHUN ZE TANG

Spring Pond Decoction

Fu Ling	*Poria*	6 - 9 g
Zhu Ling	*Polyporus*	6 - 9 g
Ze Xie	*Alisma*	6 - 9 g
Gui Zhi	*Cinnamomum*	3 - 9 g
Bai Zhu	*Atractylodes*	6 - 9 g
Chai Hu	*Bupleurum*	6 - 9 g
Mai Men Dong	*Ophiopogon*	6 - 9 g
Ren Shen	*Panax*	6 - 9 g

Summerheat with internal water and damp accumulation leading to headaches and fever. This leads to depletion of qi and yin. Symptoms include nausea and vomiting, thirst and dry mouth, diarrhea, or restlessness.

T red, sticky yellowish coat

P rapid, superficial

GUI LING GAN LU YIN

Cinnamon and Poria Sweet Dew Decoction

Hua Shi	*Talcum*	15 - 30 g
Shi Gao	*Gypsum*	15 - 30 g
Han Shui Shi	*Calcitum*	12 - 30 g
Rou Gui	*Cinnamomum*	6 - 9 g
Fu Ling	*Poria*	12 - 30 g
Ze Xie	*Alisma*	9 - 15 g
Zhu Ling	*Polyporus*	9 - 15 g
Bai Zhu	*Atractylodes*	9 - 12 g
Gan Cao	*Glycyrrhiza*	6 - 9 g
Sheng Jiang	*Zingiber*	1 - 3 g

Summer damp heat, mostly manifesting in the upper jiao with fever, chills, sweating, or dizziness.

T thin sticky coat

P rapid, slippery

LEI SHI QING LIANG DI SHU TANG

Master Lei's Decoction to Clear, Cool and Remove Summerheat

Hua Shi	*Talcum*	12 - 15 g
Qing Hao	*Artemisia*	3 - 6 g
Bian Dou	*Dolichos*	6 - 9 g
Lian Qiao	*Forsythia*	6 - 9 g
Tong Cao	*Tetrapanax*	3 - 9 g
Fu Ling	*Poria*	6 - 9 g
Gan Cao	*Glycyrrhiza*	3 - 6 g
Xi Gua	*Citrullus*	1 pc

A patient with pre-existing qi deficiency gets a summerheat and damp invasion leading to dizziness, headache, diarrhea, heaviness, and fever and chills.

T red or normal color

P rapid, weak

LI SHI QING SHU YI QI TANG

Master Li's Decoction to Clear Summerheat and Augment the Qi

Ren Shen	*Panax*	6-9 g
Cang Zhu	*Atractylodes*	3-9 g
Bai Zhu	*Atractylodes*	6-9 g
Huang Qi	*Astragalus*	6-12 g
Ge Gen	*Pueraria*	6-9 g
Mai Men Dong	*Ophiopogon*	6-9 g
Wu Wei Zi	*Schisandra*	3-9 g
Qing Pi	*Citrus*	3-6 g
Chen Pi	*Citrus*	3-6 g
Sheng Ma	*Cimicifuga*	3-6 g
Dang Gui	*Angelica*	3-6 g
Shen Qu	*Massa Fermentata*	6-9 g
Ze Xie	*Alisma*	6-9 g
Huang Bai	*Phellodendron*	6-9 g
Gan Cao	*Glycyrrhiza*	3-6 g

Summer heat with damp causing nausea and vomiting, thirst, fullness in the chest, or diarrhea.

T sticky coat

P slippery, superficial

LIU HE TANG

Harmonize the Six Decoction

Extract Formula Name: Cardamon Combination

Huo Xiang	*Agastache*	6-9 g
Sha Ren	*Amomum*	3-9 g
Hou Po	*Magnolia*	6-9 g
Dang Shen	*Codonopsis*	6-9 g
Xing Ren	*Prunus*	3-6 g
Bian Dou	*Dolichos*	6-9 g
Ban Xia	*Pinellia*	6-9 g
Mu Gua	*Chaenomeles*	6-9 g
Bai Zhu	*Atractylodes*	6-9 g
Chi Fu Ling	*Poria*	6-9 g
Gan Cao	*Glycyrrhiza*	3-6 g

Summerheat with damp causing fever, nausea, vomiting, thirst, irritability, or sweating.

T sticky yellow coat

P rapid, slippery

✪ Major Formula

LIU YI SAN

Six-to-One Powder

Hua Shi	*Talcum*	6 parts
Zhi Gan Cao	*Glycyrrhiza*	1 part

Mild summer heat invading the qi level with residual pathogens lingering causing mild superficial and damp symptoms. The patient feels thirst but can only sip fluids, and experiences diarrhea, gas, vomiting, or cold limbs.

T red, thin white coat

P rapid, maybe superficial

☞ The prepared form of Xi Gua - Citrullus is used. The outer skin of Si Gua Luo - Luffa is used.

QING LUO YIN

Clear the Collaterals Decoction

Bian Dou Hua	*Dolichos*	6 - 9 g
Xi Gua Shuang	*Citrullus*	6 - 9 g
Si Gua Pi	*Luffa*	6 - 9 g
Jin Yin Hua	*Lonicera*	6 - 9 g
He Ye	*Nelumbo*	6 g
Dan Zhu Ye	*Lophatherum*	6 - 9 g

Summerheat opens the pores so the patient sweats which leads to qi and yin deficiency; or yin deficient patient gets a summerheat invasion. Symptoms include thirst, high fever, or profuse sweating.

T red

P frail, rapid

QING SHU YI QI TANG

Clear Summerheat and Augment the Qi Decoction

Extract Formula Name: Lotus Stem and Ginseng Combination

Xi Gua Pi	*Citrullus*	20 -30 g
Xi Yang Shen	*Panax*	6 - 9 g
Mai Men Dong	*Ophiopogon*	6 - 9 g
Lian Geng	*Nelumbo*	6 - 9 g
Shi Hu	*Dendrobium*	6 - 9 g
Dan Zhu Ye	*Lophatherum*	3 - 6 g
Fu Ling	*Poria*	6 - 9 g
Huang Lian	*Coptis*	3 - 6 g
Zhi Mu	*Anemarrhena*	6 - 9 g
Gan Cao	*Glycyrrhiza*	3 - 6 g
Jing Mi	*Oryza*	10 - 15 g

Pre-existing Spleen qi deficiency leading to damp and water in the middle jiao. This creates damp heat. The formula is also used for summer heat invasions. Symptoms include fever and chills, poor appetite, and headache.

T thin white coat

P soggy, wiry, thin

SAN REN TANG

Three-Nut Decoction

Extract Formula Name: Apricot, Coix, and Cluster Combination

Xing Ren	*Prunus*	6 - 12 g
Yi Yi Ren	*Coix*	12 - 15 g
Bai Dou Kou	*Amomum*	3 - 6 g
Hou Po	*Magnolia*	6 - 9 g
Ban Xia	*Pinellia*	6 - 9 g
Dan Zhu Ye	*Lophatherum*	6 - 9 g
Tong Cao	*Tetrapanax*	3 g
Hua Shi	*Talcum*	12 - 15 g

Severe toxin, epidemic summer heat, and blood heat causing delirious speech, purpura, or red eyes. This formula opens the orifice.

T scarlet

P rapid or flooding

☞ Herbs should be made into pills. Xi Jiao - Rhinoceros should be substituted with Shui Niu Jiao - Bubalus.

SHEN XI DAN

Magical Rhinoceros Special Pill

Xi Jiao	*Rhinoceros*	60 - 90 g
Jin Yin Hua	*Lonicera*	200 - 225 g
Ban Lan Gen	*Isatis*	100 - 135 g
Huang Qin	*Scutellaria*	60 - 90 g
Sheng Di Huang	*Rehmannia*	200 - 225 g
Lian Qiao	*Forsythia*	125 - 150 g
Xuan Shen	*Scrophularia*	90 - 105 g
Dan Dou Chi	*Glycine*	100 - 120 g
Shi Chang Pu	*Acorus*	60 - 90 g
Tian Hua Fen	*Trichosanthes*	40 - 60 g
Zi Cao	*Lithospermum*	40 - 60 g

Severe early-stage summer heat (excess type) causing lack of sweating, nausea and vomiting, or high fever.

T thin sticky white coat

P superficial, rapid

XIN JIA XIANG RU YIN

Newly-Augmented Elsholtzia Decoction

Bian Dou Hua	*Dolichos*	6 - 9 g
Xiang Ru	*Elsholtzia*	6 - 9 g
Jin Yin Hua	*Lonicera*	6 - 9 g
Lian Qiao	*Forsythia*	6 - 9 g
Hou Po	*Magnolia*	6 - 12 g

Summer damp heat in all three jiaos leading to sweating, diarrhea, nausea, scanty urination, or tidal fever.

T red tip, sticky yellow coat

P superficial, rapid, slippery

XING REN HUA SHI TANG

Apricot Kernel and Talcum Decoction

Xing Ren	*Prunus*	6 - 9 g
Hua Shi	*Talcum*	9 - 12 g
Huang Lian	*Coptis*	3 - 6 g
Huang Qin	*Scutellaria*	6 - 9 g
Hou Po	*Magnolia*	6 - 12 g
Chen Pi	*Citrus*	3 - 6 g
Ban Xia	*Pinellia*	6 - 9 g
Tong Cao	*Tetrapanax*	3 - 6 g
Yu Jin	*Curcuma*	6 - 9 g

OPEN THE ORIFICE, COMA

- paralysis
- coma or delirium
- aphasia

T depends on the involved syndrome

P depends on the involved syndrome

Heart/Pericardium fire with toxic heat and fever which congeals into phlegm. This leads to delirium, coma, aphasia, or convulsions in children.

T dark red, sticky yellow coat

P rapid, forceful, wiry

☞ Herbs should be ground and made into 3 g pills. The adult dosage is one pill two to three times a day. Xi Jiao - Rhinoceros should be substituted with Shui Niu Jiao - Bubalus.

✘ Do not use during pregnancy. Do not take over a prolonged period of time. Note that Zhu Sha - Cinnabaris is toxic.

✪ Major Formula

AN GONG NIU HUANG WAN

Calm the Palace Pill with Cattle Gallstone

Extract Formula Name: Bos and Curcuma Formula

Niu Huang	*Bos*	25 - 30 g
Xi Jiao	*Rhinoceros*	25 - 30 g
She Xiang	*Moschus*	7.5 g
Huang Lian	*Coptis*	25 - 30 g
Zhi Zi	*Gardenia*	25 - 30 g
Huang Qin	*Scutellaria*	25 - 30 g
Bing Pian	*Dryobalanops*	7.5 g
Zhen Zhu Mu	*Pteria*	12 - 15 g
Yu Jin	*Curcuma*	25 - 30 g
Xiong Huang	*Realgar*	25 - 30 g
Zhu Sha	*Cinnabaris*	25 - 30 g

Qi and blood stagnation with qi deficiency and blockage in the channels leading to wind stroke, hemiplegia, and atrophy in the lower limbs. The patient has difficulty walking.

T purple, thin white coat

P wiry, weak, slow

BU YANG HUAN WU TANG

Tonify the Yang to Restore Five-tenths Decoction

Extract Formula Name: Astragalus and Peony Combination

Huang Qi	*Astragalus*	60 - 120 g
Chuan Xiong	*Ligusticum*	3 - 6 g
Chi Shao Yao	*Paeonia*	3 - 6 g
Dang Gui Wei	*Angelica*	6 - 9 g
Hong Hua	*Carthamus*	3 - 6 g
Tao Ren	*Prunus*	3 - 6 g
Di Long	*Pheretima*	3 - 6 g

Kidney yin/yang deficiency with false fire and phlegm leading to depletion of Heart qi. Symptoms include paraplegia, aphasia, and blockage of the orifice.

T red or normal color, sticky yellow coat

P slippery, slightly rapid, weak, or thin, deep

DI HUANG YIN ZI

Rehmannia Decoction

Shu Di Huang	*Rehmannia*	12 - 15 g
Shan Zhu Yu	*Cornus*	6 - 9 g
Ba Ji Tian	*Morinda*	6 - 9 g
Rou Cong Rong	*Cistanche*	6 - 9 g
Rou Gui	*Cinnamomum*	3 - 9 g
Shi Hu	*Dendrobium*	6 - 9 g
Shi Chang Pu	*Acorus*	6 - 9 g
Yuan Zhi	*Polygala*	3 - 6 g
Mai Men Dong	*Ophiopogon*	6 - 9 g
Fu Ling	*Poria*	6 - 9 g
Wu Wei Zi	*Schisandra*	6 - 9 g
Fu Zi	*Aconitum*	3 - 6 g
[Bo He	*Mentha*	1 - 3 g]
[Sheng Jiang	*Zingiber*	3 - 6 g]
[Da Zao	*Ziziphus*	1 g]

Wind and phlegm accumulation causing hypertension, vertigo, and aphasia.

T rigid, sticky white or yellowish coat

P slippery

DI TAN TANG

Scour Phlegm Decoction

Extract Formula Name: Arisaema and Acorus Combination

Ban Xia	*Pinellia*	6 - 9 g
Fu Ling	*Poria*	6 - 9 g
Zhi Shi	*Citrus*	3 - 6 g
Chen Pi	*Citrus*	3 - 6 g
Zhu Ru	*Bambusa*	1 - 3 g
Dan Nan Xing	*Arisaema*	1 - 3 g
Ren Shen	*Panax*	3 - 6 g
Shi Chang Pu	*Acorus*	6 g
Gan Cao	*Glycyrrhiza*	3 - 6 g
[Sheng Jiang	*Zingiber*	3 - 6 g]
[Da Zao	*Ziziphus*	1 - 3 pc]

Phlegm fire obstructing the orifice causing mania, severe palpitations, cough with profuse phlegm, dizziness, wheezing, anxiety, bad dreams, or lumps in the neck.

T red, thick yellow sticky coat

P wiry, rapid, forceful

☞ Herbs should be made into 6 - 9 g pills. Adults take one pill one or two times a day.

✘ Do not use during pregnancy or post-partum.

GUN TAN WAN

Vaporize Phlegm Pill

Extract Formula Name: Lapis and Scute Formula

Da Huang	*Rheum*	200 - 240 g
Huang Qin	*Scutellaria*	200 - 240 g
Meng Shi	*Lapis Micae Seu Chloriti*	20 - 30 g
Chen Xiang	*Aquilaria*	9 - 15 g

Phlegm heat invading the Pericardium giving rise to wind. Symptoms include spasms, convulsions, loss of consciousness, or nausea and vomiting from phlegm in the middle jiao. This is seen most commonly in small children and infants.

T red, sticky yellow coat

P rapid, wiry, slippery

☞ Herbs should be powdered and made into very tiny pills. For infants the dosage is one pill 2 - 3 times a day.

✘ Do not use during pregnancy. Zhu Sha - Cinnabaris is toxic. The formula should not be used over a long period of time.

HUI CHUN DAN (XIAO ER HUI CHUN DAN)

Return of the Spring Special Pill

Niu Huang	*Bos*	9 - 12 g
Dan Nan Xing	*Arisaema*	50 - 60 g
Tian Zhu Huang	*Bambusa*	35 - 40 g
Chuan Bei Mu	*Fritillaria*	35 - 40 g
Ban Xia	*Pinellia*	35 - 40 g
Chen Xiang	*Aquilaria*	35 - 40 g
Jiang Can	*Bombyx*	35 - 40 g
Quan Xie	*Buthus*	35 - 40 g
She Xiang	*Moschus*	9 - 12 g
Gou Teng	*Uncaria*	20 - 25 g
Tian Ma	*Gastrodia*	35 - 40 g
Zhu Sha	*Cinnabaris*	0.2 - 1.5 g
Bai Dou Kou	*Amomum*	35 - 40 g
Tan Xiang	*Santalum*	35 - 40 g
Da Huang	*Rheum*	50 - 60 g
Mu Xiang	*Saussurea*	35 - 40 g
Chen Pi	*Citrus*	35 - 40 g
Zhi Ke	*Citrus*	35 - 40 g
Gan Cao	*Glycyrrhiza*	25 - 27 g

Heat settles into the Pericardium causing irritability, delirious speech, or childhood convulsions.

T dark red

P rapid, wiry

☞ Herbs should be powdered and made into 3 g pills. Take one pill 2 - 3 times a day.

✘ Zhu Sha - Cinnabaris is toxic and should only be used short-term.

NIU HUANG QING XIN WAN

Cattle Gallstone Pill to Clear the Heart

Extract Formula Name: Bovis Bezoar and Coptis Formula

Niu Huang	*Bos*	0.5 - 0.75 g
Huang Lian	*Coptis*	9 - 15 g
Zhi Zi	*Gardenia*	6 - 9 g
Huang Qin	*Scutellaria*	6 - 9 g
Yu Jin	*Curcuma*	6 - 9 g
Zhu Sha	*Cinnabaris*	3 - 5 g

Wind phlegm attacking the channels, especially the head and face with pre-existing qi and yang deficiency. This leads to paralysis, facial twitches, stiff muscles, spasms, or loose stools.

T pale, swollen, teethmarks, thick sticky coat

P slippery, deep, frail

✘ The formula is toxic and should not be taken over a long period of time. Do not use during pregnancy.

QIAN ZHENG SAN

Lead to Symmetry Powder

Jiang Can	*Bombyx*	6 g
Bai Fu Zi	*Typhonium*	6 g
Quan Xie	*Buthus*	6 g

Wind heat with wind stroke causing paraplegia, or facial paralysis with severe heat symptoms.

T red, yellow coat

P rapid

✘ Caution during pregnancy.

QU FENG ZHI BAO DAN

Greatest Treasure Special Pill to Dispel Wind

Hua Shi	Talcum	12 - 15 g
Dang Gui	Angelica	9 - 12 g
Chuan Xiong	Ligusticum	9 g
Gan Cao	Glycyrrhiza	6 g
Fang Feng	Ledebouriella	6 - 9 g
Bai Shao Yao	Paeonia	6 - 9 g
Bai Zhu	Atractylodes	6 g
Du Huo	Angelica	6 g
Ren Shen	Panax	3 g
Qiang Huo	Notopterygium	3 - 6 g
Shu Di Huang	Rehmannia	6 g
Tian Ma	Gastrodia	6 g
Shi Gao	Gypsum	6 g
Huang Qin	Scutellaria	6 g
Jie Geng	Platycodon	3 g
Zhi Zi	Gardenia	1 - 3 g
Jing Jie	Schizonepeta	6 g
Bo He	Mentha	3 g
Da Huang	Rheum	6 g
Mang Xiao	Mirabilitum	6 g
Lian Qiao	Forsythia	3 - 6 g
Ma Huang	Ephedra	6 g
Huang Lian	Coptis	3 g
Huang Bai	Phellodendron	3 g
Xi Xin	Asarum	3 g
Quan Xie	Buthus	3 g

Wind stroke with phlegm accumulation causing hemiplegia, facial paralysis, aphasia, or seizures from wind phlegm.

T sticky coat

P slippery, forceful

☞ Herbs should be ground into a powder and then taken as a draft. The actual dosage of Li Lu - Veratrum depends on the constitution of the patient.

✘ This formula causes vomiting.

SAN SHENG SAN

Three-Sage Powder

Gua Di	*Cucumis*	100 - 150 g
Li Lu	*Veratrum*	6 - 25 g
Fang Feng	*Ledebouriella*	100 - 150 g

Damp cold and phlegm causing sudden collapse, clenched jaw, or coma; or qi stagnation or damp cold leading to coldness in the chest and abdomen or chest pain, coma, or qi stagnation from an epidemic manifesting in fullness in the chest. The patient feels the urge to vomit or defecate but is unable to do so, which then leads to sudden loss of consciousness.

T pale

P slow, slippery

☞ The prescription is made into pills. Xi Jiao - Rhinoceros should be substituted with Shui Niu Jiao - Bubalus.

✘ Do not use during pregnancy. Zhu Sha - Cinnabaris is toxic, and should only be used short-term.

✪ Major Formula

SU HE XIANG WAN

Liquid Styrax Pill

Extract Formula Name: Styrax Formula

Su He Xiang	*Liquidambar*	30 g
She Xiang	*Moschus*	60 g
Bing Pian	*Dryobalanops*	30 g
An Xi Xiang	*Styrax*	60 g
Ru Xiang	*Boswellia*	30 g
Tan Xiang	*Santalum*	60 g
Ding Xiang	*Eugenia*	60 g
Bi Ba	*Piper*	60 g
Xiang Fu	*Cyperus*	60 g
Xi Jiao	*Rhinoceros*	60 g
Bai Zhu	*Atractylodes*	60 g
He Zi	*Terminalia*	60 g
Zhu Sha	*Cinnabaris*	60 g
Mu Xiang	*Saussarea*	60 g
Chen Xiang	*Aguilaria*	60 g

Exposure to bad smells with phlegm obstruction causing clenched jaw, difficulty breathing, and loss of consciousness. This may be a life-threatening disorder.

T thick sticky coat

P slippery

☞ Equal amounts of the two herbs should be made into a powder. A very small amount of the powder should be blown into the nose, but inhalation into the lungs should be avoided.

✘ Do not use during pregnancy. Do not use for loss of consciousness from cerebral hemorrhage or traumatic head injuries.

TONG GUAN SAN

Open the Gate Powder

Zao Jiao	*Gleditsia*	10 g
Xi Xin	*Asarum*	10 g

Liver wind due to fire in the pericardium, or phlegm heat obstructing the orifice causing stroke, high fever, irritability, loss of consciousness, or a raspy voice.

T dark red, sticky yellow grey coat

P rapid, slippery

☞ Herbs should be ground separately, then sifted together. Make into 3 g pills. Adults take one pill 2 - 3 times a day. Xi Jiao - Rhinoceros should be substituted with Shui Niu Jiao - Bubalus or 50 - 60 g of Bai Mao Gen - Imperata.

✘ Do not use during pregnancy. Zhu Sha - Cinnabaris is toxic and should not be used over a prolonged period of time.

ZHI BAO DAN

Greatest Treasure Special Pill

Extract Formula Name: Rhinoceros and Succinum Formula

Xi Jiao	*Rhinoceros*	20 - 30 g
Niu Huang	*Bos*	12 - 15 g
She Xiang	*Moschus*	0.1 - 0.3 g
Dai Mao	*Eretmochelydis*	20 - 30 g
An Xi Xiang	*Styrax*	30 - 45 g
Hu Po	*Succinum*	20 - 30 g
Xiong Huang	*Realgar*	20 - 30 g
Zhu Sha	*Cinnabaris*	20 - 30 g
Bing Pian	*Dryobalanops*	0.1 - 0.3 g

Severe heat enters the Pericardium causing Liver wind which leads to delirious speech, fever, twitches, and convulsions.

T red, yellow coat

P wiry, rapid, forceful

☞ Available in prepared form.

✘ Do not use during pregnancy. Zhu Sha - Cinnabaris is toxic and should not be used over a long period of time.

ZI XUE DAN

Purple Snow Special Pill

Extract Formula Name: Rhinoceros and Antelope Horn Formula

Han Shui Shi	*Calcitum*	6-9 g
Hua Shi	*Talcum*	9 - 15 g
Ling Yang Jiao	*Saiga*	0.5 - 1 g
She Xiang	*Moschus*	0.3 g
Chen Xiang	*Aquilaria*	1 - 3 g
Qing Mu Xiang	*Aristolochia*	3 - 6 g
Xi Jiao	*Rhinoceros*	0.5 - 1 g
Shi Gao	*Gypsum*	6 - 9 g
Xuan Shen	*Scrophularia*	9 - 15 g
Sheng Ma	*Cimicifuga*	6 - 9 g
Zhu Sha	*Cinnabaris*	1 g
Ci Shi	*Magnetitum*	6 - 9 g
Ding Xiang	*Eugenia*	2 g
Xiao Shi	*Niter*	9 - 15 g.
Mang Xiao	*Mirabilitum*	9 - 15 g
Huang Jin	*Aurum*	9 - 15 g
Zhi Gan Cao	*Glycyrrhiza*	3 - 6 g

TUMOR OR NODULE DISSOLVING

- masses or lumps anywhere in the body
- subcutaneous nodules

T depends on the involved syndrome

P depends on the involved syndrome

Blood and phlegm stagnation in the uterus leading to masses or lumps, amenorrhea, dysmenorrhea, or restless fetus.

T purple, sticky coat

P wiry, slippery, choppy

GUI ZHI FU LING WAN

Cinnamon Twig and Poria Pill

Extract Formula Name: Cinnamon and Hoelen Formula

Gui Zhi	*Cinnamomum*	6 - 12 g
Fu Ling	*Poria*	6 - 12 g
Mu Dan Pi	*Paeonia*	6 - 12 g
Tao Ren	*Prunus*	6 - 12 g
Chi Shao Yao	*Paeonia*	9 - 12 g

Phlegm accumulation causing hardenings; or Liver qi stagnation leading to goiter or cancer.

T sticky coat

P slippery, wiry

✪ Major Formula

HAI ZAO YU HU TANG

Sargassum Decoction for the Jade Flask

Hai Zao	*Sargassum*	3 - 6 g
Kun Bu	*Laminaria*	3 - 6 g
Hai Dai	*Ecklonia*	1.5 g
Du Huo	*Angelica*	3 - 6 g
Lian Qiao	*Forsythia*	3 - 6 g
Zhe Bei Mu	*Fritillaria*	3 - 6 g
Chuan Xiong	*Ligusticum*	3 - 6 g
Ban Xia	*Pinellia*	3 - 6 g
Dang Gui	*Angelica*	3 - 6 g
Chen Pi	*Citrus*	3 - 6 g
Qing Pi	*Citrus*	3 - 6 g
Gan Cao	*Glycyrrhiza*	3 - 6 g

Blood and phlegm accumulation leading to solid scrofula due to Liver yang excess with a mild heat aspect.

T red, sticky yellow coat

P wiry, rapid

☞ Xia Ku Cao - Prunella should be decocted until it is very thick. The other herbs should be added to the strained tea and decocted until they become like syrup.

XIA KU CAO GAO

Prunella Syrup

Xia Ku Cao	*Prunella*	500 - 700 g
Wu Yao	*Lindera*	9 - 15 g
Xuan Shen	*Scrophularia*	9 - 15 g
Dang Gui	*Angelica*	9 - 15 g
Zhe Bei Mu	*Fritillaria*	9 - 15 g
Kun Bu	*Laminaria*	9 - 15 g
Jie Geng	*Platycodon*	6 - 9 g
Bai Shao Yao	*Paeonia*	9 - 15 g
Jiang Can	*Bombyx*	9 - 15 g
Chuan Xiong	*Ligusticum*	6 - 9 g
Chen Pi	*Citrus*	6 - 9 g
Xiang Fu	*Cyperus*	20 - 25 g
Hong Hua	*Carthamus*	6 - 9 g
Da Zao	*Ziziphus*	200 - 230 g
Gan Cao	*Glycyrrhiza*	6 - 9 g

Qi and blood deficiency with qi/blood and phlegm stagnation causing masses on the neck, breasts, or axilla areas.

T pale or purple

P weak or choppy

XIANG BEI YANG YING TANG

Cyperus and Fritillaria Decoction to Nourish the Nutritive Qi

Ren Shen	*Panax*	6 - 9 g
Bai Zhu	*Atractylodes*	3 - 6 g
Fu Ling	*Poria*	6 - 9 g
Chuan Xiong	*Ligusticum*	3 - 6 g
Chen Pi	*Citrus*	3 - 6 g
Dang Gui	*Angelica*	6 - 9 g
Xiang Fu	*Cyperus*	6 - 9 g
Shu Di Huang	*Rehmannia*	6 - 12 g
Bei Mu	*Fritillaria*	3 - 6 g
Bai Shao Yao	*Paeonia*	6 - 9 g
Jie Geng	*Platycodon*	3 - 6 g
Da Zao	*Ziziphus*	3 - 6 pc
Sheng Jiang	*Zingiber*	3 - 6 g
Gan Cao	*Glycyrrhiza*	1 - 3 g

Goiter, scrofula, and lumps due to yin deficieny with false heat. The false heat dries the fluids and causes phlegm accumulation.

T red, coat

P rapid, slippery, or wiry

XIAO LUO WAN

Reduce Scrofula Pill

Chuan Bei Mu	*Fritillaria*	6 - 12 g
Mu Li	*Ostrea*	6 - 12 g
Xuan Shen	*Scrophularia*	6 - 12 g

WIND ATTACKING THE CHANNELS OR SKIN

- skin rashes which move around
- itchy rashes
- muscle spasms
- various types of paralysis

T unremarkable

P superficial

Wind phlegm attacking the channels, especially the head and face with pre-existing qi and yang deficiency. This leads to paralysis, facial twitches, stiff muscles, spasms, or loose stools.

T pale, swollen, teethmarks, thick sticky coat

P slippery, deep, frail

✘ The formula is toxic and should not be taken over a long period of time. Do not use during pregnancy.

QIAN ZHENG SAN

Lead to Symmetry Powder

Jiang Can	*Bombyx*	6 g
Bai Fu Zi	*Typhonium*	6 g
Quan Xie	*Buthus*	6 g

Blood deficiency which gives rise to wind. This causes an itchy rash which is dry and pale red.

T pale or purple

P thin

SI WU XIAO FENG YIN

Eliminate Wind Decoction with the Four-Substances

Sheng Di Huang	*Rehmannia*	6 - 9 g
Dang Gui	*Angelica*	6 - 9 g
Chi Shao Yao	*Paeonia*	3 - 6 g
Chuan Xiong	*Ligusticum*	3 - 6 g
Jing Jie	*Schizonepeta*	3 - 6 g
Fang Feng	*Ledebouriella*	3 - 6 g
Bai Xian Pi	*Dictamnus*	3 - 6 g
Bo He	*Mentha*	3 - 6 g
Chai Hu	*Bupleurum*	2 g
Du Huo	*Angelica*	3 g
Chan Tui	*Cryptotympana*	3 - 6 g
Da Zao	*Ziziphus*	2 - 3 pc

Wind phlegm in the channels with severe spasms, stiffness in the jaw, or rigidity of the whole body. This formula is a strong anti-spasmodic.

T deviated, sticky white coat

P variable

☞ Zhu Sha - Cinnabaris and 60 ml of yellow wine should be added at the end to the strained tea.

✘ Do not use during pregnancy. Do not use over long periods of time. Tian Nan Xing - Arisaema is slightly toxic and Zhu Sha - Cinnabaris is very toxic.

WU HU ZHUI FENG SAN

Five-Tiger Powder to Pursue Wind

Chan Tui	*Cryptotympana*	30 g
Tian Ma	*Gastrodia*	6 g
Tian Nan Xing	*Arisaema*	3 - 6 g
Jiang Can	*Bombyx*	6 g
Quan Xie	*Buthus*	7 - 9 g
Zhu Sha	*Cinnabaris*	1 g

Liver wind or external wind with phlegm accumulation in the channels causing stroke, aphasia, cerebral hemorrhage, or numbness; or cold attacking the chest and axillae causing severe localized pain in the flanks.

T sticky white coat

P slippery or wiry

WU YAO SHUN QI SAN

Lindera Powder to Smooth the Flow of Qi

Extract Formula Name: Lindera Formula

Wu Yao	*Lindera*	9 - 15 g
Chen Pi	*Citrus*	9 - 15 g
Ma Huang	*Ephedra*	6 - 9 g
Bai Zhi	*Angelica*	3 - 9 g
Zhi Ke	*Citrus*	3 - 6 g
Jiang Can	*Bombyx*	3 g
Jie Geng	*Platycodon*	3 g
Chuan Xiong	*Ligusticum*	3 - 9 g
Pao Jiang	*Zingiber*	3 - 6 g
Gan Cao	*Glycyrrhiza*	3 - 6 g
[Da Zao	*Ziziphus*	3 - 8 pc]
[Sheng Jiang	*Zingiber*	3 - 6 g]

Wind heat and damp with preexisting damp heat lodged in the skin and muscles. This causes an itchy, weepy rash, or bleeding under the skin (purpura) with heat or wind intolerance.

T red tip or border, white or yellow coat

P superficial, rapid

✪ Major Formula

XIAO FENG SAN I

Eliminate Wind Powder from True Lineage

Extract Formula Name: Tang-Kuei and Arctium Formula

Fang Feng	*Ledebouriella*	3-6 g
Jing Jie	*Schizonepeta*	3-6 g
Chan Tui	*Cryptotympana*	3 g
Ku Shen	*Sophora*	3 g
Niu Bang Zi	*Arctium*	3 g
Hei Zhi Ma	*Sesamum*	3 g
Shi Gao	*Gypsum*	3 g
Zhi Mu	*Anemarrhena*	3 g
Cang Zhu	*Atractylodes*	3 g
Sheng Di Huang	*Rehmannia*	3 g
Dang Gui	*Angelica*	3 g
Mu Tong	*Akebia*	2 g
Gan Cao	*Glycyrrhiza*	2 g

Wind damp with qi stagnation causes a rash, dizziness, headache, and numbness of the skin.

T sticky coat

P slippery

XIAO FENG SAN II

Eliminate Wind Powder from Imperial Grace Formulary

Jing Jie	*Schizonepeta*	6-9 g
Bo He	*Mentha*	6 g
Chan Tui	*Cryptotympana*	6 g
Jiang Can	*Bombyx*	6 g
Hou Po	*Magnolia*	3-6 g
Qiang Huo	*Notopterygium*	6 g
Fang Feng	*Ledebouriella*	6 g
Ren Shen	*Panax*	6 g
Chuan Xiong	*Ligusticum*	6 g
Fu Ling	*Poria*	6 g
Chen Pi	*Citrus*	3-6 g

Wind heat with pre-existing heat and lumps leading to dizziness during pregnancy or swellings around the jaw and neck.

T red tip and body, sticky coat

P rapid

XIAO FENG SAN III

Eliminate Wind Powder from Effective Formulas

Shi Gao	*Gypsum*	20 g
Chuan Xiong	*Ligusticum*	3 - 9 g
Jing Jie	*Schizonepeta*	3 - 6 g
Ju Hua	*Chrysanthemum*	3 - 6 g
Fang Feng	*Ledebouriella*	6 - 9 g
Dang Gui	*Angelica*	6 - 9 g
Bai Zhi	*Angelica*	3 - 9 g
Qiang Huo	*Notopterygium*	6 - 9 g
Dou Juan	*Glycine*	3 - 6 g
Ling Yang Jiao	*Saiga*	6 g
Gan Cao	*Glycyrrhiza*	6 - 15 g

Wind stroke leading to paralysis and numbness; or wind cold damp in the channels resulting in wandering or fixed pain in the joints and muscles. The patient has difficulty controlling the muscles due to weakness and spasms.

T moist, white coat

P slow, slippery

☞ The formula should be taken as a powder. The prepared types of Aconite are used here.

✘ Do not use during pregnancy. It is a very strong prescription. Use only for a short period of time.

XIAO HUO LUO DAN

Minor Invigorate the Collaterals Special Pill

Cao Wu	*Aconitum*	60 g
Chuan Wu	*Aconitum*	60 g
Tian Nan Xing	*Arisaema*	60 g
Di Long	*Pheretima*	60 g
Ru Xiang	*Boswellia*	30 g
Mo Yao	*Commiphora*	30 g

Wind stroke with wind cold invasion and pre-existing qi deficiency causing fever and chills, hemiplegia, aphasia, or facial paralysis.

T pale, deviated, thin white coat

P superficial, or deep, frail

☞ Fu Zi - Aconitum should be cooked 30 - 60 minutes prior to adding the other herbs.

XIAO XU MING TANG

Minor Prolong Life Decoction

Extract Formula Name: Ma-Huang and Peony Combination

Chuan Xiong	*Ligusticum*	3 - 6 g
Ma Huang	*Ephedra*	3 - 6 g
Bai Shao Yao	*Paeonia*	6 - 12 g
Guang Fang Ji	*Aristolochia*	6 - 12 g
Fang Feng	*Ledebouriella*	9 - 12 g
Ren Shen	*Panax*	3 - 6 g
Fu Zi	*Aconitum*	3 - 6 g
Rou Gui	*Cinnamomum*	3 - 6 g
Huang Qin	*Scutellaria*	3 - 9 g
Xing Ren	*Prunus*	9 - 12 g
Sheng Jiang	*Zingiber*	9 - 12 pc
Gan Cao	*Glycyrrhiza*	3 - 6 g

External wind attacks the channels with pre-existing qi/Blood deficiency; or Liver wind with heat causing flaccid hemiplegia, aphasia, or mild fever. There may also be slight mental confusion.

T sticky yellow coat

P wiry, forceful, or rapid, slippery

XU MING TANG

Prolong Life Decoction

Extract Formula Name: Ma-Huang and Ginseng Combination

Gui Zhi	*Cinnamomum*	6 - 9 g
Ma Huang	*Ephedra*	6 - 9 g
Chuan Xiong	*Ligusticum*	3 - 6 g
Xing Ren	*Prunus*	6 - 9 g
Shi Gao	*Gypsum*	6 - 9 g
Ren Shen	*Panax*	6 - 9 g
Dang Gui	*Angelica*	6 - 9 g
Gan Jiang	*Zingiber*	6 - 9 g
Gan Cao	*Glycyrrhiza*	3 - 9 g

Wind with phlegm causing muscle spasms, lockjaw, tetanus, kyphotic arch, or spasms in the trachea.

T deviated or stiff

P tight or wiry

✘ Do not use during pregnancy. The formula is toxic and should not be taken over a long period of time.

YU ZHEN SAN

True Jade Powder

Tian Nan Xing	*Arisaema*	10 g
Bai Fu Zi	*Typhonium*	10 g
Qiang Huo	*Notopterygium*	10 g
Tian Ma	*Gastrodia*	10 g
Fang Feng	*Ledebouriella*	10 g
Bai Zhi	*Angelica*	10 g

Severe heat causing Liver wind. This causes muscle twitches, convulsions, or spasms.

T red, deviated, yellow coat

P forceful

✘ Do not use during pregnancy. The formula is toxic and should not be taken over a prolonged period of time.

ZHI JING SAN

Stop Spasms Powder

Wu Gong	*Scolopendra*	10 g
Quan Xie	*Buthus*	10 g

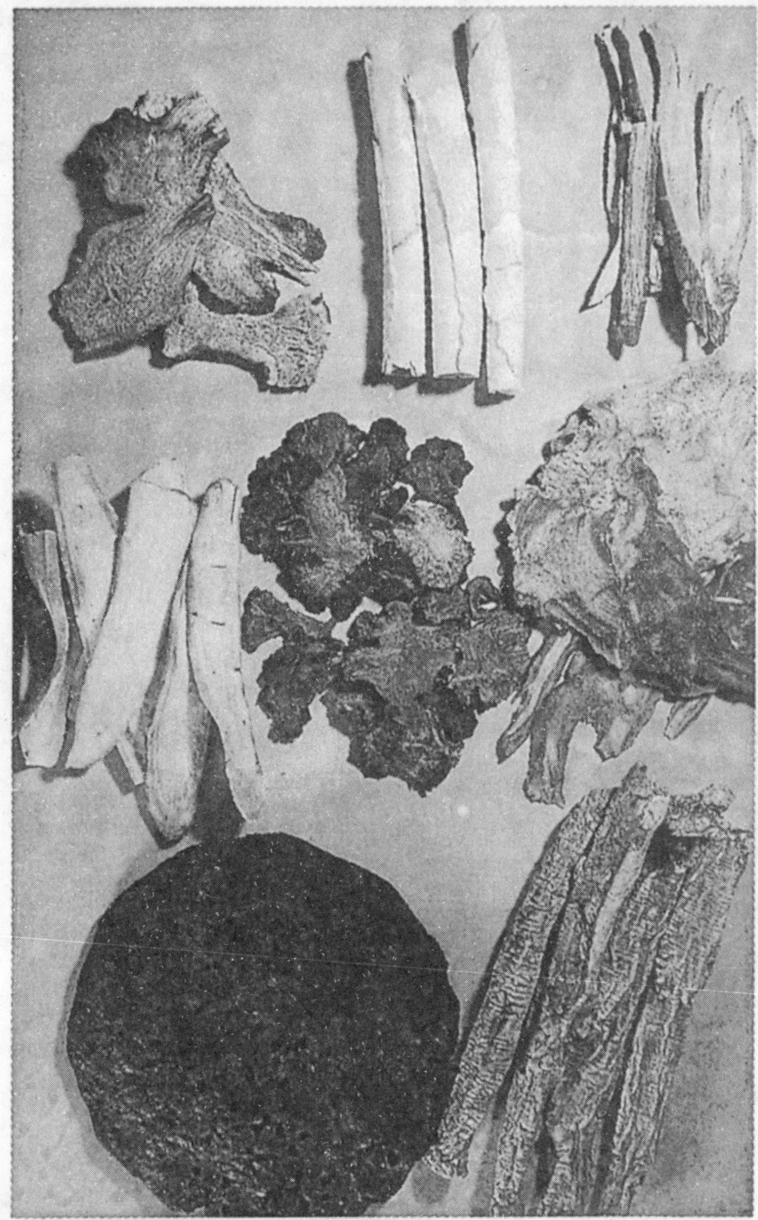

Ba Zhen Tang - Eight-Treasure Decoction

1. Row from left: Bai Zhu - Atractylodes, Fu Ling - Poria, Gan Cao - Glycyrrhiza
2. Row from left: Bai Shao - Paeonia, Chuan Xiong - Ligusticum, Dang Gui - Angelica
3. Row from left: Shu Di Huang - Rehmannia, Dang Shen - Codonopsis.

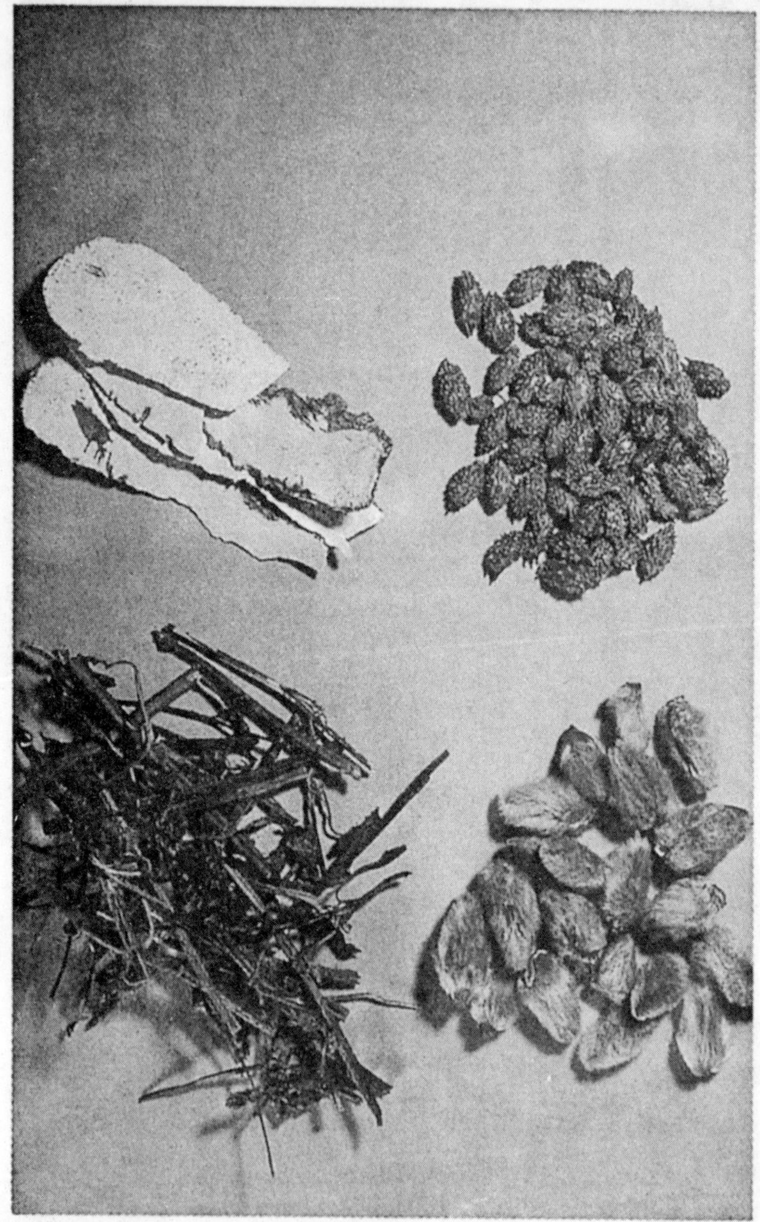

Cang Er Zi San - Xanthium Powder

1. Row from left: Bai Zhi - Angelica, Cang Er Zi - Xanthium

2. Row form left: Bo He - Mentha, Xin Yi Hua - Magnolia

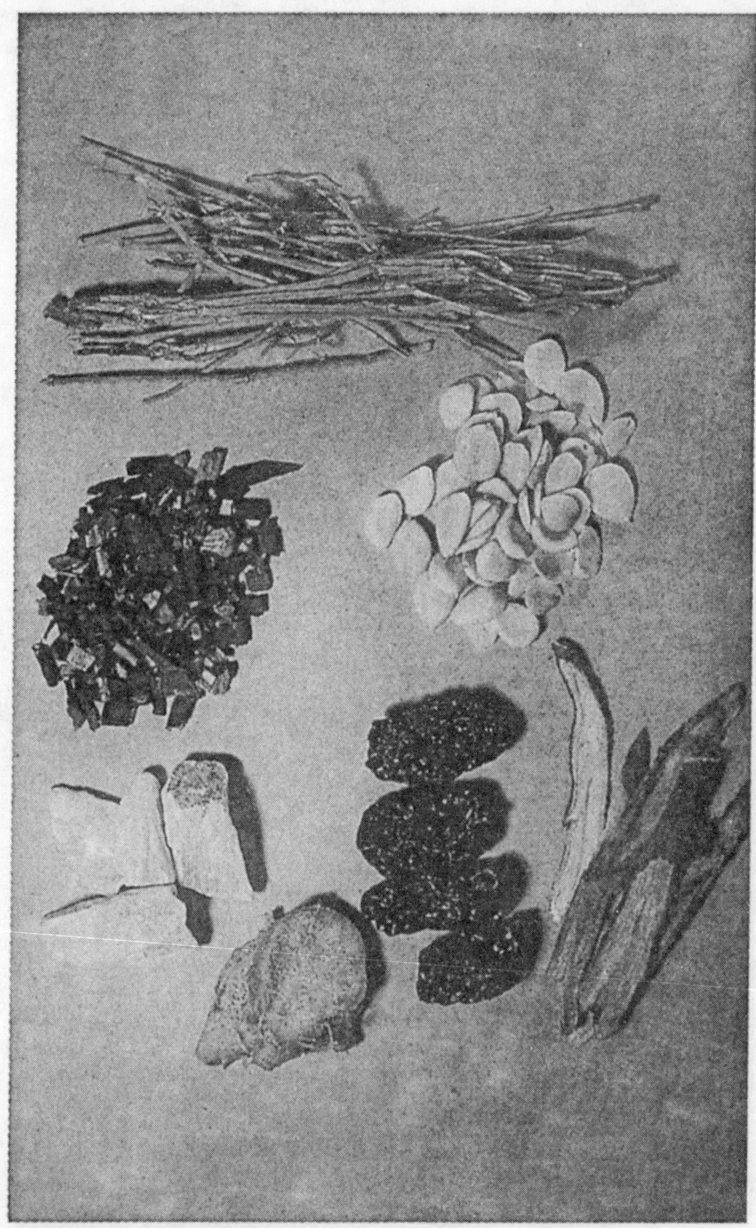

Da Qing Long Tang - Major Bluegreen Dragon Decoction

1. Row from left: Ma Huang - Ephedra

2. Row from left: Gui Zhi - Cinnamomum, Xing Ren - Prunus

3. Row from left: Shi Gao - Gypsum, Sheng Jiang - Zingiber, Da Zao - Ziziphus, Gan Cao - Glycyrrhiza

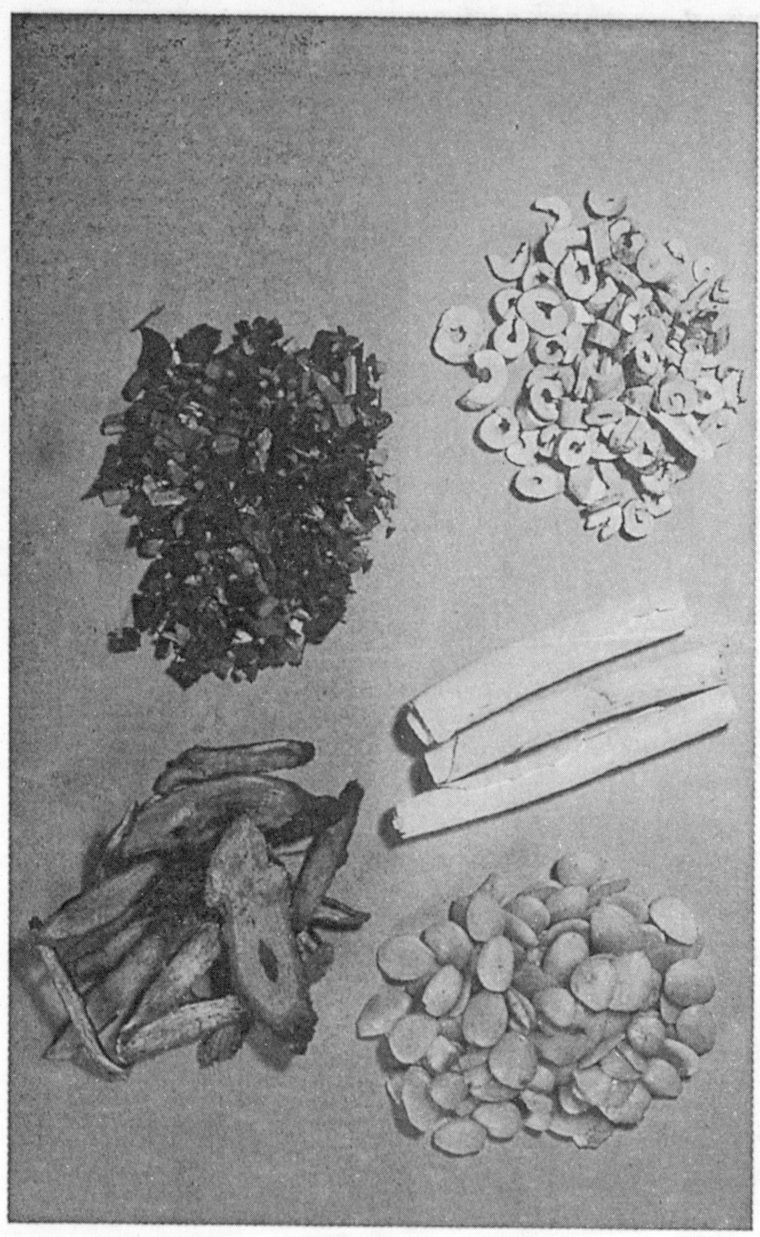

Gui Zhi Fu Ling Wan - Cinnamon Twig and Poria Pill

1. Row from left: Gui Zhi - Cinnamomum, Mu Dan Pi - Paeonia
2. Row from left: Chi Shao Yao - Paeonia, Fu Ling - Poria
3. Row right: Tao Ren - Prunus

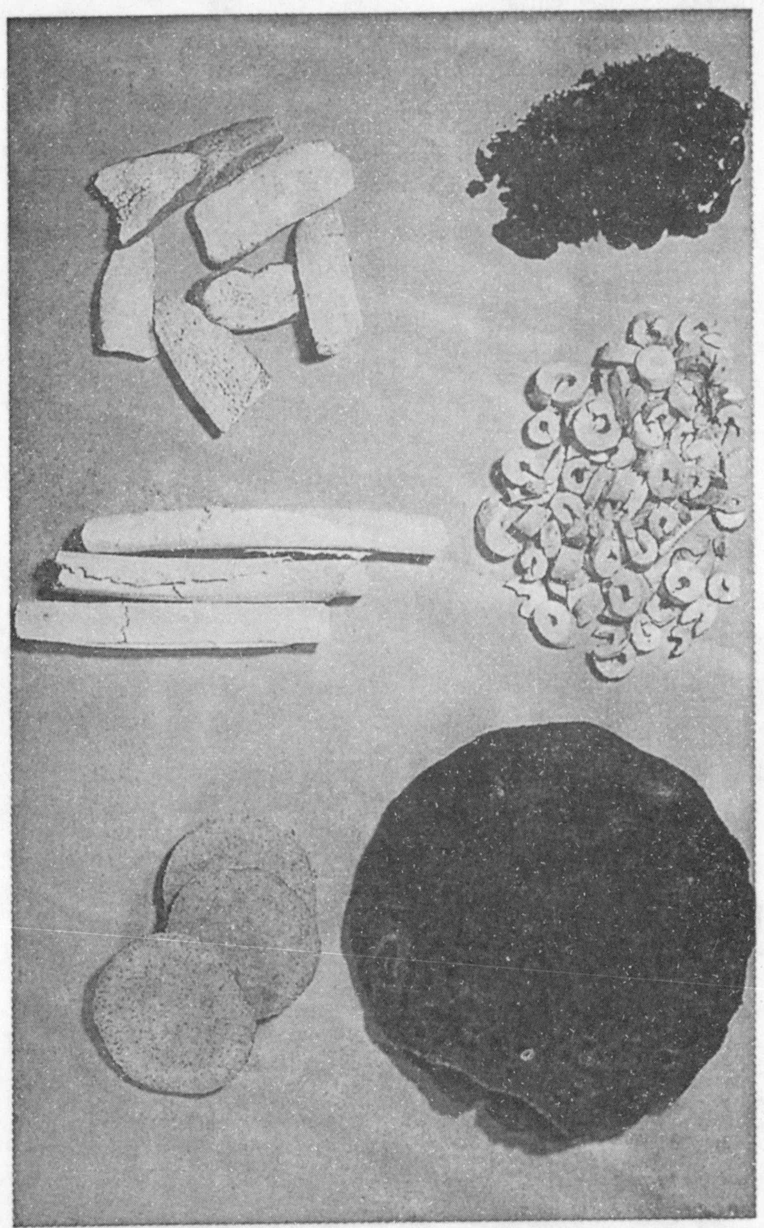

Liu Wei Di Huang Wan - Six-Ingredient with Rehmannia Pill

1. Row from left: Shan Yao - Dioscorea, Shan Zhu Yu - Cornus
2. Row from left: Fu Ling - Poria, Mu Dan Pi - Paeonia
3. Row from left: Ze Xie - Alisma, Shu Di Huang - Rehmannia

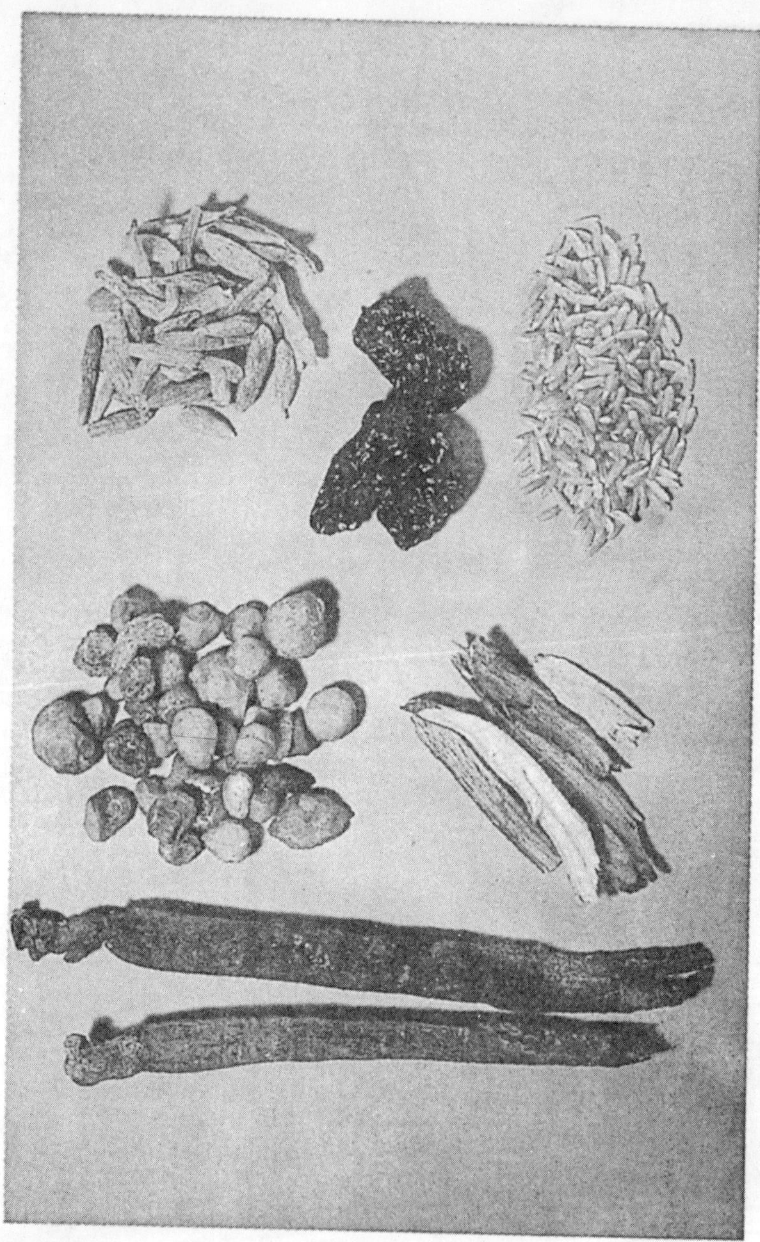

Mai Men Dong Tang - Ophiopogon Decoction

1. Row from left: Mai Men Dong - Ophiopogon, Da Zao - Ziziphus, Jing Mi - Oryza
2. Row from left: Ban Xia - Pinellia, Gan Cao - Glycyrrhiza
3. Row from left: Ren Shen - Panax

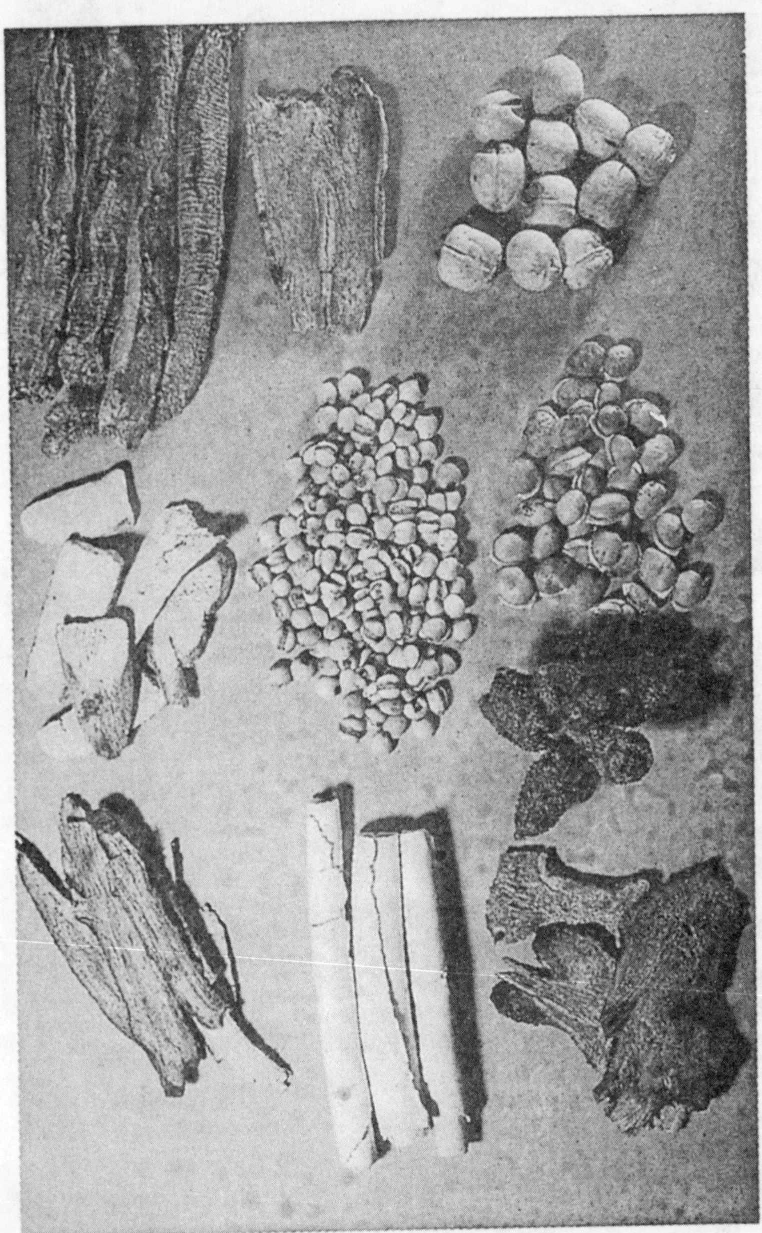

Shen Ling Bai Zhu San - Ginseng, Poria, and Atractylodes Powder

1. Row from left: Dang Shen - Codonopsis, Jie Geng - Platycodon, Lian Zi - Nelumbo
2. Row from left: Shan Yao - Dioscorea, Yi Yi Ren - Coix, Bian Dou - Dolichos
3. Row from left: Gan Cao - Glycyrrhiza, Fu Ling - Poria, Sha Ren - Amomum, Bai Zhu - Atractylodes

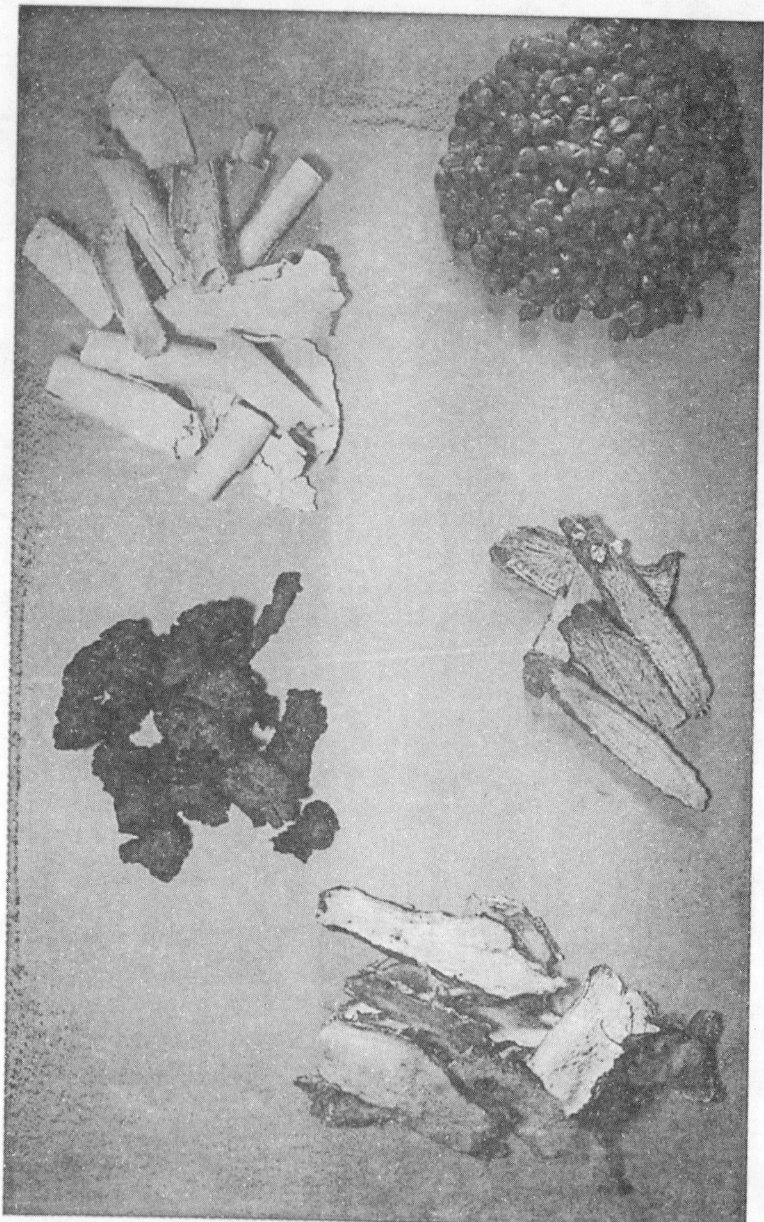

Suan Zao Ren Tang - Sour Jujube Decoction

1. Row from left: Fu Ling - Poria, Suan Zao Ren - Ziziphus
2. Row from left: Chuan Xiong - Ligusticum, Gan Cao - Glycyrrhiza
3. Row from left: Zhi Mu - Anemarrhena

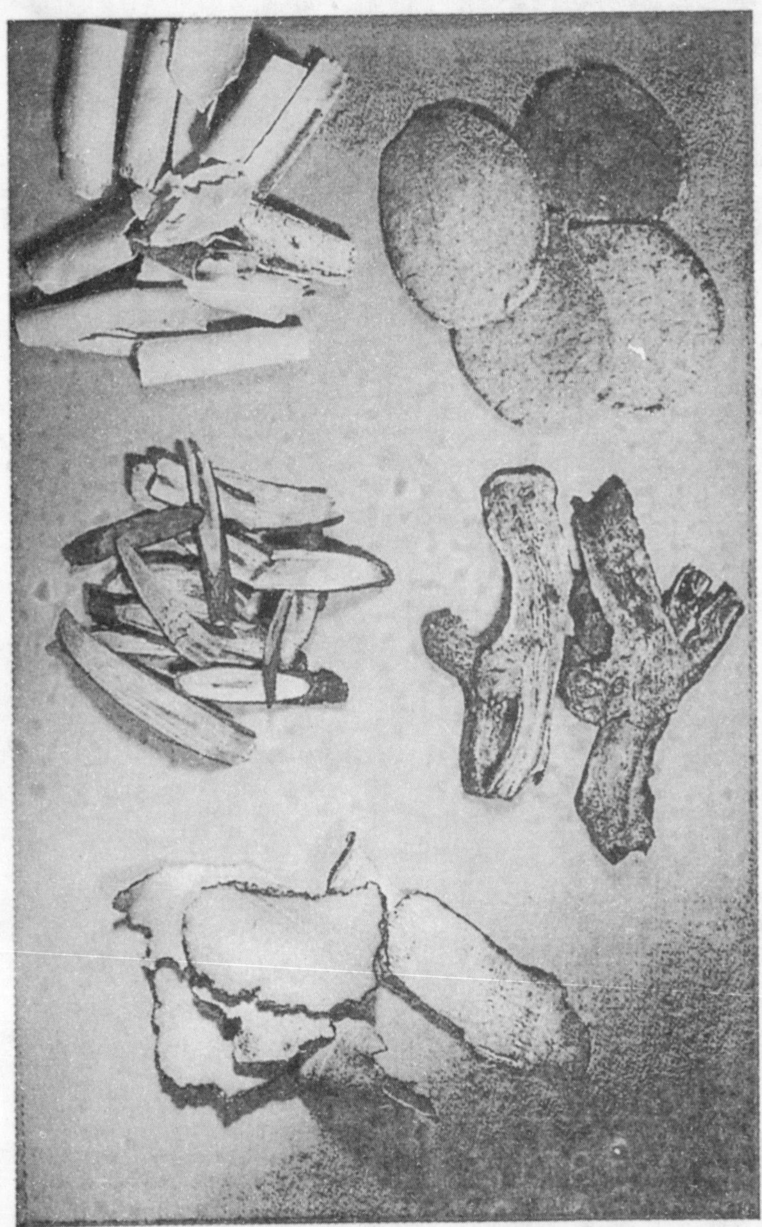

Wu Ling San - Five-Ingredient Powder with Poria

1. Row from left: Fu Ling - Poria, Ze Xie - Alisma

2. Row from left: Gui Zhi - Cinnamomum, Bai Zhu - Atractylodes

3. Row from left: Zhu Ling - Polyporus

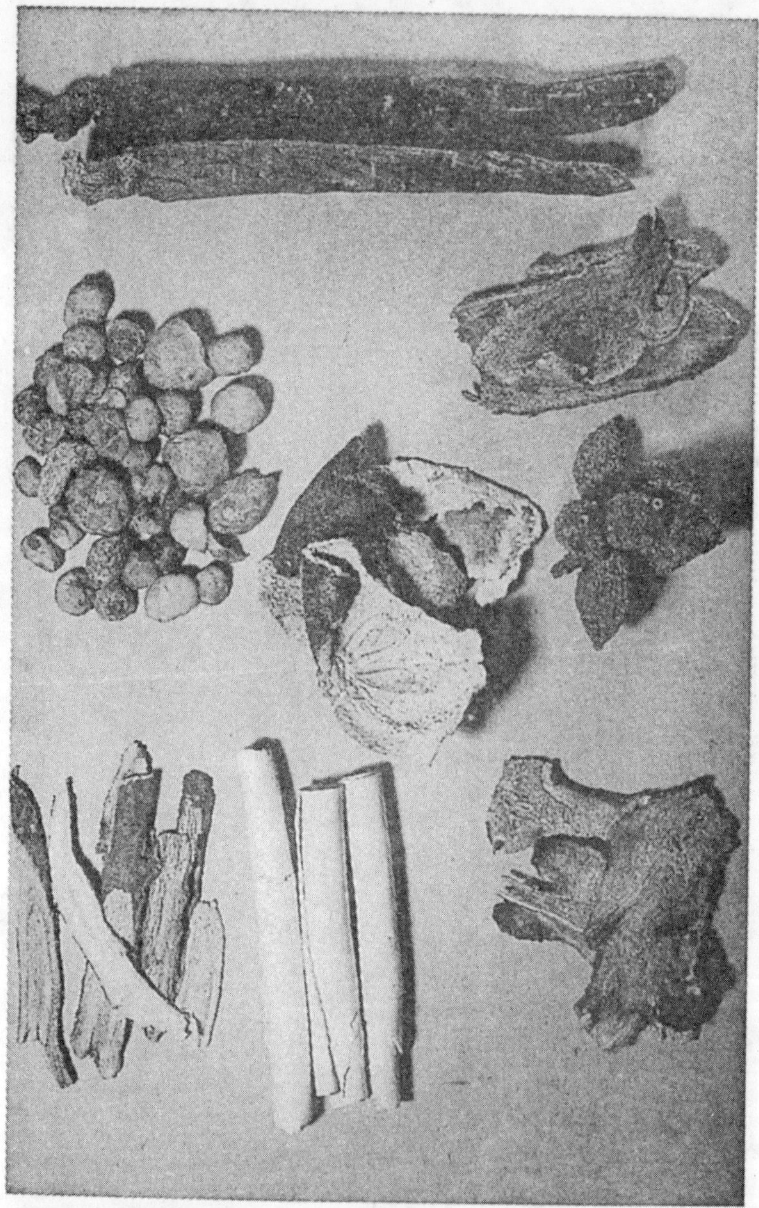

Xiang Sha Liu Jun Zi Tang - Six-Gentlemen Decoction with Aucklandia and Amomum

1. Row from left: Ren Shen - Panax
2. Row from left: Ban Xia - Pinellia, Mu Xiang - Saussurea
3. Row from left: Chen Pi - Citrus, Sha Ren - Amomum
Gan Cao - Glycyrrhiza, Fu Ling - Poria, Bai Zhu - Atractylodes

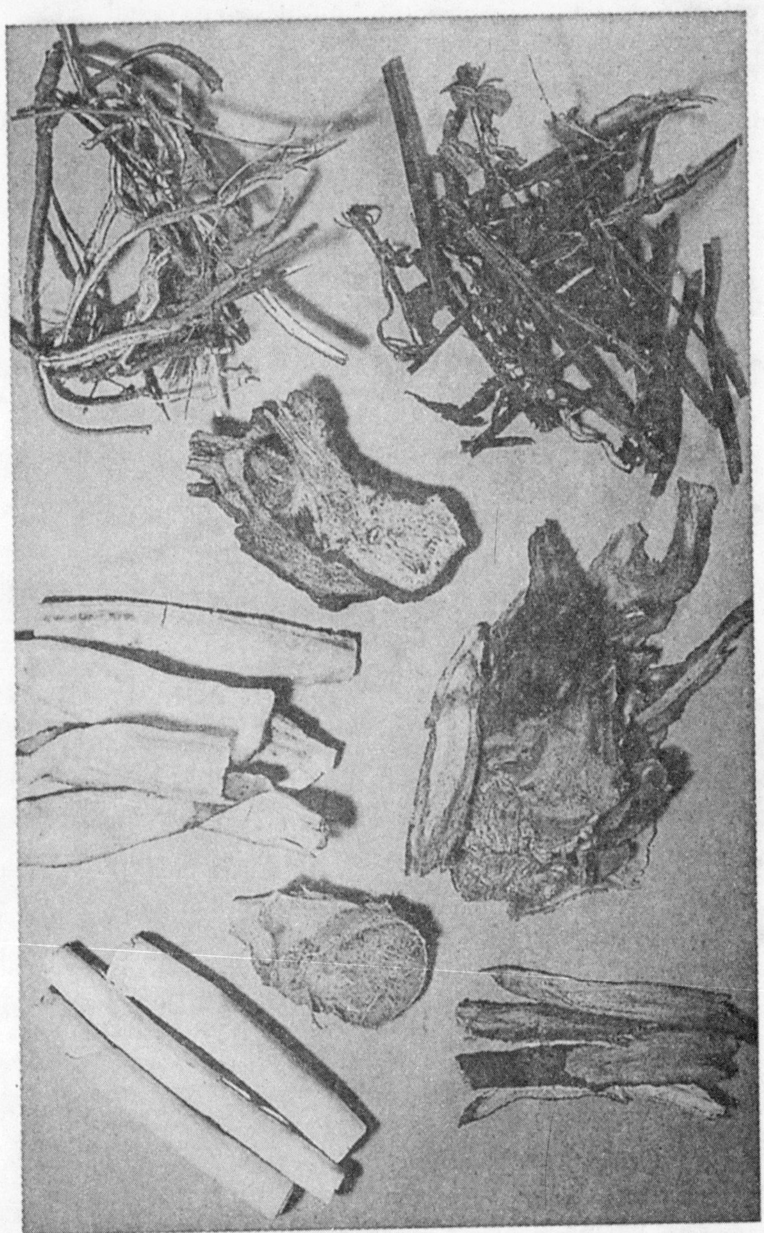

Xiao Yao San - Rambling Powder

1. Row from left: Chai Hu - Bupleurum, Bo He - Mentha
2. Row from left: Bai Shao - Paeonia, Bai Zhu - Atractylodes, Dang Gui - Angelica
3. Row from left: Fu Ling - Poria, Sheng Jiang - Zingiber, Gan Cao - Glycyrrhiza

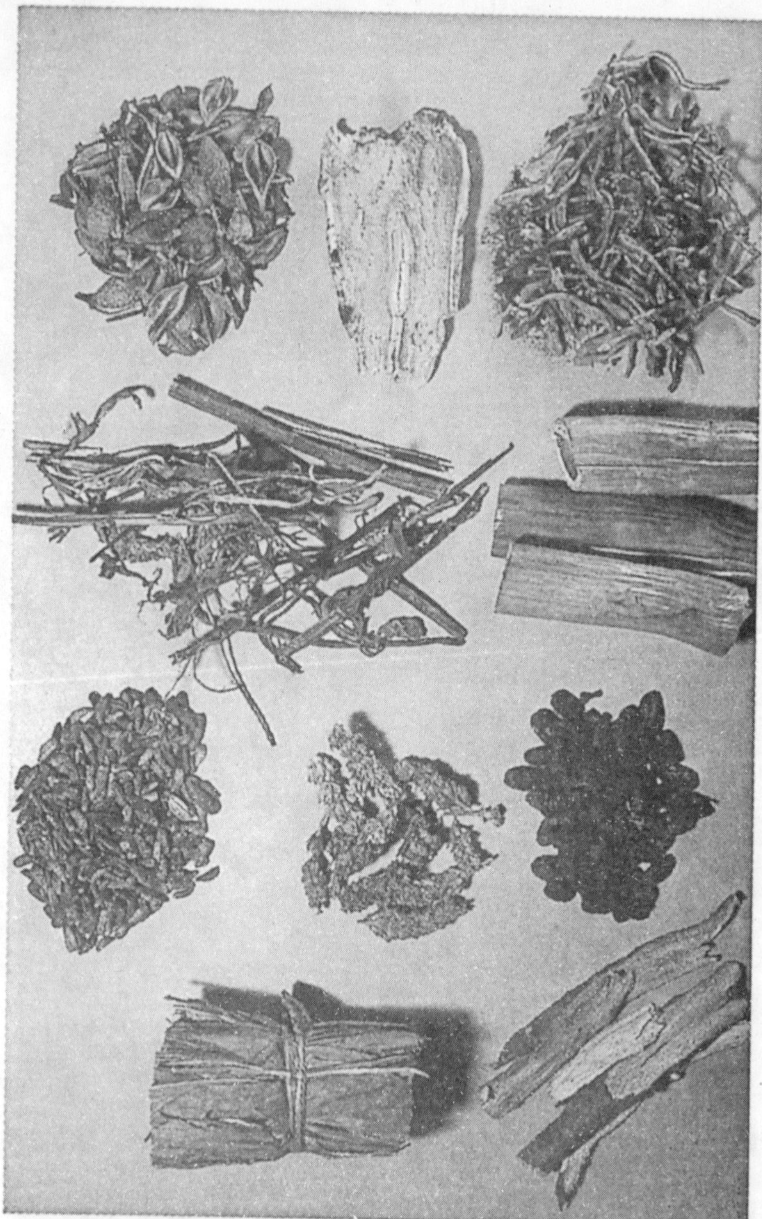

Yin Qiao San - Honeysuckle and Forsythia Powder

1. Row from left: Lian Qiao - Forsythia, Jie Geng - Platycodon, Jin Yin Hua - Lonicera
2. Row from left: Bo He - Mentha, Lu Gen - Phragmites
3. Row from left: Niu Bang Zi - Arctium, Jing Jie - Schizonepeta, Dan Dou Chi - Glycine
4. Row from left: Dan Zhu Ye - Lophatherum, Gan Cao - Glycyrrhiza

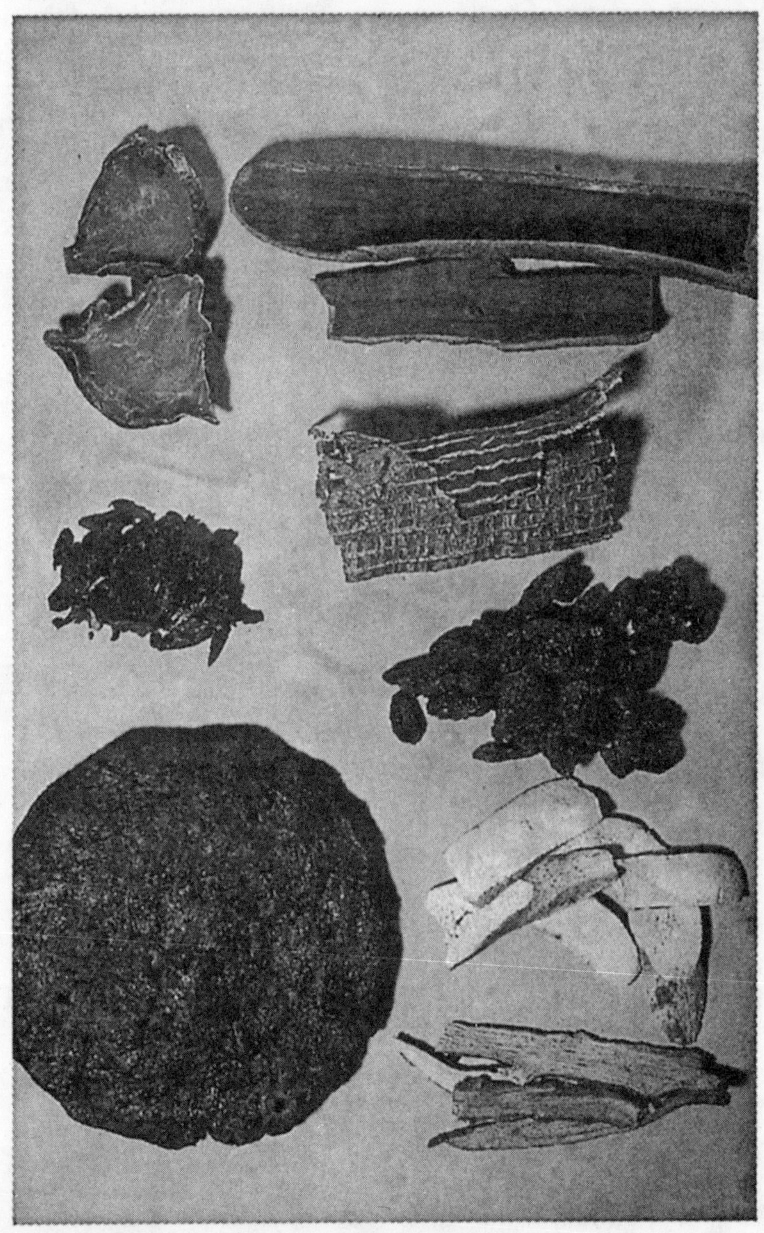

You Gui Yin - Restore the Right Decoction

1. Row from left: Fu Zi - Aconitum, Rou Gui - Cinnamomum

2. Row from left: Shan Zhu Yu - Cornus, Du Zhong - Eucommia, Gou Qi Zi - Lycium

3. Row from left: Shu Di Huang - Rehmannia, Shan Yao - Dioscorea, Gan Cao - Glycerrhiza

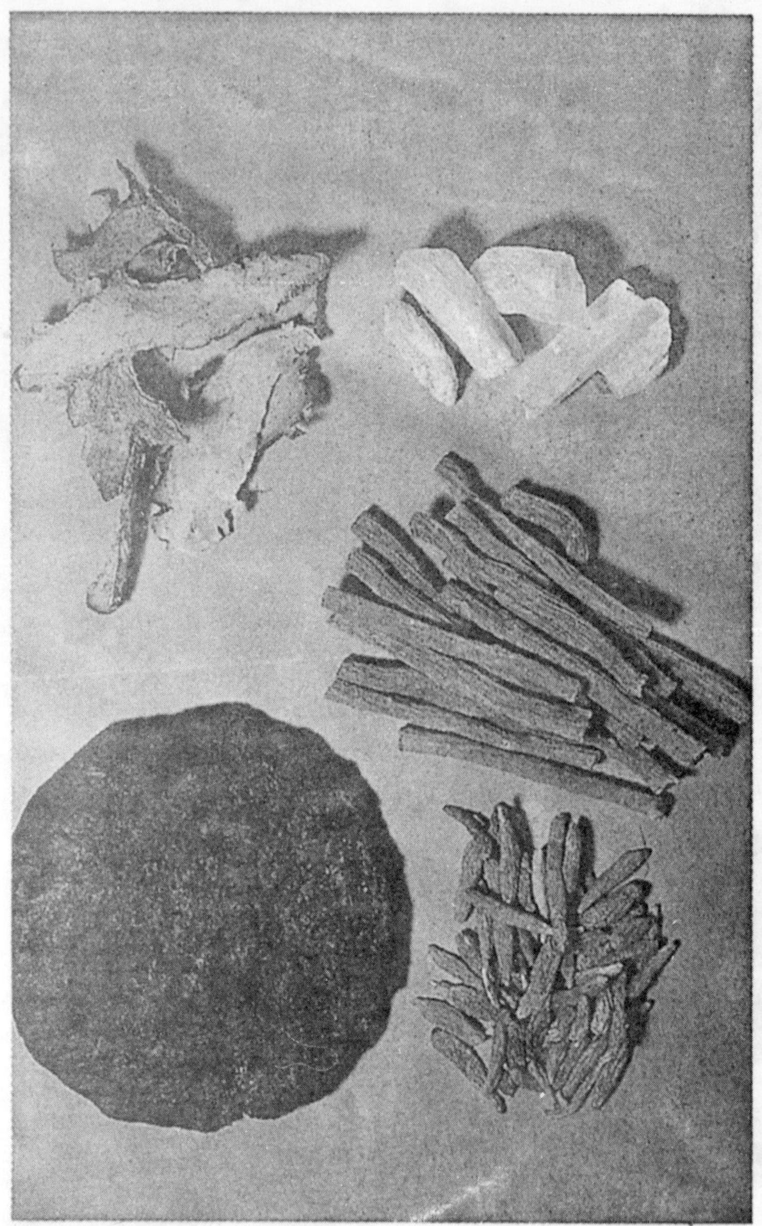

Yu Nu Jian - Jade Woman Decoction

1. Row from left: Zhi Mu - Anemarrhena, Shi Gao - Gypsum

2. Row from left: Huai Niu Xi - Achyranthes,

3. Row from left: Shụ Di Huang - Rehmannia, Mai Men Dong - Ophiopogon

Part 2

Clinical Quick Reference for Single Herbs

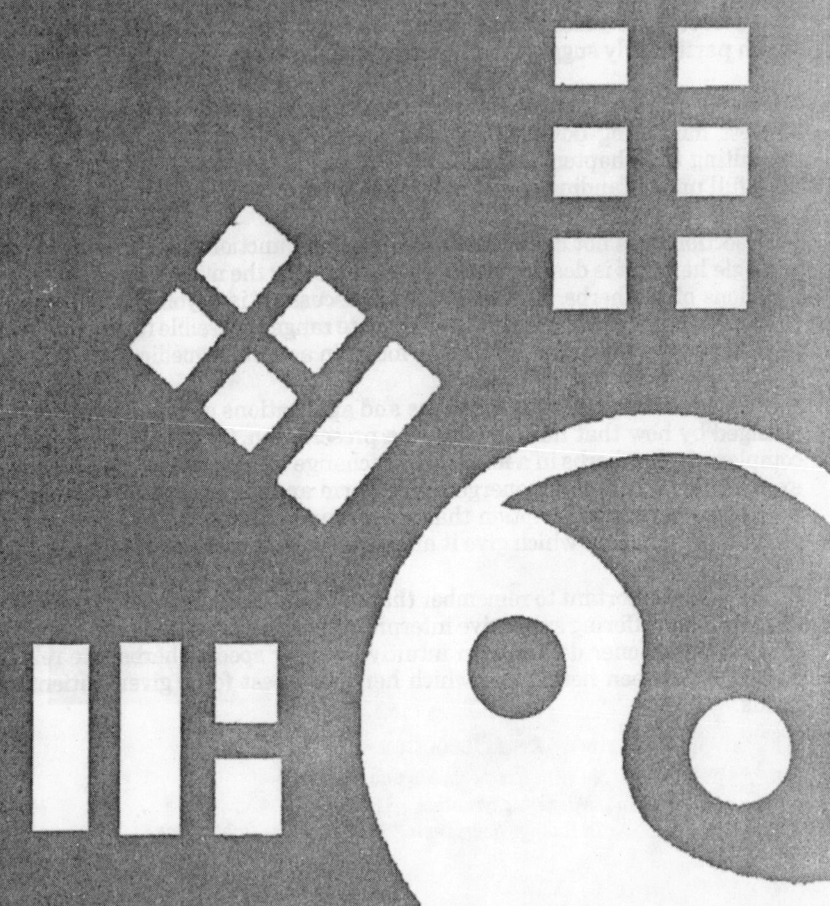

Many inexperienced practitioners of Chinese herbal medicine rely on standard formulas. This is both unfortunate and prudent. It takes solid knowledge of herbs and clinical experience to gain the confidence necessary to modify and individualize formulas. Yet customizing formulas can produce effectiveness far beyond that of standard formulas.

This chapter is a selected listing of single herbs organized by traditional categories. However, within the traditional categories, there are innovative subdivisions intended to help steer the practitioner toward choosing the most likely herbs to add or subtract from formulas.

The herb lists selected for this chapter are purposely limited in scope. The herbs within each subdivision are only the most important or commonly used herbs for a given energetic function. Furthermore, herbs are listed only in places where they have primary relevance. (Secondary uses for herbs are not covered here.) Herbs in a given category possess specific properties which particularly suggest their use for that function.

For the practitioner with limited experience using loose herbs, the authors suggest narrowing down the choices for herbs to modify a formula by consulting this chapter. Then it will be helpful to check a materia medica for a full understanding of the final few choices.

This section does not detail the many complex functions and applications of single herbs. It is designed as a learning tool for the most basic energetic functions of the herbs. A more in-depth discussion is beyond the scope of this work. An understanding of the complete range of possible functions and indications of any single herb can be found in a materia medica.

Please note that particular functions and applications of any herb may be changed by how that herb is used in a prescription. The total synergistic complex of other herbs in a formula may change the actions of an herb. For example, an herb that is energetically warm and dispels wind damp cold may be used in a prescription that treats wind damp heat if the formula contains other herbs which give it an overall cool or cold temperature.

Finally, it is important to remember that in Chinese medicine it is common to find many differing subjective interpretations on the uses of herbs. Over time, a practitioner develops an intuitive feel for specific herbs, the relationships between herbs, and which herbs are best for a given patient's needs.

Herbs that Clear Exterior Conditions (Diaphoretics)

Warm, Pungent Herbs that Clear Exterior Conditions

Treat Wind Cold Excess (Strong Wind Cold Dispersing Function)

Ma Huang / Ephedra
Xi Xin / Asarum
Zi Su Ye / Perilla
Gui Zhi / Cinnamomum

Treat Wind Cold Deficiency (Mild, Moderate Wind Cold Dispersing Function)

Jing Jie / Schizonepeta
Fang Feng / Ledebouriella
Gui Zhi / Cinnamomum

Dispel Wind Cold Damp and Alleviate Headaches

Qiang Huo / Notopterygium
Gao Ben / Ligusticum
Bai Zhi / Angelica
Xi Xin / Asarum

Dispel Wind Cold and Open the Nasal Passages

Xin Yi Hua / Magnolia
Cang Er Zi / Xanthium
Xi Xin/ Asarum

Warm Herbs with Multiple Functions and Wide Applications

Sheng Jiang / Zingiber
Cong Bai / Allium
Xiang Ru / Elsholtzia
E Bu Shi Cao / Centipeda
Sheng Liu / Tamarix

Cool, Pungent Herbs that Clear Exterior Conditions

Dispel Wind Heat and Promote the Surfacing of Rashes

Bo He / Mentha
Niu Bang Zi / Arctium
Chan Tui / Cryptotympana

Dispel Wind Heat and Clear Vision

Mu Zei / Equisetum
Gu Jing Cao / Eriocaulon

Dispel Wind Heat, Clear Vision, and Clear the Liver

Sang Ye / Morus
(Huang) Ju Hua / Chrysanthemum

Dispel Wind Heat and Raise Yang Qi

Chai Hu / Bupleurum
Sheng Ma / Cimicifuga

Dispel Wind Heat Trapped in the Muscles

Ge Gen / Pueraria

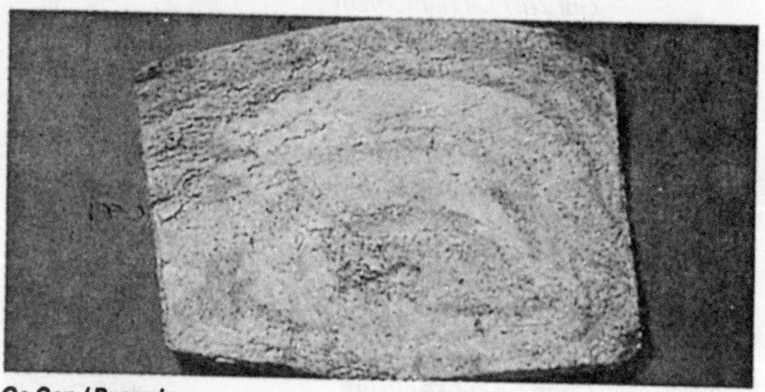

Ge Gen / Pueraria

Cool Herbs with Multiple Functions and Wide Applications

Fu Ping / Spirodela
Dan Dou Chi / Glycine
Man Jing Zi / Vitex
Chai Hu / Bupleurum
Ge Gen / Pueraria

Herbs that Clear Heat

Herbs that Extinguish Fire by Clearing Internal Heat

Clear Heat in the Qi (Yangming) Stage

Clear Lung and Stomach Heat

Shi Gao / Gypsum
Zhi Mu / Anemarrhena
Lu Gen / Phragmites
Ya Zhi Cao / Commelina

Clear Heart and Stomach Heat

Dan Zhu Ye / Lophatherum

Clear Heart Fire

Lian Xin / Nelumbo

Clear Heat (and Damp) from the Liver and Three Burners

Zhi Zi / Gardenia

Clear Fire and Summer Heat

Han Shui Shi / Calcitum

Clear Heat, Spasms, and Fire Poison

Xiong Dan / Ursus
Niu Dan / Bos

Clear Heat and Brighten the Eyes

Clear Both Excess Liver Heat and Wind Heat and Brighten Eyes

Jue Ming Zi / Cassia
Qing Xiang Zi / Celosia

Clear Both Excess and Deficient Liver Heat and Brighten the Eyes

Xia Ku Cao / Prunella
Mi Meng Hua / Buddleia
Chong Wei Zi / Leonurus
(Bai) Ju Hua / Chrysanthemum

Clear Excess Liver Heat Only

Ye Ming Sha / Vespertilio

Herbs that Clear Heat and Cool the Blood

Cool the Blood and Clear Heart Fire

Xi Jiao / Rhinoceros
Shui Niu Jiao / Bubalus

Cool the Blood and Clear Large Intestine and Liver Heat

Huai Jiao / Sophora

Cool the Blood and Detoxify Fire Poison

Zi Cao / Lithospermum
Mu Dan Pi / Paeonia

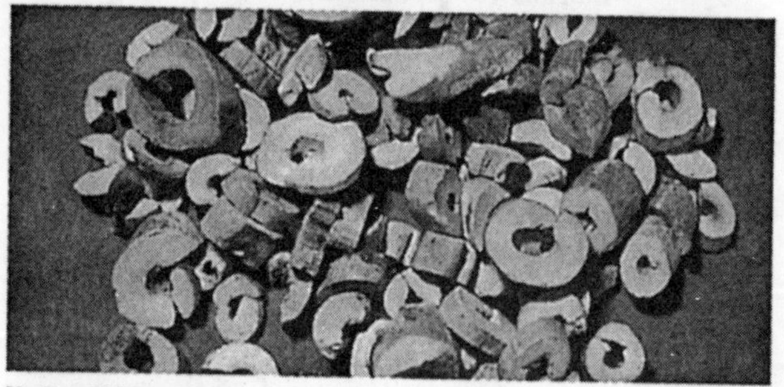

Mu Dan Pi / Paeonia

Cool the Blood and Clear Yin Deficient Heat

Di Gu Pi / Lycium
Yin Chai Hu / Stellaria
Bai Wei / Cynanchum

Cool the Blood, Nourish Yin, and Produce Fluids

Sheng Di Huang / Rehmannia
Xuan Shen / Scrophularia

Additional Herb with Multiple Functions and Wide Applications

Mu Dan Pi / Paeonia

Herbs that Clear Heat and Dry Damp

Target the Three Burners

Upper Burner

Huang Qin / Scutellaria
Tang Song Cao / Thalictrum

Middle Burner

Huang Lian / Coptis
Xiao Nie / Berberis
Shi Da Gong Lao / Mahonia

Lower Burner

Huang Bai / Phellodendron

Targets the Liver/Gallbladder

Long Dan Cao / Gentiana

Targets the Liver and Large Intestine

Qin Pi / Fraxinus

Targets the Large Intestine and Skin

Ku Shen / Sophora

Clears Heat, Dries Dampness, and Clears Yin Deficient Heat

Hu Huang Lian / Picrorhiza

Herbs that Clear Heat and Toxins

Treat Febrile Disease and Epidemic Poison

Particularly Throat and Lung Fire Poison

Da Qing Ye / Isatis
Ban Lan Gen / Isatis

Particularly Toxic Abscesses and Swellings

Jin Yin Hua / Lonicera
Lian Qiao / Forsythia

Treat a Wide Range of Heat Patterns Including Fire Poison, Toxic Abscesses and Swellings

Pu Gong Ying / Taraxacum
Chuan Xin Lian / Andrographis
Zao Xiu / Paris
Qing Mu Xiang / Aristolochia
Zi Bei Tian Kui / Begonia

Treat Toxic Swelling: Internal and External Abscesses, Nodules, Sores, Carbuncles, Boils, etc. (Including Some Tumors)

Primarily Administered Internally

Ban Zhi Lian / Scutellaria
Tu Fu Ling / Smilax

Breast Abscess

Lou Lu / Rhaponticum

Lung Abscess

Yu Xing Cao / Houttuynia

Intestinal Abscess

Bai Hua She She Cao / Oldenlandia
Hong Teng / Sargentodoxa

Administered Both Internally and Externally

Bai Xian Pi / Dictamnus
Bai Lian / Ampelopsis
Lu Jiao / Cervus
Si Ji Qing / Ilex
Zao Jiao Ci / Gleditsia

Lung Abscess

Hu Er Cao / Saxifraga

Intestinal Abscess

Bai Jiang Cao / Patrinia

Breast or Intestinal Abscess

Pu Gong Ying / Taraxacum

Benefit the Throat and Clear Throat Inflammation

Clear Heat and Fire Poison

Jin Sha Teng / Lygodium
Ma Bo / Lasiosphaera
Shan Dou Gen / Sophora
Qing Dai / Indigo
Dian Di Mei / Androsace
Zhu Sha Gen / Ardisia
Jin Guo Lan / Tinospora
Wan Nian Qing / Rhodea

Clear Heat, Fire Poison and Hot Poisonous Phlegm (such as Diptheria)

She Gan / Belamcanda
Suan Jiang / Physalis

Treat Throat Inflammation and Toxic Abscesses

Ye Ju Hua / Chrysanthemum
Zi Hua Di Ding / Viola
Tu Niu Xi / Achyranthes
Shi Shang Bai / Selaginella
Qian Li Guang / Senecio
Guan Ye Liao / Polygonum
Jin Qiao Mai / Fagopyrum

Treat Toxic Dysentery-Like Disorders

Treat Acute Disorders: Epidemic Damp Heat, Fire Poison and Bleeding

Bai Tou Weng / Pulsatilla
Ma Chi Xian / Portulaca
Tie Xian / Acalypha
Feng Wei Cao / Pteris
Fan Bai Cao / Potentilla

Treat Chronic, Recurring and Cold Stagnation Disorders

Ya Dan Zi / Brucea

Herbs that Clear and Alleviate Summerheat

Summerheat with Thirst

Lu Dou / Phaseolus
Ren Shen Ye / Panax

Summerheat with Thirst and Scanty Urine

Xi Gua / Citrullus
Dong Gua Pi / Benincasa

Summerheat with Chest Discomfort

Lian Geng / Nelumbo

Summerheat with Diarrhea

He Ye / Nelumbo

Summerheat with Diarrhea and Vomiting

Bian Dou / Dolichos

Summerheat with Multiple Signs and Symptoms of Damp Heat

Dou Juan / Glycine

Clear Summerheat, Cool the Blood and Clear Deficient Blood or Yin Fevers

Qing Hao / Artemisia

Herbs that Treat Malaria

Chang Shan / Dichroa
Shu Qi / Dichroa
Qing Hao / Artemisia
Ma Bian Cao / Verbena
Ya Dan Zi / Brucea
Yan Fu Mu / Rhus
Tian Ming Jing / Carpesium
Ba Xian Hua / Hydrangea

Herbs that Drain Downward

Purgatives

Treat Acute Excess Heat Accumulation

Da Huang / Rheum
Mang Xiao / Mirabilitum
Fan Xie Ye / Cassia

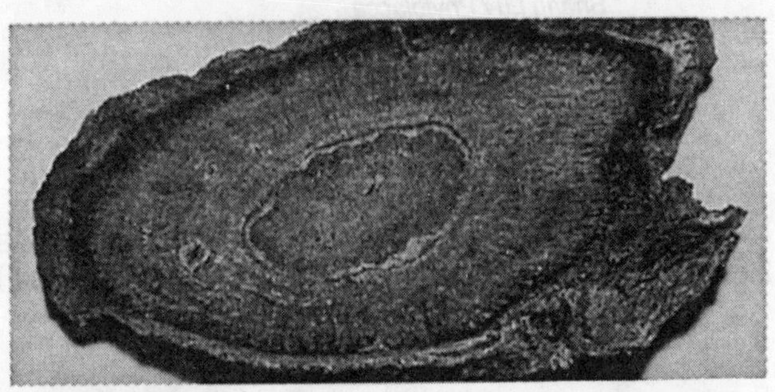

Da Huang / Rheum

Treat Chronic Accumulation of Heat

Lu Hui / Aloe

Moist Lubricants

Gentle, Nourishing Moist Laxatives for Deficient Conditions

Huo Ma Ren / Cannabis
Feng Mi / Mel

Strong Moist Laxative for Excess Conditions

Yu Li Ren / Prunus

Severe Expellants (Cathartics)

Moderate Expellant Herb that Can Be Used for a Longer Period of Time

Qian Nui Zi / Pharbitis

Severe Cathartic Herbs that Should Be Used for Short Periods of Time Only

Shang Lu / Phytolacca
Yuan Hua / Daphne
Gan Sui / Euphorbia
Jing Da Ji / Euphorbia
Xu Sui Zi / Euphorbia
Wu Jiu Gen Pi / Sapium

Severe Cathartic Herb for Cold Conditions that Should Be Used for Short Periods of Time Only

Ba Dou / Croton

Herbs that Drain Damp (Diuretics)

Anti-edemic Herbs that Regulate Water Metabolism

Promote Urination and Drain Damp

Fu Ling / Poria
Fu Ling Pi / Poria
Ze Xie / Alisma
Zhu Ling / Polyporus
Dong Gua Pi / Benincasa
Sheng Jiang Pi / Zingiber
Pu Hui / Typha

Promote Urination, Drain Damp and Fortify the Spleen

Fu Ling / Poria
Shu Yi Ren / Coix

Clear Heat and Drain Damp

Chi Fu Ling / Poria
Yi Yi Ren / Coix
Han Fang Ji / Stephania
Guang Fang Ji / Aristolochia
Dong Gua Ren / Benincasa
Chi Xiao Dou / Phaseolus
Ban Bian Lian / Lobelia
Lu Ying / Sambucus
San Bai Cao / Saururus

Urinary Soothing Herbs that Treat Painful Urinary Disorder

With Equal Heat and Damp

Mu Tong / Akebia
Tong Cao / Tetrapanax
Di Fu Zi / Kochia
Bian Xu / Polygonum

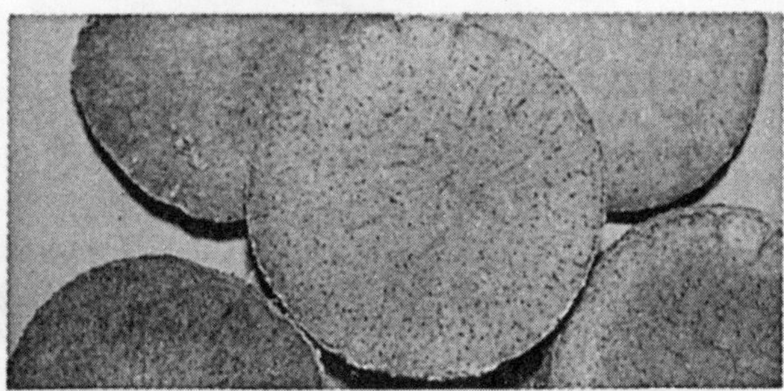

Ze Xie / Alisma

With Predominant Heat

Shi Wei / Pyrrosia
Deng Xin Cao / Juncus
Qu Mai / Dianthus
Che Qian Cao / Plantago
Hai Jin Sha / Lygodium

With Predominant Dampness

Bei Xie / Dioscorea

With Stones

Jin Qian Cao / Lysimachia
Yu Mi Xu / Zea
Hai Jin Sha / Lygodium
Lou Gu / Gryllotalpa

With Concomitant Diarrhea

Che Qian Zi / Plantago
Hua Shi / Talcum

With Concomitant Constipation

Dong Kui Zi / Abutilon

Herbs that Relieve Jaundice

Yin Chen Hao / Artemisia
Jin Qian Cao / Lysimachia
Yu Mi Xu / Zea
Hu Zhang / Polygonum
Chui Pen Cao / Sedum

Herbs that Resolve Phlegm and Stop Cough

Herbs that Resolve Phlegm

Cool Herbs that Resolve Hot Phlegm

Hot Phlegm Accumulation in the Lungs

Chuan Bei Mu / Fritillaria
Qian Hu / Peucedanum
Gua Luo / Trichosanthes
Gua Lua Ren / Trichosanthes
Tian Hua Fen / Trichosanthes
Tian Zhu Huang / Bambusa
Pang Da Hai / Sterculia
Bai Mao Xia Ku Cao / Ajuga
Gan Jie Geng / Adenophora

Hot Phlegm Accumulation in the Stomach

Zhu Ru / Bambusa

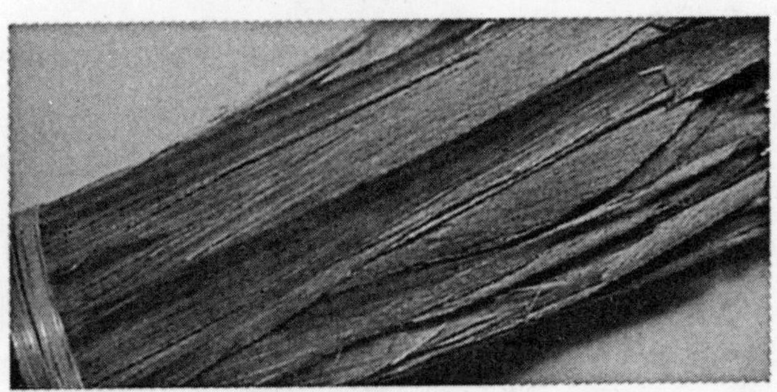

Zhu Ru / Bambusa

Turbid Phlegm Blocking the Channels

Kun Bu / Laminaria
Hai Dai / Laminaria
Hai Zao / Sargassum
Zhe Bei Mu / Fritillaria
Fu Hai Shi / Pumice
Ze Qi / Euphorbia
Huang Yao Zi / Dioscorea

Turbid Phlegm Obstructing the Orifices

Zhu Li / Bambusa
Hou Zao / Macaque

Warm Herbs that Resolve Cold Phlegm

Cold Phlegm Accumulation in the Lungs

Bai Qian / Cynanchum
Ju Hong / Citrus

Cold Damp Phlegm Accumulation in the Stomach/Spleen

(Fa) Ban Xia / Pinellia
Xuan Fu Hua / Inula
Jin Fei Cao / Inula

Turbid Phlegm Blocking the Channels

Bai Jie Zi / Brassica

Turbid Phlegm Obstructing the Orifices

Bai Fu Zi / Typhonium
Zao Jiao / Gleditsia
Zhi Nan Xing / Arisaema

Neutral Temperature Herbs that Resolve Both Hot and Cold Phlegm

Phlegm Accumulation in the Lungs

(Ku) Jie Geng / Platycodon
Han Cai / Rorippa

Turbid Phlegm Blocking the Channels

Hai Ge Ke / Cyclina
Wa Leng Zi / Arca
Mao Zhao Cao / Ranunculus

Turbid Phlegm Obstructing the Orifices

Meng Shi / Lapis Micae seu Chloriti

Herbs that Alleviate Cough and Wheezing

Cough from Many Different Etiologies

(Bei) Xing Ren / Prunus
Zi Wan / Aster
Kuan Dong Hua / Tussilago

Externally Contracted Cough

Kuan Dong Hua / Tussilago
(Bei) Xing Ren / Prunus
Gua Lou Pi / Trichosanthes

Cold Induced Cough

Zi Wan / Aster
Zi Su Zi / Perilla
Hu Tui Ye / Eleagnus
(Bei)Xing Ren / Prunus

Heat Induced Cough

Sang Bai Pi / Morus
Pi Pa Ye / Eriobotrya
Ma Dou Ling / Aristolochia
Bao Ma Zi / Syringa
(Bei) Xing Ren / Prunus
Da Juan Hua Ye / Rhododendron
Ji Ning / Salvia

Cough with Phlegm Accumulation in the Lungs

Kuan Dong Hua / Tussilago
Zi Su Zi / Perilla
Zi Wan / Aster
(Bei) Xing Ren / Prunus
Zi Jin Niu / Ardisia
Da Juan Hua Ye / Rhododendron
Ji Ning / Salvia
Bao Ma Zi / Syringa

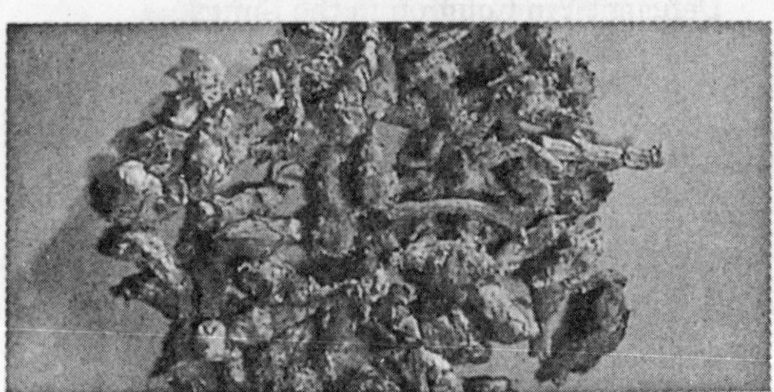

Kuan Dong Hua / Tussilago

Cough with Phlegm Accumulation in the Stomach and/or Lungs

Pi Pa Ye / Eriobotrya

Dry Cough

Kuan Dong Hua / Tussilago
Pi Pa Ye / Eriobotrya
(Nan) Xing Ren / Prunus
Gua Lou Pi / Trichosanthes

Nan Wu Wei Zi / Schisandra

Cough with Wheezing

Kuan Dong Hua / Tussilago
Zi Su Zi / Perilla
Sang Bai Pi / Morus
Ma Dou Ling / Aristolochia
(Bei) Xing Ren / Prunus
Sha Ren Hua / Amomum
Fo Shou Hua / Citrus
Ting Li Zi / Lepidium

Chronic, Deficient Cough Stemming from Internal Damage

Cold Deficient Cough

Zi Wan / Aster
Bai Bu / Stemona
Hu Tui Ye / Eleagnus

Lung Deficient Cough with Phlegm Heat

Ma Dou Ling / Aristolochia
Ba Mao Zi / Syringa

Deficient Yin Cough

Bai Bu / Stemona
Nan Sha Shen / Adenophora

Cough with Hoarseness

Mu Hu Die / Oroxylum
Ren Shen Ye / Panax

Cough with a Sensation of Chest Constriction

Zi Su Zi / Perilla
Zi Su Geng / Perilla

Cough accompanied by Edema

Sang Bai Pi / Morus
Zi Jin Niu / Ardisia
Jiao Mu / Zanthoxylum

Herbs that Expel Phlegm Through Vomiting (Emetics)

Li Lu / Veratrum
Gua Di / Cucumis
Chang Shan / Dichroa
Shu Qi / Dichroa
Ren Shen Lu / Panax

Herbs that Expel Wind Damp (Anti-rheumatics)

Pain Relieving Herbs that Target the Muscle Layer

Wind Damp Cold in the Upper Body

Qiang Huo / Notopterygium

Wind Damp Cold in the Lower Body

Du Huo / Angelica
Can Sha / Bombyx

Wind Damp Cold in Both the Upper and Lower Body

Fang Feng / Ledebouriella
Wei Ling Xian / Clematis
Cang Er Zi / Xanthium
Song Jie / Pinus
Cang Er Cao / Xanthium
Chuan Wu / Aconitum
Wu Tou / Aconitum
Cao Wu / Aconitum

Wind Damp Heat in Both the Upper and Lower Body

Guang Fang Ji / Aristolochia

Neutral Temperature Herbs that Dispel Wind Damp in Both the Upper and Lower Body

Qin Jiao / Gentiana
She Tui / Zaocys
Chuan Shan Long / Dioscorea
Xun Gu Feng / Aristolochia
Ba Qia / Smilax

Invigorating Herbs that Target the Channel Layer

Wind Damp Cold in the Lower Body

Mu Gua / Chaenomeles

Wind Damp Cold in Both the Upper and Lower Body

Hai Feng Teng / Piper
Wei Ling Xian / Clematis
Bai Hua She / Agkistrodon
Shen Jin Cao / Lycopodium

Wind Damp Heat in Both the Upper and Lower Body

Xi Xian Cao / Siegesbeckia
Luo Shi Teng / Trachelospermum
Kuan Jin Teng / Tinospora
Si Gua Luo / Luffa
Chou Wu Tong / Clerodendron
Ren Dong Teng/ Lonicera

Neutral Temperature Herbs that Dispel Wind Damp in the Upper Body

Sang Zhi / Morus

Neutral Temperature Herbs that Dispel Wind Damp in the Lower Body

Lu Lu Tong / Liquidambar
Chuan Niu Xi / Cyathula
Hai Tong Pi / Erythrina

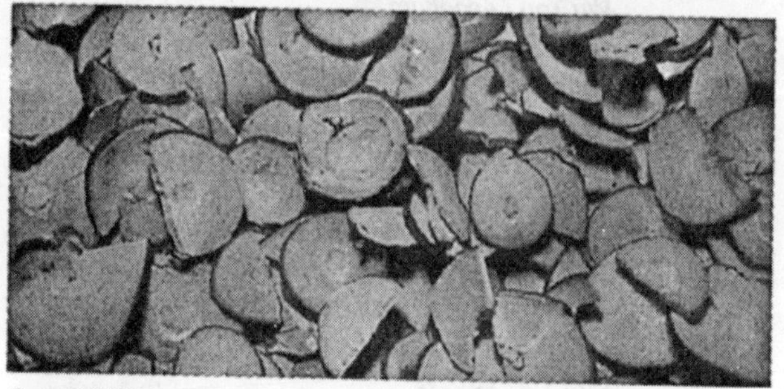

Sang Zhi / Morus

Neutral Temperature Herbs that Dispel Wind Damp in Both the Upper and Lower Body

Wu Shao She / Zaocys
Lao Guan Cao / Erodium

Strengthening Herbs that Target the Bone and Tendon Layer

Wind Damp Cold in the Lower Body

Xu Duan / Dipsacus
Lu Xian Cao / Pyrola
Gou Ji / Cibotium
Sang Ji Sheng / Loranthus
Du Huo / Angelica

Wind Damp Cold in Both the Upper and Lower Body

Wu Jia Pi / Acanthopanax
Hu Gu / Panthera
Bao Gu / Panthera
Gou Gu / Canis
Qian Nian Jian / Homalomena
Chang Chun Teng / Hedera

Aromatic Herbs that Resolve Middle Jiao Damp

Release Exterior Damp Summerheat Patterns with Digestive Symptoms

Huo Xiang / Agastache
Pei Lan / Eupatorium

Dispel Damp which Distresses the Middle Jiao

Huo Xiang / Agastache
Hou Po / Magnolia
Hou Po Hua / Magnolia
Cang Zhu / Atractylodes
Bai Dou Kou / Amomum
Sha Ren / Amomum
Sha Ren Ke / Amomum

Dispel Cold and Dry Damp Due to Cold, Deficient Middle Jiao

Cao Guo / Amomum
Cao Dou Kou / Alpinia

Herbs that Alleviate Food Stagnation

Alleviate Food Stagnation and Accumulation Due to Meat

Shan Zha / Crataegus

Alleviate Food Stagnation and Accumulation Due to Grains

Hot Food Stagnation

Gu Ya / Oryza

Cold Food Stagnation and Deficient Middle Jiao

Mai Ya / Hordeum

Treat Cold Food Stagnation Due to Cold, Deficient Middle Jiao

Shen Qu / Massa Fermentata
Ji Nei Jin / Gallus
E Wei / Ferula
Ji Shi Teng / Paederia
Ge Shan Xiang / Cynanchum

Treat Food and Phlegm Stagnation

Lai Fu Zi / Raphanus

Herbs that Warm the Interior and Dispel Cold

Warm Endogenous Spleen Cold Deficiency

Fu Zi / Aconitum
Rou Gui / Cinnamomum
Gan Jiang / Zingiber

Warm Kidneys and Tonify Yang

Fu Zi / Aconitum
Rou Gui / Cinnamomum

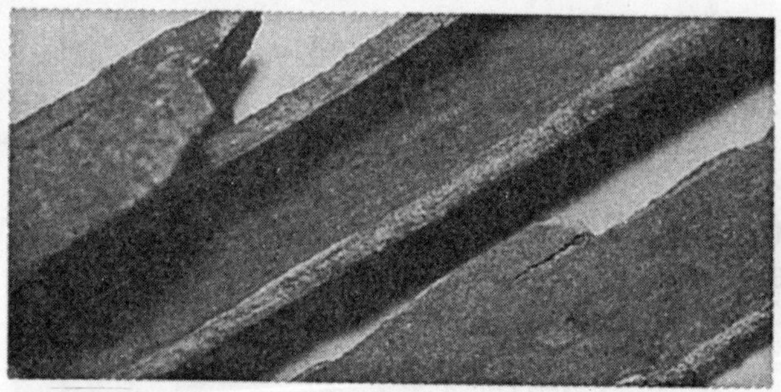

Rou Gui / Cinnamomum

Dispel Cold Pathogenic Influence in the Stomach

Bi Ba / Piper
Hu Jiao / Piper
Bi Cheng Qie / Piper

Dispel Cold Pathogenic Influence in the Middle Jiao

Chuan Jiao / Zanthoxylum
Ding Xiang / Caryophyllum
Gao Liang Jiang / Alpinia
Ba Jiao Hui Xiang / Illicium

Dispel Cold Pathogenic Influence in the Stomach/Liver and their Respective Channels

Wu Zhu Yu / Evodia
Xiao Hui Xiang / Foeniculum

Alleviate the Pain of Cold Pathogenic Influence in the Low Back and Lower Abdomen

Dou Chi Jiang / Litsea

Herbs that Rectify Qi

Rectify Middle Jiao Qi Stagnation

Zhi Shi / Citrus
Zhi Ke / Citrus
Da Fu Pi / Areca
Bing Lang / Areca
Shi Di / Diospyros

Course Liver Qi Stagnation

Qing Pi / Citrus
Ju He / Citrus
Mei Gui Hua / Rosa
Xiang Fu / Cyperus
Chuan Lian Zi / Melia

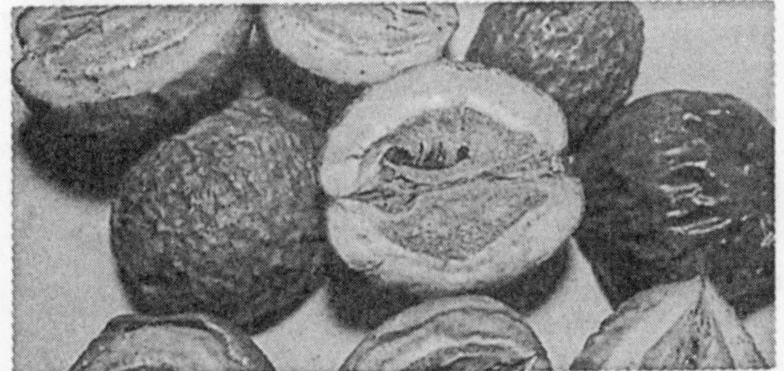

Chuan Lian Zi / Melia

Rectify Mixed Qi Stagnation

Lung, Spleen and Stomach Qi Stagnation

Chen Pi / Citrus
Chen Xiang / Aquilaria

Liver and Stomach Qi Stagnation

Li Zhi He / Litchi
Ba Yue Zha / Akebia

Liver and Spleen/Stomach Qi Stagnation

Mu Xiang / Saussurea
Fo Shou / Citrus

Multiple Mixed Qi Stagnation

Tan Xiang / Santalum
Xie Bai / Allium
Wu Yao / Lindera
Yan Hu Suo / Corydalis

Herbs that Regulate the Blood

Herbs that Arrest Bleeding (Hemostatics)

Hemostatic Herbs with Astringent Action

Stop Coughing and Vomiting of Blood

Bai Ji / Bletilla

Arrest Excessive Uterine Bleeding

Xue Yu Tan / Homo Sapiens

Arrest Urinary Bleeding

Zi Zhu / Callicarpa

Arrest the Bleeding Diarrhea of Chronic Dysentery-like Disorders

Shan Zha Tan / Crataegus
Shi Bing / Diospyros

Arrest Bleeding in Miscellaneous Locations

Xian He Cao / Agrimonia
Zong Lu Pi Tan / Trachycarpus
Hua Sheng Yi / Arachis
Ji Mu / Loropetalum

Hemostatic Herbs with Astringent and Invigorating Actions that Dispel Congealed Blood Stasis

Stop Coughing and Vomiting of Blood

Ou Jie / Nelumbo

Stop Excessive Menstrual or Uterine Bleeding

Chong Wei Zi / Leonurus

Stop Bleeding Due to Trauma

Jiang Xiang / Dalbergia

Arrest Bleeding in Miscellaneous Locations

Pu Huang Tan / Typha
Lian Fang / Nelumbo
Hua Rui Shi / Ophicalcitum
Jing Tian San Qi / Sedum
Mao Mei / Rubus

Hemostatic Herbs that are Unobstructing and Dispel Congealed Blood Stasis

San Qi / Panax
Ju Ye San Qi / Gynura

Blood Cooling Hemostatic Herbs

Arrest Nasal Bleeding

Bai Mao Gen / Imperata
Bai Mao Hua / Imperata

Stop Coughing and Vomiting of Blood

Qian Cao Gen / Rubia

Arrest Excessive Uterine Bleeding

Zhu Ma Gen / Boehmeria

Arrest Urinary Bleeding

Xiao Ji / Cephalanoplos

Stop Bloody Stool

Di Yu / Sanguisorba
Huai Hua Mi / Sophora
Ji Guan Hua / Celosia

Arrest Bleeding in Miscellaneous Locations

Ce Bai Ye / Biota
Da Ji / Cirsium
Ji Cai / Capsella

Warming Hemostatic Herbs that Arrest Cold Induced Bleeding

Cold Induced Stomach and Intestinal Bleeding

Pao Jiang / Zingiber
Fu Long Gan / Terra Flava Usta

Cold Deficient Uterine Bleeding

Lu Jiao Shuang / Cervus

Channel Warming Hemostatic for Cold Induced Uterine and Menstrual Bleeding

Ai Ye / Artemisia

Herbs Quicken the Blood

Quicken the Blood and Promote Menses

Ji Xue Teng / Millettia

Move the Blood and Promote Menses

Chuan Xiong / Ligusticum
Yi Mu Cao / Leonurus
Wang Bu Liu Xing / Vaccaria
Yue Ji Hua / Rosa
(Sheng) Pu Huang / Typha

Dispel Congealed Blood and Promote Menses

Dan Shen / Salvia
Ze Lan / Lycopus
Chi Shao Yao / Paeonia
Tao Ren / Prunus
Hong Hua / Carthamus
Huai Niu Xi / Achyranthes

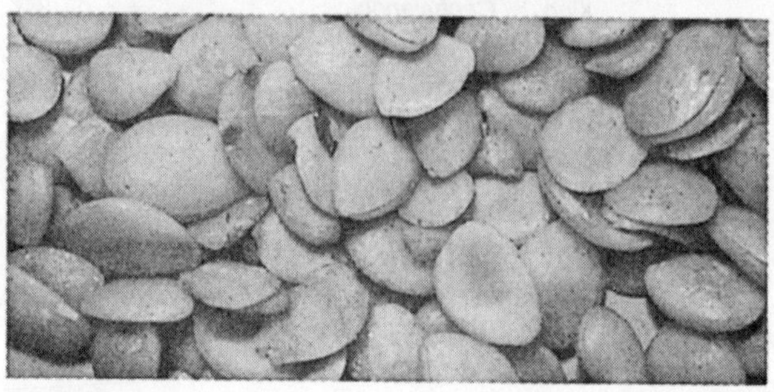

Tao Ren / Prunus

Resolve Congealed Blood and Masses and Move Qi

Yu Jin / Curcuma
Jiang Huang / Curcuma
San Leng / Sparganium
E Zhu / Curcuma
Gan Qi / Rhus

Strong Animal Substances that Break Up Congealed Blood Stasis and Masses

Shui Zhi / Hirudo
Tu Bie Chong / Eupolyphaga
Meng Chong / Tabanus

Alleviate Internal Pain

Yan Hu Suo / Corydalis
Wu Ling Zhi / Trogopterus
Lu Jiao / Cervus

Reduce Swelling and Pain due to Trauma

Ru Xiang / Boswellia
Mo Yao / Commiphora
Zi Ran Tong / Pyritum
Xue Jie / Dracaena
Su Mu / Caesalpinia
Liu Ji Nu / Artemisia

Blood Quickening Herbs with Multiple Functions

Wa Leng Zi / Arca
Chuan Niu Xi / Cyathula
Lu Lu Tong / Liquidambar
Chuan Shan Jia / Manis
Mao Dong Qing / Ilex
Hu Zhang / Polygonum

Herbs that Supplement

Herbs that Boost Qi

Boost Qi of the Middle Jiaos (Spleen/Stomach)

Bai Zhu / Atractylodes
Da Zao / Ziziphus
Hong Zao / Ziziphus
Zhi Gan Cao / Glycyrrhiza
Jing Mi / Oryza

Boost Qi of the Middle and Upper Jiaos (Spleen/Lungs)

Dang Shen / Codonopsis
Huang Qi / Astragalus
Gan Cao / Glycyrrhiza
Yi Tang / Saccharum Granorum
Feng Mi / Mel
Mian Hua Gen / Gossypium

Qi and Yang of the Middle and Upper Jiaos

(Hong) Ren Shen / Panax
Ye Shan Shen / Panax
Ji Lin Shen / Panax

Qi and Yin of the Middle and Upper Jiaos

Tai Zi Shen / Pseudostellaria
Huang Jing / Polygonatum
Bai Shen / Panax
Shen Xu / Panax

Boost Qi of the Upper, Middle and Lower Jiaos (Lungs/Stomach/Spleen/Kidney)

Shan Yao / Dioscorea

Herbs that Nourish the Blood

Nourish Blood and Tonify the Heart and Spleen

Long Yan Rou / Euphoria

Nourish Liver Blood

He Shou Wu / Polygonum

Nourish Blood and Kidney Yin

Shu Di Huang / Rehmannia

Nourish Liver and Kidney Blood and Yin

Gou Qi Zi / Lycium
Sang Shen / Morus
Chu Shi Zi / Broussonetia

Nourish, Quicken and Harmonize the Blood

Dang Gui / Angelica
Dang Gui Tou / Angelica
Dang Gui Wei / Angelica

Nourish Blood, Retain Yin and Soothe the Liver

Bai Shao Yao / Paeonia

Nourish Blood, Nourish Yin or Essence and Arrest Bleeding

E Jiao / Equus
Lu Jiao Jiao / Cervus

Herbs that Nourish Yin

Nourish Lung Yin

Bai He / Lilium
Luo Han Guo / Momordica
Luo Han Ye / Momordica

Nourish Lung and Stomach Yin

Bei Sha Shen / Glehnia
Mai Men Dong / Ophiopogon
Yu Zhu / Polygonatum
Shi Hu / Dendrobium
Ming Dang Shen / Changium
Tian Hua Fen / Trichosanthes

Nourish Lung and Kidney Yin

Tian Men Dong / Asparagus

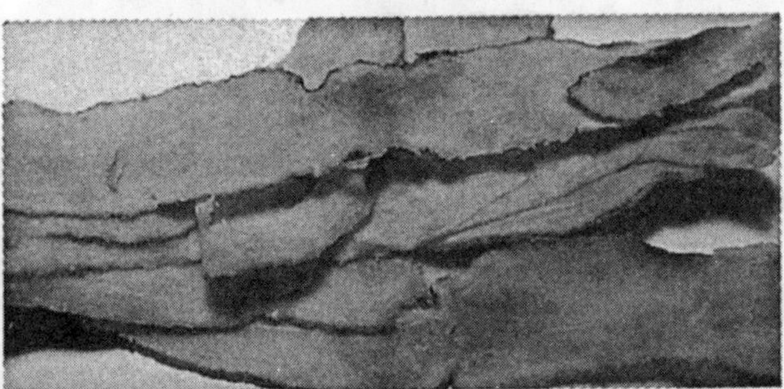

Yu Zhu / Polygonatum

Nourish Liver and Kidney Yin

Nu Zhen Zi / Ligustrum
Han Lian Cao / Eclipta
Sang Ji Sheng / Loranthus
Hei Zhi Ma / Sesamum
Gui Ban Jiao / Chinemys
Bie Jia Jiao / Amyda

Nourish Yin and Qi

Xi Yang Shen / Panax
Sheng Shai Shen / Panax
Nan Sha Shen / Adenophora

Nourish Yin, Subdue Ascending Yang

Gui Ban / Chinemys
Bie Jia / Amyda
Bai Mu Er / Tremella
Huai Niu Xi / Achyranthes

Herbs that Supplement Yang

Supplement Kidney and Lung

Dong Chong Xia Cao / Cordyceps
Hu Tao Ren / Juglans
Ge Jie / Gekko
E Guan Shi / Stalactitum
Zi He Che / Placenta Hominis

Supplement Kidneys, Warm Spleen Yang and Treat Urinary Incontinence and Diarrhea due to Cold Deficiency

Bu Gu Zhi / Psoralea
Yi Zhi Ren / Alpinia
Jiu Xiang Chong / Aspongopus

Warm Cold Deficient Kidneys

Hu Lu Ba / Trigonella
Jiu Zi / Allium
Yang Qi Shi / Actinolitum

Supplement Kidney Yang, Benefit the Essence and Moisten the Intestines

Rou Cong Rong / Cistanche
Suo Yang / Cynomorium

Supplement Kidney Yang, Strengthen the Sinews and Expel Wind Cold Damp

Ba Ji Tian / Morinda
Yin Yang Huo / Epimedium
Xian Mao / Curculigo

Nourish the Liver and Kidneys, Strengthen the Sinews and Bones and Treat Pain and Weakness in Low Back and Knees

Du Zhong / Eucommia
Xu Duan / Dipsacus
Gou Ji / Cibotium
Gu Sui Bu / Drynaria

Nourish Liver and Kidney Essence and Brighten the Eyes

Tu Si Zi / Cuscuta
Sha Yuan Ji Li / Astragalus

Animal Substances that Supplement the Kidneys, Fortify the Yang and Essence, and Strengthen Sexual Functioning

Guang Gou Shen / Canis
Hai Gou Shen / Phoca
Hei Lu Shen / Equus
Hua Lu Shen / Cervus
Hai Ma / Hippocampus
Hai Long / Solenognathus
Hai Shen / Strichopus

Animal Substances that Strongly Supplement the Yang, Essence, Blood and Qi

Lu Rong / Cervus
Zi He Che / Homo Sapiens

Astringents

Primarily for the Upper Jiao

Prevent and Stop Abnormal Sweating

Fu Xiao Mai / Triticum
Ma Huang Gen / Ephedra
Nuo Dao Gen / Oryza

Restrain Lung Qi and Repress Coughing

Bai Guo / Ginkgo
Yin Guo Ye/ Ginkgo

Primarily for the Middle Jiao

Stop Chronic Diarrhea

Rou Dou Kou / Myristica
Chun Pi / Ailanthus
Shi Liu Pi / Punica

Stop Chronic Diarrhea, Restrain Lung Qi and Repress Cough

He Zi / Terminalia
Wu Mei / Prunus
Ying Su Ke / Papaver
Wu Bei Zi / Rhus/Melaphis

Stop Chronic Diarrhea, Stabilize the Menses and Arrest Abnormal Uterine Bleeding

Chi Shi Zhi / Halloysitum Rubrum
Yu Liang Shi / Limonite

Primarily for the Lower Jiao

Preserve the Essence, Stabilize the Menses and Arrest Abnormal Uterine Bleeding

Hai Piao Xiao / Sepia

Benefit and Stabilize the Kidney, Preserve the Essence and Stop Frequent Urination and Incontinence

Sang Piao Xiao / Paratenodera
Fu Pen Zi / Rubus
Lian Xu / Nelumbo

Preserve the Essence and Stop Chronic Diarrhea

Qian Shi / Euryale
Jin Ying Zi / Rosa
Lian Zi / Nelumbo

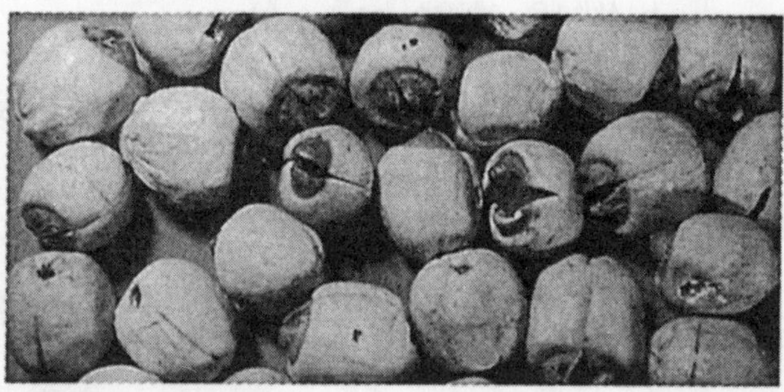

Lian Zi / Nelumbo

Astringents with Multiple Functions and Wide Applications

Shan Zhu Yu / Cornus
Wu Wei Zi / Schisandra

Substances that Calm the Shen (Tranquilizers)

Herbs that Nurture the Heart, Calm the Shen and:

Nourish Heart Blood

Bai Zi Ren / Biota

Nourish Liver Yin

Suan Zao Ren / Ziziphus

Nourish Blood and Yin and Balance Yin and Yang

Ye Jiao Teng / Polygonum

Boost Qi and Nourish Blood

Ling Zhi / Ganoderma

Drain Damp

Fu Shen / Poria

Release Constrained Emotions Due to Liver Qi Stagnation

He Huan Pi / Albizzia
He Huan Hua / Albizzia

Release Constrained Emotions and Expel Phlegm

Yuan Zhi / Polygala

Substances that Calm the Shen, Subdue Liver Yang and:

Subdue Rising Liver Yang

Dai Zhe Shi / Hematitum
Ci Shi / Magnetitum
Zhen Zhu Mu / Pteria
Sheng Tie Luo / Frusta Ferri

Subdue Rising Liver Yang and Possess Astringent Properties

Long Gu / Os Draconis
Mu Li / Ostrea
Long Chi / Dens Draconis
Duan Mu Li / Ostrea
Duan Long Gu / Os Draconis

Sedate the Heart and Treat Palpitations, Emotional Distress, Seizures and Convulsions

Zi Shi Ying / Fluoritum
Hu Po / Succinum
Zhen Zhu / Pteria
Zhu Sha / Cinnabaris

Herbs that Subdue Wind, Stop Tremors and Sedate Liver Yang

Strongly Calm and Suppress Convulsions, Seizures and Spasms

Treat Wind, Convulsions and Seizures due to Extreme Heat

Clear Blazing Heat, Soothe the Liver and Subdue Rising Liver Yang

Ling Yang Jiao / Saiga
Shan Yang Jiao / Naemorhedis
Gou Teng / Uncaria
Dai Mao / Eretmochelydis
Ren Gong Niu Huang / Bos

Clear Blazing Heat, Dispel Wind and Open the Channels in Windstroke Patterns

Di Long / Pheretima

Treat Wind and Spasms in Wind Phlegm Heat Patterns

Quan Xie / Buthus
Jiang Can / Bombyx
Meng Shi / Lapis Micae seu Chloriti
Dan Nan Xing / Arisaema

Treat Wind and Spasms in Wind Cold Patterns

Wu Gong / Scolopendra

Soothe the Liver and Subdue Rising Liver Yang and Fire

Bai Ji Li / Tribulus
Shi Jue Ming / Haliotis
San Qi Hua / Panax
Luo Bu Ma / Apocynum

Pacify the Liver and Subdue Wind in Patterns of Heat, Deficient Blood, Wind Phlegm and Windstroke

Tian Ma / Gastrodia

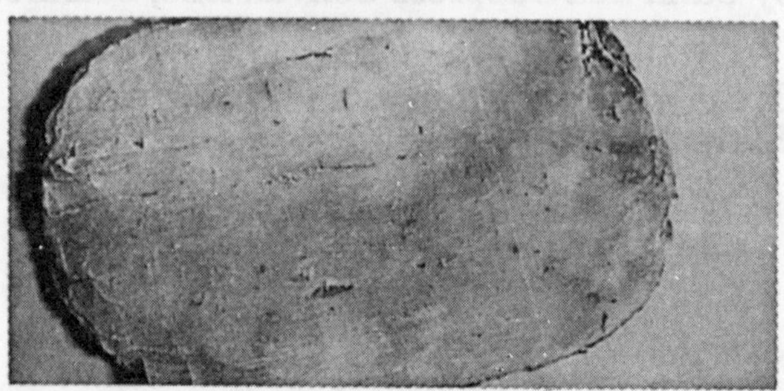

Tian Ma / Gastrodia

Aromatic Substances that Open the Orifices

Particularly Strong for Opening the Orifices

She Xiang / Moschus

Open Orifices and Clear Heat

Niu Huang / Bos
Bing Pian / Dryobalanops

Open Orifices and Penetrate Turbid Phlegm

Su He Xiang / Liquidambar
Shi Chang Pu / Acorus
Jiu Jie Chang Pu / Anemone

Open Orifices and Invigorate Qi and Blood

An Xi Xiang / Styrax

Herbs that Expel Parasites (Anti-helminthics)

Roundworms

Shi Jun Zi / Quisqualis
Ku Lian Gen Pi / Melia
Ku Lian Mu Pi / Melia
Wu Yi / Ulmus
Nan Gua Zi / Cucurbita
Shi Liu Gen Pi / Punica
Fei Zi / Torreya
He Shi / Carpesium

Tapeworms

Bing Lang / Areca
Lei Wan / Omphalia
Wu Yi / Ulmus
Nan Gua Zi / Cucurbita
Shi Liu Gen Pi / Punica
Fei Zi / Torreya
He Shi / Carpesium

Hookworms

Guan Zhong / Dryopteris
Da Suan / Allium
Fei Zi / Torreya
He Shi / Carpesium

Pinworms

Da Suan / Allium
Fei Zi / Torreya
He Shi / Carpesium

Substances For Topical Use

Kill Parasites and Treat Damp Skin Rash

Ming Fan / Alumen
Ku Fan / Alumen

Dry Damp, Kill Parasites and Strengthen the Yang

Liu Huang / Sulphur
She Chuang Zi / Cnidium

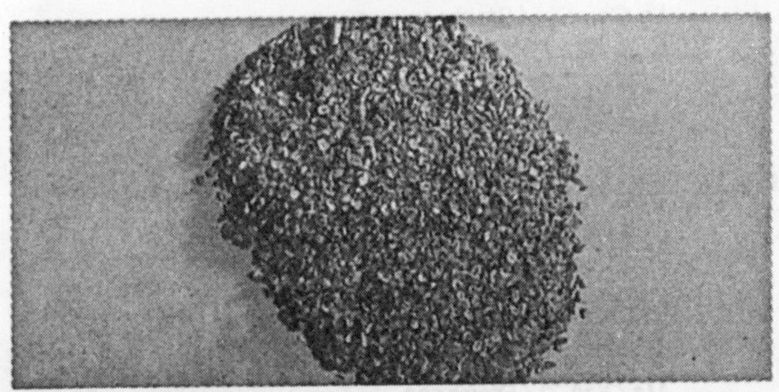

She Chuang Zi / Cnidium

Expel Wind Damp and Kill Parasites

Da Feng Zi / Hydnocarpus
Zhang Nao / Cinnamomum
Zao Jiao Ci / Gleditsia

Detoxify Poison and Kill Parasites

Qing Fen / Calomelas
Xiong Huang / Realgar
Shui Yin / Hydrargyrum

Detoxify Poison and Invigorate Blood

Mu Bie Zi / Momordica
Ban Mao / Mylabris

Detoxify Poison and Diminish Swelling

Peng Sha / Borax
Chan Su / Bufo
Xuan Ming Fan / Mirabilitum
(Sheng) Ban Xia / Pinellia
(Sheng) Tian Nan Xing / Arisaema

Detoxify Poison, Expel Wind and Damp, and Stop Pain

Lu Feng Fang / Polistes

Drain Poison and Regenerate Flesh

Lu Gan Shi / Smithsonitum
Qian Dan / Minium
Pi Shi / Arsenolite
Dan Fan / Chalcanthitum

Clear Heat, Detoxify Fire Toxin and Treat Nodules

Shan Ci Gu / Tulipa

Activate the Channels, Stop Pain, Move Blood and Diminish Swelling

Ma Qian Zi / Strychnos

Absorb Fluid Leakage and Alleviate Bleeding and Chronic Dysentery

Mi Tuo Seng / Lithargyrum
Er Cha / Acacia
Chen Shi Huei / Calcaria

Part 3

Table of Herbal Preparation Procedures

Part Three is a quick reference table of herbal preparation methods for the clinical setting. The herbs are categorized alphabetically by Pinyin herb name followed by the botanical name, zoological or pharmaceutical names. For further cross-referencing of names please consult Part Four.

Preparation methods listed here are easily applicable in the clinical setting. Complex Pao Zhi methods, the traditional processing and preparation methods to enhance certain medicinal functions by a Chinese herbal pharmacist, are not included here.

The second to last column of the table numbers lists the 18 incompatibilities and the 19 antagonists. The last three pages of this chapter summarize these combining cautions for those herbs.

The last column lists standard adult dosages. In cases where medicinals have no dosage the standard dosage was either unavailable or the herb is used externally.

Name of herb or substance	Decoction	Powder/Pills taken internally: ○ may be ◉ commonly ● always	Used with wine or extracted	Whole substance often eaten separately	External use: ○ possible ◉ mainly (internal caution) ● only	◉ Do not cook substance ● Refrigerate	Add near end of cooking: ○ last 5 min ◉ 10 min ● 15 min	Cook 30 - 60 minutes before adding other herbs	Dissolve/steep in strained previously cooked decoction	Wrap in separate porous bag (cheesecloth)	Slice or Crush: ◉ small pieces ● powder	May be used: ◉ fresh or dried ● fresh only	May be available in prepared form - less toxic or stronger this way	Available in charred form	Toxic: ◉ slightly ● very toxic	Contraindicated in pregnancy: ◉ caution ● never use	Combining Cautions... See page 620	Standard Dosage Range in Grams
Ai Ye/ Artemisia	✓				○									✓				*3-8*
An Xi Xiang/ Styrax	✓	◉																*0.3-1*
Ba Dou/ Croton		●													●	◉	*2*	*0.1-0.3*
Ba Jiao Hui Xiang/ Illicium	✓	○																*3-8*
Ba Ji Tian/ Morinda	✓																	*6-15*
Ba Qia/ Smilax	✓				○													*12-30*
Ba Xian Hua/ Hydrangea	✓														◉			*9-12*
Bai Bu/ Stemona	✓				○													*3-9*
Bai Dou Kou/ Amomum	✓	◉					◉				◉							*1.5-10*
Bai Fu Zi/ Typhonium	✓				○										●	●		*1.5-5*
Bai Guo/ Ginkgo	✓														◉			*4.5-9*
Bai He/ Lilium	✓																	*15-30*
Bai Hua She/ Agkistrodon	✓	○	✓	✓											◉			*1-10*
Bai Hua She She Cao/ Oldenlandia	✓											◉				◉		*15-60*
Bai Ji/ Bletilla	✓				○												*1*	*5-15*
Bai Ji Li/ Tribulus	✓															◉		*5-12*
Bai Jiang Cao/ Patrinia	✓				○							◉						*6-15*

A, B

Name of herb or substance	Decoction	Powder/Pills taken internally: ○ may be ◎ commonly ● always	Used with wine or extracted	Whole substance often eaten separately	External use: ○ possible ◎ mainly (internal caution) ● only	◎ Do not cook substance ● Refrigerate	Add near end of cooking: ○ last 5 min ◎ 10 min ● 15 min	Cook 30 - 60 minutes before adding other herbs	Dissolve/steep in strained previously cooked decoction	Wrap in separate porous bag (cheesecloth)	Slice or Crush: ◎ small pieces ● powder	May be used: ◎ fresh or dried ● fresh only	May be available in prepared form - less toxic or stronger this way	Available in charred form	Toxic: ◎ slightly ● very toxic	Contraindicated in pregnancy: ◎ caution ● never use	Combining Cautions... See page 620	Standard Dosage Range in Grams
Bai Jie Zi/ Brassica	✓																	*3-9*
Bai Lian/ Ampelopsis	✓				○												*9*	*3-10*
Bai Mao Gen/ Imperata	✓											◎						*15-30*
Bai Mao Hua/ Imperata	✓																	*10-20*
Bai Mao Xia Ku Cao/ Ajuga	✓																	*15-30*
Bai Mu Er/ Tremella	✓			✓														*5-10*
Bai Qian/ Cynanchum	✓																	*3-9*
Bai Shao Yao/ Paeonia	✓																*28*	*9-18*
Bai Tou Weng/ Pulsatilla	✓				○													*6-15*
Bai Wei/ Cynanchum	✓		✓														*39*	*3-9*
Bai Xian Pi/ Dictamnus	✓				○													*4-10*
Bai Zhi/ Angelica	✓	○			○												*34*	*3-10*
Bai Zhu/ Atractylodes	✓																	*3-12*
Bai Zi Ren/ Biota	✓				○	●												*9-18*
Ban Bian Lian/ Lobelia	✓				○							◎						*9-30*

Name of herb or substance	Decoction	Powder/Pills taken internally: ○ may be ◎ commonly ● always	Used with wine or extracted	Whole substance often eaten separately	External use: ○ possible ◎ mainly (internal caution) ● only	◎ Do not cook substance ● Refrigerate	Add near end of cooking: ○ last 5 min ◎ 10 min ● 15 min	Cook 30 - 60 minutes before adding other herbs	Dissolve/steep in strained previously cooked decoction	Wrap in separate porous bag (cheesecloth)	Slice or Crush: ◎ small pieces ● powder	May be used: ◎ fresh or dried ● fresh only	May be available in prepared form - less toxic or stronger this way	Available in charred form	Toxic: ◎ slightly ● very toxic	Contraindicated in pregnancy: ◎ caution ● never use	Combining Cautions... See page 620	Standard Dosage Range in Grams
Ban Lan Gen/ Isatis	✓																	*15-30*
Ban Mao/ Mylabris	✓	◎			◎										●	●	*8*	*0.03-0.06*
(Fa) Ban Xia/ Pinellia	✓												✓		◎	●	*9*	*5-9*
(Sheng) Ban Xia/ Pinellia					●										●			
Ban Zhi Lian/ Scutellaria	✓				○							◎				◎		*15-60*
Bao Gu/ Panthera	✓	◎	✓	✓							◎							*9-15*
Bao Ma Zi/ Syringa	✓											◎						*20-50*
Bei Sha Shen/ Glehnia	✓																*4*	*9-30*
Bei Xie/ Dioscorea	✓																	*9-15*
Bi Ba/ Piper	✓	◎			○						◎							*2-5*
Bi Cheng Qie/ Litsea	✓																	*2-5*
Bian Dou/ Dolichos	✓											◎						*9-18*
Bian Xu/ Polygonum	✓				○													*9-15*
Bie Jia/ Amyda	✓							✓			◎					●	*63*	*9-30*
Bing Lang/ Areca	✓			✓											◎	◎		*6-15*
Bing Pian/ Dryobalanops		●			○											◎		*0.3-0.9*

Name of herb or substance	Decoction	Powder/Pills taken internally: ○ may be ◎ commonly ● always	Used with wine or extracted	Whole substance often eaten separately	External use: ○ possible ◎ mainly (internal caution) ● only	◎ Do not cook substance ● Refrigerate	Add near end of cooking: ○ last 5 min ◎ 10 min ● 15 min	Cook 30 - 60 minutes before adding other herbs	Dissolve/steep in strained previously cooked decoction	Wrap in separate porous bag (cheesecloth)	Slice or Crush: ◎ small pieces ● powder	May be used: ◎ fresh or dried ● fresh only	May be available in prepared form - less toxic or stronger this way	Available in charred form	Toxic: ◎ slightly ● very toxic	Contraindicated in pregnancy: ◎ caution ● never use	Combining Cautions... See page 620	Standard Dosage Range in Grams
Bo He/ Mentha	✓						○											*2-10*
Bu Gu Zhi/ Psoralea	✓				○												*8*	*3-10*
Can Sha/ Bombyx	✓			✓	○					✓								*3-10*
Cang Er Zi/ Xanthium	✓				○										◎			*3-10*
Cang Zhu/ Atractylodes	✓																	*3-10*
Cao Dou Kou/ Alpinia	✓						◎				◎							*2-6*
Cao Guo/ Amomum	✓						◎				◎				◎			*3-6*
Ce Bai Ye/ Biota	✓				○									✓				*10-15*
Chai Hu/ Bupleurum	✓																	*3-10*
Chan Su/ Bufo		●			◎										●	●		*0.02-0.03*
Chan Tui/ Cryptotympana	✓															◎		*3-10*
Chang Chun Teng/ Hedera	✓				○													*9-15*
Chang Shan/ Dichroa	✓												✓		●	◎		*4-9*
Che Qian Cao/ Plantago	✓			✓	○							◎						*9-20*
Che Qian Zi/ Plantago	✓									✓						●		*3-12*
Chen Pi/ Citrus	✓						●											*3-9*

Name of herb or substance	Decoction	Powder/Pills taken internally: ○ may be ◉ commonly ● always	Used with wine or extracted	Whole substance often eaten separately	External use: ○ possible ◉ mainly (internal caution) ● only	◉ Do not cook substance ● Refrigerate	Add near end of cooking: ○ last 5 min ◉ 10 min ● 15 min	Cook 30 - 60 minutes before adding other herbs	Dissolve/steep in strained previously cooked decoction	Wrap in separate porous bag (cheesecloth)	Slice or Crush: ◉ small pieces ● powder	May be used: ◉ fresh or dried ● fresh only	May be available in prepared form - less toxic or stronger this way	Available in charred form	Toxic: ◉ slightly ● very toxic	Contraindicated in pregnancy: ◉ caution ● never use	Combining Cautions... See page 620	Standard Dosage Range in Grams
Chen Shi Huei/ Calcaria		○			◉										●			
Chen Xiang/ Aquilaria		◉							✓		◉							*1-3*
Cheng Liu/ Tamarix	✓																	*3-10*
Chi Fu Ling/ Poria	✓																	*6-18*
Chi Shao Yao/ Paeonia	✓																*4*	*6-9*
Chi Shi Zhi/ Halloysitum Rubrum	✓				○			✓			◉		✓			◉	*66*	*9-30*
Chi Xiao Dou/ Phaseolus	✓			✓	○													*9-30*
Chong Wei Zi/ Leonurus	✓															●		*3-9*
Chou Wu Tong/ Clerodendron	✓						○											*10-30*
Chu Shi Zi/ Broussonetia	✓																	*9-15*
Chuan Bei Mu/ Fritillaria	✓	○							✓		◉						*30*	*3-9*
Chuan Jiao/ Zanthoxylum	✓				○										◉	◉	*56*	*2-5*
Chuan Lian Zi/ Melia	✓				○						◉				◉			*3-9*
Chuan Niu Xi/ Cyathula	✓															●		*6-12*

C

Name of herb or substance	Decoction	Powder/Pills taken internally: ○ may be ◎ commonly ● always	Used with wine or extracted	Whole substance often eaten separately	External use: ○ possible ◎ mainly (internal caution) ● only	◎ Do not cook substance ● Refrigerate	Add near end of cooking: ○ last 5 min ◎ 10 min ● 15 min	Cook 30 - 60 minutes before adding other herbs	Dissolve/steep in strained previously cooked decoction	Wrap in separate porous bag (cheesecloth)	Slice or Crush: ◎ small pieces ● powder	May be used: ◎ fresh or dried ● fresh only	May be available in prepared form - less toxic or stronger this way	Available in charred form	Toxic: ◎ slightly ● very toxic	Contraindicated in pregnancy: ◎ caution ● never use	Combining Cautions... See page 620	Standard Dosage Range in Grams
Chuan Shan Jia/ Manis	✓	◎			○											●		*1-9*
Chuan Shan Long/ Dioscorea	✓																	*9-20*
Chuan Xin Lian/ Andrographis	✓	○			○							◎						*1-15*
Chuan Xiong/ Ligusticum	✓															●		*3-9*
Chui Pen Cao/ Sedum	✓				○							◎						*15-30*
Chun Pi/ Ailanthus	✓				○													*3-15*
Ci Shi/ Magnetitum	✓							✓			●		✓					*9-30*
Cong Bai/ Allium	✓				○	●	●					◎						*3-10*
Da Feng Zi/ Hydnocarpus	✓	○			◎										●			*0.3-0.9*
Da Fu Pi/ Areca	✓																	*3-9*
Da Huang/ Rheum	✓	○			○		○									◎		*3-12*
Da Ji/ Cirsium	✓				○							◎						*4.5-15*
Da Qing Ye/ Isatis	✓											◎						*10-30*
Da Suan/ Allium	✓				○							◎						*5-15*
Da Zao/ Ziziphus	✓																	*10-30*
Dai Mao/ Eretmochelys	✓							✓			◎							*3-6*

Name of herb or substance	Decoction	Powder/Pills taken internally: ○ may be ◎ commonly ● always	Used with wine or extracted	Whole substance often eaten separately	External use: ○ possible ◎ mainly (internal caution) ● only	◎ Do not cook substance ● Refrigerate	Add near end of cooking: ○ last 5 min ◎ 10 min ● 15 min	Cook 30 - 60 minutes before adding other herbs	Dissolve/steep in strained previously cooked decoction	Wrap in separate porous bag (cheesecloth)	Slice or Crush: ◎ small pieces ● powder	May be used: ◎ fresh or dried ● fresh only	May be available in prepared form - less toxic or stronger this way	Available in charred form	Toxic: ◎ slightly ● very toxic	Contraindicated in pregnancy: ◎ caution ● never use	Combining Cautions... See page 620	Standard Dosage Range in Grams
Dai Zhe Shi/ Haematitum	✓							✓			◎		✓			◎		*10-30*
Dan Dou Chi/ Glycine	✓												✓					*10-15*
Dan Fan/ Chalcanthitum					●										●			*0.1-0.3*
Dan Nan Xing/ Arisaema	✓												✓		◎	●		*3-6*
Dan Shen/ Salvia	✓																*4*	*3-15*
Dan Zhu Ye/ Lophatherum	✓															◎		*10-15*
Dang Gui/ Angelica	✓																	*3-15*
Dang Gui Tou/ Angelica	✓																	*3-15*
Dang Gui Wei/ Angelica	✓																	*3-15*
Dang Shen/ Codonopsis	✓																*4*	*9-15*
Deng Xin Cao/ Juncus	✓																	*1.5-3*
Di Er Cao/ Hypericum	✓				○							◎						*20-50*
Di Feng/ Illicium	✓																	
Di Fu Zi/ Kochia	✓				○												*46*	*6-15*
Di Gu Pi/ Lycium	✓				○													*6-15*
Di Long/ Pheretima	✓	○									●							*5-15*

Name of herb or substance	Decoction	Powder/Pills taken internally: ○ may be ⊙ commonly ● always	Used with wine or extracted	Whole substance often eaten separately	External use: ○ possible ⊙ mainly (internal caution) ● only	⊙ Do not cook substance ● Refrigerate	Add near end of cooking: ○ last 5 min ⊙ 10 min ● 15 min	Cook 30 - 60 minutes before adding other herbs	Dissolve/steep in strained previously cooked decoction	Wrap in separate porous bag (cheesecloth)	Slice or Crush: ⊙ small pieces ● powder	May be used: ⊙ fresh or dried ● fresh only	May be available in prepared form - less toxic or stronger this way	Available in charred form	Toxic: ⊙ slightly ● very toxic	Contraindicated in pregnancy: ⊙ caution ● never use	Combining Cautions... See page 620	Standard Dosage Range in Grams
Di Yu/ Sanguisorba	✓				○									✓				*10-15*
Dian Di Mai/ Androsace	✓																	*3-9*
Ding Xiang/ Eugenia	✓	○															*3*	*0.5-4.5*
Dong Bei Guan Zhong/ Dryopteris	✓														⊙	●		*6-15*
Dong Chong Xia Cao/ Cordyceps	✓	○		✓														*3-9*
Dong Gua Pi/ Benincasa	✓																	*15-30*
Dong Gua Ren/ Benincasa	✓										⊙							*3-12*
Dong Kui Zi/ Malva	✓															⊙		*9-15*
Dou Chi Jiang/ Litsea	✓																	*1.5-6*
Dou Juan/ Glycine	✓																*5*	*9-15*
Du Huo/ Angelica	✓																	*3-9*
Du Zhong/ Eucommia	✓																	*9-15*
E Bu Shi Cao/ Centipeda	✓																	*3-6*
E Guan Shi/ Stalactitum	✓							✓			⊙							*9-30*
E Jiao/ Equus		○	✓			⊙			✓		●						*57*	*6-15*

Name of herb or substance	Decoction	Powder/Pills taken internally: ○ may be ⊙ commonly ● always	Used with wine or extracted	Whole substance often eaten separately	External use: ○ possible ⊙ mainly (internal caution) ● only	⊙ Do not cook substance ● Refrigerate	Add near end of cooking: ○ last 5 min ⊙ 10 min ● 15 min	Cook 30 - 60 minutes before adding other herbs	Dissolve/steep in strained previously cooked decoction	Wrap in separate porous bag (cheesecloth)	Slice or Crush: ⊙ small pieces ● powder	May be used: ⊙ fresh or dried ● fresh only	May be available in prepared form - less toxic or stronger this way	Available in charred form	Toxic: ⊙ slightly ● very toxic	Contraindicated in pregnancy: ⊙ caution ● never use	Combining Cautions... See page 620	Standard Dosage Range in Grams
E Wei/ Ferula	✓															●		1-2
E Zhu/ Curcuma	✓															●		3-9
Er Cha/ Acacia		●			⊙						●							0.1-0.9
Fan Bai Cao/ Potentilla	✓				○							⊙						9-15
Fan Xie Ye/ Cassia	✓						●									●		3-9
Fang Feng/ Ledebouriella	✓																33	5-9
Fei Zi/ Torreya	✓	⊙																9-15
Feng Mi/ Mel	✓			✓														15-50
Feng Wei Cao/ Pteris	✓				○							⊙						9-18
Fo Shou/ Citrus	✓																	3-9
Fo Shou Hua/ Citrus	✓																	3-6
Fu Hai Shi/ Pumice	✓	○								✓								9-15
Fu Ling/ Poria	✓																44	9-15
Fu Ling Pi/ Poria	✓																	9-15
Fu Long Gan/ Terra Flava Usta	✓									✓								15-60
Fu Pen Zi/ Rubus	✓																	4.5-9
Fu Ping/ Spirodela	✓				○													3-6

Name of herb or substance	Decoction	Powder/Pills taken internally: ○ may be ❂ commonly ● always	Used with wine or extracted	Whole substance often eaten separately	External use: ○ possible ❂ mainly (internal caution) ● only	❂ Do not cook substance ● Refrigerate	Add near end of cooking: ○ last 5 min ❂ 10 min ● 15 min	Cook 30 - 60 minutes before adding other herbs	Dissolve/steep in strained previously cooked decoction	Wrap in separate porous bag (cheesecloth)	Slice or Crush: ❂ small pieces ● powder	May be used: ❂ fresh or dried ● fresh only	May be available in prepared form - less toxic or stronger this way	Available in charred form	Toxic: ❂ slightly ● very toxic	Contraindicated in pregnancy: ❂ caution ● never use	Combining Cautions... See page 620	Standard Dosage Range in Grams
Fu Shen/ Poria	✓																	*9-15*
Fu Xiao Mai/ Triticum	✓																	*9-30*
(Hei) Fu Zi/ Aconitum	✓							✓					✓		●	●	*6*	*3-15*
Gan Cao/ Glycyrrhiza	✓				○												*7*	*3-9*
Gan Jiang/ Zingiber	✓															❂		*3-9*
Gan Sui/ Euphorbia	✓	❂			○								✓		●	●	*43*	*0.5-1*
Gao Ben/ Ligusticum	✓																	*2-10*
Gao Liang Jiang/ Alpinia	✓																	*1.5-9*
Ge Gen/ Pueraria	✓																	*5-20*
Ge Hua/ Pueraria	✓																	*5-9*
Ge Jie/ Gekko	✓	❂																*3-15*
Ge Shan Xiang/ Cynanchum	✓																	
Gou Gu/ Canis	✓	❂	✓	✓				✓										*9-15*
Gou Ji/ Cibotium	✓																*59*	*5-9*
Gou Qi Zi/ Lycium	✓																	*6-18*
Gou Teng/ Uncaria	✓						❂											*6-15*

Name of herb or substance	Decoction	Powder/Pills taken internally: ○ may be ◎ commonly ● always	Used with wine or extracted	Whole substance often eaten separately	External use: ○ possible ◎ mainly (internal caution) ● only	◎ Do not cook substance ● Refrigerate	Add near end of cooking: ○ last 5 min ◎ 10 min ● 15 min	Cook 30 - 60 minutes before adding other herbs	Dissolve/steep in strained previously cooked decoction	Wrap in separate porous bag (cheesecloth)	Slice or Crush: ◎ small pieces ● powder	May be used: ◎ fresh or dried ● fresh only	May be available in prepared form - less toxic or stronger this way	Available in charred form	Toxic: ◎ slightly ● very toxic	Contraindicated in pregnancy: ◎ caution ● never use	Combining Cautions... See page 620	Standard Dosage Range in Grams
Gu Jing Cao/ Eriocaulon	✓																	*6-15*
Gu Sui Bu/ Drynaria	✓				○													*9-15*
Gu Ya/ Oryza						◎			✓		●							*9-15*
Gua Di/ Cucumis	✓	○			○										◎	●		*0.3-1.0*
Gua Lou/ Trichosanthes	✓										◎						*10*	*9-30*
Gua Lou Pi/ Trichosanthes	✓																*10*	*6-12*
Gua Lou Ren/ Trichosanthes	✓										◎						*10*	*9-15*
Guan Ye Liao/ Polygonum	✓																	
Guan Zhong/ Dryopteris	✓														◎	●		*6-16*
Guang Fang Ji/ Aristolochia	✓																	*3-15*
Guang Gou Shen/ Canis		●		✓							●							*3-15*
Gui Ban/ Chinemys	✓							✓			◎					●	*62*	*9-30*
Gui Zhi/ Cinnamomum	✓															◎		*3-15*
Hai Dai/ Laminaria	✓																	*5-15*
Hai Feng Teng/ Piper	✓															●		*6-15*
Hai Ge Ke/ Cyclina	✓	○								✓	●		✓					*1-15*

Name of herb or substance	Decoction	Powder/Pills taken internally: ○ may be ◎ commonly ● always	Used with wine or extracted	Whole substance often eaten separately	External use: ○ possible ◎ mainly (internal caution) ● only	◎ Do not cook substance ● Refrigerate	Add near end of cooking: ○ last 5 min ◎ 10 min ● 15 min	Cook 30 - 60 minutes before adding other herbs	Dissolve/steep in strained previously cooked decoction	Wrap in separate porous bag (cheesecloth)	Slice or Crush: ◎ small pieces ● powder	May be used: ◎ fresh or dried ● fresh only	May be available in prepared form - less toxic or stronger this way	Available in charred form	Toxic: ◎ slightly ● very toxic	Contraindicated in pregnancy: ◎ caution ● never use	Combining Cautions... See page 620	Standard Dosage Range in Grams
Hai Gou Shen/ Phoca		●		✓							●							*3-15*
Hai Jin Sha/ Lygodium	✓									✓								*6-15*
Hai Long/ Solenognathus	✓	◎		✓							◎					●		*1.5-2.4*
Hai Ma/ Hippocampus	✓	◎	✓	✓							◎					●		*3-9*
Hai Piao Xiao/ Sepia	✓				○						◎						*11*	*5-9*
Hai Tong Pi/ Erythrina	✓				○						◎							*6-12*
Hai Zao/ Sargassum	✓																*8*	*5-15*
Han Cai/ Rorippa	✓			✓								◎					*27*	*20-50*
Han Fang Ji/ Stephania	✓																	*5-9*
Han Lian Cao/ Eclipta	✓											◎						*9-30*
Han Shui Shi/ Calcitum	✓				○			✓			●							*9-30*
He Huan Hua/ Albizzia	✓																	*3-9*
He Huan Pi/ Albizzia	✓																	*9-15*
He Shi/ Carpesium	✓	◎													◎			*9-15*
He Shou Wu/ Polygonum	✓																*12*	*9-30*

Name of herb or substance	Decoction	Powder/Pills taken internally: ○ may be ◎ commonly ● always	Used with wine or extracted	Whole substance often eaten separately	External use: ○ possible ◎ mainly (internal caution) ● only	◎ Do not cook substance ● Refrigerate	Add near end of cooking: ○ last 5 min ◎ 10 min ● 15 min	Cook 30 - 60 minutes before adding other herbs	Dissolve/steep in strained previously cooked decoction	Wrap in separate porous bag (cheesecloth)	Slice or Crush: ◎ small pieces ● powder	May be used: ◎ fresh or dried ● fresh only	May be available in prepared form - less toxic or stronger this way	Available in charred form	Toxic: ◎ slightly ● very toxic	Contraindicated in pregnancy: ◎ caution ● never use	Combining Cautions... See page 620	Standard Dosage Range in Grams
He Zi/ Terminalia	✓										◎							*3-9*
Hei Lu Shen/ Equus		●		✓							●							*3-15*
Hei Zhi Ma/ Sesamum	✓																	*9-30*
Hong Hua/ Carthamus	✓						●									●		*3-9*
Hong Teng/ Sargentodoxa	✓		✓													◎		*15-30*
Hou Po/ Magnolia	✓															◎	*50*	*3-9*
Hou Po Hua/ Magnolia	✓																	*3-6*
Hou Zao/ Macaca		●		✓							●							*0.3-1*
Hu Er Cao/ Saxifraga	✓				○							◎			◎			*9-15*
Hu Gu/ Panthera	✓	◎	✓	✓	○						◎							*3-6*
Hu Huang Lian/ Picrorhiza	✓																	*3-9*
Hu Jiao/ Piper	✓																	*2-3*
Hu Lu Ba/ Trigonella	✓															●		*3-9*
Hu Po/ Succinum		●			○						●							*1.5-3*
Hu Tao Ren/ Juglans	✓			✓														*9-30*
Hu Tui Ye/ Eleagnus	✓																	*9-15*

Name of herb or substance	Decoction	Powder/Pills taken internally: ○ may be ◎ commonly ● always	Used with wine or extracted	Whole substance often eaten separately	External use: ○ possible ◎ mainly (internal caution) ● only	◎ Do not cook substance ● Refrigerate	Add near end of cooking: ○ last 5 min ◎ 10 min ● 15 min	Cook 30 - 60 minutes before adding other herbs	Dissolve/steep in strained previously cooked decoction	Wrap in separate porous bag (cheesecloth)	Slice or Crush: ◎ small pieces ● powder	May be used: ◎ fresh or dried ● fresh only	May be available in prepared form - less toxic or stronger this way	Available in charred form	Toxic: ◎ slightly ● very toxic	Contraindicated in pregnancy: ◎ caution ● never use	Combining Cautions... See page 620	Standard Dosage Range in Grams
Hu Zhang/ Polygonum	✓				○							◎				●		6-12
Hua Lu Shen/ Cervus		●		✓							●							6-15
Hua Rui Shi/ Ophicalcitum		◎	✓		○	◎					●					●		3-9
Hua Sheng Yi/ Arachis	✓																	6-10
Hua Shi/ Talcum	✓				○					✓	●					◎		9-12
Huai Hua Mi/ Sophora	✓													✓				6-15
Huai Jiao/ Sophora	✓															●		6-15
Huai Niu Xi/ Achyranthes	✓	○	✓													●	54	9-15
Huang Bai/ Phellodendron	✓				○													3-12
Huang Jing/ Polygonatum	✓																	9-15
Huang Lian/ Coptis	✓	○			○												41	1.5-9
Huang Qi/ Astragalus	✓				○													9-25
Huang Qin/ Scutellaria	✓																40	6-15
Huang Yao Zi/ Dioscorea	✓	◎	✓		○										◎			4.5-9
Huo Ma Ren/ Cannabis	✓										◎							9-15

Name of herb or substance	Decoction	Powder/Pills taken internally: ○ may be ❂ commonly ● always	Used with wine or extracted	Whole substance often eaten separately	External use: ○ possible ❂ mainly (internal caution) ● only	❂ Do not cook substance ● Refrigerate	Add near end of cooking: ○ last 5 min ❂ 10 min ● 15 min	Cook 30 - 60 minutes before adding other herbs	Dissolve/steep in strained previously cooked decoction	Wrap in separate porous bag (cheesecloth)	Slice or Crush: ❂ small pieces ● powder	May be used: ❂ fresh or dried ● fresh only	May be available in prepared form - less toxic or stronger this way	Available in charred form	Toxic: ❂ slightly ● very toxic	Contraindicated in pregnancy: ❂ caution ● never use	Combining Cautions... See page 620	Standard Dosage Range in Grams
Huo Xiang/ Agastache	✓						●											*4.5-9*
Ji Cai/ Capsella	✓											❂						*9-15*
Ji Gu Cao/ Abrus	✓											❂						*9-15*
Ji Guan Hua/ Celosia	✓																	*10-15*
Ji Mu/ Loropetalum	✓																	*20-100*
Ji Nei Jin/ Gallus	✓	❂																*1.5-9*
Ji Ning/ Salvia	✓																	*9-15*
Ji Shi Teng/ Paederia	✓				○													*9-15*
Ji Xue Teng/ Millettia	✓																	*9-15*
Jiang Can/ Bombyx	✓	❂									●							*1-9*
Jiang Huang/ Curcuma	✓				○											❂		*3-9*
Jiang Xiang/ Dalbergia	✓	○			○													*1.5-9*
(Ku) Jie Geng/ Platycodon	✓																5	*3-6*
Jin Guo Lan/ Tinospora	✓				○													*3-9*
Jin Qian Cao/ Lysimachia	✓			✓								❂						*15-60*
Jin Sha Teng/ Lygodium	✓				○													*15-60*

Name of herb or substance	Decoction	Powder/Pills taken internally: ○ may be ◎ commonly ● always	Used with wine or extracted	Whole substance often eaten separately	External use: ○ possible ◎ mainly (internal caution) ● only	◎ Do not cook substance ● Refrigerate	Add near end of cooking: ○ last 5 min ◎ 10 min ● 15 min	Cook 30 - 60 minutes before adding other herbs	Dissolve/steep in strained previously cooked decoction	Wrap in separate porous bag (cheesecloth)	Slice or Crush: ◎ small pieces ● powder	May be used: ◎ fresh or dried ● fresh only	May be available in prepared form - less toxic or stronger this way	Available in charred form	Toxic: ◎ slightly ● very toxic	Contraindicated in pregnancy: ◎ caution ● never use	Combining Cautions... See page 620	Standard Dosage Range in Grams
Jin Yin Hua/ Lonicera	✓																	*9-15*
Jin Yin Teng/ Lonicera	✓																	*15-30*
Jin Ying Zi/ Rosa	✓																	*5-9*
Jing Da Ji/ Euphorbia	✓	◎													●	●	*13*	*1-3*
Jing Jie/ Schizonepeta	✓						◎											*4.5-9*
Jing Mi/ Oryza	✓			✓														*50-100*
Jing Tian San Qi/ Sedum	✓				○							◎						*9-15*
Jiu Jie Chang Pu/ Anemone	✓																	*2-4.5*
Jiu Xiang Chong/ Aspongopus	✓										●							*3-6*
Jiu Zi/ Allium	✓																	*3-9*
Ju He/ Citrus	✓																	*3-9*
Ju Hong/ Citrus	✓																	*2-4.5*
Ju Hua/ Chrysanthemum	✓																	*4.5-15*
Ju Ye San Qi/ Gynura	✓	○			○													*6-9*
Jue Ming Zi/ Cassia	✓																*14*	*9-15*
Ku Lian Gen Pi/ Melia	✓				○										◎			*6-15*

Name of herb or substance	Decoction	Powder/Pills taken internally: ○ may be ⊙ commonly ● always	Used with wine or extracted	Whole substance often eaten separately	External use: ○ possible ⊙ mainly (internal caution) ● only	⊙ Do not cook substance ● Refrigerate	Add near end of cooking: ○ last 5 min ⊙ 10 min ● 15 min	Cook 30 - 60 minutes before adding other herbs	Dissolve/steep in strained previously cooked decoction	Wrap in separate porous bag (cheesecloth)	Slice or Crush: ⊙ small pieces ● powder	May be used: ⊙ fresh or dried ● fresh only	May be available in prepared form - less toxic or stronger this way	Available in charred form	Toxic: ⊙ slightly ● very toxic	Contraindicated in pregnancy: ⊙ caution ● never use	Combining Cautions... See page 620	Standard Dosage Range in Grams
Ku Lian Mu Pi/ Melia	✓				○										⊙			*6-15*
Ku Shen/ Sophora	✓	⊙	✓		○												*42*	*3-15*
Kuan Dong Hua/ Tussilago	✓																*49*	*3-9*
Kuan Jin Teng/ Tinospora	✓				○											●		*15-30*
Kun Bu/ Laminaria	✓																	*4.5-15*
Lai Fu Zi/ Raphanus	✓																	*6-12*
Lao Guan Cao/ Geranium	✓				○													*9-30*
Lei Wan/ Omphalia		⊙		✓							●				⊙		*68*	*6-9*
Li Lu/ Veratrum		●			⊙										●	●	*15*	*0.3-0.9*
Li Pi/ Pyrus	✓		✓									⊙						*9-15*
Li Zhi He/ Litchi	✓										⊙							*6-15*
Lian Fang/ Nelumbo	✓											⊙		✓				*4.5-9*
Lian Geng/ Nelumbo	✓																	*9-15*
Lian Qiao/ Forsythia	✓																	*6-16*
Lian Xin/ Nelumbo	✓																	*1.5-6*
Lian Xu/ Nelumbo	✓																*16*	*1.5-9*

Name of herb or substance	Decoction	Powder/Pills taken internally: ○ may be ◎ commonly ● always	Used with wine or extracted	Whole substance often eaten separately	External use: ○ possible ◎ mainly (internal caution) ● only	◎ Do not cook substance ● Refrigerate	Add near end of cooking: ○ last 5 min ◎ 10 min ● 15 min	Cook 30 - 60 minutes before adding other herbs	Dissolve/steep in strained previously cooked decoction	Wrap in separate porous bag (cheesecloth)	Slice or Crush: ◎ small pieces ● powder	May be used: ◎ fresh or dried ● fresh only	May be available in prepared form - less toxic or stronger this way	Available in charred form	Toxic: ◎ slightly ● very toxic	Contraindicated in pregnancy: ◎ caution ● never use	Combining Cautions... See page 620	Standard Dosage Range in Grams
Lian Zi/ Nelumbo	✓										◎							*6-15*
Ling Yang Jiao/ Saiga	✓	◎						✓			◎							*1.5-3*
Ling Zhi/ Ganoderma	✓	◎	✓	✓							◎							*3-15*
Liu Huang/ Sulphur		●			◎	◎									◎	●	*52*	*0.15-0.6*
Liu Ji Nu/ Artemisia	✓				○													*5-9*
Long Chi/ Dens Draconis	✓							✓			◎							*9-15*
Long Dan Cao/ Gentiana	✓																	*3-9*
Long Gu/ Os Draconis	✓				○			✓			◎		✓					*9-30*
Long Yan Rou/ Euphoria	✓			✓														*6-15*
Lou Gu/ Gryllotalpa	✓	○	✓								●				◎			*3-4.5*
Lou Lu/ Rhaponticum	✓															●		*3-12*
Lu Dou/ Phaseolus	✓			✓	○													*25-50*
Lu Feng Fang/ Polistes	✓				◎										●		*65*	*1.5-3*
Lu Gan Shi/ Smithsonitum					●								✓		●			
Lu Gen/ Phragmites	✓											◎						*15-30*
Lu Hui/ Aloe		●			○	◎					●					●		*0.3-1.5*

Name of herb or substance	Decoction	Powder/Pills taken internally: ○ may be ◎ commonly ● always	Used with wine or extracted	Whole substance often eaten separately	External use: ○ possible ◎ mainly (internal caution) ● only	◎ Do not cook substance ● Refrigerate	Add near end of cooking: ○ last 5 min ◎ 10 min ● 15 min	Cook 30 - 60 minutes before adding other herbs	Dissolve/steep in strained previously cooked decoction	Wrap in separate porous bag (cheesecloth)	Slice or Crush: ◎ small pieces ● powder	May be used: ◎ fresh or dried ● fresh only	May be available in prepared form - less toxic or stronger this way	Available in charred form	Toxic: ◎ slightly ● very toxic	Contraindicated in pregnancy: ○ caution ● never use	Combining Cautions... See page 620	Standard Dosage Range in Grams
Lu Jiao/ Cervus	✓	◎		✓	○			✓			◎							*4.5-9*
Lu Jiao Jiao/ Cervus		◎	✓	✓		◎			✓		●							*6-12*
Lu Jiao Shuang/ Cervus	✓				○						●		✓					*15-30*
Lu Lu Tong/ Liquidambar	✓				○											●		*3-9*
Lu Rong/ Cervus	✓	◎	✓	✓							◎							*1-4.5*
Lu Xian Cao/ Pyrola	✓				○													*15-30*
Lu Ying/ Sambucus	✓				○													*9-15*
Luo Bu Ma/ Apocynum	✓																	*6-9*
Luo Han Guo/ Momordica	✓			✓														*9-15*
Luo Han Ye/ Momordica																		
Luo Shi Teng/ Trachelo-spermum	✓																*47*	*6-15*
Ma Bian Cao/ Verbena	✓				○							◎				●		*9-30*
Ma Bo/ Lasiosphaera	✓				○					✓								*1.5-3*
Ma Chi Xian/ Portulaca	✓				○							◎				●		*15-60*
Ma Dou Ling/ Aristolochia	✓																	*3-9*

Name of herb or substance	Decoction	Powder/Pills taken internally: ○ may be ◉ commonly ● always	Used with wine or extracted	Whole substance often eaten separately	External use: ○ possible ◉ mainly (internal caution) ● only	◉ Do not cook substance ● Refrigerate	Add near end of cooking: ○ last 5 min ◉ 10 min ● 15 min	Cook 30 - 60 minutes before adding other herbs	Dissolve/steep in strained previously cooked decoction	Wrap in separate porous bag (cheesecloth)	Slice or Crush: ◉ small pieces ● powder	May be used: ◉ fresh or dried ● fresh only	May be available in prepared form - less toxic or stronger this way	Available in charred form	Toxic: ◉ slightly ● very toxic	Contraindicated in pregnancy: ◉ caution ● never use	Combining Cautions... See page 620	Standard Dosage Range in Grams
Ma Huang/ Ephedra	✓																	*3-9*
Ma Huang Gen/ Ephedra	✓																	*3-9*
Ma Qian Zi/ Strychnos		○			◉						●				●	●		*0.3-0.6*
Mai Men Dong/ Ophiopogon	✓																*61*	*6-12*
Mai Ya/ Hordeum	✓	◉							✓									*9-30*
Man Jing Zi/ Vitex	✓		✓														*36*	*6-9*
Man Shan Hong/ Rhododendron	✓				○													*25-50*
Mang Xiao/ Mirabilitum	✓	○			○				✓							●		*4.5-9*
Mao Dong Qing/ Ilex	✓																	*30-60*
Mao Mei/ Rubus	✓				○							◉						*15-60*
Mao Zhao Cao/ Ranunculus	✓																	*20-50*
Mei Gui Hua/ Rosa	✓		✓															*3-6*
Meng Chong/ Tabanus	✓	○									●				◉	●		*1.5-3*
Meng Shi/ Lapis Micae seu Chloriti	✓	○						✓		✓	●		✓			●		*1.5-3*

Name of herb or substance	Decoction	Powder/Pills taken internally: ○ may be ◎ commonly ● always	Used with wine or extracted	Whole substance often eaten separately	External use: ○ possible ◎ mainly (internal caution) ● only	◎ Do not cook substance ● Refrigerate	Add near end of cooking: ○ last 5 min ◎ 10 min ● 15 min	Cook 30 - 60 minutes before adding other herbs	Dissolve/steep in strained previously cooked decoction	Wrap in separate porous bag (cheesecloth)	Slice or Crush: ◎ small pieces ● powder	May be used: ◎ fresh or dried ● fresh only	May be available in prepared form - less toxic or stronger this way	Available in charred form	Toxic: ◎ slightly ● very toxic	Contraindicated in pregnancy: ◎ caution ● never use	Combining Cautions... See page 620	Standard Dosage Range in Grams
Mi Meng Hua/ Buddleia	✓																	*3-9*
Mi Tuo Seng/ Lithargyrum		○			◎										●			*0.3-1*
Mian Hua Gen/ Gossypium	✓															●		*50-100*
Ming Dang Shen/ Changium	✓															●		*6-9*
Ming Fan/ Alumen		○			◎						●				◎		*67*	*0.5-3*
Mo Yao/ Commiphora	✓				○											●		*3-12*
Mu Bie Zi/ Momordica		○			◎										●	●		*0.6-1.2*
Mu Dan Pi/ Paeonia	✓															●	*38*	*6-12*
Mu Gua/ Chaenomeles	✓																	*4.5-12*
Mu Hu Die/ Oroxylum	✓				○													*1.5-6*
Mu Li/ Ostrea	✓							✓			◎		✓				*17*	*15-30*
Mu Tong/ Akebia	✓															●		*3-9*
Mu Xiang/ Saussurea	✓						○											*1.5-9*
Mu Zei/ Equisetum	✓				○											◎		*3-9*
Nan Gua Zi/ Cucurbita	✓	○										◎						*30-60*

Name of herb or substance	Decoction	Powder/Pills taken internally: ○ may be ◎ commonly ● always	Used with wine or extracted	Whole substance often eaten separately	External use: ○ possible ◎ mainly (internal caution) ● only	◎ Do not cook substance ● Refrigerate	Add near end of cooking: ○ last 5 min ◎ 10 min ● 15 min	Cook 30 - 60 minutes before adding other herbs	Dissolve/steep in strained previously cooked decoction	Wrap in separate porous bag (cheesecloth)	Slice or Crush: ◎ small pieces ● powder	May be used: ◎ fresh or dried ● fresh only	May be available in prepared form - less toxic or stronger this way	Available in charred form	Toxic: ◎ slightly ● very toxic	Contraindicated in pregnancy: ◎ caution ● never use	Combining Cautions... See page 620	Standard Dosage Range in Grams
Nan Sha Shen/ Adenophora	✓																4	9-15
Niu Bang Zi/ Arctium	✓																	4.5-9
Niu Dan/ Bos		●			○													
Niu Huang/ Bos		●		✓	○	◎					●					●	20	0.15-1
Nu Zhen Zi/ Ligustrum	✓																	4.5-15
Nuo Dao Gen/ Oryza	✓																	25-50
Ou Jie/ Nelumbo	✓											◎						9-15
Pang Da Hai/ Sterculia	✓				○													4.5-9
Pao Jiang/ Zingiber	✓															◎		3-6
Pei Lan/ Eupatorium	✓																	5-9
Peng Sha/ Borax		○			◎						●					●		1.5-3
Pi Pa Ye/ Eriobotrya	✓											◎						4.5-9
Pi Shi/ Arsenolite					●										●	●		0.03-0.08
Pu Gong Ying/ Taraxacum	✓				○							◎						9-30
Pu Huang/ Typha	✓			✓	○					✓	●			✓		◎		4.5-9
Pu Hui/ Typha	✓													✓				

Name of herb or substance	Decoction	Powder/Pills taken internally: ○ may be ◉ commonly ● always	Used with wine or extracted	Whole substance often eaten separately	External use: ○ possible ◉ mainly (internal caution) ● only	◉ Do not cook substance ● Refrigerate	Add near end of cooking: ○ last 5 min ◉ 10 min ● 15 min	Cook 30 - 60 minutes before adding other herbs	Dissolve/steep in strained previously cooked decoction	Wrap in separate porous bag (cheesecloth)	Slice or Crush: ◉ small pieces ● powder	May be used: ◉ fresh or dried ● fresh only	May be available in prepared form - less toxic or stronger this way	Available in charred form	Toxic: ◉ slightly ● very toxic	Contraindicated in pregnancy: ◉ caution ● never use	Combining Cautions... See page 620	Standard Dosage Range in Grams
Qian Cao Gen/ Rubia	✓																	6-9
Qian Dan/ Minium		○			◉										●			0.3-0.6
Qian Hu/ Peucedanum	✓																4	4.5-9
Qian Li Guang/ Senecio	✓											◉						9-15
Qian Niu Zi/ Pharbitis	✓	○													◉	●		1.5-9
Qian Shi/ Euryale	✓										◉							9-15
Qiang Huo/ Notopterygium	✓																	6-15
Qiao Mai/ Fagopyrum	✓																	3-50
Qin Jiao/ Gentiana	✓																	4.5-9
Qin Pi/ Fraxinus	✓																	4.5-9
Qing Dai/ Indigo		◉			○				✓									1.5-2.5
Qing Fen/ Calomelas		○			◉						●				●	●		0.06-0.15
Qing Hao/ Artemisia	✓																18	4.5-9
Qing Mu Xiang/ Aristolochia	✓																	3-9
Qing Pi/ Citrus	✓						●											3-9
Qing Xiang Zi/ Celosia	✓																	9-15

Name of herb or substance	Decoction	Powder/Pills taken internally: ○ may be ʘ commonly ● always	Used with wine or extracted	Whole substance often eaten separately	External use: ○ possible ʘ mainly (internal caution) ● only	ʘ Do not cook substance ● Refrigerate	Add near end of cooking: ○ last 5 min ʘ 10 min ● 15 min	Cook 30 - 60 minutes before adding other herbs	Dissolve/steep in strained previously cooked decoction	Wrap in separate porous bag (cheesecloth)	Slice or Crush: ʘ small pieces ● powder	May be used: ʘ fresh or dried ● fresh only	May be available in prepared form - less toxic or stronger this way	Available in charred form	Toxic: ʘ slightly ● very toxic	Contraindicated in pregnancy: ʘ caution ● never use	Combining Cautions... See page 620	Standard Dosage Range in Grams
Qu Mai/ Dianthus	✓															●	45	6-12
Quan Xie/ Buthus	✓	ʘ			○						●				●			0.6-0.9
Ren Shen/ Panax	✓	○		✓									✓				19	1.5-9
Ren Shen Lu/ Panax	✓																	3-9
Ren Shen Ye/ Panax	✓																	3-9
Rou Cong Rong/ Cistanche	✓																	9-21
Rou Dou Kou/ Myristica	✓										ʘ				ʘ			1.5-9
Rou Gui/ Cinnamomum	✓	ʘ	✓				○		✓		●					ʘ	31	1.5-4.5
Ru Xiang/ Boswellia	✓				○											●		3-9
San Bai Cao/ Saururus	✓				○													9-15
San Leng/ Sparganium	✓															●	53	4.5-9
San Qi/ Panax	✓	ʘ		✓	○											●		1-9
San Qi Hua/ Panax	✓																	6-15
Sang Bai Pi/ Morus	✓																	6-15
Sang Ji Sheng/ Loranthus	✓																	9-30

Name of herb or substance	Decoction	Powder/Pills taken internally: ○ may be ◎ commonly ● always	Used with wine or extracted	Whole substance often eaten separately	External use: ○ possible ◎ mainly (internal caution) ● only	◎ Do not cook substance ● Refrigerate	Add near end of cooking: ○ last 5 min ◎ 10 min ● 15 min	Cook 30 - 60 minutes before adding other herbs	Dissolve/steep in strained previously cooked decoction	Wrap in separate porous bag (cheesecloth)	Slice or Crush: ◎ small pieces ● powder	May be used: ◎ fresh or dried ● fresh only	May be available in prepared form - less toxic or stronger this way	Available in charred form	Toxic: ◎ slightly ● very toxic	Contraindicated in pregnancy: ◎ caution ● never use	Combining Cautions... See page 620	Standard Dosage Range in Grams
Sang Piao Xiao/ Paratenodera	✓	◎															34	*5-9*
Sang Shen/ Morus	✓																	*9-15*
Sang Ye/ Morus	✓				○													*5-15*
Sang Zhi/ Morus	✓																	*10-30*
Sha Ren/ Amomum	✓						○				◎							*1.5-6*
Sha Ren Ke/ Amomum	✓				○		○				◎							*2.5-4.5*
Sha Yuan Ji Li/ Astragalus	✓																	*6-15*
Shan Ci Gu/ Tulipa	✓				◎						◎				●			*3-9*
Shan Dou Gen/ Sophora	✓				○													*3-9*
Shan Li Hong/ Crataegus	✓																	*3-9*
Shan Yang Jiao/ Naemorhedis	✓	◎		✓				✓			◎							*9-15*
Shan Yao/ Dioscorea	✓																	*9-30*
Shan Zha/ Crataegus	✓																	*9-15*
Shan Zha Rou/ Crataegus	✓																	*12-15*
Shan Zha Tan/ Crataegus	✓														✓			*12-15*

Name of herb or substance	Decoction	Powder/Pills taken internally: ○ may be ◉ commonly ● always	Used with wine or extracted	Whole substance often eaten separately	External use: ○ possible ◉ mainly (internal caution) ● only	◉ Do not cook substance ● Refrigerate	Add near end of cooking: ○ last 5 min ◉ 10 min ● 15 min	Cook 30 - 60 minutes before adding other herbs	Dissolve/steep in strained previously cooked decoction	Wrap in separate porous bag (cheesecloth)	Slice or Crush: ◉ small pieces ● powder	May be used: ◉ fresh or dried ● fresh only	May be available in prepared form - less toxic or stronger this way	Available in charred form	Toxic: ◉ slightly ● very toxic	Contraindicated in pregnancy: ◉ caution ● never use	Combining Cautions... See page 620	Standard Dosage Range in Grams
Shan Zhu Yu/ Cornus	✓																*64*	*3-12*
Shang Lu/ Phytolacca	✓				○							◉			●	●		*4.5-9*
She Chuang Zi/ Cnidium	✓	○			◉												*69*	*3-9*
She Gan/ Belamcanda	✓															●		*1.5-9*
She Xiang/ Moschus		●		✓	○	◉					●					●		*0.06-0.15*
She Tui/ Zaocys	✓	○														●		*0.3-3*
Shen Jin Cao/ Lycopodium	✓															●		*9-15*
Shen Qu/ Massa Fermentata	✓	○											✓			◉		*6-12*
Sheng Di Huang/ Rehmannia	✓											◉				◉		*9-30*
Sheng Jiang/ Zingiber	✓				○							●						*3-9*
Sheng Jiang Pi/ Zingiber	✓											●						*3-9*
Sheng Ma/ Cimicifuga	✓																	*1.5-9*
Sheng Tie Luo/ Frusta Ferri	✓							✓			◉							*9-30*
Shi Chang Pu/ Acorus	✓	○			○							◉					*67*	*3-9*
Shi Da Gong Lao/ Mahonia	✓																	*6-9*

Name of herb or substance	Decoction	Powder/Pills taken internally: ○ may be ◎ commonly ● always	Used with wine or extracted	Whole substance often eaten separately	External use: ○ possible ◎ mainly (internal caution) ● only	◎ Do not cook substance ● Refrigerate	Add near end of cooking: ○ last 5 min ◎ 10 min ● 15 min	Cook 30 - 60 minutes before adding other herbs	Dissolve/steep in strained previously cooked decoction	Wrap in separate porous bag (cheesecloth)	Slice or Crush: ◎ small pieces ● powder	May be used: ◎ fresh or dried ● fresh only	May be available in prepared form - less toxic or stronger this way	Available in charred form	Toxic: ◎ slightly ● very toxic	Contraindicated in pregnancy: ◎ caution ● never use	Combining Cautions... See page 620	Standard Dosage Range in Grams
Shi Di/ Diospyros	✓																	6-12
Shi Gao/ Gypsum	✓				○			✓			◎							9-30
Shi Hu/ Dendrobium	✓																32	6-15
Shi Jue Ming/ Haliotis	✓	○			○			✓			◎						34	9-30
Shi Jun Zi/ Quisqualis	✓										◎	◎			◎			4.5-12
Shi Liu Gen Pi/ Punica	✓														◎			1.5-9
Shi Liu Pi/ Punica	✓														◎		21	3-9
Shi Shang Bai/ Selaginella	✓			✓														15-30
Shi Wei/ Pyrrosia	✓																	4.5-9
Shu Di Huang/ Rehmannia	✓																	9-30
Shu Qi/ Dichroa	✓														◎			3-6
Shu Yi Ren/ Coix	✓																	9-30
Shui Niu Jiao/ Bubalus	✓	◎		✓				✓								◎		6-120
Shui Yin/ Hydrargyrum					●										●	●	22	
Shui Zhi/ Hirudo		●									●				◎	●		1.5-3
Si Gua Luo/ Luffa	✓																	6-12

S

Name of herb or substance	Decoction	Powder/Pills taken internally: ○ may be ◎ commonly ● always	Used with wine or extracted	Whole substance often eaten separately	External use: ○ possible ◎ mainly (internal caution) ● only	◎ Do not cook substance ● Refrigerate	Add near end of cooking: ○ last 5 min ◎ 10 min ● 15 min	Cook 30 - 60 minutes before adding other herbs	Dissolve/steep in strained previously cooked decoction	Wrap in separate porous bag (cheesecloth)	Slice or Crush: ◎ small pieces ● powder	May be used: ◎ fresh or dried ● fresh only	May be available in prepared form - less toxic or stronger this way	Available in charred form	Toxic: ◎ slightly ● very toxic	Contraindicated in pregnancy: ◎ caution ● never use	Combining Cautions... See page 620	Standard Dosage Range in Grams
Song Jie/ Pinus	✓										◎							*9-15*
Su He Xiang/ Liquidambar		●			○													*0.3-1*
Su Mu/ Caesalpinia	✓										◎					●		*3-9*
Suan Jiang/ Physalis	✓				○							◎				◎		*9-15*
Suan Zao Ren/ Ziziphus	✓	○									◎							*1.5-18*
Suo Yang/ Cynomorium	✓	○																*5-15*
Tai Zi Shen/ Pseudostellaria	✓																*4*	*9-30*
Tan Xiang/ Santalum	✓	○					●				◎							*1.5-9*
Tang Song Cao/ Thalictrum	✓																	*3-9*
Tao Ren/ Prunus	✓										◎					●		*5-9*
Tian Hua Fen/ Trichosanthes	✓				○											●		*9-15*
Tian Ma/ Gastrodia	✓	○																*0.9-9*
Tian Men Dong/ Asparagus	✓																	*6-15*
Tian Nan Xing/ Arisaema	✓	●			◎						●				●	●	*23*	*0.3-1*
Tian Zhu Huang/ Bambusa	✓	○																*0.6-9*

Name of herb or substance	Decoction	Powder/Pills taken internally: ○ may be ◉ commonly ● always	Used with wine or extracted	Whole substance often eaten separately	External use: ○ possible ◉ mainly (internal caution) ● only	◉ Do not cook substance ● Refrigerate	Add near end of cooking: ○ last 5 min ◉ 10 min ● 15 min	Cook 30 - 60 minutes before adding other herbs	Dissolve/steep in strained previously cooked decoction	Wrap in separate porous bag (cheesecloth)	Slice or Crush: ◉ small pieces ● powder	May be used: ◉ fresh or dried ● fresh only	May be available in prepared form - less toxic or stronger this way	Available in charred form	Toxic: ◉ slightly ● very toxic	Contraindicated in pregnancy: ◉ caution ● never use	Combining Cautions... See page 620	Standard Dosage Range in Grams
Tie Xian/ Acalypha	✓				○							◉				●		*9-15*
Ting Li Zi/ Lepidium	✓									✓								*4.5-9*
Tong Cao/ Tetrapanax	✓															◉		*3-6*
Tu Bie Chong/ Eupolyphaga	✓	○			○						●				◉	●		*1-6*
Tu Fu Ling/ Smilax	✓																	*15-60*
Tu Niu Xi/ Achyranthes	✓															●		*15-30*
Tu Si Zi/ Cuscuta	✓															◉		*9-15*
Wa Leng Zi/ Arca	✓							✓			◉							*9-15*
Wan Nian Qing/ Rhodea	✓											◉			◉			*3-9*
Wang Bu Liu Xing/ Vaccaria	✓															●		*4.5-9*
Wei Jiang/ Zingiber	✓															◉		*6-12*
Wei Ling Xian/ Clematis	✓		✓															*6-12*
Wu Bei Zi/ Rhus/ Melaphis	✓	◉			○													*1-6*
Wu Gong/ Scolopendra	✓	◉			○						●				●	●		*0.6-3*
Wu Jia Pi/ Acanthopanax	✓		✓															*4.5-15*

Name of herb or substance	Decoction	Powder/Pills taken internally: ○ may be ◎ commonly ● always	Used with wine or extracted	Whole substance often eaten separately	External use: ○ possible ◎ mainly (internal caution) ● only	◎ Do not cook substance ● Refrigerate	Add near end of cooking: ○ last 5 min ◎ 10 min ● 15 min	Cook 30 - 60 minutes before adding other herbs	Dissolve/steep in strained previously cooked decoction	Wrap in separate porous bag (cheesecloth)	Slice or Crush: ◎ small pieces ● powder	May be used: ◎ fresh or dried ● fresh only	May be available in prepared form - less toxic or stronger this way	Available in charred form	Toxic: ◎ slightly ● very toxic	Contraindicated in pregnancy: ◎ caution ● never use	Combining Cautions... See page 620	Standard Dosage Range in Grams
Wu Jiu Gen Pi/ Sapium	✓														◎	●		*4.5-9*
Wu Ling Zhi/ Trogopterus	✓									✓						◎	*24*	*4.5-9*
Wu Mei/ Prunus	✓				○													*3-9*
Wu Shao She/ Zaocys	✓	◎		✓														*3-9*
Wu Tou/ Aconitum	✓				○			✓					✓		●	●	*25*	*3-9*
Wu Wei Zi/ Schisandra	✓		✓															*1.5-9*
Wu Yao/ Lindera	✓																	*4.5-9*
Wu Zhi Mao Tao/ Ficus	✓																	
Wu Zhu Yu/ Evodia	✓														◎		*55*	*3-9*
Xi Gua/ Citrullus	✓					◎						●						*1 cup juice*
Xi Hong Hua/ Crocus	✓															●		*0.9-1.5*
Xi Jiao/ Rhinoceros		●		✓												◎	*9*	*1-2*
Xi Xian Cao/ Siegesbeckia	✓		✓															*9-15*
Xi Xin/ Asarum	✓				○												*35*	*1-3*
Xi Yang Shen/ Panax	✓			✓													*4*	*2.5-9*
Xia Ku Cao/ Prunella	✓																	*6-15*

Name of herb or substance	Decoction	Powder/Pills taken internally: ○ may be ◎ commonly ● always	Used with wine or extracted	Whole substance often eaten separately	External use: ○ possible ◎ mainly (internal caution) ● only	◎ Do not cook substance ● Refrigerate	Add near end of cooking: ○ last 5 min ◎ 10 min ● 15 min	Cook 30 - 60 minutes before adding other herbs	Dissolve/steep in strained previously cooked decoction	Wrap in separate porous bag (cheesecloth)	Slice or Crush: ◎ small pieces ● powder	May be used: ◎ fresh or dried ● fresh only	May be available in prepared form - less toxic or stronger this way	Available in charred form	Toxic: ◎ slightly ● very toxic	Contraindicated in pregnancy: ◎ caution ● never use	Combining Cautions... See page 620	Standard Dosage Range in Grams
Xian He Cao/ Agrimonia	✓				○							◎						*9-15*
Xian Mao/ Curculigo	✓		✓												◎			*4.5-9*
Xiang Fu/ Cyperus	✓																	*4.5-12*
Xiang Ru/ Elsholtzia	✓						○											*3-9*
Xiao Hui Xiang/ Foeniculum	✓				○													*3-9*
Xiao Ji/ Cephalanoplos	✓				○							◎						*10-15*
Xie Bai/ Allium	✓											◎						*4.5-9*
Xin Yi Hua/ Magnolia	✓	○			○					✓								*3-9*
(Ku) Xing Ren/ Prunus	✓										◎				◎		*48*	*3-9*
(Tian) Xing Ren/ Prunus	✓										◎				◎			*3-9*
Xiong Dan/ Ursus		●		✓	○						●						*26*	*1-2.5*
Xiong Huang/ Realgar		●			◎						●				●	●		*0.15-0.6*
Xu Duan/ Dipsacus	✓				○												*58*	*6-21*
Xu Sui Zi/ Euphorbia		●													◎	●		*1.5-3*
Xuan Fu Hua/ Inula	✓									✓								*3-12*
Xuan Ming Fen/ Mirabilitum					●	◎												

X, Y

Name of herb or substance	Decoction	Powder/Pills taken internally: ○ may be ◎ commonly ● always	Used with wine or extracted	Whole substance often eaten separately	External use: ○ possible ◎ mainly (internal caution) ● only	◎ Do not cook substance ● Refrigerate	Add near end of cooking: ○ last 5 min ◎ 10 min ● 15 min	Cook 30 - 60 minutes before adding other herbs	Dissolve/steep in strained previously cooked decoction	Wrap in separate porous bag (cheesecloth)	Slice or Crush: ◎ small pieces ● powder	May be used: ◎ fresh or dried ● fresh only	May be available in prepared form - less toxic or stronger this way	Available in charred form	Toxic: ◎ slightly ● very toxic	Contraindicated in pregnancy: ◎ caution ● never use	Combining Cautions... See page 620	Standard Dosage Range in Grams
Xuan Shen/ Scrophularia	✓																29	*9-30*
Xue Jie/ Dracaena		●			○											●		*0.3-1.5*
Xue Yu Tan/ HomoSapiens	✓	◎			○									✓				*1.5-9*
Xun Gu Feng/ Aristolochia	✓																	*9-15*
Ya Dan Zi/ Brucea		●			○										●	◎		*10-30 pieces*
Ya Zhi Cao/ Commelina	✓				○							◎						*9-15*
Yan Fu Mu/ Rhus	✓				○													*9-15*
Yan Hu Suo/ Corydalis	✓	○														●		*4.5-12*
Yang Qi Shi/ Actinolitum		●											✓				60	*3-4.5*
Ye Jiao Teng/ Polygonum	✓				○													*9-30*
Ye Ju Hua/ Chrysanthemum	✓				○													*6-12*
Ye Ming Sha/ Vespertilio	✓															◎	37	*3 0*
Yi Mu Cao/ Leonurus	✓															●		*9-30*
Yi Tang/ Saccharum Granorum						◎			✓									*30-60*
Yi Yi Ren/ Coix	✓										◎					◎		*9-30*

Name of herb or substance	Decoction	Powder/Pills taken internally: ○ may be ◎ commonly ● always	Used with wine or extracted	Whole substance often eaten separately	External use: ○ possible ◎ mainly (internal caution) ● only	◎ Do not cook substance ● Refrigerate	Add near end of cooking: ○ last 5 min ◎ 10 min ● 15 min	Cook 30 - 60 minutes before adding other herbs	Dissolve/steep in strained previously cooked decoction	Wrap in separate porous bag (cheesecloth)	Slice or Crush: ◎ small pieces ● powder	May be used: ◎ fresh or dried ● fresh only	May be available in prepared form - less toxic or stronger this way	Available in charred form	Toxic: ◎ slightly ● very toxic	Contraindicated in pregnancy: ◎ caution ● never use	Combining Cautions... See page 620	Standard Dosage Range in Grams
Yi Zhi Ren/ Alpinia	✓										◎							*3-9*
Yin Chai Hu/ Stellaria	✓																	*3-9*
Yin Chen Hao/ Artemisia	✓																	*9-15*
Yin Yang Huo/ Epimedium	✓		✓															*6-15*
Ying Su Ke/ Papaver	✓														●			*1.5-6*
Yu Jin/ Curcuma	✓															◎	*51*	*4.5-9*
Yu Li Ren/ Prunus	✓										◎					◎		*3-9*
Yu Mi Xu/ Zea	✓																	*15-30*
Yu Xing Cao/ Houttuynia	✓				○							◎						*15-30*
Yu Zhu/ Polygonatum	✓																	*9-15*
Yuan Hua/ Daphne	✓	◎			○										◎	●	*8*	*1.5-3*
Yuan Zhi/ Polygala	✓		✓		○													*3-9*
Yue Ji Hua/ Rosa	✓		✓													●		*3-6*
Zao Jiao/ Gleditsia		●			○						●				◎	●		*0.6-1.5*
Zao Jiao Ci/ Gleditsia	✓	○			○										◎	●		*3-9*
Zao Xiu/ Paris	✓				○										◎	●		*3-9*

Name of herb or substance	Decoction	Powder/Pills taken internally: ○ may be ◎ commonly ● always	Used with wine or extracted	Whole substance often eaten separately	External use: ○ possible ◎ mainly (internal caution) ● only	◎ Do not cook substance ● Refrigerate	Add near end of cooking: ○ last 5 min ◎ 10 min ● 15 min	Cook 30 - 60 minutes before adding other herbs	Dissolve/steep in strained previously cooked decoction	Wrap in separate porous bag (cheesecloth)	Slice or Crush: ◎ small pieces ● powder	May be used: ◎ fresh or dried ● fresh only	May be available in prepared form - less toxic or stronger this way	Available in charred form	Toxic: ◎ slightly ● very toxic	Contraindicated in pregnancy: ◎ caution ● never use	Combining Cautions... See page 620	Standard Dosage Range in Grams
Ze Lan/ Lycopus	✓				○											◎		4.5-9
Ze Qi/ Euphorbia	✓				○										◎			3-15
Ze Xie/ Alisma	✓																	6-15
Zhang Nao/ Cinnamomum		○	✓		◎										●	●		0.06-0.15
Zhe Bei Mu/ Fritillaria	✓																9	4.5-9
Zhen Zhu/ Pteria		●		✓	○			✓			●							0.6-1
Zhen Zhu Mu/ Pteria	✓	○						✓			◎							15-30
Zhi Gan Cao/ Glycyrrhiza	✓												✓					2-12
Zhi Ke/ Citrus	✓															◎		3-9
Zhi Mu/ Anemarrhena	✓																	6-15
Zhi Shi/ Citrus	✓															◎		3-9
Zhi Nan Xing/ Arisaema	✓														◎	●		4.5-9
Zhi Zi/ Gardenia	✓				○						◎							6-12
Zhu Ling/ Polyporus	✓																	6-15
Zhu Li/ Bambusa		◎		✓								◎						9-60
Zhu Ma Gen/ Boehmeria	✓				○													5-15
Zhu Ru/ Bambusa	✓																	4.5-9

Name of herb or substance	Decoction	Powder/Pills taken internally: ○ may be ⊙ commonly ● always	Used with wine or extracted	Whole substance often eaten separately	External use: ○ possible ⊙ mainly (internal caution) ● only	⊙ Do not cook substance ● Refrigerate	Add near end of cooking: ○ last 5 min ⊙ 10 min ● 15 min	Cook 30 - 60 minutes before adding other herbs	Dissolve/steep in strained previously cooked decoction	Wrap in separate porous bag (cheesecloth)	Slice or Crush: ⊙ small pieces ● powder	May be used: ⊙ fresh or dried ● fresh only	May be available in prepared form - less toxic or stronger this way	Available in charred form	Toxic: ⊙ slightly ● very toxic	Contraindicated in pregnancy: ⊙ caution ● never use	Combining Cautions... See page 620	Standard Dosage Range in Grams
Zhu Sha/ Cinnabaris		⊙			○	⊙			✓		●				●	●		*0.3-1*
Zhu Sha Gen/ Ardisia	✓				○													*9-15*
Zi Cao/ Lithospermum	✓				○													*3-9*
Zi He Che/ Homo Sapiens		⊙		✓							●							*2.5-4.5*
Zi Hua Di Ding/ Viola	✓				○							⊙						*10-16*
Zi Ran Tong/ Pyritum	✓	○			○			✓			⊙							*0.3-9*
Zi Shi Ying/ Fluoritum	✓							✓			●							*6-15*
Zi Su Geng/ Perilla	✓																	*4.5-9*
Zi Su Ye/ Perilla	✓						●											*6-9*
Zi Su Zi/ Perilla	✓										●							*4.5-9*
Zi Wan/ Aster	✓																	*1.5-9*
Zi Zhu / Callicarpa	✓	○			○													*1.5-30*
Zong Lu Pi Tan/ Trachycarpus	✓	○												✓				*1-15*

Combining Cautions as Listed in Column 17

1. Do not use with *Fu Zi / Aconitum* or *Wu Tou / Aconitum*.
2. Do not use with *Qian Niu Zi / Pharbitis*.
3. Do not use with *Yu Jin / Curcuma*.
4. Do not use with *Li Lu / Veratrum*.
5. Do not use with *Long Dan Cao / Gentiana*.
6. Do not use with *Bai Ji / Bletilla, (Fa) Ban Xia / Pinellia, Bei Mu / Fritillaria, Gua Lou / Trichosanthes, Xi Jiao / Rhinoceros, Wu Gong / Scolopendra, Bai Wei / Cynanchum* or *Lu Dou / Phaseolus*.
7. Do not use with *Jing Da Ji / Euphorbia, Yuan Hua / Daphne, Gan Sui / Euphorbia, Hai Zao / Sargassum* or *Yuan Zhi / Polygala*.
8. Do not use with *Gan Cao / Glycyrrhiza*.
9. Do not use with *Wu Tou / Aconitum*.
10. Do not use with *Gan Jiang / Zingiber, Huai Niu Xi / Achyranthes* or *Wu Tou / Aconitum*.
11. Do not use with *Fu Zi / Aconitum* or *Bai Ji / Bletilla*.
12. Do not cook in steel or iron pot.
13. Do not use with *Gan Cao / Glycyrrhiza, Yuan Hua / Daphne*, or *Hai Zao / Sargassum*.
14. Do not use with *Huo Ma Ren / Cannabis* or *Li Lu / Veratrum*.
15. Do not use with *Xi Xin / Asarum, Bai Shao Yao / Paeonia, Dan Shen / Salvia, Dang Shen / Codonopsis, Ren Shen / Panax, Ku Shen / Sophora, Nan Sha Shen / Adenophora* or *Bei Sha Shen / Glehnia*.
16. Do not use with *Sheng Di Huang / Rehmannia, Cong Bai / Allium* or *Da Suan / Allium*.
17. Do not use with *Ma Huang / Ephedra, Wu Zhu Yu / Evodia*, or *Xi Xin / Asarum*.
18. Do not use with *Sheng Di Huang / Rehmannia* or *Dang Gui / Angelica*.
19. Do not use with *Wu Ling Zhi / Trogopterus* or *Li Lu / Veratrum*. Note: this herb is usually decocted separately.
20. Do not use with *Long Dan Cao / Gentiana, Huai Niu Xi / Achyranthes, Chang Shan / Dichroa, Long Gu / Os Draconis* or *Sheng Di Huang / Rehmannia*.
21. Do not use with fat or oil.
22. Do not use with *Pi Shi / Arsenolite*.
23. Do not use with *Fu Zi / Aconitum, Gan Jiang / Zingiber*, or *Sheng Jiang / Zingiber*.
24. Do not use with *Ren Shen / Panax*.
25. Do not use with *Gua Lou / Trichosanthes, Bai Lian / Ampelopsis, Bei Mu / Fritillaria, Bai Ji / Bletilla* or *(Fa) Ban Xia / Pinellia*.
26. Do not use with *Sheng Di Huang / Rehmannia* or *Han Fang Ji / Stephania*.

27. Do not use with *Huang Jing Ye / Polygonatum.*
28. Do not use with *Shi Hu / Dendrobium, Mang Xiao / Mirabilitum, Bie Jia / Amyda, Xiao Ji / Cephalanoplos* or *Li Lu / Veratrum.*
29. Do not use with *Gan Jiang / Zingiber, Li Lu / Veratrum, Huang Qi / Astragalus, Da Zao / Ziziphus* or *Shan Zhu Yu / Cornus.*
30. Do not use with *Wu Tou / Aconitum* or *Qin Jiao / Gentiana.*
31. Do not use with *Chi Shi Zi / Halloysitum Rubrum.*
32. Do not use with *Ba Dou / Croton* or *Lei Wan / Omphalia.*
33. Do not use with *Li Lu / Veratrum, Gan Jiang / Zingiber* or *Bei Xie / Dioscorea.*
34. Do not use with *Xuan Fu Hua / Inula.*
35. Do not use with *Hua Shi / Talcum, Shan Zhu Yu / Cornus,* or *Huang Qi / Astragalus.*
36. Do not use with *Shi Gao / Gypsum* or *Wu Tou / Aconitum.*
37. Do not use with *Bai Wei / Cynanchum.*
38. Do not use with *Tu Si Zi / Cuscuta, Bei Mu / Fritillaria,* or *Da Huang / Rheum.*
39. Do not use with *Jing Da Ji / Euphorbia, Da Huang / Rheum, Huang Qi / Astragalus, Da Zao / Ziziphus, Shan Zhu Yu / Cornus,* or *Gan Jiang / Zingiber.*
40. Do not use with *Li Lu / Veratrum* or *Mu Dan Pi / Paeonia.*
41. Do not use with *Huai Niu Xi / Achyranthes, Bai Xian Pi / Dictamnus, Ju Hua / Chrysanthemum, Xuan Shen / Scrophularia, Jiang Can / Bombyx,* or *Kuan Dong Hua / Tussilago.*
42. Do not use with *Li Lu / Veratrum, Bei Mu / Fritillaria* or *Tu Si Zi / Cuscuta.*
43. Do not use with *Gan Cao / Glycyrrhiza* or *Yuan Zhi / Polygala.*
44. Do not use with *Bie Jia / Amyda, Qin Jiao / Gentiana,* or *Di Yu / Sanguisorba.*
45. Do not use with *Sang Piao Xiao / Paratenodera.*
46. Do not use with *Hai Piao Xiao / Sepia.*
47. Do not use with *Bei Mu / Fritillaria* or *Shi Chang Pu / Acorus.*
48. Do not use with *Huang Qin / Scutellaria, Ge Gen / Pueraria* or *Huang Qi / Astragalus.*
49. Do not use with *Ma Huang / Ephedra, Huang Qin / Scutellaria, Xuan Shen / Scrophularia, Bei Mu / Fritillaria, Huang Lian / Coptis, Huang Qi / Astragalus,* or *Xin Yi Hua / Magnolia.*
50. Do not use with *Ze Xie / Alisma* or *Han Shui Shi / Calcitum.*
51. Do not use with *Ding Xiang / Eugenia.*
52. Do not use with *Po Xiao / Sal Glauberis.*
53. Do not use with *Ya Xiao / Nitrum.*
54. Do not use with *Bai Qian / Cynanchum.*
55. Do not use with *Dan Shen / Salvia* or *Zi Shi Ying / Fluoritum.*
56. Do not use with *Kuan Dong Hua / Tussilago, Gua Lou / Trichosanthes, Fang Feng / Ledebouriella* or *Fu Zi / Aconitum.*
57. Do not use with *Da Huang / Rheum.*

58. Do not use with *Lei Wan / Omphalia.*

59. Do not use with *Bai Jiang Cao / Patrinia.*

60. Do not use with *Lei Wan / Omphalia, Ze Xie / Alisma, Tu Si Zi / Cuscuta*, or *Chan Tui / Cryptotympana.*

61. Do not use with *Bai Mu Er / Tremella, Ku Shen / Sophora*, or *Kuan Dong Hua / Tussilago.*

62. Do not use with *Ren Shen / Panax, Nan Sha Shen / Adenophora*, or *Bei Sha Shen / Glehnia.*

63. Do not use with *Ming Fan / Alumen.*

64. Do not use with *Fang Feng / Ledebouriella, Guang Fang Ji / Aristolochia*, or *Jie Geng / Platycodon.*

65. Do not use with *Dan Shen / Salvia, Mu Li / Ostrea, Shao Yao / Paeonia*, or *Gan Jiang / Zingiber.*

66. Do not use with *Rou Gui / Cinnamomum, Huang Qin / Scutellaria, Yuan Hua / Daphne*, or *Da Huang / Rheum.*

67. Do not use with *Ma Huang / Ephedra.*

68. Do not use with *Ge Gen / Pueraria* or *Bian Xu / Polygonum.*

69. Do not use with *Mu Dan Pi / Paeonia, Ba Dou / Croton*, or *Bei Mu / Fritillaria.*

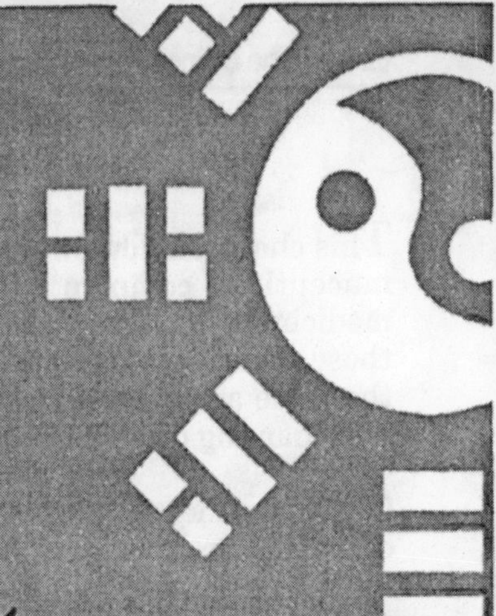

Part 4

Naming Convention Cross Reference

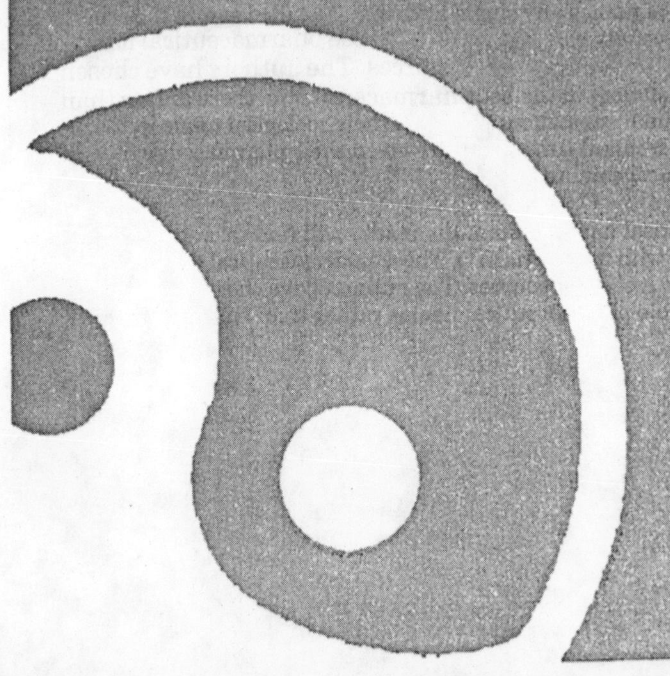

This chapter allows instant cross-referencing by botanical, pharmaceutical, common, and Pinyin names of over 480 Chinese medicinals. It contains tables of the herbs listed alphabetically by those four naming conventions. The herbs in the first column of the table are alphabetized and then re-sorted four times, so that each naming convention appears in the first column once.

Generally, there is consensus regarding Pinyin names. The botanical names are shortened to their genus form and do not necessarily indicate differences in species. For plant substances, the pharmaceutical nomenclature represents the genus, the part of the plant used, and usually the species, as well as adjectival information, such as location of discovery. As the most specific nomenclature, the pharmaceutical name may be considered the most useful, but it is not necessarily the most widely used. There are often two or three common names for an herb, representing geographical and folkloric diversity.

For non-plant substances in the botanical name column, there are some points to note: animal substances are listed with their zoological name in the botanical column whereas mineral substances are given their pharmaceutical name in that same column.

In the pharmaceutical name column, the reader will find that some herbs are marked with an asterisk (*). These pharmaceutical names are disputed or are from obscure sources. The authors have chosen to include and mark disputable pharmaceutical names rather than omit those herbs altogether.

Herb Name Cross Reference Keyed to Pinyin Names

Pinyin	Botanical	Pharmaceutical	Common
Ai Ye	Artemisia	Folium Artemisiae Argyi	Mugwort Leaf
An Xi Xiang	Styrax	Benzoinum	Processed Resin of Styrax Benzoin
Ba Dou	Croton	Semen Croton Tiglii	Croton Seed
Ba Ji Tian	Morinda	Radix Morindae Officinalis	Morinda Root
Ba Jiao Hui Xiang	Illicium	Fructus Illicii*	Star Anise Fruit
Ba Qia	Smilax	Rhizoma Smilacis China*	Smilax Rhizome
Ba Xian Hua	Hydrangea	Flos Hydrangeae Macrophyllae*	Hydrangea Flower
Ba Yue Zha	Akebia	Fructus Akebiae	Akebia Fruit
Bai Bu	Stemona	Radix Stemonae	Stemona Root
Bai Dou Kou	Amomum	Fructus Amomi Kravanh	Round Cardamon Fruit; Cluster Fruit
Bai Fu Zi	Typhonium	Rhizoma Typhonii Gigantei	Typhonium Rhizome
Bai Guo	Ginkgo	Semen Ginkgo Bilobae	Ginkgo Nut
Bai He	Lilium	Bulbus Lilii	Lily Bulb
Bai Hua She	Agkistrodon	Agkistrodon seu Bungarus	Long-noded Pit Viper Snake
Bai Hua She She Cao	Oldenlandia	Herba Oldenlandiae Diffusae	Oldenlandia
Bai Ji	Bletilla	Rhizoma Bletillae Striatae	Bletilla Rhizome
Bai Ji Li	Tribulus	Fructus Tribuli Terrestris	Puncture Vine Fruit; Caltrop Fruit
Bai Jiang Cao	Patrinia or Thiaspi	Herba cum Radice Patriniae	Patrinia; Thiaspi
Bai Jie Zi	Brassica	Semen Sinapsis Albae	White Mustard Seed
Bai Lian	Ampelopsis	Radix Ampelopsis Japonicae*	Ampelopsis Root
Bai Mao Gen	Imperata	Rhizoma Imperatae Cylindricae	Woolly Grass Rhizome; White Grass Rhizome
Bai Mao Hua	Imperata	Flos Imperatae Cylindricae	Wooly Grass Flower; White Grass Flower
Bai Mao Xia Ku Cao	Ajuga	Herba Ajugae Decumbentis*	Ajuga
Bai Mu Er	Tremella	Fructificatio Tremellae Fuciformis	Tremella Fungus Fruiting Body
Bai Qian	Cynanchum	Rhizoma et Radix Cynanchi Baiqian	Cynanchum Rhizome and Root
Bai Shao	Paeonia	Radix Paeoniae Lactiflorae	White Peony Root
Bai Shen	Panax	Radix Ginseng	Rock Candy cured White Ginseng Root
Bai Tou Weng	Pulsatilla	Radix Pulsatillae Chinensis	Pulsatilla Root; Anemone Root

Pinyin	Botanical	Pharmaceutical	Common
Bai Wei	Cynanchum	Radix Cynanchi Baiwei	Swallowort Root
Bai Xian Pi	Dictamnus	Cortex Dictamni Dasycarpi Radicis	Dittany Root Bark
Bai Zhi	Angelica	Radix Angelicae Dahuricae	Angelica Root
Bai Zhu	Atractylodes	Rhizoma Atractylodis Macrocephalae	White Atractylodes Rhizome
Bai Zi Ren	Biota	Semen Biotae Orientalis	Arbor-Vitae Seed
Ban Bian Lian	Lobelia	Herba Lobeliae Chinensis cum Radice	Chinese Lobelia
Ban Lan Gen	Isatis	Radix Isatidis seu Baphicacanthi	Isatis Root; Woad Root
Ban Mao	Mylabris	Mylabris	Cantharides; Chinese Blistering Beetle
(Fa) Ban Xia	Pinellia	Rhizoma Pinelliae Ternatae	Prepared Pinellia Rhizome
(Sheng) Ban Xia	Pinellia	Rhizoma Pinelliae Ternatae	Raw Pinellia Rhizome
Ban Zhi Lian	Scutellaria	Herba Scutellariae Barbatae	Barbat Scullcap
Bao Gu	Panthera	Os Leopardis	Leopard Bone
Bao Ma Zi	Syringa	Cortex Syringae*	Manchurian Lilac Bark
Bei Sha Shen	Glehnia	Radix Glehniae Littoralis	Beech Silver-top Root; Northern Sand Root
Bei Xie	Dioscorea	Rhizoma Dioscoreae Hypoglaucae	Hypoglauca Yam Rhizome; Fish-poison Yam Rhizome
Bi Ba	Piper	Fructus Piperis Longi	Long Pepper Fruit
Bi Cheng Qie	Piper	Fructus Cubebae	Cubeba Fruit
Bian Dou	Dolichos	Semen Dolichoris Lablab	Hyacinth Bean
Bian Dou Hua	Dolichos	Flos Dolichoris Lablab	Hyacinth Bean Flower
Bian Xu	Polygonum	Herba Polygoni Avicularis	Avicularis; Knotweed
Bie Jia	Amyda	Carapax Amydae Sinensis	Chinese Soft-shell Turtle Shell
Bing Lang	Areca	Semen Arecae Catechu	Betel Nut
Bing Pian	Dryobalanops	Borneol	Processed Resin of Borneol Camphor
Bo He	Mentha	Herba Menthae Haplocalycis	Peppermint; Spearmint; Field Mint
Bu Gu Zhi	Psoralea	Fructus Psoraleae Corylifoliae	Scurfy Pea Fruit
Can Sha	Bombyx	Excrementum Bombycis Mori	Silkworm Feces
Cang Er Zi	Xanthium	Fructus Xanthii Sibirici	Xanthium Fruit; Cocklebur Fruit
Cang Zhu	Atractylodes	Rhizoma Atractylodis	Atractylodes Rhizome
Cao Dou Kou	Alpinia	Semen Alpiniae Katsumadai	Wild Cardamon Seed; Katsumada's Galangal Seed
Cao Guo	Amomum	Fructus Amomi Tsao-Ko	Chinese Cardamon Fruit

Pinyin	Botanical	Pharmaceutical	Common
Cao Wu	Aconitum	Radix Aconiti Kusnezoffii	Wild Aconite
Ce Bai Ye	Biota	Cacumen Biotae Orientalis	Arborvitae Leafy Twig
Chai Hu	Bupleurum	Radix Bupleuri	Thorowax Root; Hare's Ear Root
Chan Su	Bufo	Secretio Bufonis	Dried Skin Secretion of Toad
Chan Tui	Cryptotympana	Periostracum Cicadae	Cicada Skin; Cicada Moulting
Chang Chun Teng	Hedera	Herba Hederae Nepalensis*	Ivy
Chang Shan	Dichroa	Radix Dichroae Febrifugae	Dichroa Root
Che Qian Cao	Plantago	Herba Plantaginis	Plantago; Plantain
Che Qian Zi	Plantago	Semen Plantaginis	Plantago Seed; Plantain Seed
Chen Pi	Citrus	Pericarpium Citri Reticulatae	Tangerine Peel
Chen Shi Huei	Calcaria	Calcaria*	Calcium Hydroxide
Chen Xiang	Aquilaria	Lignum Aquilariae	Aloeswood Secretion or Sap
Cheng Liu	Tamarix	Cacumen Tamaricis Chinensis*	Tamarisk
Chi Fu Ling	Poria	Sclerotium Poriae Cocos Rubrae	Red Hoelen; Red Tuckahoe
Chi Shao	Paeonia	Radix Paeoniae Rubra	Red Peony Root
Chi Shi Zhi	Halloysitum Rubrum	Halloysitum Rubrum	Halloysite; Red Kaolin
Chi Xiao Dou	Phaseolus	Semen Phaseoli Calcarati	Aduki Bean
Chong Wei Zi	Leonurus	Semen Leonuri Heterophylli	Motherwort Seed
Chou Wu Tong	Clerodendron	Folium Clerodendri Trichotomi	Glorybower Leaf
Chu Shi Zi	Broussonetia	Semen Broussonetiae Papyriferae*	Broussonetia Seed
Chuan Bei Mu	Fritillaria	Bulbus Fritillariae Cirrhosae	Tendrilled Fritillary Bulb
Chuan Jiao	Zanthoxylum	Pericarpum Zanthoxyli Bungeani	Sichuan Pepper Fruit
Chuan Jiao Mu	Zanthoxylum	Semen Zanthoxyli Bungeani	Sichuan Pepper Seed
Chuan Lian Zi	Melia	Fructus Meliae Toosendan	Sichuan Chinaberry Fruit; Sichuan Pagoda Tree Fruit; Neem Fruit
Chuan Niu Xi	Cyathula	Radix Cyathulae Officinalis	Cyathula Root
Chuan Shan Jia	Manis	Squama Manitis Pentadactylae	Anteater-Scales; Pangolin Scales
Chuan Shan Long	Dioscorea	Rhizoma Dioscoreae Nipponicae*	Japanese Dioscorea Rhizome
Chuan Wu	Aconitum	Radix Aconite Carmichaeli	Sichuan Aconite
Chuan Xin Lian	Andrographis	Herba Andrographitis Paniculatae	Kariyat; Green Chiretta
Chuan Xiong	Ligusticum	Radix Ligustici Chuan Xiong	Sichuan Lovage Root
Chui Pen Cao	Sedum	Herba Sedii Sarmentosi*	Stonecrop

Pinyin	Botanical	Pharmaceutical	Common
Chun Pi	Ailanthus	Cortex Ailanthi Altissimae	Tree of Heaven Bark
Ci Shi	Magnetitum	Magnetitum	Magnetite; Magnetic Iron Ore; Loadstone
Cong Bai	Allium	Bulbus Allii Fistulosi	White Bulb of Green Onion or Scallion
Da Feng Zi	Hydnocarpus	Semen Hydnocarpi Anthelminticae	Chaulmoogra Seed
Da Fu Pi	Areca	Pericarpium Arecae Catechu	Betelnut Husk
Da Huang	Rheum	Radix et Rhizoma Rhei	Rhubarb Root and Rhizome
Da Ji	Cirsium	Herba seu Radix Cirsii Japonici	Japanese Thistle
Da Qing Ye	Isatis	Folium Isatidis Daqingye	Isatis Leaf; Woad Leaf
Da Suan	Allium	Bulbus Allii Sativi	Garlic Bulb
Da Zao	Ziziphus	Fructus Ziziphi Jujubae	Jujube Fruit; Chinese Black Date
Dai Mao	Eretmochelys	Carapax Eretmochelydis Imbricatae*	Hawksbill Turtle Shell
Dai Zhe Shi	Haematitum	Haematitum	Hematite; Iron Ore
Dan Dou Chi	Glycine	Semen Glycinis Praeparatum	Prepared (Fermented) Soybean
Dan Fan	Chalcanthitum	Chalcanthitum*	Copper Sulphate; Blue Vitriol
Dan Nan Xing	Arisaema	Pulvis Arisaemae cum Felle Bovis	Powdered Jack-in-the-Pulpit Rhizome mixed with Cow Bile
Dan Shen	Salvia	Radix Salviae Miltiorrhizae	Red Sage Root
Dan Zhu Ye	Lophatherum	Herba Lophatheri Gracilis	Bland Bamboo Leaf and Stem
Dang Gui	Angelica	Radix Angelicae Sinensis	Tangkuei Root
Dang Gui Tou	Angelica	Caput Radicis Angelicae Sinensis	Tangkuei Head
Dang Gui Wei	Angelica	Extremas Radicis Angelicae Sinensis	Tangkuei Tail
Dang Shen	Codonopsis	Radix Codonopsitis Pilosulae	Asiabell Root
Deng Xin Cao	Juncus	Medulla Junci Effusi	Rush Pith
Di Fu Zi	Kochia	Fructus Kochiae Scopariae	Broom Cyperus Seed
Di Gu Pi	Lycium	Cortex Lycii Radicis	Matrimony-vine Rootbark, Wolfberry Bark
Di Long	Pheretima	Lumbricus	Earthworm
Di Yu	Sanguisorba	Radix Sanguisorbae Officinalis	Burnet-bloodwort Root
Dian Di Mei	Androsace	Herba Androsacae Umbellatae*	Androsace
Ding Xiang	Eugenia	Flos Caryophylli	Clove Flower-bud
Dong Bei Guan Zhong	Dryopteris	Rhizoma Dryopteridis	Dryopteris Rhizome

Pinyin	Botanical	Pharmaceutical	Common
Dong Chong Xia Cao	Cordyceps	Cordyceps Sinensis	Chinese Caterpillar Fungus
Dong Gua Pi	Benincasa	Epicarpium Benincasae Hispidae	Wintermelon Fruit Peel; Wax Gourd Fruit Peel
Dong Gua Ren	Benincasa	Semen Benincasae Hispidae	Wintermelon Seed; Wax Gourd Seed
Dong Kui Zi	Malva or Abutilon	Semen Albutili seu Malvae	Musk Mallow Seed; Malva Seed
Dou Chi Jiang	Litsea	Radix et Ramus Litseae Cubebae	Aromatic Litsea Root and Stem
Dou Juan	Glycine	Semen Glycinis Germinatum	Young Soybean Sprout
Du Huo	Angelica	Radix Angelicae Pubescentis	Pubescent Angelica Root
Du Zhong	Eucommia	Cortex Eucommiae Ulmoidis	Eucommia Bark
Duan Long Gu	Os Draconis	Os Draconis	Calcined Dragon Bone; Calcined Fossilized Bone
Duan Mu Li	Ostrea	Concha Ostreae	Calcined Oyster Shell
E Bu Shi Cao	Centipeda	Herba Centipedae Minimae*	Centipeda Herb
E Guan Shi	Stalactitum	Stalactitum	Stalactite Tubular Tip
E Jiao	Equus	Gelatinum Corii Asini	Donkey Hide Gelatin; Ass Skin Glue
E Wei	Ferula	Resina Asafoetidae*	Asafoetida Gum-resin; Devil's Dung
E Zhu	Curcuma	Rhizoma Curcumae	Zedoary Tumeric Rhizome
Er Cha	Acacia or Uncaria	Pasta Acacia seu Uncaria	Dried Paste of Concentrated Decoction of Black or White Cutch
Fan Bai Cao	Potentilla	Herba Potentillae Discoloris*	Potentilla
Fan Xie Ye	Cassia	Folium Sennae	Senna Leaf
Fang Feng	Ledebouriella	Radix Ledebouriella Divaricatae	Siler Root; Ledebouriella Root
Fei Zi	Torreya	Semen Torreyae Grandis	Torreya Seed
Feng Mi	Mel	Mel*	Honey
Feng Wei Cao	Pteris	Herba Pterii*	Pteris
Fo Shou	Citrus	Fructus Citri Sarcodactylis	Finger Citron Fruit
Fo Shou Hua	Citrus	Flos Citri Sarcodactylis	Finger Citron Flower
Fu Hai Shi	Pumice	Pumice	Pumice
Fu Ling	Poria	Sclerotium Poriae Cocos	Hoelen; China Root; Tuckahoe; Indian Bread
Fu Ling Pi	Poria	Cortex Poriae Cocos	Tuckahoe Skin
Fu Long Gan	Terra Flava Usta	Terra Flava Usta	Ignited Wood Stove Earth
Fu Pen Zi	Rubus	Fructus Rubi Chingii	Raspberry Fruit Bud
Fu Ping	Spirodela or Lemna	Herba Lemnae seu Spirodelae	Duckweed

Pinyin	Botanical	Pharmaceutical	Common
Fu Shen	Poria Cocos	Sclerotium Poriae Cocos Pararadicis	Tuckahoe Spirit
Fu Xiao Mai	Triticum	Semen Tritici Aestivi Levis	Wheat Chaff/Grain
(Hei)Fu Zi	Aconitum	Radix Lateralis Aconiti Carmichaeli Praeparata	Prepared Sichuan Aconite Root
Gan Cao	Glycyrhiza	Radix Glycyrrhizae Uralensis	Licorice Root
Gan Jiang	Zingiber	Rhizoma Zingiberis Officinalis	Dried Ginger Rhizome
Gan Jie Geng	Adenophora	Radix Adenophorae Trachelioidis	Sweet Jie Geng
Gan Qi	Rhus	Lacca Sinica Exsiccatae	Laquer
Gan Sui	Euphorbia	Radix Euphorbiae Kansui	Kansui Spurge Root
Gao Ben	Ligusticum	Rhizoma et Radix Ligustici	Straw Weed Rhizome and Root; Chinese Lovage Rhizome and Root
Gao Liang Jiang	Alpinia	Rhizoma Alpiniae Officinari	Lesser Galangal Rhizome
Ge Gen	Pueraria	Radix Puerariae	Kudzu Root
Ge Hua	Pueraria	Flos Puerariae	Kudzu Flower
Ge Jie	Gekko	Gekko	Gecko Lizard
Ge Shan Xiang	Cynanchum	Radix Cynanchi Auriculati	Cynanchum Root
Gou Gu	Canis	Os Canine	Dog Bone
Gou Ji	Cibotium	Rhizoma Cibotii Barometz	Chain Fern Rhizome
Gou Qi Zi	Lycium	Fructus Lycii	Matrimony Vine Fruit; Wolfberry Fruit
Gou Teng	Uncaria	Ramulus cum Uncis Uncariae	Gambir vine Stems and Hooks
Gu Jing Cao	Eriocaulon	Scapus et Inflorescentia Eriocaulonis Buergeriani	Pipewort Scapus
Gu Sui Bu	Drynaria	Rhizoma Drynariae	Drynaria Rhizome
Gu Ya	Oryza	Fructus Oryzae Sativae Germinatus	Rice Sprout
Gua Di	Cucumis	Pedicellus Cucumeris	Melon Pedicle
Gua Lou	Trichosanthes	Fructus Trichosanthis	Snakegourd Fruit
Gua Lou Pi	Trichosanthes	Pericarpium Trichosanthis	Snakegourd Peel
Gua Lou Ren	Trichosanthes	Semen Trichosanthis	Snakegourd Seed
Guan Gui	Cinnamomum	Cortex Tubiformis Cinnamomi Cassiae	Thin Cinnamon Bark from Young Trees
Guan Ye Liao	Polygonum	Herba Polygoni Perfoliati*	Polygonum
Guan Zhong	Dryopteris	Rhizoma Guanzhong	Shield-fern Rhizome
Guang Fang Ji	Aristolochia or Cocculus	Radix Aristolochiae Fangchi	Aristolochia Root
Guang Gou Shen	Canis	Testis et Penis Canis*	Male Dog Sexual Organs
Gui Ban	Chinemys	Plastrum Testudinis	Fresh Water Turtle Shell
Gui Zhi	Cinnamomum	Ramulus Cinnamomi Cassiae	Cinnamon Twig

Pinyin	Botanical	Pharmaceutical	Common
Hai Dai	*Laminaria*	*Herba Laminaria Japonicae*	*Algae*
Hai Feng Teng	*Piper*	*Caulis Piperis Futokadsurae*	*Kadsura Stem*
Hai Ge Ke	*Cyclina*	*Concha Cyclinae Sinensis*	*Clam Shell*
Hai Gou Shen	*Phoca*	*Testis et Penis Otariae**	*Male Seal Sexual Organs*
Hai Jin Sha	*Lygodium*	*Spora Lygodii Japonici*	*Japanese Climbing Fern Spore*
Hai Long	*Solenognathus*	*Hailong*	*Pipe-fish*
Hai Ma	*Hippocampus*	*Hippocampus*	*Sea Horse*
Hai Piao Xiao	*Sepia or Sepiella*	*Os Sepiae seu Sepiellae*	*Cuttle-fish Bone*
Hai Shen	*Strichopus*	*Strichopus Japonicus*	*Sea Cucumber, Sea Slug*
Hai Tong Pi	*Erythrina*	*Cortex Erythrinae*	*Coral-bean Bark*
Hai Zao	*Sargassum*	*Herba Sargassii*	*Sargassum Seaweed*
Han Cai	*Rorippa*	*Herba Rorippae**	*Rorippa*
Han Fang Ji	*Stephania*	*Radix Stephaniae Tetrandrae*	*Stephania Root*
Han Lian Cao	*Eclipta*	*Herba Ecliptae Prostratae*	*Eclipta*
Han Shui Shi	*Calcitum*	*Calcitum*	*Calcite*
He Huan Hua	*Albizzia*	*Flos Albizziae Julibrissin**	*Mimosa Tree Flower; Silktree Flower*
He Huan Pi	*Albizzia*	*Cortex Albizziae Julibrissin*	*Mimosa Tree Bark; Silktree Bark*
He Shi	*Carpesium or Daucus*	*Fructus Carpesii seu Daucusi*	*Carpesium Fruit*
He Shou Wu	*Polygonum*	*Radix Polygoni Multiflori*	*Fleeceflower Root; Fo-Ti Root*
He Ye	*Nelumbo*	*Folium Nelumbinis Nuciferae*	*Lotus Leaf*
He Zi	*Terminalia*	*Fructus Terminaliae Chebulae*	*Myrobalan Fruit*
Hei Lu Shen	*Equus*	*Testis et Penis Equii**	*Male Horse Sexual Organs*
Hei Zhi Ma	*Sesamum*	*Semen Sesami Indici*	*Black Sesame Seed*
Hong Hua	*Carthamus*	*Flos Carthami Tinctorii*	*Safflower*
Hong Teng	*Sargentodoxa*	*Caulis Sargentodoxae Cuneatae*	*Sargentodoxa Stem*
Hong Zao	*Ziziphus*	*Fructus Ziziphi Jujubae*	*Jujube Fruit; Chinese Red Date*
Hou Po	*Magnolia*	*Cortex Magnoliae Officinalis*	*Magnolia Bark*
Hou Po Hua	*Magnolia*	*Flos Magnoliae Officinalis*	*Magnolia Flower*
Hou Zao	*Macaca*	*Calculus Macacae Mulattae*	*Macaque Gallstone*
Hu Er Cao	*Saxifrage*	*Herba Saxifragae Stoloniferae**	*Saxifrage*
Hu Gu	*Panthera*	*Os Tigris*	*Tiger Bone*
Hu Huang Lian	*Picrorhiza*	*Rhizoma Picrorhizae*	*Picrorhiza Rhizome*
Hu Jiao	*Piper*	*Fructus Piperis Nigri*	*Black Pepper Fruit*

Pinyin	Botanical	Pharmaceutical	Common
Hu Lu Ba	Trigonella	Semen Trigonellae Foeni-graeci	Fenugreek Seed
Hu Po	Succinum	Succinum	Amber; Fossilized Resin of Pine Tree
Hu Tao Ren	Juglans	Semen Juglandis Regiae	Walnut
Hu Tui Ye	Eleagnus	Folium Eleagni Pungens	Eleagnus Leaf
Hu Zhang	Polygonum	Radix et Rhizoma Polygoni Cuspidati	Giant Knotweed Rhizome
Hua Lu Shen	Cervus	Testis et Penis Cervi*	Male Deer Sexual Organs
Hua Rui Shi	Ophicalcitum	Ophicalcitum	Ophicalcite
Hua Sheng Yi	Arachis	Pericarpium Arachi*	Peanut Skin
Hua Shi	Talcum	Talcum	Talc; Soapstone
Huai Hua Mi	Sophora	Flos Sophorae Japonicae Immaturus	Pagoda Tree Flower Bud
Huai Jiao	Sophora	Fructus Sophorae Japonicae	Pagoda Tree Fruit
Huai Niu Xi	Achyranthes	Radix Achyranthis Bidentatae	Achyranthes Root
Huang Bai	Phellodendron	Cortex Phellodendri	Amur Cork-tree Bark
Huang Jin	Aurum	Aurum*	Gold
Huang Jing	Polygonatum	Rhizoma Polygonati	Siberian Solomon Seal Rhizome
Huang Lian	Coptis	Rhizoma Coptidis	Coptis; Golden Thread Rhizome
Huang Qi	Astragalus	Radix Astragali Membranaceus	Yellow Milk-vetch Root
Huang Qin	Scutellaria	Radix Scutellariae Baicalensis	Scute; Baical Skullcap Root
Huang Yao Zi	Dioscorea	Tuber Dioscoreae Bulbiferae	Dioscorea Tuber
Huo Ma Ren	Cannabis	Semen Cannabis Sativae	Hemp Seed; Marihuana Seed
Huo Xiang	Agastache or Pogostemon	Herba Agastaches seu Pogostemi	Patchouli, Agastache
Ji Cai	Capsella	Herba Capsellae*	Shepherd's Purse
Ji Guan Hua	Celosia	Flos Celosiae Cristatae	Cockscomb Flower
Ji Lin Shen	Panax	Radix Ginseng	Jilin Wild Ginseng
Ji Mu	Loropetalum	Cortex Loropetali*	Loropetalum Bark
Ji Nei Jin	Gallus	Endothelium Corneum Gigeriae Galli	Chicken Gizard Lining
Ji Ning	Salvia	Herba Salviae Plebeia*	Salvia
Ji Shi Teng	Paederia	Caulis Paederiae*	Paederia Stem
Ji Xue Teng	Millettia	Radix et Caulis Jixueteng	Millettia Root and Vine; Chicken Blood Vine
Jiang Can	Bombyx	Bombyx Batryticatus	Dead Stiff Body of Sick Silkworm Larvae

Pinyin	Botanical	Pharmaceutical	Common
Jiang Huang	Curcuma	Rhizoma Curcumae Longae	Tumeric Rhizome
Jiang Xiang	Dalbergia	Lignum Dalbergiae Odoriferae	Dalbergia Heartwood
(Chuan) Jiao Mu	Zanthoxylum	Semen Zanthoxyli Bungeani	Sichuan Pepper Seed
(Ku) Jie Geng	Platycodon	Radix Platycodi Grandiflori	Ballonflower Root; Bellflower Root; Bitter Jie Geng
Jin Fei Cao	Inula	Herba Inulae	Elecampane
Jin Guo Lan	Tinospora	Radix Tinosporae Capillipes*	Tinospora Root
Jin Qian Cao	Lysimachia	Herba Lysimachiae	Lysimachia
Jin Qiao Mai	Fagopyrum	Rhizoma Fagopyri Cynosi*	Wild Buckwheat Rhizome
Jin Sha Teng	Lygodium	Herba Lygodii Japonici	Japanese Climbing Fern
Jin Yin Hua	Lonicera	Flos Lonicerae Japonicae	Honeysuckle Flower
Jin Yin Teng	Lonicera	Ramus Lonicerae Japonicae	Honeysuckle Stem
Jin Ying Zi	Rosa	Fructus Rosae Laevigatae	Cherokee Rose Fruit / Rosehip
Jing Da Ji	Euphorbia or Knoxia	Radix Euphorbiae seu Knoxiae	Peking Spurge Root
Jing Jie	Schizonepeta	Herba Schizonepetae Tenuifoliae	Schizonepeta Stem or Bud
Jing Mi	Oryza	Semen Oryzae Sativae*	Rice Grain
Jing Tian San Qi	Sedum	Herba Sedi*	Sedum
Jiu Jie Chang Pu	Anemone	Rhizoma Anemoni Altaicae*	Altaica Rhizome
Jiu Xiang Chong	Aspongopus	Aspongopus*	Stink Bug
Jiu Zi	Allium	Semen Allii Tuberosi	Chinese Leek Seed
Ju He	Citrus	Semen Citri Reticulatae*	Tangerine Seed
Ju Hong	Citrus	Pars Rubra Epicarpii Citri Erythrocarpae	Red Tangerine Peel
(Bai) Ju Hua	Chrysanthemum	Flos Chrysanthemi Morifolii	White Chrysanthemum Flower
(Huang) Ju Hua	Chrysanthemum	Flos Chrysanthemi Morifolii	Yellow Chrysanthemum Flower
Ju Ye San Qi	Gynura	Folium Gynurae*	Gynura Leaf
Jue Ming Zi	Cassia	Semen Cassiae	Cassia Seed
Ku Fan	Alumen Praeparatum	Alumen Praeparatum	Prepared Alum
Ku Lian Gen Pi	Melia	Cortex Meliae Radicis	Sichuan Chinaberry Root Bark; Sichuan Pagoda Tree Root Bark; Neem Root Bark
Ku Lian Mu Pi	Melia	Cortex Meliae	Sichuan Chinaberry Tree Bark; Sichuan Pagoda Tree Bark; Neem Tree Bark
Ku Shen	Sophora	Radix Sophorae Flavenscentis	Bitter Ginseng Root
Kuan Dong Hua	Tussilago	Flos Tussilaginis Farfarae	Coltsfoot Flower

Pinyin	Botanical	Pharmaceutical	Common
Kuan Jin Teng	*Tinospora*	*Ramus Tinosporae Sinensis*	*Tinospora Stem*
Kun Bu	*Laminaria or Ecklonia*	*Thallus Algae*	*Kelp Thallus; Kombu Thallus*
Lai Fu Zi	*Raphanus*	*Semen Raphani Satavi*	*Radish Seed*
Lao Guan Cao	*Erodium or Geranium*	*Herba Erodii seu Geranii**	*Geranium; Heronbill; Cranebill*
Lei Wan	*Omphalia*	*Sclerotium Omphaliae Lapidescens*	*Omphalia Fungus Fruiting Body*
Li Lu	*Veratrum*	*Radix et Rhizoma Veratri*	*Veratrum Root*
Li Pi	*Pyrus*	*Pericarpium Pyri**	*Pear Peel*
Li Zhi He	*Litchi*	*Semen Litchi Chinensis*	*Leechee Nut*
Lian Fang	*Nelumbo*	*Receptaculum Nelumbinis Nuciferae*	*Mature Lotus Receptacle*
Lian Geng	*Nelumbo*	*Ramulus Nelumbinis Nuciferae*	*Lotus Stem*
Lian Qiao	*Forsythia*	*Fructus Forsythiae Suspensae*	*Forsythia Fruit; Golden Bells*
Lian Xin	*Nelumbo*	*Plumula Nelumbinis Nuciferae*	*Lotus Plumule*
Lian Xu	*Nelumbo*	*Stamen Nelumbinis Nuciferae*	*Lotus Stamen*
Lian Zi	*Nelumbo*	*Semen Nelumbinis Nuciferae*	*Lotus Seed*
Ling Yang Jiao	*Saiga*	*Cornu Antelopis*	*Antelope Horn*
Ling Zhi	*Ganoderma*	*Fructificatio Ganodermae Lucidi**	*Lucid Ganoderma; Reishi*
Liu Huang	*Sulphur*	*Sulphur*	*Sulphur*
Liu Ji Nu	*Artemisia*	*Herba Artemisiae Anomalae*	*Artemisia*
Long Chi	*Dens Draconis*	*Dens Draconis*	*Dragon Tooth; Fossilized Tooth*
Long Dan Cao	*Gentiana*	*Radix Gentianae Longdancao*	*Chinese Gentian Root*
Long Gu	*Os Draconis*	*Os Draconis*	*Dragon Bone; Fossilized Bone*
Long Yan Rou	*Euphoria*	*Arillus Euphoriae Longanae*	*Longan Fruit Flesh*
Lou Lu	*Rhaponticum or Echinops*	*Radix Rhapontici seu Echinops*	*Rhaponticum Root, Echinops Root*
Lu Dou	*Phaseolus*	*Semen Phaseoli Radiati*	*Mung Bean*
Lu Feng Fang	*Polistes*	*Nidus Vespae*	*Hornet Nest; Wasp Nest*
Lu Gan Shi	*Smithsonitum*	*Smithsonitum*	*Smithsonite; Calamine*
Lu Gen	*Phragmites*	*Rhizoma Phragmitis Communis*	*Reed Rhizome; Corrizo Rhizome*
Lu Hui	*Aloe*	*Herba Aloes*	*Aloe Vera Leaf*
Lu Jiao	*Cervus*	*Cornu Cervi*	*Antler; Deerhorn; Ossified Horn of the Mature Male Deer*

Pinyin	Botanical	Pharmaceutical	Common
Lu Jiao Jiao	Cervus	Colla Cornu Cervi	Mature Antler Glue; Mature Antler Gelatin
Lu Jiao Shuang	Cervus	Cornu Cervi Degelatinatium	Antler Powder from the dregs of cooking Antler Glue
Lu Lu Tong	Liquidambar	Fructus Liquidambaris Taiwanianae	Sweetgum Fruit
Lu Rong	Cervus	Cornu Cervi Parvum	Young Deer Antler Velvet
Lu Xian Cao	Pyrola	Herba Pyrolae*	Pyrola
Lu Ying	Sambucus	Cortex Sambuci*	Japanese Elder Bark
Luo Bu Ma	Apocynum	Herba seu Folium Apocyni Veneti*	Red Dogbane Whole Herb or Leaf
Luo Han Guo	Momordica	Fructus Momordicae Grosvenori	Momordica Fruit
Luo Huo Guo Ye	Momordica	Folium Momordicae Grosvenori	Momordica Leaf
Luo Shi Teng	Trachelospermum	Caulis Trachelospermi Jasminoidis	Star Jasmine Stem
Ma Bian Cao	Verbena	Herba Verbenae*	Vervain
Ma Bo	Lasiosphaera	Fructificatio Lasiosphaerae seu Calvatiae	Puffball Fruiting Body
Ma Chi Xian	Portulaca	Herba Portulacae Oleraceae	Purslane
Ma Dou Ling	Aristolochia	Fructus Aristolochiae	Birthwort Fruit
Ma Huang	Ephedra	Herba Ephedrae	Ephedra Stem
Ma Huang Gen	Ephedra	Radix Ephedrae	Ephedra Root
Ma Qian Zi	Strychnos	Semen Strychni	Nux-vomica Seed
Mai Men Dong	Ophiopogon	Tuber Ophiopogonis Japonici	Creeping Lily-turf Tuber
Mai Ya	Hordeum	Fructus Hordei Vulgaris Germinatus	Barley Sprout, Malted Barley
Man Jing Zi	Vitex	Fructus Viticis	Vitex Fruit
Man Shan Hong	Rhododendron	Folium Rhododendri*	Rhododendron Leaf
Mang Xiao	Mirabilitum	Mirabilitum	Mirabilite; Glauber's Salt
Mao Dong Qing	Ilex	Radix Ilicis Pubescentis*	Pubescent Holly Root
Mao Mei	Rubus	Herba Rubi Parvifolii*	Thimbleberry
Mao Zhao Cao	Ranunculus	Radix Ranunculi Ternati*	Buttercup Root
Mei Gui Hua	Rosa	Flos Rosae Rugosae	Young Chinese Rose Flower
Meng Chong	Tabanus	Tabani Bivittati*	Gadfly
Meng Shi	Lapis Micae seu Chloriti	Lapis Micae seu Chloriti	Chlorite Schist; Lapis
Mi Meng Hua	Buddleia	Flos Buddleiae Officinalis Immaturus	Buddleia Flower
Mi Tuo Seng	Lithargyrum	Lithargyrum	Litharge; Galena
Mian Hua Gen	Gossypium	Radix Gossypii Hirsuti*	Cotton Root
Ming Dang Shen	Changium	Radix Changii*	Changium Root

Pinyin	Botanical	Pharmaceutical	Common
Ming Fan	Alumen	Alumen	Alum; Potassium Aluminum Sulfate
Mo Yao	Commiphora	Resinae Myrrhae	Myrrh Gum-resin
Mu Bie Zi	Momordica	Semen Momordicae Cochinchinensis	Momordica Seed
Mu Dan Pi	Paeonia	Cortex Moutan Radicis	Tree Peony Rootbark
Mu Gua	Chaenomeles	Fructus Chaenomelis	Chinese Quince Fruit
Mu Hu Die	Oroxylum	Semen Oroxyli Indici	Oroxylum Seed
Mu Li	Ostrea	Concha Ostreae	Oyster Shell
Mu Tong	Akebia	Caulis Mutong	Akebia Stem
Mu Xiang	Saussurea	Radix Saussureae Lappae	Costus Root, Aucklandia
Mu Zei	Equisetum	Herba Equiseti Hiemalis	Horsetail, Scouring Rush; Shavegrass
Nan Gua Zi	Cucurbita	Semen Cucurbitae Moschatae	Pumpkin Seed and Husk
Nan Sha Shen	Adenophora	Radix Adenophorae	Ladybell Root, Southern Sand Root
Nan Wu Wei Zi	Schisandra	Fructus Schisandrae Sphenantherae	Southern Schisandra Fruit
Niu Bang Zi	Arctium	Fructus Arctii Lappae	Burdock Seed
Niu Dan	Bos	Vesica Fellea Bovus	Cow Gallbladder
Niu Huang	Bos or Bubalis	Calculus Bovis seu Calculus Bubali	Ox or Water Buffalo Gallstone
Nu Zhen Zi	Ligustrum	Fructus Ligustri Lucidi	Privet Fruit; Waxtree Fruit
Nuo Dao Gen Xu	Oryza	Radix et Rhizoma Oryzae Glutinosae	Sweet Rice Root and Rhizome
Ou Jie	Nelumbo	Nodus Nelumbinis Nuciferae Rhizomatis	Lotus Rhizome Node
Pang Da Hai	Sterculia	Semen Sterculiae Scaphigerae	Sterculia Seed
Pao Jiang	Zingiber	Rhizoma Zingiberis*	Quick-fried Ginger Rhizome
Pei Lan	Eupatorium	Herba Eupatorii Fortunei	Boneset; Thoroughwort; Feverwort
Peng Sha	Borax	Borax	Borax; Sodium Tetraborate
Pi Pa Ye	Eriobotrya	Folium Eriobotryae Japonicae	Loquat Leaf
Pi Shi	Arsenolith	Arseolitum	White Arsenic
Pu Gong Ying	Taraxacum	Herba Taraxaci Mongolici cum Radice	Dandelion
(Sheng) Pu Huang	Typha	Pollen Typhae	Raw Cattail Pollen
Pu Huang Tan	Typha	Pollen Typhae Carbonisatus	Charred Cattail Pollen
Pu Hui	Typha	Folium Typhae	Cattail Leaves
Qian Cao Gen	Rubia	Radix Rubiae Cordifoliae	Madder Root
Qian Dan	Minium	Minium	Red Lead Oxide

Pinyin	Botanical	Pharmaceutical	Common
Qian Hu	Peucedanum	Radix Peucedani	Hogfennel Root
Qian Li Guang	Senecio	Herba Senecionis Scandentis*	Groundsel
Qian Nian Jian	Homalomena	Rhizoma Homalomenae Occultae	Homalomena Rhizome
Qian Niu Zi	Pharbitis	Semen Pharbitidis	Morning Glory Seed
Qian Shi	Euryale	Semen Euryales Ferocis	Euryale Seed
Qiang Huo	Notopterygium	Rhizoma et Radix Notopterygii	Notopterygium Rhizome and Root
Qin Jiao	Gentiana	Radix Gentianae Qinjiao	Large-Leaf Gentian Root
Qin Pi	Fraxinus	Cortex Fraxini	Korean Ash Bark
Qing Dai	Indigo	Indigo Pulverata Levis	Indigo
Qing Fen	Calomelas	Calomelas	Calomel; Mercurous Chloride
Qing Hao	Artemisia	Herba Artemisiae Annuae	Sweet Wormwood; Southernwood
Qing Mu Xiang	Aristolochia	Radix Aristolochiae	Birthwort Root
Qing Pi	Citrus	Pericarpium Citri Reticulatae Viride	Immature (Green) Tangerine Peel
Qing Xiang Zi	Celosia	Semen Celosiae Argenteae	Celosia Seed
Qu Mai	Dianthus	Herba Dianthi	Pink Flower Herb
Quan Xie	Buthus	Buthus Martensi	Scorpion
Ren Gong Niu Huang	Bos	Calculus Artificialis	Artificially Induced Cow Gallstons
(Hong) Ren Shen	Panax	Radix Ginseng	Ginseng Root steamed until red
Ren Shen Lu	Panax	Cervix Ginseng	Ginseng Root Neck
Ren Shen Ye	Panax	Folium Ginseng	Ginseng Leaf
Rou Cong Rong	Cistanche	Herba Cistanches Deserticolae	Broomrape Fleshy Stem
Rou Dou Kou	Myristica	Semen Myristicae Fragrantis	Nutmeg Seed
Rou Gui	Cinnamomum	Cortex Cinnamomi Cassiae	Cinnamon Bark
Ru Xiang	Boswellia	Gummi Olibanum	Frankincense Gum-resin
San Bai Cao	Saururus	Herba Saururi Chinensis*	Saururus
San Leng	Sparganium	Rhizoma Sparganii Stoloniferi	Bur-reed Rhizome
San Qi	Panax	Radix Pseudoginseng	Pseudoginseng Root; Notoginseng Root
San Qi Hua	Panax	Flos Pseudoginseng	Pseudoginseng Flower; Notoginseng Flower
Sang Bai Pi	Morus	Cortex Mori Albae Radicis	Mulberry Rootbark
Sang Ji Sheng	Loranthus or Viscum	Ramulus Sangjishang	Mulberry Mistletoe Stem
Sang Piao Xiao	Paratenodera	Ootheca Mantidis	Praying Mantis Egg Case
Sang Shen	Morus	Fructus Mori Albae	Mulberry Fruit Bud

Pinyin	Botanical	Pharmaceutical	Common
Sang Ye	*Morus*	*Folium Mori Albae*	*Mulberry Leaf*
Sang Zhi	*Morus*	*Ramulus Mori Albae*	*Mulberry Twig*
Sha Ren	*Amomum*	*Fructus seu Semen Amomi*	*Grains-of-Paradise Fruit or Seeds*
Sha Ren Hua	*Amomum*	*Flos Amomi*	*Grains-of-Paradise Flower*
Sha Ren Ke	*Amomum*	*Pericarpium Amomi*	*Grains-of-Paradise Shell*
Sha Yuan Ji Li	*Astragalus*	*Semen Astragali Complanati*	*Flattened Milk-vetch Seed*
Shan Ci Gu	*Tulipa*	*Pseudobulbus Shancigu*	*Chinese Tulip Bulb*
Shan Dou Gen	*Sophora*	*Radix Sophorae Tonkinensis*	*Pigeon Pea Root*
Shan Yang Jiao	*Naemorhedis*	*Cornu Naemorhedis*	*Goat Horn*
Shan Yao	*Dioscorea*	*Radix Dioscoreae Oppositae*	*Chinese Wild Yam Root*
Shan Zha	*Crataegus*	*Fructus Crataegi*	*Hawthorn Unripe Fruit or Berry*
Shan Zha Rou	*Crataegus*	*Fructus Crataegi*	*Hawthorn Ripe Fruit or Berry*
Shan Zha Tan	*Crataegus*	*Fructus Crataegi Carbonisatus*	*Charred Hawthorn Fruit or Berry*
Shan Zhu Yu	*Cornus*	*Fructus Corni Officinalis*	*Dogwood Fruit; Asiatic Cornelian Cherry Fruit*
Shang Lu	*Phytolacca*	*Radix Phytolaccae*	*Poke Root*
She Chuang Zi	*Cnidium*	*Fructus Cnidii Monnieri*	*Cnidium Seed*
She Gan	*Belamcanda*	*Rhizoma Belamcandae Chinensis*	*Belamcanda Rhizome; Blackberry Lily Rhizome*
She Tui	*Zaocys*	*Exuviae Serpentis*	*Snake Skin Slough*
She Xiang	*Moschus*	*Secretio Moschus*	*Musk; Musk Deer Navel Gland Secretion*
Shen Jin Cao	*Lycopodium*	*Herba Lycopodii Clavati**	*Clubmoss*
Shen Qu	*Massa Fermentata*	*Massa Fermentata*	*Medicated Leaven*
Shen Xu	*Panax*	*Radix Ginseng*	*Rock Candy cured White Ginseng Root Tail*
Sheng Di Huang	*Rehmannia*	*Radix Rehmanniae Glutinosae*	*Fresh Chinese Foxglove Root*
Sheng Jiang	*Zingiber*	*Rhizoma Zingiberis Officinalis Recens*	*Fresh Ginger Rhizome*
Sheng Jiang Pi	*Zingiber*	*Cortex Zingiberis Officinalis Recens*	*Fresh Ginger Skin*
Sheng Ma	*Cimicifuga*	*Rhizoma Cimicifugae*	*Black Cohosh Rhizome; Bugbane Rhizome*
Sheng Shai Shen	*Panax*	*Radix Ginseng*	*Dried Ginseng Root*
Sheng Tie Luo	*Frusta Ferri*	*Frusta Ferri*	*Iron Filing*
Shi Bing	*Diospyros*	*Fructus Diospyri Kaki**	*Dried Persimmon Fruit*
Shi Chang Pu	*Acorus*	*Rhizoma Acori Graminei*	*Sweetflag Rhizome*
Shi Da Gong Lao	*Mahonia*	*Folium Mahoniae**	*Mahonia Leaf*
Shi Di	*Diospyros*	*Calyx Diospyri Kaki*	*Persimmon Calyx*

Pinyin	Botanical	Pharmaceutical	Common
Shi Gao	Gypsum	Gypsum Fibrosum	Gypsum; Calcium Sulphate
Shi Hu	Dendrobium	Herba Dendrobii	Dendrobium Stem
Shi Jue Ming	Haliotis	Concha Haliotidis	Abalone Shell
Shi Jun Zi	Quisqualis	Fructus Quisqualis Indicae	Rangoon Creeper Fruit
Shi Liu Gen Pi	Punica	Cortex Punicae Granati Radicis	Pomegranate Root Bark
Shi Liu Pi	Punica	Pericarpium Punicae Granati	Pomegranate Husk or Rind
Shi Shang Bai	Selaginella	Herba Selaginellae Doederleinii	Selaginella
Shi Wei	Pyrrosia	Folium Pyrrosiae	Pyrrosia Leaf
Shu Di Huang	Rehmannia	Radix Rehmanniae Glutinosae Conquitae	Wine-cooked Chinese Foxglove Root
Shu Qi	Dichroa	Folium Dichroae Febrifugae	Dichroa Leaf
Shu Yi Ren	Coix	Semen Coicis Lachryma-jobi	Dry-Fried Coix Seed
Shui Niu Jiao	Bubalus	Cornu Bubali	Waterbuffalo Horn
Shui Yin	Hydrargyrum	Hydrargyrum	Mercury
Shui Zhi	Hirudo	Hirudo seu Whitmania	Leech
Si Gua Lou	Luffa	Fasciculus Vascularis Luffae	Dried Skeleton of Luffa Sponge
Si Gua Pi	Luffa	Pericarpium Luffae Acutangulae	Luffa Skin
Si Ji Qing	Ilex	Folium Ilicis Chinensis*	Holly Leaf
Song Jie	Pinus	Lignum Pini Nodi	Knotty Pine Wood
Su He Xiang	Liquidambar	Styrax Liquidis	Rose Maloes Resin
Su Mu	Caesalpinia	Lignum Sappan	Sappan Heartwood
Suan Jiang	Physalis	Calyx seu Fructus Physalis*	Wintercherry Calyx or Fruit
Suan Zao Ren	Ziziphus	Semen Ziziphi Spinosae	Sour Jujube Seed; Zizyphus
Suo Yang	Cynomorium	Herba Cynomorii Songarici	Cynomorium Fleshy Stem
Tai Zi Shen	Pseudostellaria	Radix Pseudostellariae Heterophyllae	Prince Ginseng Root
Tan Xiang	Santalum	Lignum Santali Albi	Sandalwood Heartwood
Tang Song Cao	Thalictrum	Herba Thalictri Foliolosi*	Thalictrum
Tao Ren	Prunus	Semen Persicae	Peach Seed (Kernel)
Tian Hua Fen	Trichosanthes	Radix Trichosanthis Kirilowii	Snakegourd Root
Tian Ma	Gastrodia	Rhizoma Gastrodiae Elatae	Gastrodia Rhizome
Tian Men Dong	Asparagus	Tuber Asparagi Cochinchinensis	Chinese Asparagus Tuber
Tian Ming Jing	Carpesium	Herba Carpesii	Carpesium
(Sheng) Tian Nan Xing	Arisaema	Rhizoma Arisaematis	Raw Jack-in-the-Pulpit Rhizome
Tian Zhu Huang	Bambusa	Concretio Silicea Bambusae Textillis	Siliceous Secretions of Bamboo

Pinyin	Botanical	Pharmaceutical	Common
Tie Xian	Acalypha	Herba Acalypae Australis*	Acalypha
Ting Li Zi	Lepidium or Descurainia	Semen Lepidii seu Descurainiae	Tansy Mustard Seed
Tong Cao	Tetrapanax	Medulla Tetrapanacis Papyriferi	Rice Paper Pith
Tu Bie Chong	Eupolyphaga	Eupolyphaga seu Opisthoplatia	Wingless Cockroach
Tu Fu Ling	Smilax	Rhizoma Smilacis Glabrae	Glabrous Greenbrier Rhizome
Tu Niu Xi	Achyranthes	Radix Achyranthis Aspera	Achyranthes Root
Tu Si Zi	Cuscuta	Semen Cuscutae Chinensis	Dodder Seed
Wa Leng Zi	Arca	Concha Arcae	Cockle Shell; Ark Shell
Wan Nian Qing	Rhodea	Herba Rhodeae Japonicae*	Rhodea
Wang Bu Liu Xing	Vaccaria	Semen Vaccariae Segetalis	Cow Soapwort Seed
Wei Ling Xian	Clematis	Radix Clematidis	Clematis Root
Wu Bei Zi	Rhus/Melaphis	Galla Rhois Chinensis	Gallnut of Chinese Sumac
Wu Gong	Scolopendra	Scolopendra Subspinipes	Centipede
Wu Jia Pi	Acanthopanax	Cortex Acanthopanacis Gracilistyli Radicis	Acanthopanax Rootbark.
Wu Jiu Gen Pi	Sapium	Cortex Sappii Sebiferi Radicis*	Tallow Tree Root Bark
Wu Ling Zhi	Trogopterus or Pteromys	Excrementum Trogopteri seu Pteromi	Flying Squirrel Feces
Wu Mei	Prunus	Fructus Pruni Mume	Ume Plum Fruit; Black Plum Fruit
Wu Shao She	Zaocys	Zaocys Dhumnades	Black-striped Snake
Wu Tou	Aconitum	Radix Aconiti	Aconite Root
Wu Wei Zi	Schisandra	Fructus Schisandrae Chinensis	Northern Schisandra Fruit
Wu Yao	Lindera	Radix Linderae Strychnifoliae	Spicebush Root
Wu Yi	Ulmus	Praepartio Fructus Ulmi Macrocarpi	Stinking Elm Fruit Paste
Wu Zhu Yu	Evodia	Fructus Evodiae Rutaecarpae	Evodia Fruit
Xi Gua	Citrullus	Fructus Citrulli Vulgaris	Watermelon Fruit and Peel or Rind
Xi Hong Hua	Crocus	Stigma Crocus Sativae	Stigma of the True Saffron Flower
Xi Jiao	Rhinoceros	Cornu Rhinoceri	Rhinoceros Horn
Xi Xian Cao	Siegesbeckia	Herba Siegesbeckiae	St. Paul's Wort

Pinyin	Botanical	Pharmaceutical	Common
Xi Xin	Asarum	Herba cum Radice Asari	Asarum; Chinese Wild Ginger
Xi Yang Shen	Panax	Radix Panacis Quinquefolii	American Ginseng Root
Xia Ku Cao	Prunella	Spica Prunellae Vulgaris	Selfheal Spike; Heal all Spike
Xian He Cao	Agrimonia	Herba Agrimoniae Pilosae	Agrimony
Xian Mao	Curculigo	Rhizoma Curculiginis Orchioidis	Golden Eye-grass Rhizome
Xiang Fu	Cyperus	Rhizoma Cyperi Rotundi	Cyperus Rhizome; Nut-grass Rhizome; Sedge Rhizome
Xiang Ru	Elsholtzia	Herba Elsholtziae seu Moslae	Aromatic Madder
Xiao Hui Xiang	Foeniculum	Fructus Foeniculi Vulgaris	Fennel Fruit
Xiao Ji	Cephalanoplos	Herba Cephalanoplos	Small Thistle; Field Thistle
Xiao Shi	Niter	Niter*	Silver
Xie Bai	Allium	Bulbus Allii	Chinese Chive Bulb
Xin Yi Hua	Magnolia	Flos Magnoliae	Magnolia Flower
(Bei) Xing Ren	Prunus	Semen Pruni Armeniacae	(Northern) Apricot Seed
(Nan) Xing Ren	Prunus	Semen Pruni Armeniacae	(Southern) Apricot Seed
Xiong Dan	Ursus	Vesica Fellea Ursi	Bear Gallbladder
Xiong Huang	Realgar	Realgar	Realgar; Arsenic Disulfide
Xu Duan	Dipsacus	Radix Dipsaci Asperi	Teasel Root
Xu Sui Zi	Euphorbia	Semen Euphorbiae Lathyridis*	Caper Spurge Seed; Moleplant Seed
Xuan Fu Hua	Inula	Flos Inulae	Elecampane Flower
Xuan Ming Fen	Mirabilitum	Mirabilitum Purum	Pure Mirabilite; Pure Sodium Sulphate; Pure Glauber's Salt
Xuan Shen	Scrophularia	Radix Scrophulariae Ningpoensis	Figwort Root
Xue Jie	Dracaena	Sanguis Draconis	Dragon's Blood Resin
Xue Yu Tan	Homo Sapiens	Crinis Carbonisatus Hominis	Charred Human Hair
Ya Dan Zi	Brucea	Fructus Bruceae Javanicae	Brucea Fruit
Ya Zhi Cao	Commelina	Herba Commelinae*	Commelina
Yan Fu Mu	Rhus	Cortex Rhois Chinensis*	Chinese Sumac Bark
Yan Hu Suo	Corydalis	Rhizoma Corydalis Yanhusuo	Corydalis Rhizome
Yang Qi Shi	Actinolitum	Actinolitum	Actinolite
Ye Jiao Teng	Polygonum	Caulis Polygoni Multiflori	Fleeceflower Stem; Fo-Ti Stem
Ye Ju Hua	Chrysanthemum	Flos Chrysanthemi Indici	Wild Chrysanthemum Flower
Ye Ming Sha	Vespertilio	Excrementum Vespertilionis Murini	Bat Dung or Feces

Pinyin	Botanical	Pharmaceutical	Common
Ye Shan Shen	Panax	Radix Ginseng	Wild Ginseng
Yi Mu Cao	Leonurus	Herba Leonuri Heterophylli	Motherwort
Yi Tang	Saccharum Granorum	Saccharum Granorum	Barley Malt Sugar/Syrup
Yi Yi Ren	Coix	Semen Coicis Lachryma-jobi	Coix Seed; Job's Tears Seed
Yi Zhi Ren	Alpinia	Fructus Alpiniae Oxyphyllae	Black Cardamon Fruit
Yin Chai Hu	Stellaria	Radix Stellariae Dichotomae	Stellaria Root
Yin Chen Hao	Artemisia	Herba Artemisiae Yinchenhao	Oriental Wormwood
Yin Guo Ye	Ginkgo	Folium Ginkgo Bilobae	Ginkgo Leaf
Yin Yang Huo	Epimedium	Herba Epimedii	Epimedium
Ying Su Ke	Papaver	Pericarpium Papaveris Somniferi	Opium Poppy Husk
Yu Jin	Curcuma	Tuber Curcumae	Tumeric Tuber
Yu Li Ren	Prunus	Semen Pruni	Bush Cherry Seed
Yu Liang Shi	Limonite	Limonite	Limonite
Yu Mi Xu	Zea	Stylus Zeae Mays	Cornsilk
Yu Xing Cao	Houttuynia	Herba cum Radice Houttuyniae Cordatae	Houttuynia; Fish Smell Plant
Yu Zhu	Polygonatum	Rhizoma Polygonati Odorati	Fragrant Solomon's Seal Rhizome; Polygonatum
Yuan Hua	Daphne	Flos Daphnes Genkwa	Daphne Flower
Yuan Zhi	Polygala	Radix Polygalae Tenuifoliae	Chinese Senega Root; Seneca Snakeroot
Yue Ji Hua	Rosa	Flos et Fructus Rosae Chinensis	Partially-blossoming Chinese Tea Rose Flower
Zao Jiao	Gleditsia	Fructus Gleditsiae Sinensis	Honeylocust Fruit; Soap Bean Fruit
Zao Jiao Ci	Gleditsia	Spina Gleditsiae Sinensis	Honeylocust Spine; Soap Bean Spine
Zao Xiu	Paris	Rhizoma Paridis Polyphyllae*	Paris Rhizome
Ze Lan	Lycopus	Herba Lycopi Lucidi	Bugleweed
Ze Qi	Euphorbia	Herba Euphorbiae Helioscopiae	Pill-bearing Spurge
Ze Xie	Alisma	Rhizoma Alismatis Orientalitis	Water Plantain Rhizome
Zhang Nao	Cinnamomum	Camphora	Crystalized Volatile Oil of the Camphor Tree
Zhe Bei Mu	Fritillaria	Bulbus Fritillariae Thunbergii	Thunberg Fritillary Bulb
Zhen Zhu	Pteria	Margarita	Pearl
Zhen Zhu Mu	Pteria	Concha Margaritiferae	Mother-of-Pearl Shell
Zhi Gan Cao	Glycyrrhiza	Radix Glycyrrhizae Praeparata*	Honey-fried Licorice Root

Pinyin	Botanical	Pharmaceutical	Common
Zhi Ke	Citrus or Poncirus	Fructus Citri Aurantii	Bitter Orange Fruit
Zhi Mu	Anemarrhena	Radix Anemarrhenae Asphodeloidis	Anemarrhena Root
Zhi Nan Xing	Arisaema	Rhizoma Arisaematis Praeparatae	Prepared Jack-in-the-Pulpit Rhizome
Zhi Shi	Citrus or Poncirus	Fructus Immaturus Citri Aurantii	Immature Bitter Orange Fruit
Zhi Zi	Gardenia	Fructus Gardeniae Jasminoidis	Gardenia Fruit
Zhu Li	Bambusa	Succus Bambusae	Dried Bamboo Sap
Zhu Ling	Polyporus	Sclerotium Polypori Umbellati	Polyporus Sclerotium
Zhu Ma Gen	Boehmeria	Radix Boehmeriae Niveae*	Ramie Root
Zhu Ru	Bambusa	Caulis Bambusae in Taeniis	Bamboo Shavings
Zhu Sha	Cinnabaris	Cinnabaris	Cinnabar; Red Mercury Sulfide
Zhu Sha Gen	Ardisia	Radix Ardisiae Crenatae*	Ardisia Root
Zi Bei Tian Kuei	Begonia	Herba Begoniae Fimbristipulatae	Begonia
Zi Cao	Lithospermum	Radix Lithospermi seu Arnebiae	Groomwell Root
Zi He Che	Homo Sapiens	Placenta Hominis	Human Placenta
Zi Hua Di Ding	Viola	Herba cum Radice Violae Yedoensitis	Viola
Zi Ran Tong	Pyritum	Pyritum	Pyrite
Zi Shi Ying	Fluoritum	Fluoritum	Fluorite
Zi Su Geng	Perilla	Ramulus Perillae*	Perilla Stem
Zi Su Ye	Perilla	Folium Perillae Frutescentis	Perilla Leaf
Zi Su Zi	Perilla	Semen Perillae Frutescentis	Perilla Seed
Zi Wan	Aster	Radix Asteris Tatarici	Purple Aster Root
Zi Zhu	Callicarpa	Folium Callicarpae	Callicarpa Leaf
Zong Lu Pi Tan	Trachycarpus	Fibra Stipulae Trachycarpi Carbonisatus	Charred Windmill Palm Petiole

Herb Name Cross Reference Keyed to Botanical Names

Botanical	Pinyin	Pharmaceutical	Common
Abrus	Ji Gu Cao	Herba Abri*	Chicken Bone Vine
Acacia or Uncaria	Er Cha	Pasta Acacia seu Uncaria	Dried Paste of Concentrated Decoction of Black or White Cutch
Acalypha	Tie Xian	Herba Acalypae Australis*	Acalypha
Acanthopanax	Wu Jia Pi	Cortex Acanthopanacis Gracilistyli Radicis	Acanthopanax Rootbark.
Achyranthes	Huai Niu Xi	Radix Achyranthis Bidentatae	Achyranthes Root
Achyranthes	Tu Niu Xi	Radix Achyranthis Aspera	Achyranthes Root
Aconitum	Cao Wu	Radix Aconiti Kusnezoffii	Wild Aconite
Aconitum	Chuan Wu	Radix Aconite Carmichaeli	Sichuan Aconite
Aconitum	(Hei)Fu Zi	Radix Lateralis Aconiti Carmichaeli Praeparata	Prepared Sichuan Aconite Root
Aconitum	Wu Tou	Radix Aconiti	Aconite Root
Acorus	Shi Chang Pu	Rhizoma Acori Graminei	Sweetflag Rhizome
Actinolitum	Yang Qi Shi	Actinolitum	Actinolite
Adenophora	Gan Jie Geng	Radix Adenophorae Trachelioidis	Sweet Jie Geng
Adenophora	Nan Sha Shen	Radix Adenophorae	Ladybell Root; Southern Sand Root
Agastache or Pogostemon	Huo Xiang	Herba Agastaches seu Pogostemi	Patchouli; Agastache
Agkistrodon	Bai Hua She	Agkistrodon seu Bungarus	Long-noded Pit Viper Snake
Agrimonia	Xian He Cao	Herba Agrimoniae Pilosae	Agrimony
Ailanthus	Chun Pi	Cortex Ailanthi Altissimae	Tree of Heaven Bark
Ajuga	Bai Mao Xia Ku Cao	Herba Ajugae Decumbentis*	Ajuga
Akebia	Ba Yue Zha	Fructus Akebiae	Akebia Fruit
Akebia	Mu Tong	Caulis Mutong	Akebia Stem
Albizzia	He Huan Hua	Flos Albizziae Julibrissin*	Mimosa Tree Flower; Silktree Flower
Albizzia	He Huan Pi	Cortex Albizziae Julibrissin	Mimosa Tree Bark; Silktree Bark
Alisma	Ze Xie	Rhizoma Alismatis Orientalitis	Water Plantain Rhizome

Botanical	Pinyin	Pharmaceutical	Common
Allium	Cong Bai	Bulbus Allii Fistulosi	White Bulb of Green Onion or Scallion
Allium	Da Suan	Bulbus Allii Sativi	Garlic Bulb
Allium	Jiu Zi	Semen Allii Tuberosi	Chinese Leek Seed
Allium	Xie Bai	Bulbus Allii	Chinese Chive Bulb
Aloe	Lu Hui	Herba Aloes	Aloe Vera Leaf
Alpinia	Cao Dou Kou	Semen Alpiniae Katsumadai	Wild Cardamon Seed; Katsumada's Galangal Seed
Alpinia	Gao Liang Jiang	Rhizoma Alpiniae Officinari	Lesser Galangal Rhizome
Alpinia	Yi Zhi Ren	Fructus Alpiniae Oxyphyllae	Black Cardamon Fruit
Alumen	Ming Fan	Alumen	Alum; Potassium Aluminum Sulfate
Alumen Praeparatum	Ku Fan	Alumen Praeparatum	Prepared Alum
Amomum	Bai Dou Kou	Fructus Amomi Kravanh	Round Cardamon Fruit; Cluster Fruit
Amomum	Cao Guo	Fructus Amomi Tsao-Ko	Chinese Cardamon Fruit
Amomum	Sha Ren	Fructus seu Semen Amomi	Grains-of-Paradise Fruit or Seeds
Amomum	Sha Ren Hua	Flos Amomi	Grains-of-Paradise Flower
Amomum	Sha Ren Ke	Pericarpium Amomi	Grains-of-Paradise Shell
Ampelopsis	Bai Lian	Radix Ampelopsis Japonicae*	Ampelopsis Root
Amyda	Bie Jia	Carapax Amydae Sinensis	Chinese Soft-shell Turtle Shell
Andrographis	Chuan Xin Lian	Herba Andrographitis Paniculatae	Kariyat; Green Chiretta
Androsace	Dian Di Mei	Herba Androsacae Umbellatae*	Androsace
Anemarrhena	Zhi Mu	Radix Anemarrhenae Asphodeloidis	Anemarrhena Root
Anemone	Jiu Jie Chang Pu	Rhizoma Anemoni Altaicae*	Altaica Rhizome
Angelica	Bai Zhi	Radix Angelicae Dahuricae	Angelica Root
Angelica	Dang Gui	Radix Angelicae Sinensis	Tangkuei Root
Angelica	Dang Gui Tou	Caput Radicis Angelicae Sinensis	Tangkuei Head
Angelica	Dang Gui Wei	Extremas Radicis Angelicae Sinensis	Tangkuei Tail
Angelica	Du Huo	Radix Angelicae Pubescentis	Pubescent Angelica Root
Apocynum	Luo Bu Ma	Herba seu Folium Apocyni Veneti*	Red Dogbane Whole Herb or Leaf
Aquilaria	Chen Xiang	Lignum Aquilariae	Aloeswood Secretion or Sap
Arachis	Hua Sheng Yi	Pericarpium Arachi*	Peanut Skin
Arca	Wa Leng Zi	Concha Arcae	Cockle Shell; Ark Shell

Botanical	Pinyin	Pharmaceutical	Common
Arctium	Niu Bang Zi	Fructus Arctii Lappae	Burdock Seed
Ardisia	Zhu Sha Gen	Radix Ardisiae Crenatae*	Ardisia Root
Areca	Bing Lang	Semen Arecae Catechu	Betel Nut
Areca	Da Fu Pi	Pericarpium Arecae Catechu	Betelnut Husk
Arisaema	Dan Nan Xing	Pulvis Arisaemae cum Felle Bovis	Powdered Jack-in-the-Pulpit Rhizome mixed with Cow Bile
Arisaema	(Sheng) Tian Nan Xing	Rhizoma Arisaematis	Raw Jack-in-the-Pulpit Rhizome
Arisaema	Zhi Nan Xing	Rhizoma Arisaematis Praeparatae	Prepared Jack-in-the-Pulpit Rhizome
Aristolochia	Ma Dou Ling	Fructus Aristolochiae	Birthwort Fruit
Aristolochia	Qing Mu Xiang	Radix Aristolochiae	Birthwort Root
Aristolochia or Cocculus	Guang Fang Ji	Radix Aristolochiae Fangchi	Aristolochia Root
Arsenolith	Pi Shi	Arseolitum	White Arsenic
Artemisia	Ai Ye	Folium Artemisiae Argyi	Mugwort Leaf
Artemisia	Liu Ji Nu	Herba Artemisiae Anomalae	Artemisia
Artemisia	Qing Hao	Herba Artemisiae Annuae	Sweet Wormwood; Southernwood
Artemisia	Yin Chen Hao	Herba Artemisiae Yinchenhao	Oriental Wormwood
Asarum	Xi Xin	Herba cum Radice Asari	Asarum; Chinese Wild Ginger
Asparagus	Tian Men Dong	Tuber Asparagi Cochinchinensis	Chinese Asparagus Tuber
Aspongopus	Jiu Xiang Chong	Aspongopus*	Stink Bug
Aster	Zi Wan	Radix Asteris Tatarici	Purple Aster Root
Astragalus	Huang Qi	Radix Astragali Membranaceus	Yellow Milk-vetch Root
Astragalus	Sha Yuan Ji Li	Semen Astragali Complanati	Flattened Milk-vetch Seed
Atractylodes	Bai Zhu	Rhizoma Atractylodis Macrocephalae	White Atractylodes Rhizome
Atractylodes	Cang Zhu	Rhizoma Atractylodis	Atractylodes Rhizome
Aurum	Huang Jin	Aurum*	Gold
Bambusa	Tian Zhu Huang	Concretio Silicea Bambusae Textillis	Siliceous Secretions of Bamboo
Bambusa	Zhu Li	Succus Bambusae	Dried Bamboo Sap
Bambusa	Zhu Ru	Caulis Bambusae in Taeniis	Bamboo Shavings
Begonia	Zi Bei Tian Kuei	Herba Begoniae Fimbristipulatae	Begonia
Belamcanda	She Gan	Rhizoma Belamcandae Chinensis	Belamcanda Rhizome; Blackberry Lily Rhizome
Benincasa	Dong Gua Pi	Epicarpium Benincasae Hispidae	Wintermelon Fruit Peel; Wax Gourd Fruit Peel

Botanical	Pinyin	Pharmaceutical	Common
Benincasa	*Dong Gua Ren*	*Semen Benincasae Hispidae*	*Wintermelon Seed; Wax Gourd Seed*
Biota	*Bai Zi Ren*	*Semen Biotae Orientalis*	*Arbor-Vitae Seed*
Biota	*Ce Bai Ye*	*Cacumen Biotae Orientalis*	*Arborvitae Leafy Twig*
Bletilla	*Bai Ji*	*Rhizoma Bletillae Striatae*	*Bletilla Rhizome*
Boehmeria	*Zhu Ma Gen*	*Radix Boehmeriae Niveae**	*Ramie Root*
Bombyx	*Can Sha*	*Excrementum Bombycis Mori*	*Silkworm Feces*
Bombyx	*Jiang Can*	*Bombyx Batryticatus*	*Dead Stiff Body of Sick Silkworm Larvae*
Borax	*Peng Sha*	*Borax*	*Borax; Sodium Tetraborate*
Bos	*Niu Dan*	*Vesica Fellea Bovus*	*Cow Gallbladder*
Bos	*Ren Gong Niu Huang*	*Calculus Artificialis*	*Artificially Induced Cow Gallstons*
Bos or Bubalis	*Niu Huang*	*Calculus Bovis seu Calculus Bubali*	*Ox or Water Buffalo Gallstone*
Boswellia	*Ru Xiang*	*Gummi Olibanum*	*Frankincense Gum-resin*
Brassica	*Bai Jie Zi*	*Semen Sinapsis Albae*	*White Mustard Seed*
Broussonetia	*Chu Shi Zi*	*Semen Broussonetiae Papyriferae**	*Broussonetia Seed*
Brucea	*Ya Dan Zi*	*Fructus Bruceae Javanicae*	*Brucea Fruit*
Bubalus	*Shui Niu Jiao*	*Cornu Bubali*	*Waterbuffalo Horn*
Buddleia	*Mi Meng Hua*	*Flos Buddleiae Officinalis Immaturus*	*Buddleia Flower*
Bufo	*Chan Su*	*Secretio Bufonis*	*Dried Skin Secretion of Toad*
Bupleurum	*Chai Hu*	*Radix Bupleuri*	*Thorowax Root; Hare's Ear Root*
Buthus	*Quan Xie*	*Buthus Martensi*	*Scorpion*
Caesalpinia	*Su Mu*	*Lignum Sappan*	*Sappan Heartwood*
Calcaria	*Chen Shi Huei*	*Calcaria**	*Calcium Hydroxide*
Calcitum	*Han Shui Shi*	*Calcitum*	*Calcite*
Callicarpa	*Zi Zhu*	*Folium Callicarpae*	*Callicarpa Leaf*
Calomelas	*Qing Fen*	*Calomelas*	*Calomel; Mercurous Chloride*
Canis	*Gou Gu*	*Os Canine*	*Dog Bone*
Canis	*Guang Gou Shen*	*Testis et Penis Canis**	*Male Dog Sexual Organs*
Cannabis	*Huo Ma Ren*	*Semen Cannabis Sativae*	*Hemp Seed; Marihuana Seed*
Capsella	*Ji Cai*	*Herba Capsellae**	*Shepherd's Purse*
Carpesium	*Tian Ming Jing*	*Herba Carpesii*	*Carpesium*
Carpesium or Daucus	*He Shi*	*Fructus Carpesii seu Daucusi*	*Carpesium Fruit*
Carthamus	*Hong Hua*	*Flos Carthami Tinctorii*	*Safflower*

Botanical	Pinyin	Pharmaceutical	Common
Cassia	Fan Xie Ye	Folium Sennae	Senna Leaf
Cassia	Jue Ming Zi	Semen Cassiae	Cassia Seed
Celosia	Ji Guan Hua	Flos Celosiae Cristatae	Cockscomb Flower
Celosia	Qing Xiang Zi	Semen Celosiae Argenteae	Celosia Seed
Centipeda	E Bu Shi Cao	Herba Centipedae Minimae*	Centipeda Herb
Cephalanoplos	Xiao Ji	Herba Cephalanoplos	Small Thistle; Field Thistle
Cervus	Hua Lu Shen	Testis et Penis Cervi*	Male Deer Sexual Organs
Cervus	Lu Jiao	Cornu Cervi	Antler; Deerhorn; Ossified Horn of the Mature Male Deer
Cervus	Lu Jiao Jiao	Colla Cornu Cervi	Mature Antler Glue; Mature Antler Gelatin
Cervus	Lu Jiao Shuang	Cornu Cervi Degelatinatium	Antler Powder from the dregs of cooking Antler Glue
Cervus	Lu Rong	Cornu Cervi Parvum	Young Deer Antler Velvet
Chaenomeles	Mu Gua	Fructus Chaenomelis	Chinese Quince Fruit
Chalcanthitum	Dan Fan	Chalcanthitum*	Copper Sulphate; Blue Vitriol
Changium	Ming Dang Shen	Radix Changii*	Changium Root
Chinemys	Gui Ban	Plastrum Testudinis	Fresh Water Turtle Shell
Chrysanthemum	(Bai) Ju Hua	Flos Chrysanthemi Morifolii	White Chrysanthemum Flower
Chrysanthemum	(Huang) Ju Hua	Flos Chrysanthemi Morifolii	Yellow Chrysanthemum Flower
Chrysanthemum	Ye Ju Hua	Flos Chrysanthemi Indici	Wild Chrysanthemum Flower
Cibotium	Gou Ji	Rhizoma Cibotii Barometz	Chain Fern Rhizome
Cimicifuga	Sheng Ma	Rhizoma Cimicifugae	Black Cohosh Rhizome; Bugbane Rhizome
Cinnabaris	Zhu Sha	Cinnabaris	Cinnabar; Red Mercury Sulfide
Cinnamomum	Guan Gui	Cortex Tubiformis Cinnamomi Cassiae	Thin Cinnamon Bark from Young Trees
Cinnamomum	Gui Zhi	Ramulus Cinnamomi Cassiae	Cinnamon Twig
Cinnamomum	Rou Gui	Cortex Cinnamomi Cassiae	Cinnamon Bark
Cinnamomum	Zhang Nao	Camphora	Crystalized Volatile Oil of the Camphor Tree
Cirsium	Da Ji	Herba seu Radix Cirsii Japonici	Japanese Thistle
Cistanche	Rou Cong Rong	Herba Cistanches Deserticolae	Broomrape Fleshy Stem
Citrullus	Xi Gua	Fructus Citrulli Vulgaris	Watermelon Fruit and Peel or Rind
Citrus	Chen Pi	Pericarpium Citri Reticulatae	Tangerine Peel
Citrus	Fo Shou	Fructus Citri Sarcodactylis	Finger Citron Fruit

Botanical

Botanical	Pinyin	Pharmaceutical	Common
Citrus	Fo Shou Hua	Flos Citri Sarcodactylis	Finger Citron Flower
Citrus	Ju He	Semen Citri Reticulatae*	Tangerine Seed
Citrus	Ju Hong	Pars Rubra Epicarpii Citri Erythrocarpae	Red Tangerine Peel
Citrus	Qing Pi	Pericarpium Citri Reticulatae Viride	Immature (Green) Tangerine Peel
Citrus or Poncirus	Zhi Ke	Fructus Citri Aurantii	Bitter Orange Fruit
Citrus or Poncirus	Zhi Shi	Fructus Immaturus Citri Aurantii	Immature Bitter Orange Fruit
Clematis	Wei Ling Xian	Radix Clematidis	Clematis Root
Clerodendron	Chou Wu Tong	Folium Clerodendri Trichotomi	Glorybower Leaf
Cnidium	She Chuang Zi	Fructus Cnidii Monnieri	Cnidium Seed
Codonopsis	Dang Shen	Radix Codonopsitis Pilosulae	Asiabell Root
Coix	Shu Yi Ren	Semen Coicis Lachryma-jobi	Dry-Fried Coix Seed
Coix	Yi Yi Ren	Semen Coicis Lachryma-jobi	Coix Seed; Job's Tears Seed
Commelina	Ya Zhi Cao	Herba Commelinae*	Commelina
Commiphora	Mo Yao	Resinae Myrrhae	Myrrh Gum-resin
Coptis	Huang Lian	Rhizoma Coptidis	Coptis; Golden Thread Rhizome
Cordyceps	Dong Chong Xia Cao	Cordyceps Sinensis	Chinese Caterpillar Fungus
Cornus	Shan Zhu Yu	Fructus Corni Officinalis	Dogwood Fruit; Asiatic Cornelian Cherry Fruit
Corydalis	Yan Hu Suo	Rhizoma Corydalis Yanhusuo	Corydalis Rhizome
Crataegus	Shan Zha	Fructus Crataegi	Hawthorn Unripe Fruit or Berry
Crataegus	Shan Zha Rou	Fructus Crataegi	Hawthorn Ripe Fruit or Berry
Crataegus	Shan Zha Tan	Fructus Crataegi Carbonisatus	Charred Hawthorn Fruit or Berry
Crocus	Xi Hong Hua	Stigma Crocus Sativae	Stigma of the True Saffron Flower
Croton	Ba Dou	Semen Croton Tiglii	Croton Seed
Cryptotympana	Chan Tui	Periostracum Cicadae	Cicada Skin; Cicada Moulting
Cucumis	Gua Di	Pedicellus Cucumeris	Melon Pedicle
Cucurbita	Nan Gua Zi	Semen Cucurbitae Moschatae	Pumpkin Seed and Husk
Curculigo	Xian Mao	Rhizoma Curculiginis Orchioidis	Golden Eye-grass Rhizome
Curcuma	E Zhu	Rhizoma Curcumae	Zedoary Tumeric Rhizome
Curcuma	Jiang Huang	Rhizoma Curcumae Longae	Tumeric Rhizome
Curcuma	Yu Jin	Tuber Curcumae	Tumeric Tuber

Botanical	Pinyin	Pharmaceutical	Common
Cuscuta	Tu Si Zi	Semen Cuscutae Chinensis	Dodder Seed
Cyathula	Chuan Niu Xi	Radix Cyathulae Officinalis	Cyathula Root
Cyclina	Hai Ge Ke	Concha Cyclinae Sinensis	Clam Shell
Cynanchum	Bai Qian	Rhizoma et Radix Cynanchi Baiqian	Cynanchum Rhizome and Root
Cynanchum	Bai Wei	Radix Cynanchi Baiwei	Swallowort Root
Cynanchum	Ge Shan Xiang	Radix Cynanchi Auriculati	Cynanchum Root
Cynomorium	Suo Yang	Herba Cynomorii Songarici	Cynomorium Fleshy Stem
Cyperus	Xiang Fu	Rhizoma Cyperi Rotundi	Cyperus Rhizome; Nut-grass Rhizome; Sedge Rhizome
Dalbergia	Jiang Xiang	Lignum Dalbergiae Odoriferae	Dalbergia Heartwood
Daphne	Yuan Hua	Flos Daphnes Genkwa	Daphne Flower
Dendrobium	Shi Hu	Herba Dendrobii	Dendrobium Stem
Dens Draconis	Long Chi	Dens Draconis	Dragon Tooth; Fossilized Tooth
Dianthus	Qu Mai	Herba Dianthi	Pink Flower Herb
Dichroa	Chang Shan	Radix Dichroae Febrifugae	Dichroa Root
Dichroa	Shu Qi	Folium Dichroae Febrifugae	Dichroa Leaf
Dictamnus	Bai Xian Pi	Cortex Dictamni Dasycarpi Radicis	Dittany Root Bark
Dioscorea	Bei Xie	Rhizoma Dioscoreae Hypoglaucae	Hypoglauca Yam Rhizome; Fish-poison Yam Rhizome
Dioscorea	Chuan Shan Long	Rhizoma Dioscoreae Nipponicae*	Japanese Dioscorea Rhizome
Dioscorea	Huang Yao Zi	Tuber Dioscoreae Bulbiferae	Dioscorea Tuber
Dioscorea	Shan Yao	Radix Dioscoreae Oppositae	Chinese Wild Yam Root
Diospyros	Shi Bing	Fructus Diospyri Kaki*	Dried Persimmon Fruit
Diospyros	Shi Di	Calyx Diospyri Kaki	Persimmon Calyx
Dipsacus	Xu Duan	Radix Dipsaci Asperi	Teasel Root
Dolichos	Bian Dou	Semen Dolichoris Lablab	Hyacinth Bean
Dolichos	Bian Dou Hua	Flos Dolichoris Lablab	Hyacinth Bean Flower
Dracaena	Xue Jie	Sanguis Draconis	Dragon's Blood Resin
Drynaria	Gu Sui Bu	Rhizoma Drynariae	Drynaria Rhizome
Dryobalanops	Bing Pian	Borneol	Processed Resin of Borneol Camphor
Dryopteris	Dong Bei Guan Zhong	Rhizoma Dryopteridis	Dryopteris Rhizome
Dryopteris	Guan Zhong	Rhizoma Guanzhong	Shield-fern Rhizome
Eclipta	Han Lian Cao	Herba Ecliptae Prostratae	Eclipta
Eleagnus	Hu Tui Ye	Folium Eleagni Pungens	Eleagnus Leaf
Elsholtzia	Xiang Ru	Herba Elsholtziae seu Moslae	Aromatic Madder

Botanical	Pinyin	Pharmaceutical	Common
Ephedra	Ma Huang	Herba Ephedrae	Ephedra Stem
Ephedra	Ma Huang Gen	Radix Ephedrae	Ephedra Root
Epimedium	Yin Yang Huo	Herba Epimedii	Epimedium
Equisetum	Mu Zei	Herba Equiseti Hiemalis	Horsetail; Scouring Rush; Shavegrass
Equus	E Jiao	Gelatinum Corii Asini	Donkey Hide Gelatin; Ass Skin Glue
Equus	Hei Lu Shen	Testis et Penis Equii*	Male Horse Sexual Organs
Eretmochelys	Dai Mao	Carapax Eretmochelydis Imbricatae*	Hawksbill Turtle Shell
Eriobotrya	Pi Pa Ye	Folium Eriobotryae Japonicae	Loquat Leaf
Eriocaulon	Gu Jing Cao	Scapus et Inflorescentia Eriocaulonis Buergeriani	Pipewort Scapus
Erodium or Geranium	Lao Guan Cao	Herba Erodii seu Geranii*	Geranium; Heronbill; Cranebill
Erythrina	Hai Tong Pi	Cortex Erythrinae	Coral-bean Bark
Eucommia	Du Zhong	Cortex Eucommiae Ulmoidis	Eucommia Bark
Eugenia	Ding Xiang	Flos Caryophylli	Clove Flower-bud
Eupatorium	Pei Lan	Herba Eupatorii Fortunei	Boneset; Thoroughwort; Feverwort
Euphorbia	Gan Sui	Radix Euphorbiae Kansui	Kansui Spurge Root
Euphorbia	Xu Sui Zi	Semen Euphorbiae Lathyridis*	Caper Spurge Seed; Moleplant Seed
Euphorbia	Ze Qi	Herba Euphorbiae Helioscopiae	Pill-bearing Spurge
Euphorbia or Knoxia	Jing Da Ji	Radix Euphorbiae seu Knoxiae	Peking Spurge Root
Euphoria	Long Yan Rou	Arillus Euphoriae Longanae	Longan Fruit Flesh
Eupolyphaga	Tu Bie Chong	Eupolyphaga seu Opisthoplatia	Wingless Cockroach
Euryale	Qian Shi	Semen Euryales Ferocis	Euryale Seed
Evodia	Wu Zhu Yu	Fructus Evodiae Rutaecarpae	Evodia Fruit
Fagopyrum	Jin Qiao Mai	Rhizoma Fagopyri Cynosi*	Wild Buckwheat Rhizome
Ferula	E Wei	Resina Asafoetidae*	Asafoetida Gum-resin; Devil's Dung
Fluoritum	Zi Shi Ying	Fluoritum	Fluorite
Foeniculum	Xiao Hui Xiang	Fructus Foeniculi Vulgaris	Fennel Fruit
Forsythia	Lian Qiao	Fructus Forsythiae Suspensae	Forsythia Fruit; Golden Bells
Fraxinus	Qin Pi	Cortex Fraxini	Korean Ash Bark
Fritillaria	Chuan Bei Mu	Bulbus Fritillariae Cirrhosae	Tendrilled Fritillary Bulb
Fritillaria	Zhe Bei Mu	Bulbus Fritillariae Thunbergii	Thunberg Fritillary Bulb

Botanical	Pinyin	Pharmaceutical	Common
Frusta Ferri	Sheng Tie Luo	Frusta Ferri	Iron Filing
Gallus	Ji Nei Jin	Endothelium Corneum Gigeriae Galli	Chicken Gizard Lining
Ganoderma	Ling Zhi	Fructificatio Ganodermae Lucidi*	Lucid Ganoderma; Reishi
Gardenia	Zhi Zi	Fructus Gardeniae Jasminoidis	Gardenia Fruit
Gastrodia	Tian Ma	Rhizoma Gastrodiae Elatae	Gastrodia Rhizome
Gekko	Ge Jie	Gekko	Gecko Lizard
Gentiana	Long Dan Cao	Radix Gentianae Longdancao	Chinese Gentian Root
Gentiana	Qin Jiao	Radix Gentianae Qinjiao	Large-Leaf Gentian Root
Ginkgo	Bai Guo	Semen Ginkgo Bilobae	Ginkgo Nut
Ginkgo	Yin Guo Ye	Folium Ginkgo Bilobae	Ginkgo Leaf
Gleditsia	Zao Jiao	Fructus Gleditsiae Sinensis	Honeylocust Fruit; Soap Bean Fruit
Gleditsia	Zao Jiao Ci	Spina Gleditsiae Sinensis	Honeylocust Spine; Soap Bean Spine
Glehnia	Bei Sha Shen	Radix Glehniae Littoralis	Beech Silver-top Root; Northern Sand Root
Glycine	Dan Dou Chi	Semen Glycinis Praeparatum	Prepared (Fermented) Soybean
Glycine	Dou Juan	Semen Glycinis Germinatum	Young Soybean Sprout
Glycyrhiza	Gan Cao	Radix Glycyrrhizae Uralensis	Licorice Root
Glycyrrhiza	Zhi Gan Cao	Radix Glycyrrhizae Praeparata*	Honey-fried Licorice Root
Gossypium	Mian Hua Gen	Radix Gossypii Hirsuti*	Cotton Root
Gynura	Ju Ye San Qi	Folium Gynurae*	Gynura Leaf
Gypsum	Shi Gao	Gypsum Fibrosum	Gypsum; Calcium Sulphate
Haematitum	Dai Zhe Shi	Haematitum	Hematite; Iron Ore
Haliotis	Shi Jue Ming	Concha Haliotidis	Abalone Shell
Halloysitum Rubrum	Chi Shi Zhi	Halloysitum Rubrum	Halloysite; Red Kaolin
Hedera	Chang Chun Teng	Herba Hederae Nepalensis*	Ivy
Hippocampus	Hai Ma	Hippocampus	Sea Horse
Hirudo	Shui Zhi	Hirudo seu Whitmania	Leech
Homalomena	Qian Nian Jian	Rhizoma Homalomenae Occultae	Homalomena Rhizome
Homo Sapiens	Xue Yu Tan	Crinis Carbonisatus Hominis	Charred Human Hair
Homo Sapiens	Zi He Che	Placenta Hominis	Human Placenta
Hordeum	Mai Ya	Fructus Hordei Vulgaris Germinatus	Barley Sprout; Malted Barley
Houttuynia	Yu Xing Cao	Herba cum Radice Houttuyniae Cordatae	Houttuynia; Fish Smell Plant

Botanical	Pinyin	Pharmaceutical	Common
Hydnocarpus	Da Feng Zi	Semen Hydnocarpi Anthelminticae	Chaulmoogra Seed
Hydrangea	Ba Xian Hua	Flos Hydrangeae Macrophyllae*	Hydrangea Flower
Hydrargyrum	Shui Yin	Hydrargyrum	Mercury
Ilex	Mao Dong Qing	Radix Ilicis Pubescentis*	Pubescent Holly Root
Ilex	Si Ji Qing	Folium Ilicis Chinensis*	Holly Leaf
Illicium	Ba Jiao Hui Xiang	Fructus Illicii*	Star Anise Fruit
Imperata	Bai Mao Gen	Rhizoma Imperatae Cylindricae	Woolly Grass Rhizome; White Grass Rhizome
Imperata	Bai Mao Hua	Flos Imperatae Cylindricae	Wooly Grass Flower; White Grass Flower
Indigo	Qing Dai	Indigo Pulverata Levis	Indigo
Inula	Jin Fei Cao	Herba Inulae	Elecampane
Inula	Xuan Fu Hua	Flos Inulae	Elecampane Flower
Isatis	Ban Lan Gen	Radix Isatidis seu Baphicacanthi	Isatis Root; Woad Root
Isatis	Da Qing Ye	Folium Isatidis Daqingye	Isatis Leaf; Woad Leaf
Juglans	Hu Tao Ren	Semen Juglandis Regiae	Walnut
Juncus	Deng Xin Cao	Medulla Junci Effusi	Rush Pith
Kochia	Di Fu Zi	Fructus Kochiae Scopariae	Broom Cyperus Seed
Laminaria	Hai Dai	Herba Laminaria Japonicae	Algae
Laminaria or Ecklonia	Kun Bu	Thallus Algae	Kelp Thallus; Kombu Thallus
Lapis Micae seu Chloriti	Meng Shi	Lapis Micae seu Chloriti	Chlorite Schist; Lapis
Lasiosphaera	Ma Bo	Fructificatio Lasiosphaerae seu Calvatiae	Puffball Fruiting Body
Ledebouriella	Fang Feng	Radix Ledebouriella Divaricatae	Siler Root; Ledebouriella Root
Leonurus	Chong Wei Zi	Semen Leonuri Heterophylli	Motherwort Seed
Leonurus	Yi Mu Cao	Herba Leonuri Heterophylli	Motherwort
Lepidium or Descurainia	Ting Li Zi	Semen Lepidii seu Descurainiae	Tansy Mustard Seed
Ligusticum	Chuan Xiong	Radix Ligustici Chuan Xiong	Sichuan Lovage Root
Ligusticum	Gao Ben	Rhizoma et Radix Ligustici	Straw Weed Rhizome and Root; Chinese Lovage Rhizome and Root
Ligustrum	Nu Zhen Zi	Fructus Ligustri Lucidi	Privet Fruit; Waxtree Fruit
Lilium	Bai He	Bulbus Lilii	Lily Bulb
Limonite	Yu Liang Shi	Limonite	Limonite
Lindera	Wu Yao	Radix Linderae Strychnifoliae	Spicebush Root
Liquidambar	Lu Lu Tong	Fructus Liquidambaris Taiwanianae	Sweetgum Fruit
Liquidambar	Su He Xiang	Styrax Liquidis	Rose Maloes Resin

Botanical	Pinyin	Pharmaceutical	Common
Litchi	Li Zhi He	Semen Litchi Chinensis	Leechee Nut
Lithargyrum	Mi Tuo Seng	Lithargyrum	Litharge; Galena
Lithospermum	Zi Cao	Radix Lithospermi seu Arnebiae	Groomwell Root
Litsea	Dou Chi Jiang	Radix et Ramus Litseae Cubebae	Aromatic Litsea Root and Stem
Lobelia	Ban Bian Lian	Herba Lobeliae Chinensis cum Radice	Chinese Lobelia
Lonicera	Jin Yin Hua	Flos Lonicerae Japonicae	Honeysuckle Flower
Lonicera	Jin Yin Teng	Ramus Lonicerae Japonicae	Honeysuckle Stem
Lophatherum	Dan Zhu Ye	Herba Lophatheri Gracilis	Bland Bamboo Leaf and Stem
Loranthus or Viscum	Sang Ji Sheng	Ramulus Sangjishang	Mulberry Mistletoe Stem
Loropetalum	Ji Mu	Cortex Loropetali*	Loropetalum Bark
Luffa	Si Gua Lou	Fasciculus Vascularis Luffae	Dried Skeleton of Luffa Sponge
Luffa	Si Gua Pi	Pericarpium Luffae Acutangulae	Luffa Skin
Lycium	Di Gu Pi	Cortex Lycii Radicis	Matrimony-vine Rootbark; Wolfberry Bark
Lycium	Gou Qi Zi	Fructus Lycii	Matrimony Vine Fruit; Wolfberry Fruit
Lycopodium	Shen Jin Cao	Herba Lycopodii Clavati*	Clubmoss
Lycopus	Ze Lan	Herba Lycopi Lucidi	Bugleweed
Lygodium	Hai Jin Sha	Spora Lygodii Japonici	Japanese Climbing Fern Spore
Lygodium	Jin Sha Teng	Herba Lygodii Japonici	Japanese Climbing Fern
Lysimachia	Jin Qian Cao	Herba Lysimachiae	Lysimachia
Macaca	Hou Zao	Calculus Macacae Mulattae	Macaque Gallstone
Magnetitum	Ci Shi	Magnetitum	Magnetite; Magnetic Iron Ore; Loadstone
Magnolia	Hou Po	Cortex Magnoliae Officinalis	Magnolia Bark
Magnolia	Hou Po Hua	Flos Magnoliae Officinalis	Magnolia Flower
Magnolia	Xin Yi Hua	Flos Magnoliae	Magnolia Flower
Mahonia	Shi Da Gong Lao	Folium Mahoniae*	Mahonia Leaf
Malva or Abutilon	Dong Kui Zi	Semen Albutili seu Malvae	Musk Mallow Seed; Malva Seed
Manis	Chuan Shan Jia	Squama Manitis Pentadactylae	Anteater-Scales; Pangolin Scales
Massa Fermentata	Shen Qu	Massa Fermentata	Medicated Leaven
Mel	Feng Mi	Mel*	Honey
Melia	Chuan Lian Zi	Fructus Meliae Toosendan	Sichuan Chinaberry Fruit; Sichuan Pagoda Tree Fruit; Neem Fruit

Botanical	Pinyin	Pharmaceutical	Common
Melia	*Ku Lian Gen Pi*	*Cortex Meliae Radicis*	*Sichuan Chinaberry Root Bark; Sichuan Pagoda Tree Root Bark; Neem Root Bark*
Melia	*Ku Lian Mu Pi*	*Cortex Meliae*	*Sichuan Chinaberry Tree Bark; Sichuan Pagoda Tree Bark; Neem Tree Bark*
Mentha	*Bo He*	*Herba Menthae Haplocalycis*	*Peppermint; Spearmint; Field Mint*
Millettia	*Ji Xue Teng*	*Radix et Caulis Jixueteng*	*Millettia Root and Vine; Chicken Blood Vine*
Minium	*Qian Dan*	*Minium*	*Red Lead Oxide*
Mirabilitum	*Mang Xiao*	*Mirabilitum*	*Mirabilite; Glauber's Salt*
Mirabilitum	*Xuan Ming Fen*	*Mirabilitum Purum*	*Pure Mirabilite; Pure Sodium Sulphate; Pure Glauber's Salt*
Momordica	*Luo Han Guo*	*Fructus Momordicae Grosvenori*	*Momordica Fruit*
Momordica	*Luo Huo Guo Ye*	*Folium Momordicae Grosvenori*	*Momordica Leaf*
Momordica	*Mu Bie Zi*	*Semen Momordicae Cochinchinensis*	*Momordica Seed*
Morinda	*Ba Ji Tian*	*Radix Morindae Officinalis*	*Morinda Root*
Morus	*Sang Bai Pi*	*Cortex Mori Albae Radicis*	*Mulberry Rootbark*
Morus	*Sang Shen*	*Fructus Mori Albae*	*Mulberry Fruit Bud*
Morus	*Sang Ye*	*Folium Mori Albae*	*Mulberry Leaf*
Morus	*Sang Zhi*	*Ramulus Mori Albae*	*Mulberry Twig*
Moschus	*She Xiang*	*Secretio Moschus*	*Musk; Musk Deer Navel Gland Secretion*
Mylabris	*Ban Mao*	*Mylabris*	*Cantharides; Chinese Blistering Beetle*
Myristica	*Rou Dou Kou*	*Semen Myristicae Fragrantis*	*Nutmeg Seed*
Naemorhedis	*Shan Yang Jiao*	*Cornu Naemorhedis*	*Goat Horn*
Nelumbo	*He Ye*	*Folium Nelumbinis Nuciferae*	*Lotus Leaf*
Nelumbo	*Lian Fang*	*Receptaculum Nelumbinis Nuciferae*	*Mature Lotus Receptacle*
Nelumbo	*Lian Geng*	*Ramulus Nelumbinis Nuciferae*	*Lotus Stem*
Nelumbo	*Lian Xin*	*Plumula Nelumbinis Nuciferae*	*Lotus Plumule*
Nelumbo	*Lian Xu*	*Stamen Nelumbinis Nuciferae*	*Lotus Stamen*
Nelumbo	*Lian Zi*	*Semen Nelumbinis Nuciferae*	*Lotus Seed*
Nelumbo	*Ou Jie*	*Nodus Nelumbinis Nuciferae Rhizomatis*	*Lotus Rhizome Node*
Niter	*Xiao Shi*	*Niter**	*Silver*

Botanical	Pinyin	Pharmaceutical	Common
Notopterygium	Qiang Huo	Rhizoma et Radix Notopterygii	Notopterygium Rhizome and Root
Oldenlandia	Bai Hua She She Cao	Herba Oldenlandiae Diffusae	Oldenlandia
Omphalia	Lei Wan	Sclerotium Omphaliae Lapidescens	Omphalia Fungus Fruiting Body
Ophicalcitum	Hua Rui Shi	Ophicalcitum	Ophicalcite
Ophiopogon	Mai Men Dong	Tuber Ophiopogonis Japonici	Creeping Lily-turf Tuber
Oroxylum	Mu Hu Die	Semen Oroxyli Indici	Oroxylum Seed
Oryza	Gu Ya	Fructus Oryzae Sativae Germinatus	Rice Sprout
Oryza	Jing Mi	Semen Oryzae Sativae*	Rice Grain
Oryza	Nuo Dao Gen Xu	Radix et Rhizoma Oryzae Glutinosae	Sweet Rice Root and Rhizome
Os Draconis	Duan Long Gu	Os Draconis	Calcined Dragon Bone; Calcined Fossilized Bone
Os Draconis	Long Gu	Os Draconis	Dragon Bone; Fossilized Bone
Ostrea	Duan Mu Li	Concha Ostreae	Calcined Oyster Shell
Ostrea	Mu Li	Concha Ostreae	Oyster Shell
Paederia	Ji Shi Teng	Caulis Paederiae*	Paederia Stem
Paeonia	Bai Shao	Radix Paeoniae Lactiflorae	White Peony Root
Paeonia	Chi Shao	Radix Paeoniae Rubra	Red Peony Root
Paeonia	Mu Dan Pi	Cortex Moutan Radicis	Tree Peony Rootbark
Panax	Bai Shen	Radix Ginseng	Rock Candy cured White Ginseng Root
Panax	Ji Lin Shen	Radix Ginseng	Jilin Wild Ginseng
Panax	(Hong) Ren Shen	Radix Ginseng	Ginseng Root steamed until red
Panax	Ren Shen Lu	Cervix Ginseng	Ginseng Root Neck
Panax	Ren Shen Ye	Folium Ginseng	Ginseng Leaf
Panax	San Qi	Radix Pseudoginseng	Pseudoginseng Root; Notoginseng Root
Panax	San Qi Hua	Flos Pseudoginseng	Pseudoginseng Flower; Notoginseng Flower
Panax	Shen Xu	Radix Ginseng	Rock Candy cured White Ginseng Root Tail
Panax	Sheng Shai Shen	Radix Ginseng	Dried Ginseng Root
Panax	Xi Yang Shen	Radix Panacis Quinquefolii	American Ginseng Root
Panax	Ye Shan Shen	Radix Ginseng	Wild Ginseng
Panthera	Bao Gu	Os Leopardis	Leopard Bone
Panthera	Hu Gu	Os Tigris	Tiger Bone
Papaver	Ying Su Ke	Pericarpium Papaveris Somniferi	Opium Poppy Husk

Botanical	Pinyin	Pharmaceutical	Common
Paratenodera	Sang Piao Xiao	Ootheca Mantidis	Praying Mantis Egg Case
Paris	Zao Xiu	Rhizoma Paridis Polyphyllae*	Paris Rhizome
Patrinia or Thiaspi	Bai Jiang Cao	Herba cum Radice Patriniae	Patrinia; Thiaspi
Perilla	Zi Su Geng	Ramulus Perillae*	Perilla Stem
Perilla	Zi Su Ye	Folium Perillae Frutescentis	Perilla Leaf
Perilla	Zi Su Zi	Semen Perillae Frutescentis	Perilla Seed
Peucedanum	Qian Hu	Radix Peucedani	Hogfennel Root
Pharbitis	Qian Niu Zi	Semen Pharbitidis	Morning Glory Seed
Phaseolus	Chi Xiao Dou	Semen Phaseoli Calcarati	Aduki Bean
Phaseolus	Lu Dou	Semen Phaseoli Radiati	Mung Bean
Phellodendron	Huang Bai	Cortex Phellodendri	Amur Cork-tree Bark
Pheretima	Di Long	Lumbricus	Earthworm
Phoca	Hai Gou Shen	Testis et Penis Otariae*	Male Seal Sexual Organs
Phragmites	Lu Gen	Rhizoma Phragmitis Communis	Reed Rhizome; Corrizo Rhizome
Physalis	Suan Jiang	Calyx seu Fructus Physalis*	Wintercherry Calyx or Fruit
Phytolacca	Shang Lu	Radix Phytolaccae	Poke Root
Picrorhiza	Hu Huang Lian	Rhizoma Picrorhizae	Picrorhiza Rhizome
Pinellia	(Fa) Ban Xia	Rhizoma Pinelliae Ternatae	Prepared Pinellia Rhizome
Pinellia	(Sheng) Ban Xia	Rhizoma Pinelliae Ternatae	Raw Pinellia Rhizome
Pinus	Song Jie	Lignum Pini Nodi	Knotty Pine Wood
Piper	Bi Ba	Fructus Piperis Longi	Long Pepper Fruit
Piper	Bi Cheng Qie	Fructus Cubebae	Cubeba Fruit
Piper	Hai Feng Teng	Caulis Piperis Futokadsurae	Kadsura Stem
Piper	Hu Jiao	Fructus Piperis Nigri	Black Pepper Fruit
Plantago	Che Qian Cao	Herba Plantaginis	Plantago; Plantain
Plantago	Che Qian Zi	Semen Plantaginis	Plantago Seed; Plantain Seed
Platycodon	(Ku) Jie Geng	Radix Platycodi Grandiflori	Ballonflower Root; Bellflower Root; Bitter Jie Geng
Polistes	Lu Feng Fang	Nidus Vespae	Hornet Nest; Wasp Nest
Polygala	Yuan Zhi	Radix Polygalae Tenuifoliae	Chinese Senega Root; Seneca Snakeroot
Polygonatum	Huang Jing	Rhizoma Polygonati	Siberian Solomon Seal Rhizome
Polygonatum	Yu Zhu	Rhizoma Polygonati Odorati	Fragrant Solomon's Seal Rhizome; Polygonatum
Polygonum	Bian Xu	Herba Polygoni Avicularis	Avicularis; Knotweed
Polygonum	Guan Ye Liao	Herba Polygoni Perfoliati*	Polygonum

Botanical	Pinyin	Pharmaceutical	Common
Polygonum	Hu Zhang	Radix et Rhizoma Polygoni Cuspidati	Giant Knotweed Rhizome
Polygonum	Ye Jiao Teng	Caulis Polygoni Multiflori	Fleeceflower Stem; Fo-Ti Stem
Polygonum	He Shou Wu	Radix Polygoni Multiflori	Fleeceflower Root; Fo-Ti Root
Polyporus	Zhu Ling	Sclerotium Polypori Umbellati	Polyporus Sclerotium
Poria	Chi Fu Ling	Sclerotium Poriae Cocos Rubrae	Red Hoelen; Red Tuckahoe
Poria	Fu Ling	Sclerotium Poriae Cocos	Hoelen; China Root; Tuckahoe; Indian Bread
Poria	Fu Ling Pi	Cortex Poriae Cocos	Tuckahoe Skin
Poria Cocos	Fu Shen	Sclerotium Poriae Cocos Pararadicis	Tuckahoe Spirit
Portulaca	Ma Chi Xian	Herba Portulacae Oleraceae	Purslane
Potentilla	Fan Bai Cao	Herba Potentillae Discoloris*	Potentilla
Prunella	Xia Ku Cao	Spica Prunellae Vulgaris	Selfheal Spike; Heal all Spike
Prunus	Tao Ren	Semen Persicae	Peach Seed (Kernel)
Prunus	Wu Mei	Fructus Pruni Mume	Ume Plum Fruit; Black Plum Fruit
Prunus	(Bei) Xing Ren	Semen Pruni Armeniacae	(Northern) Apricot Seed
Prunus	(Nan) Xing Ren	Semen Pruni Armeniacae	(Southern) Apricot Seed
Prunus	Yu Li Ren	Semen Pruni	Bush Cherry Seed
Pseudostellaria	Tai Zi Shen	Radix Pseudostellariae Heterophyllae	Prince Ginseng Root
Psoralea	Bu Gu Zhi	Fructus Psoraleae Corylifoliae	Scurfy Pea Fruit
Pteria	Zhen Zhu	Margarita	Pearl
Pteria	Zhen Zhu Mu	Concha Margaritiferae	Mother-of-Pearl Shell
Pteris	Feng Wei Cao	Herba Pterii*	Pteris
Pueraria	Ge Gen	Radix Puerariae	Kudzu Root
Pueraria	Ge Hua	Flos Puerariae	Kudzu Flower
Pulsatilla	Bai Tou Weng	Radix Pulsatillae Chinensis	Pulsatilla Root; Anemone Root
Pumice	Fu Hai Shi	Pumice	Pumice
Punica	Shi Liu Gen Pi	Cortex Punicae Granati Radicis	Pomegranate Root Bark
Punica	Shi Liu Pi	Pericarpium Punicae Granati	Pomegranate Husk or Rind
Pyritum	Zi Ran Tong	Pyritum	Pyrite
Pyrola	Lu Xian Cao	Herba Pyrolae*	Pyrola
Pyrrosia	Shi Wei	Folium Pyrrosiae	Pyrrosia Leaf
Pyrus	Li Pi	Pericarpium Pyri*	Pear Peel

Botanical

Botanical	Pinyin	Pharmaceutical	Common
Quisqualis	Shi Jun Zi	Fructus Quisqualis Indicae	Rangoon Creeper Fruit
Ranunculus	Mao Zhao Cao	Radix Ranunculi Ternati*	Buttercup Root
Raphanus	Lai Fu Zi	Semen Raphani Satavi	Radish Seed
Realgar	Xiong Huang	Realgar	Realgar; Arsenic Disulfide
Rehmannia	Sheng Di Huang	Radix Rehmanniae Glutinosae	Fresh Chinese Foxglove Root
Rehmannia	Shu Di Huang	Radix Rehmanniae Glutinosae Conquitae	Wine-cooked Chinese Foxglove Root
Rhaponticum or Echinops	Lou Lu	Radix Rhapontici seu Echinops	Rhaponticum Root; Echinops Root
Rheum	Da Huang	Radix et Rhizoma Rhei	Rhubarb Root and Rhizome
Rhinoceros	Xi Jiao	Cornu Rhinoceri	Rhinoceros Horn
Rhodea	Wan Nian Qing	Herba Rhodeae Japonicae*	Rhodea
Rhododendron	Man Shan Hong	Folium Rhododendri*	Rhododendron Leaf
Rhus	Gan Qi	Lacca Sinica Exsiccatae	Laquer
Rhus	Yan Fu Mu	Cortex Rhois Chinensis*	Chinese Sumac Bark
Rhus/Melaphis	Wu Bei Zi	Galla Rhois Chinensis	Gallnut of Chinese Sumac
Rorippa	Han Cai	Herba Rorippae*	Rorippa
Rosa	Jin Ying Zi	Fructus Rosae Laevigatae	Cherokee Rose Fruit / Rosehip
Rosa	Mei Gui Hua	Flos Rosae Rugosae	Young Chinese Rose Flower
Rosa	Yue Ji Hua	Flos et Fructus Rosae Chinensis	Partially-blossoming Chinese Tea Rose Flower
Rubia	Qian Cao Gen	Radix Rubiae Cordifoliae	Madder Root
Rubus	Fu Pen Zi	Fructus Rubi Chingii	Raspberry Fruit Bud
Rubus	Mao Mei	Herba Rubi Parvifolii*	Thimbleberry
Saccharum Granorum	Yi Tang	Saccharum Granorum	Barley Malt Sugar/Syrup
Saiga	Ling Yang Jiao	Cornu Antelopis	Antelope Horn
Salvia	Dan Shen	Radix Salviae Miltiorrhizae	Red Sage Root
Salvia	Ji Ning	Herba Salviae Plebeia*	Salvia
Sambucus	Lu Ying	Cortex Sambuci*	Japanese Elder Bark
Sanguisorba	Di Yu	Radix Sanguisorbae Officinalis	Burnet-bloodwort Root
Santalum	Tan Xiang	Lignum Santali Albi	Sandalwood Heartwood
Sapium	Wu Jiu Gen Pi	Cortex Sappii Sebiferi Radicis*	Tallow Tree Root Bark
Sargassum	Hai Zao	Herba Sargassii	Sargassum Seaweed
Sargentodoxa	Hong Teng	Caulis Sargentodoxae Cuneatae	Sargentodoxa Stem
Saururus	San Bai Cao	Herba Saururi Chinensis*	Saururus
Saussurea	Mu Xiang	Radix Saussureae Lappae	Costus Root; Aucklandia

Botanical	Pinyin	Pharmaceutical	Common
Saxifrage	Hu Er Cao	Herba Saxifragae Stoloniferae*	Saxifrage
Schisandra	Nan Wu Wei Zi	Fructus Schisandrae Sphenantherae	Southern Schisandra Fruit
Schisandra	Wu Wei Zi	Fructus Schisandrae Chinensis	Northern Schisandra Fruit
Schizonepeta	Jing Jie	Herba Schizonepetae Tenuifoliae	Schizonepeta Stem or Bud
Scolopendra	Wu Gong	Scolopendra Subspinipes	Centipede
Scrophularia	Xuan Shen	Radix Scrophulariae Ningpoensis	Figwort Root
Scutellaria	Ban Zhi Lian	Herba Scutellariae Barbatae	Barbat Scullcap
Scutellaria	Huang Qin	Radix Scutellariae Baicalensis	Scute; Baical Skullcap Root
Sedum	Chui Pen Cao	Herba Sedii Sarmentosi*	Stonecrop
Sedum	Jing Tian San Qi	Herba Sedi*	Sedum
Selaginella	Shi Shang Bai	Herba Selaginellae Doederleinii	Selaginella
Senecio	Qian Li Guang	Herba Senecionis Scandentis*	Groundsel
Sepia or Sepiella	Hai Piao Xiao	Os Sepiae seu Sepiellae	Cuttle-fish Bone
Sesamum	Hei Zhi Ma	Semen Sesami Indici	Black Sesame Seed
Siegesbeckia	Xi Xian Cao	Herba Siegesbeckiae	St. Paul's Wort
Smilax	Ba Qia	Rhizoma Smilacis China*	Smilax Rhizome
Smilax	Tu Fu Ling	Rhizoma Smilacis Glabrae	Glabrous Greenbrier Rhizome
Smithsonitum	Lu Gan Shi	Smithsonitum	Smithsonite; Calamine
Solenognathus	Hai Long	Hailong	Pipe-fish
Sophora	Huai Hua Mi	Flos Sophorae Japonicae Immaturus	Pagoda Tree Flower Bud
Sophora	Huai Jiao	Fructus Sophorae Japonicae	Pagoda Tree Fruit
Sophora	Ku Shen	Radix Sophorae Flavenscentis	Bitter Ginseng Root
Sophora	Shan Dou Gen	Radix Sophorae Tonkinensis	Pigeon Pea Root
Sparganium	San Leng	Rhizoma Sparganii Stoloniferi	Bur-reed Rhizome
Spirodela or Lemna	Fu Ping	Herba Lemnae seu Spirodelae	Duckweed
Stalactitum	E Guan Shi	Stalactitum	Stalactite Tubular Tip
Stellaria	Yin Chai Hu	Radix Stellariae Dichotomae	Stellaria Root
Stemona	Bai Bu	Radix Stemonae	Stemona Root
Stephania	Han Fang Ji	Radix Stephaniae Tetrandrae	Stephania Root
Sterculia	Pang Da Hai	Semen Sterculiae Scaphigerae	Sterculia Seed

Botanical	Pinyin	Pharmaceutical	Common
Strichopus	Hai Shen	Strichopus Japonicus	Sea Cucumber; Sea Slug
Strychnos	Ma Qian Zi	Semen Strychni	Nux-vomica Seed
Styrax	An Xi Xiang	Benzoinum	Processed Resin of Styrax Benzoin
Succinum	Hu Po	Succinum	Amber; Fossilized Resin of Pine Tree
Sulphur	Liu Huang	Sulphur	Sulphur
Syringa	Bao Ma Zi	Cortex Syringae*	Manchurian Lilac Bark
Tabanus	Meng Chong	Tabani Bivittati*	Gadfly
Talcum	Hua Shi	Talcum	Talc; Soapstone
Tamarix	Cheng Liu	Cacumen Tamaricis Chinensis*	Tamarisk
Taraxacum	Pu Gong Ying	Herba Taraxaci Mongolici cum Radice	Dandelion
Terminalia	He Zi	Fructus Terminaliae Chebulae	Myrobalan Fruit
Terra Flava Usta	Fu Long Gan	Terra Flava Usta	Ignited Wood Stove Earth
Tetrapanax	Tong Cao	Medulla Tetrapanacis Papyriferi	Rice Paper Pith
Thalictrum	Tang Song Cao	Herba Thalictri Foliolosi*	Thalictrum
Tinospora	Jin Guo Lan	Radix Tinosporae Capillipes*	Tinospora Root
Tinospora	Kuan Jin Teng	Ramus Tinosporae Sinensis	Tinospora Stem
Torreya	Fei Zi	Semen Torreyae Grandis	Torreya Seed
Trachelospermum	Luo Shi Teng	Caulis Trachelospermi Jasminoidis	Star Jasmine Stem
Trachycarpus	Zong Lu Pi Tan	Fibra Stipulae Trachycarpi Carbonisatus	Charred Windmill Palm Petiole
Tremella	Bai Mu Er	Fructificatio Tremellae Fuciformis	Tremella Fungus Fruiting Body
Tribulus	Bai Ji Li	Fructus Tribuli Terrestris	Puncture Vine Fruit; Caltrop Fruit
Trichosanthes	Gua Lou	Fructus Trichosanthis	Snakegourd Fruit
Trichosanthes	Gua Lou Pi	Pericarpium Trichosanthis	Snakegourd Peel
Trichosanthes	Gua Lou Ren	Semen Trichosanthis	Snakegourd Seed
Trichosanthes	Tian Hua Fen	Radix Trichosanthis Kirilowii	Snakegourd Root
Trigonella	Hu Lu Ba	Semen Trigonellae Foeni-graeci	Fenugreek Seed
Triticum	Fu Xiao Mai	Semen Tritici Aestivi Levis	Wheat Chaff/Grain
Trogopterus or Pteromys	Wu Ling Zhi	Excrementum Trogopteri seu Pteromi	Flying Squirrel Feces
Tulipa	Shan Ci Gu	Pseudobulbus Shancigu	Chinese Tulip Bulb
Tussilago	Kuan Dong Hua	Flos Tussilaginis Farfarae	Coltsfoot Flower
Typha	(Sheng) Pu Huang	Pollen Typhae	Raw Cattail Pollen
Typha	Pu Huang Tan	Pollen Typhae Carbonisatus	Charred Cattail Pollen

Botanical	Pinyin	Pharmaceutical	Common
Typha	*Pu Hui*	*Folium Typhae*	*Cattail Leaves*
Typhonium	*Bai Fu Zi*	*Rhizoma Typhonii Gigantei*	*Typhonium Rhizome*
Ulmus	*Wu Yi*	*Praepartio Fructus Ulmi Macrocarpi*	*Stinking Elm Fruit Paste*
Uncaria	*Gou Teng*	*Ramulus cum Uncis Uncariae*	*Gambir vine Stems and Hooks*
Ursus	*Xiong Dan*	*Vesica Fellea Ursi*	*Bear Gallbladder*
Vaccaria	*Wang Bu Liu Xing*	*Semen Vaccariae Segetalis*	*Cow Soapwort Seed*
Veratrum	*Li Lu*	*Radix et Rhizoma Veratri*	*Veratrum Root*
Verbena	*Ma Bian Cao*	*Herba Verbenae**	*Vervain*
Vespertilio	*Ye Ming Sha*	*Excrementum Vespertilionis Murini*	*Bat Dung or Feces*
Viola	*Zi Hua Di Ding*	*Herba cum Radice Violae Yedoensitis*	*Viola*
Vitex	*Man Jing Zi*	*Fructus Viticis*	*Vitex Fruit*
Xanthium	*Cang Er Zi*	*Fructus Xanthii Sibirici*	*Xanthium Fruit; Cocklebur Fruit*
Zanthoxylum	*Chuan Jiao*	*Pericarpum Zanthoxyli Bungeani*	*Sichuan Pepper Fruit*
Zanthoxylum	*Chuan Jiao Mu*	*Semen Zanthoxyli Bungeani*	*Sichuan Pepper Seed*
Zanthoxylum	*(Chuan) Jiao Mu*	*Semen Zanthoxyli Bungeani*	*Sichuan Pepper Seed*
Zaocys	*She Tui*	*Exuviae Serpentis*	*Snake Skin Slough*
Zaocys	*Wu Shao She*	*Zaocys Dhumnades*	*Black-striped Snake*
Zea	*Yu Mi Xu*	*Stylus Zeae Mays*	*Cornsilk*
Zingiber	*Gan Jiang*	*Rhizoma Zingiberis Officinalis*	*Dried Ginger Rhizome*
Zingiber	*Pao Jiang*	*Rhizoma Zingiberis**	*Quick-fried Ginger Rhizome*
Zingiber	*Sheng Jiang*	*Rhizoma Zingiberis Officinalis Recens*	*Fresh Ginger Rhizome*
Zingiber	*Sheng Jiang Pi*	*Cortex Zingiberis Officinalis Recens*	*Fresh Ginger Skin*
Ziziphus	*Da Zao*	*Fructus Ziziphi Jujubae*	*Jujube Fruit; Chinese Black Date*
Ziziphus	*Hong Zao*	*Fructus Ziziphi Jujubae*	*Jujube Fruit; Chinese Red Date*
Ziziphus	*Suan Zao Ren*	*Semen Ziziphi Spinosae*	*Sour Jujube Seed; Zizyphus*

Herb Name Cross Reference Keyed to Pharmaceutical Names

Pharmaceutical	Pinyin	Botanical	Common
Actinolitum	Yang Qi Shi	Actinolitum	Actinolite
Agkistrodon seu Bungarus	Bai Hua She	Agkistrodon	Long-noded Pit Viper Snake
Alumen	Ming Fan	Alumen	Alum; Potassium Aluminum Sulfate
Alumen Praeparatum	Ku Fan	Alumen Praeparatum	Prepared Alum
Arillus Euphoriae Longanae	Long Yan Rou	Euphoria	Longan Fruit Flesh
Arseolitum	Pi Shi	Arsenolith	White Arsenic
Aspongopus*	Jiu Xiang Chong	Aspongopus	Stink Bug
Aurum*	Huang Jin	Aurum	Gold
Benzoinum	An Xi Xiang	Styrax	Processed Resin of Styrax Benzoin
Bombyx Batryticatus	Jiang Can	Bombyx	Dead Stiff Body of Sick Silkworm Larvae
Borax	Peng Sha	Borax	Borax; Sodium Tetraborate
Borneol	Bing Pian	Dryobalanops	Processed Resin of Borneol Camphor
Bulbus Allii	Xie Bai	Allium	Chinese Chive Bulb
Bulbus Allii Fistulosi	Cong Bai	Allium	White Bulb of Green Onion or Scallion
Bulbus Allii Sativi	Da Suan	Allium	Garlic Bulb
Bulbus Fritillariae Cirrhosae	Chuan Bei Mu	Fritillaria	Tendrilled Fritillary Bulb
Bulbus Fritillariae Thunbergii	Zhe Bei Mu	Fritillaria	Thunberg Fritillary Bulb
Bulbus Lilii	Bai He	Lilium	Lily Bulb
Buthus Martensi	Quan Xie	Buthus	Scorpion
Cacumen Biotae Orientalis	Ce Bai Ye	Biota	Arborvitae Leafy Twig
Cacumen Tamaricis Chinensis*	Cheng Liu	Tamarix	Tamarisk
Calcaria*	Chen Shi Huei	Calcaria	Calcium Hydroxide
Calcitum	Han Shui Shi	Calcitum	Calcite
Calculus Artificialis	Ren Gong Niu Huang	Bos	Artificially Induced Cow Gallstons
Calculus Bovis seu Calculus Bubali	Niu Huang	Bos or Bubalis	Ox or Water Buffalo Gallstone
Calculus Macacae Mulattae	Hou Zao	Macaca	Macaque Gallstone
Calomelas	Qing Fen	Calomelas	Calomel; Mercurous Chloride
Calyx Diospyri Kaki	Shi Di	Diospyros	Persimmon Calyx
Calyx seu Fructus Physalis*	Suan Jiang	Physalis	Wintercherry Calyx or Fruit

Pharmaceutical

Pharmaceutical	Pinyin	Botanical	Common
Camphora	Zhang Nao	Cinnamomum	Crystalized Volatile Oil of the Camphor Tree
Caput Radicis Angelicae Sinensis	Dang Gui Tou	Angelica	Tangkuei Head
Carapax Amydae Sinensis	Bie Jia	Amyda	Chinese Soft-shell Turtle Shell
Carapax Eretmochelydis Imbricatae*	Dai Mao	Eretmochelys	Hawksbill Turtle Shell
Caulis Bambusae in Taeniis	Zhu Ru	Bambusa	Bamboo Shavings
Caulis Mutong	Mu Tong	Akebia	Akebia Stem
Caulis Paederiae*	Ji Shi Teng	Paederia	Paederia Stem
Caulis Piperis Futokadsurae	Hai Feng Teng	Piper	Kadsura Stem
Caulis Polygoni Multiflori	Ye Jiao Teng	Polygonum	Fleeceflower Stem; Fo-Ti Stem
Caulis Sargentodoxae Cuneatae	Hong Teng	Sargentodoxa	Sargentodoxa Stem
Caulis Trachelospermi Jasminoidis	Luo Shi Teng	Trachelospermum	Star Jasmine Stem
Cervix Ginseng	Ren Shen Lu	Panax	Ginseng Root Neck
Chalcanthitum*	Dan Fan	Chalcanthitum	Copper Sulphate; Blue Vitriol
Cinnabaris	Zhu Sha	Cinnabaris	Cinnabar; Red Mercury Sulfide
Colla Cornu Cervi	Lu Jiao Jiao	Cervus	Mature Antler Glue; Mature Antler Gelatin
Concha Arcae	Wa Leng Zi	Arca	Cockle Shell; Ark Shell
Concha Cyclinae Sinensis	Hai Ge Ke	Cyclina	Clam Shell
Concha Haliotidis	Shi Jue Ming	Haliotis	Abalone Shell
Concha Margaritiferae	Zhen Zhu Mu	Pteria	Mother-of-Pearl Shell
Concha Ostreae	Mu Li	Ostrea	Oyster Shell
Concha Ostreae	Duan Mu Li	Ostrea	Calcined Oyster Shell
Concretio Silicea Bambusae Textillis	Tian Zhu Huang	Bambusa	Siliceous Secretions of Bamboo
Cordyceps Sinensis	Dong Chong Xia Cao	Cordyceps	Chinese Caterpillar Fungus
Cornu Antelopis	Ling Yang Jiao	Saiga	Antelope Horn
Cornu Bubali	Shui Niu Jiao	Bubalus	Waterbuffalo Horn
Cornu Cervi	Lu Jiao	Cervus	Antler; Deerhorn; Ossified Horn of the Mature Male Deer
Cornu Cervi Degelatinatium	Lu Jiao Shuang	Cervus	Antler Powder from the dregs of cooking Antler Glue
Cornu Cervi Parvum	Lu Rong	Cervus	Young Deer Antler Velvet
Cornu Naemorhedis	Shan Yang Jiao	Naemorhedis	Goat Horn
Cornu Rhinoceri	Xi Jiao	Rhinoceros	Rhinoceros Horn

Pharmaceutical	Pinyin	Botanical	Common
Cortex Acanthopanacis Gracilistyli Radicis	Wu Jia Pi	Acanthopanax	Acanthopanax Rootbark.
Cortex Ailanthi Altissimae	Chun Pi	Ailanthus	Tree of Heaven Bark
Cortex Albizziae Julibrissin	He Huan Pi	Albizzia	Mimosa Tree Bark; Silktree Bark
Cortex Cinnamomi Cassiae	Rou Gui	Cinnamomum	Cinnamon Bark
Cortex Dictamni Dasycarpi Radicis	Bai Xian Pi	Dictamnus	Dittany Root Bark
Cortex Erythrinae	Hai Tong Pi	Erythrina	Coral-bean Bark
Cortex Eucommiae Ulmoidis	Du Zhong	Eucommia	Eucommia Bark
Cortex Fraxini	Qin Pi	Fraxinus	Korean Ash Bark
Cortex Loropetali*	Ji Mu	Loropetalum	Loropetalum Bark
Cortex Lycii Radicis	Di Gu Pi	Lycium	Matrimony-vine Rootbark; Wolfberry Bark
Cortex Magnoliae Officinalis	Hou Po	Magnolia	Magnolia Bark
Cortex Meliae	Ku Lian Mu Pi	Melia	Sichuan Chinaberry Tree Bark; Sichuan Pagoda Tree Bark; Neem Tree Bark
Cortex Meliae Radicis	Ku Lian Gen Pi	Melia	Sichuan Chinaberry Root Bark; Sichuan Pagoda Tree Root Bark; Neem Root Bark
Cortex Mori Albae Radicis	Sang Bai Pi	Morus	Mulberry Rootbark
Cortex Moutan Radicis	Mu Dan Pi	Paeonia	Tree Peony Rootbark
Cortex Phellodendri	Huang Bai	Phellodendron	Amur Cork-tree Bark
Cortex Poriae Cocos	Fu Ling Pi	Poria	Tuckahoe Skin
Cortex Punicae Granati Radicis	Shi Liu Gen Pi	Punica	Pomegranate Root Bark
Cortex Rhois Chinensis*	Yan Fu Mu	Rhus	Chinese Sumac Bark
Cortex Sambuci*	Lu Ying	Sambucus	Japanese Elder Bark
Cortex Sappii Sebiferi Radicis*	Wu Jiu Gen Pi	Sapium	Tallow Tree Root Bark
Cortex Syringae*	Bao Ma Zi	Syringa	Manchurian Lilac Bark
Cortex Tubiformis Cinnamomi Cassiae	Guan Gui	Cinnamomum	Thin Cinnamon Bark from Young Trees
Cortex Zingiberis Officinalis Recens	Sheng Jiang Pi	Zingiber	Fresh Ginger Skin
Crinis Carbonisatus Hominis	Xue Yu Tan	Homo Sapiens	Charred Human Hair
Dens Draconis	Long Chi	Dens Draconis	Dragon Tooth; Fossilized Tooth
Endothelium Corneum Gigeriae Galli	Ji Nei Jin	Gallus	Chicken Gizard Lining

Pharmaceutical	Pinyin	Botanical	Common
Epicarpium Benincasae Hispidae	*Dong Gua Pi*	*Benincasa*	*Wintermelon Fruit Peel; Wax Gourd Fruit Peel*
Eupolyphaga seu Opisthoplatia	*Tu Bie Chong*	*Eupolyphaga*	*Wingless Cockroach*
Excrementum Bombycis Mori	*Can Sha*	*Bombyx*	*Silkworm Feces*
Excrementum Trogopteri seu Pteromi	*Wu Ling Zhi*	*Trogopterus or Pteromys*	*Flying Squirrel Feces*
Excrementum Vespertilionis Murini	*Ye Ming Sha*	*Vespertilio*	*Bat Dung or Feces*
Extremas Radicis Angelicae Sinensis	*Dang Gui Wei*	*Angelica*	*Tangkuei Tail*
Exuviae Serpentis	*She Tui*	*Zaocys*	*Snake Skin Slough*
Fasciculus Vascularis Luffae	*Si Gua Lou*	*Luffa*	*Dried Skeleton of Luffa Sponge*
Fibra Stipulae Trachycarpi Carbonisatus	*Zong Lu Pi Tan*	*Trachycarpus*	*Charred Windmill Palm Petiole*
*Flos Albizziae Julibrissin**	*He Huan Hua*	*Albizzia*	*Mimosa Tree Flower; Silktree Flower*
Flos Amomi	*Sha Ren Hua*	*Amomum*	*Grains-of-Paradise Flower*
Flos Buddleiae Officinalis Immaturus	*Mi Meng Hua*	*Buddleia*	*Buddleia Flower*
Flos Carthami Tinctorii	*Hong Hua*	*Carthamus*	*Safflower*
Flos Caryophylli	*Ding Xiang*	*Eugenia*	*Clove Flower-bud*
Flos Celosiae Cristatae	*Ji Guan Hua*	*Celosia*	*Cockscomb Flower*
Flos Chrysanthemi Indici	*Ye Ju Hua*	*Chrysanthemum*	*Wild Chrysanthemum Flower*
Flos Chrysanthemi Morifolii	*(Bai) Ju Hua*	*Chrysanthemum*	*White Chrysanthemum Flower*
Flos Chrysanthemi Morifolii	*(Huang) Ju Hua*	*Chrysanthemum*	*Yellow Chrysanthemum Flower*
Flos Citri Sarcodactylis	*Fo Shou Hua*	*Citrus*	*Finger Citron Flower*
Flos Daphnes Genkwa	*Yuan Hua*	*Daphne*	*Daphne Flower*
Flos Dolichoris Lablab	*Bian Dou Hua*	*Dolichos*	*Hyacinth Bean Flower*
Flos et Fructus Rosae Chinensis	*Yue Ji Hua*	*Rosa*	*Partially-blossoming Chinese Tea Rose Flower*
*Flos Hydrangeae Macrophyllae**	*Ba Xian Hua*	*Hydrangea*	*Hydrangea Flower*
Flos Imperatae Cylindricae	*Bai Mao Hua*	*Imperata*	*Wooly Grass Flower; White Grass Flower*
Flos Inulae	*Xuan Fu Hua*	*Inula*	*Elecampane Flower*
Flos Lonicerae Japonicae	*Jin Yin Hua*	*Lonicera*	*Honeysuckle Flower*
Flos Magnoliae	*Xin Yi Hua*	*Magnolia*	*Magnolia Flower*
Flos Magnoliae Officinalis	*Hou Po Hua*	*Magnolia*	*Magnolia Flower*
Flos Pseudoginseng	*San Qi Hua*	*Panax*	*Pseudoginseng Flower; Notoginseng Flower*
Flos Puerariae	*Ge Hua*	*Pueraria*	*Kudzu Flower*

Pharmaceutical	Pinyin	Botanical	Common
Flos Rosae Rugosae	Mei Gui Hua	Rosa	Young Chinese Rose Flower
Flos Sophorae Japonicae Immaturus	Huai Hua Mi	Sophora	Pagoda Tree Flower Bud
Flos Tussilaginis Farfarae	Kuan Dong Hua	Tussilago	Coltsfoot Flower
Fluoritum	Zi Shi Ying	Fluoritum	Fluorite
Folium Artemisiae Argyi	Ai Ye	Artemisia	Mugwort Leaf
Folium Callicarpae	Zi Zhu	Callicarpa	Callicarpa Leaf
Folium Clerodendri Trichotomi	Chou Wu Tong	Clerodendron	Glorybower Leaf
Folium Isatidis Daqingye	Da Qing Ye	Isatis	Isatis Leaf; Woad Leaf
Folium Dichroae Febrifugae	Shu Qi	Dichroa	Dichroa Leaf
Folium Eleagni Pungens	Hu Tui Ye	Eleagnus	Eleagnus Leaf
Folium Eriobotryae Japonicae	Pi Pa Ye	Eriobotrya	Loquat Leaf
Folium Ginkgo Bilobae	Yin Guo Ye	Ginkgo	Ginkgo Leaf
Folium Ginseng	Ren Shen Ye	Panax	Ginseng Leaf
Folium Gynurae*	Ju Ye San Qi	Gynura	Gynura Leaf
Folium Ilicis Chinensis*	Si Ji Qing	Ilex	Holly Leaf
Folium Mahoniae*	Shi Da Gong Lao	Mahonia	Mahonia Leaf
Folium Momordicae Grosvenori	Luo Huo Guo Ye	Momordica	Momordica Leaf
Folium Mori Albae	Sang Ye	Morus	Mulberry Leaf
Folium Nelumbinis Nuciferae	He Ye	Nelumbo	Lotus Leaf
Folium Perillae Frutescentis	Zi Su Ye	Perilla	Perilla Leaf
Folium Pyrrosiae	Shi Wei	Pyrrosia	Pyrrosia Leaf
Folium Rhododendri*	Man Shan Hong	Rhododendron	Rhododendron Leaf
Folium Sennae	Fan Xie Ye	Cassia	Senna Leaf
Folium Typhae	Pu Hui	Typha	Cattail Leaves
Fructificatio Ganodermae Lucidi*	Ling Zhi	Ganoderma	Lucid Ganoderma; Reishi
Fructificatio Lasiosphaerae seu Calvatiae	Ma Bo	Lasiosphaera	Puffball Fruiting Body
Fructificatio Tremellae Fuciformis	Bai Mu Er	Tremella	Tremella Fungus Fruiting Body
Fructus Akebiae	Ba Yue Zha	Akebia	Akebia Fruit
Fructus Alpiniae Oxyphyllae	Yi Zhi Ren	Alpinia	Black Cardamon Fruit
Fructus Amomi Kravanh	Bai Dou Kou	Amomum	Round Cardamon Fruit; Cluster Fruit
Fructus Amomi Tsao-Ko	Cao Guo	Amomum	Chinese Cardamon Fruit
Fructus Arctii Lappae	Niu Bang Zi	Arctium	Burdock Seed
Fructus Aristolochiae	Ma Dou Ling	Aristolochia	Birthwort Fruit
Fructus Bruceae Javanicae	Ya Dan Zi	Brucea	Brucea Fruit

Pharmaceutical	Pinyin	Botanical	Common
Fructus Carpesii seu Daucusi	*He Shi*	*Carpesium or Daucus*	*Carpesium Fruit*
Fructus Citri Aurantii	*Zhi Ke*	*Citrus or Poncirus*	*Bitter Orange Fruit*
Fructus Citri Sarcodactylis	*Fo Shou*	*Citrus*	*Finger Citron Fruit*
Fructus Citrulli Vulgaris	*Xi Gua*	*Citrullus*	*Watermelon Fruit and Peel or Rind*
Fructus Cnidii Monnieri	*She Chuang Zi*	*Cnidium*	*Cnidium Seed*
Fructus Corni Officinalis	*Shan Zhu Yu*	*Cornus*	*Dogwood Fruit; Asiatic Cornelian Cherry Fruit*
Fructus Crataegi	*Shan Zha*	*Crataegus*	*Hawthorn Unripe Fruit or Berry*
Fructus Crataegi	*Shan Zha Rou*	*Crataegus*	*Hawthorn Ripe Fruit or Berry*
Fructus Crataegi Carbonisatus	*Shan Zha Tan*	*Crataegus*	*Charred Hawthorn Fruit or Berry*
Fructus Cubebae	*Bi Cheng Qie*	*Piper*	*Cubeba Fruit*
*Fructus Diospyri Kaki**	*Shi Bing*	*Diospyros*	*Dried Persimmon Fruit*
Fructus Evodiae Rutaecarpae	*Wu Zhu Yu*	*Evodia*	*Evodia Fruit*
Fructus Foeniculi Vulgaris	*Xiao Hui Xiang*	*Foeniculum*	*Fennel Fruit*
Fructus Forsythiae Suspensae	*Lian Qiao*	*Forsythia*	*Forsythia Fruit; Golden Bells*
Fructus Gardeniae Jasminoidis	*Zhi Zi*	*Gardenia*	*Gardenia Fruit*
Fructus Gleditsiae Sinensis	*Zao Jiao*	*Gleditsia*	*Honeylocust Fruit; Soap Bean Fruit*
Fructus Hordei Vulgaris Germinatus	*Mai Ya*	*Hordeum*	*Barley Sprout; Malted Barley*
*Fructus Illicii**	*Ba Jiao Hui Xiang*	*Illicium*	*Star Anise Fruit*
Fructus Immaturus Citri Aurantii	*Zhi Shi*	*Citrus or Poncirus*	*Immature Bitter Orange Fruit*
Fructus Kochiae Scopariae	*Di Fu Zi*	*Kochia*	*Broom Cyperus Seed*
Fructus Ligustri Lucidi	*Nu Zhen Zi*	*Ligustrum*	*Privet Fruit; Waxtree Fruit*
Fructus Liquidambaris Taiwanianae	*Lu Lu Tong*	*Liquidambar*	*Sweetgum Fruit*
Fructus Lycii	*Gou Qi Zi*	*Lycium*	*Matrimony Vine Fruit; Wolfberry Fruit*
Fructus Meliae Toosendan	*Chuan Lian Zi*	*Melia*	*Sichuan Chinaberry Fruit; Sichuan Pagoda Tree Fruit; Neem Fruit*
Fructus Momordicae Grosvenori	*Luo Han Guo*	*Momordica*	*Momordica Fruit*
Fructus Mori Albae	*Sang Shen*	*Morus*	*Mulberry Fruit Bud*
Fructus Oryzae Sativae Germinatus	*Gu Ya*	*Oryza*	*Rice Sprout*
Fructus Piperis Longi	*Bi Ba*	*Piper*	*Long Pepper Fruit*
Fructus Piperis Nigri	*Hu Jiao*	*Piper*	*Black Pepper Fruit*

Pharmaceutical	Pinyin	Botanical	Common
Fructus Pruni Mume	Wu Mei	Prunus	Ume Plum Fruit; Black Plum Fruit
Fructus Psoraleae Corylifoliae	Bu Gu Zhi	Psoralea	Scurfy Pea Fruit
Fructus Quisqualis Indicae	Shi Jun Zi	Quisqualis	Rangoon Creeper Fruit
Fructus Rosae Laevigatae	Jin Ying Zi	Rosa	Cherokee Rose Fruit / Rosehip
Fructus Rubi Chingii	Fu Pen Zi	Rubus	Raspberry Fruit Bud
Fructus Schisandrae Chinensis	Wu Wei Zi	Schisandra	Northern Schisandra Fruit
Fructus Schisandrae Sphenantherae	Nan Wu Wei Zi	Schisandra	Southern Schisandra Fruit
Fructus seu Semen Amomi	Sha Ren	Amomum	Grains-of-Paradise Fruit or Seeds
Fructus Sophorae Japonicae	Huai Jiao	Sophora	Pagoda Tree Fruit
Fructus Terminaliae Chebulae	He Zi	Terminalia	Myrobalan Fruit
Fructus Tribuli Terrestris	Bai Ji Li	Tribulus	Puncture Vine Fruit; Caltrop Fruit
Fructus Trichosanthis	Gua Lou	Trichosanthes	Snakegourd Fruit
Fructus Viticis	Man Jing Zi	Vitex	Vitex Fruit
Fructus Xanthii Sibirici	Cang Er Zi	Xanthium	Xanthium Fruit; Cocklebur Fruit
Fructus Ziziphi Jujubae	Da Zao	Ziziphus	Jujube Fruit; Chinese Black Date
Fructus Ziziphi Jujubae	Hong Zao	Ziziphus	Jujube Fruit; Chinese Red Date
Frusta Ferri	Sheng Tie Luo	Frusta Ferri	Iron Filing
Fructus Chaenomelis	Mu Gua	Chaenomeles	Chinese Quince Fruit
Galla Rhois Chinensis	Wu Bei Zi	Rhus/Melaphis	Gallnut of Chinese Sumac
Gekko	Ge Jie	Gekko	Gecko Lizard
Gelatinum Corii Asini	E Jiao	Equus	Donkey Hide Gelatin; Ass Skin Glue
Gummi Olibanum	Ru Xiang	Boswellia	Frankincense Gum-resin
Gypsum Fibrosum	Shi Gao	Gypsum	Gypsum; Calcium Sulphate
Haematitum	Dai Zhe Shi	Haematitum	Hematite; Iron Ore
Hailong	Hai Long	Solenognathus	Pipe-fish
Halloysitum Rubrum	Chi Shi Zhi	Halloysitum Rubrum	Halloysite; Red Kaolin
Herba Acalypae Australis*	Tie Xian	Acalypha	Acalypha
Herba Agastaches seu Pogostemi	Huo Xiang	Agastache or Pogostemon	Patchouli; Agastache
Herba Agrimoniae Pilosae	Xian He Cao	Agrimonia	Agrimony
Herba Ajugae Decumbentis*	Bai Mao Xia Ku Cao	Ajuga	Ajuga
Herba Aloes	Lu Hui	Aloe	Aloe Vera Leaf

Pharmaceutical	Pinyin	Botanical	Common
Herba Andrographitis Paniculatae	Chuan Xin Lian	Andrographis	Kariyat; Green Chiretta
Herba Androsacae Umbellatae*	Dian Di Mei	Androsace	Androsace
Herba Artemisiae Annuae	Qing Hao	Artemisia	Sweet Wormwood; Southernwood
Herba Artemisiae Anomalae	Liu Ji Nu	Artemisia	Artemisia
Herba Artemisiae Yinchenhao	Yin Chen Hao	Artemisia	Oriental Wormwood
Herba Begoniae Fimbristipulatae	Zi Bei Tian Kuei	Begonia	Begonia
Herba Capsellae*	Ji Cai	Capsella	Shepherd's Purse
Herba Carpesii	Tian Ming Jing	Carpesium	Carpesium
Herba Centipedae Minimae*	E Bu Shi Cao	Centipeda	Centipeda Herb
Herba Cephalanoplos	Xiao Ji	Cephalanoplos	Small Thistle; Field Thistle
Herba Cistanches Deserticolae	Rou Cong Rong	Cistanche	Broomrape Fleshy Stem
Herba Commelinae*	Ya Zhi Cao	Commelina	Commelina
Herba cum Radice Asari	Xi Xin	Asarum	Asarum; Chinese Wild Ginger
Herba cum Radice Houttuyniae Cordatae	Yu Xing Cao	Houttuynia	Houttuynia; Fish Smell Plant
Herba cum Radice Patriniae	Bai Jiang Cao	Patrinia or Thiaspi	Patrinia; Thiaspi
Herba cum Radice Violae Yedoensitis	Zi Hua Di Ding	Viola	Viola
Herba Cynomorii Songarici	Suo Yang	Cynomorium	Cynomorium Fleshy Stem
Herba Dendrobii	Shi Hu	Dendrobium	Dendrobium Stem
Herba Dianthi	Qu Mai	Dianthus	Pink Flower Herb
Herba Ecliptae Prostratae	Han Lian Cao	Eclipta	Eclipta
Herba Elsholtziae seu Moslae	Xiang Ru	Elsholtzia	Aromatic Madder
Herba Ephedrae	Ma Huang	Ephedra	Ephedra Stem
Herba Epimedii	Yin Yang Huo	Epimedium	Epimedium
Herba Equiseti Hiemalis	Mu Zei	Equisetum	Horsetail; Scouring Rush; Shavegrass
Herba Erodii seu Geranii*	Lao Guan Cao	Erodium or Geranium	Geranium; Heronbill; Cranebill
Herba Eupatorii Fortunei	Pei Lan	Eupatorium	Boneset; Thoroughwort; Feverwort
Herba Euphorbiae Helioscopiae	Ze Qi	Euphorbia	Pill-bearing Spurge
Herba Hederae Nepalensis*	Chang Chun Teng	Hedera	Ivy
Herba Inulae	Jin Fei Cao	Inula	Elecampane
Herba Laminaria Japonicae	Hai Dai	Laminaria	Algae

Pharmaceutical	Pinyin	Botanical	Common
Herba Lemnae seu Spirodelae	*Fu Ping*	*Spirodela or Lemna*	*Duckweed*
Herba Leonuri Heterophylli	*Yi Mu Cao*	*Leonurus*	*Motherwort*
Herba Lobeliae Chinensis cum Radice	*Ban Bian Lian*	*Lobelia*	*Chinese Lobelia*
Herba Lophatheri Gracilis	*Dan Zhu Ye*	*Lophatherum*	*Bland Bamboo Leaf and Stem*
Herba Lycopi Lucidi	*Ze Lan*	*Lycopus*	*Bugleweed*
*Herba Lycopodii Clavati**	*Shen Jin Cao*	*Lycopodium*	*Clubmoss*
Herba Lygodii Japonici	*Jin Sha Teng*	*Lygodium*	*Japanese Climbing Fern*
Herba Lysimachiae	*Jin Qian Cao*	*Lysimachia*	*Lysimachia*
Herba Menthae Haplocalycis	*Bo He*	*Mentha*	*Peppermint; Spearmint; Field Mint*
Herba Oldenlandiae Diffusae	*Bai Hua She She Cao*	*Oldenlandia*	*Oldenlandia*
Herba Plantaginis	*Che Qian Cao*	*Plantago*	*Plantago; Plantain*
Herba Polygoni Avicularis	*Bian Xu*	*Polygonum*	*Avicularis; Knotweed*
*Herba Polygoni Perfoliati**	*Guan Ye Liao*	*Polygonum*	*Polygonum*
Herba Portulacae Oleraceae	*Ma Chi Xian*	*Portulaca*	*Purslane*
*Herba Potentillae Discoloris**	*Fan Bai Cao*	*Potentilla*	*Potentilla*
*Herba Pterii**	*Feng Wei Cao*	*Pteris*	*Pteris*
*Herba Pyrolae**	*Lu Xian Cao*	*Pyrola*	*Pyrola*
*Herba Rhodeae Japonicae**	*Wan Nian Qing*	*Rhodea*	*Rhodea*
*Herba Rorippae**	*Han Cai*	*Rorippa*	*Rorippa*
*Herba Rubi Parvifolii**	*Mao Mei*	*Rubus*	*Thimbleberry*
*Herba Salviae Plebeia**	*Ji Ning*	*Salvia*	*Salvia*
Herba Sargassii	*Hai Zao*	*Sargassum*	*Sargassum Seaweed*
*Herba Saururi Chinensis**	*San Bai Cao*	*Saururus*	*Saururus*
*Herba Saxifragae Stoloniferae**	*Hu Er Cao*	*Saxifrage*	*Saxifrage*
Herba Schizonepetae Tenuifoliae	*Jing Jie*	*Schizonepeta*	*Schizonepeta Stem or Bud*
Herba Scutellariae Barbatae	*Ban Zhi Lian*	*Scutellaria*	*Barbat Scullcap*
*Herba Sedi**	*Jing Tian San Qi*	*Sedum*	*Sedum*
*Herba Sedii Sarmentosi**	*Chui Pen Cao*	*Sedum*	*Stonecrop*
Herba Selaginellae Doederleinii	*Shi Shang Bai*	*Selaginella*	*Selaginella*
*Herba Senecionis Scandentis**	*Qian Li Guang*	*Senecio*	*Groundsel*
*Herba seu Folium Apocyni Veneti**	*Luo Bu Ma*	*Apocynum*	*Red Dogbane Whole Herb or Leaf*
Herba seu Radix Cirsii Japonici	*Da Ji*	*Cirsium*	*Japanese Thistle*
Herba Siegesbeckiae	*Xi Xian Cao*	*Siegesbeckia*	*St. Paul's Wort*

Pharmaceutical	Pinyin	Botanical	Common
Herba Taraxaci Mongolici cum Radice	Pu Gong Ying	Taraxacum	Dandelion
Herba Thalictri Foliolosi*	Tang Song Cao	Thalictrum	Thalictrum
Herba Verbenae*	Ma Bian Cao	Verbena	Vervain
Hippocampus	Hai Ma	Hippocampus	Sea Horse
Hirudo seu Whitmania	Shui Zhi	Hirudo	Leech
Hydrargyrum	Shui Yin	Hydrargyrum	Mercury
Indigo Pulverata Levis	Qing Dai	Indigo	Indigo
Lacca Sinica Exsiccatae	Gan Qi	Rhus	Laquer
Lapis Micae seu Chloriti	Meng Shi	Lapis Micae seu Chloriti	Chlorite Schist; Lapis
Lignum Aquilariae	Chen Xiang	Aquilaria	Aloeswood Secretion or Sap
Lignum Dalbergiae Odoriferae	Jiang Xiang	Dalbergia	Dalbergia Heartwood
Lignum Pini Nodi	Song Jie	Pinus	Knotty Pine Wood
Lignum Santali Albi	Tan Xiang	Santalum	Sandalwood Heartwood
Lignum Sappan	Su Mu	Caesalpinia	Sappan Heartwood
Limonite	Yu Liang Shi	Limonite	Limonite
Lithargyrum	Mi Tuo Seng	Lithargyrum	Litharge; Galena
Lumbricus	Di Long	Pheretima	Earthworm
Magnetitum	Ci Shi	Magnetitum	Magnetite; Magnetic Iron Ore; Loadstone
Margarita	Zhen Zhu	Pteria	Pearl
Massa Fermentata	Shen Qu	Massa Fermentata	Medicated Leaven
Medulla Junci Effusi	Deng Xin Cao	Juncus	Rush Pith
Medulla Tetrapanacis Papyriferi	Tong Cao	Tetrapanax	Rice Paper Pith
Mel*	Feng Mi	Mel	Honey
Minium	Qian Dan	Minium	Red Lead Oxide
Mirabilitum	Mang Xiao	Mirabilitum	Mirabilite; Glauber's Salt
Mirabilitum Purum	Xuan Ming Fen	Mirabilitum	Pure Mirabilite; Pure Sodium Sulphate; Pure Glauber's Salt
Mylabris	Ban Mao	Mylabris	Cantharides; Chinese Blistering Beetle
Nidus Vespae	Lu Feng Fang	Polistes	Hornet Nest; Wasp Nest
Niter*	Xiao Shi	Niter	Silver
Nodus Nelumbinis Nuciferae Rhizomatis	Ou Jie	Nelumbo	Lotus Rhizome Node
Ootheca Mantidis	Sang Piao Xiao	Paratenodera	Praying Mantis Egg Case
Ophicalcitum	Hua Rui Shi	Ophicalcitum	Ophicalcite
Os Canine	Gou Gu	Canis	Dog Bone
Os Draconis	Duan Long Gu	Os Draconis	Calcined Dragon Bone; Calcined Fossilized Bone

Pharmaceutical	Pinyin	Botanical	Common
Os Draconis	Long Gu	Os Draconis	Dragon Bone; Fossilized Bone
Os Leopardis	Bao Gu	Panthera	Leopard Bone
Os Sepiae seu Sepiellae	Hai Piao Xiao	Sepia or Sepiella	Cuttle-fish Bone
Os Tigris	Hu Gu	Panthera	Tiger Bone
Pars Rubra Epicarpii Citri Erythrocarpae	Ju Hong	Citrus	Red Tangerine Peel
Pasta Acacia seu Uncaria	Er Cha	Acacia or Uncaria	Dried Paste of Concentrated Decoction of Black or White Cutch
Pedicellus Cucumeris	Gua Di	Cucumis	Melon Pedicle
Pericarpium Amomi	Sha Ren Ke	Amomum	Grains-of-Paradise Shell
Pericarpium Arachi*	Hua Sheng Yi	Arachis	Peanut Skin
Pericarpium Arecae Catechu	Da Fu Pi	Areca	Betelnut Husk
Pericarpium Citri Reticulatae	Chen Pi	Citrus	Tangerine Peel
Pericarpium Citri Reticulatae Viride	Qing Pi	Citrus	Immature (Green) Tangerine Peel
Pericarpium Luffae Acutangulae	Si Gua Pi	Luffa	Luffa Skin
Pericarpium Papaveris Somniferi	Ying Su Ke	Papaver	Opium Poppy Husk
Pericarpium Punicae Granati	Shi Liu Pi	Punica	Pomegranate Husk or Rind
Pericarpium Pyri*	Li Pi	Pyrus	Pear Peel
Pericarpium Trichosanthis	Gua Lou Pi	Trichosanthes	Snakegourd Peel
Pericarpum Zanthoxyli Bungeani	Chuan Jiao	Zanthoxylum	Sichuan Pepper Fruit
Periostracum Cicadae	Chan Tui	Cryptotympana	Cicada Skin; Cicada Moulting
Placenta Hominis	Zi He Che	Homo Sapiens	Human Placenta
Plastrum Testudinis	Gui Ban	Chinemys	Fresh Water Turtle Shell
Plumula Nelumbinis Nuciferae	Lian Xin	Nelumbo	Lotus Plumule
Pollen Typhae	(Sheng) Pu Huang	Typha	Raw Cattail Pollen
Pollen Typhae Carbonisatus	Pu Huang Tan	Typha	Charred Cattail Pollen
Praepartio Fructus Ulmi Macrocarpi	Wu Yi	Ulmus	Stinking Elm Fruit Paste
Pseudobulbus Shancigu	Shan Ci Gu	Tulipa	Chinese Tulip Bulb
Pulvis Arisaemae cum Felle Bovis	Dan Nan Xing	Arisaema	Powdered Jack-in-the-Pulpit Rhizome mixed with Cow Bile
Pumice	Fu Hai Shi	Pumice	Pumice
Pyritum	Zi Ran Tong	Pyritum	Pyrite
Radix Achyranthis Aspera	Tu Niu Xi	Achyranthes	Achyranthes Root
Radix Achyranthis Bidentatae	Huai Niu Xi	Achyranthes	Achyranthes Root

Pharmaceutical

Pharmaceutical	Pinyin	Botanical	Common
Radix Aconite Carmichaeli	Chuan Wu	Aconitum	Sichuan Aconite
Radix Aconiti	Wu Tou	Aconitum	Aconite Root
Radix Aconiti Kusnezoffii	Cao Wu	Aconitum	Wild Aconite
Radix Adenophorae	Nan Sha Shen	Adenophora	Ladybell Root; Southern Sand Root
Radix Adenophorae Trachelioidis	Gan Jie Geng	Adenophora	Sweet Jie Geng
Radix Ampelopsis Japonicae*	Bai Lian	Ampelopsis	Ampelopsis Root
Radix Anemarrhenae Asphodeloidis	Zhi Mu	Anemarrhena	Anemarrhena Root
Radix Angelicae Dahuricae	Bai Zhi	Angelica	Angelica Root
Radix Angelicae Pubescentis	Du Huo	Angelica	Pubescent Angelica Root
Radix Angelicae Sinensis	Dang Gui	Angelica	Tangkuei Root
Radix Ardisiae Crenatae*	Zhu Sha Gen	Ardisia	Ardisia Root
Radix Aristolochiae	Qing Mu Xiang	Aristolochia	Birthwort Root
Radix Aristolochiae Fangchi	Guang Fang Ji	Aristolochia or Cocculus	Aristolochia Root
Radix Asteris Tatarici	Zi Wan	Aster	Purple Aster Root
Radix Astragali Membranaceus	Huang Qi	Astragalus	Yellow Milk-vetch Root
Radix Boehmeriae Niveae*	Zhu Ma Gen	Boehmeria	Ramie Root
Radix Bupleuri	Chai Hu	Bupleurum	Thorowax Root; Hare's Ear Root
Radix Changii*	Ming Dang Shen	Changium	Changium Root
Radix Clematidis	Wei Ling Xian	Clematis	Clematis Root
Radix Codonopsitis Pilosulae	Dang Shen	Codonopsis	Asiabell Root
Radix Cyathulae Officinalis	Chuan Niu Xi	Cyathula	Cyathula Root
Radix Cynanchi Auriculati	Ge Shan Xiang	Cynanchum	Cynanchum Root
Radix Cynanchi Baiwei	Bai Wei	Cynanchum	Swallowort Root
Radix Dichroae Febrifugae	Chang Shan	Dichroa	Dichroa Root
Radix Dioscoreae Oppositae	Shan Yao	Dioscorea	Chinese Wild Yam Root
Radix Dipsaci Asperi	Xu Duan	Dipsacus	Teasel Root
Radix Ephedrae	Ma Huang Gen	Ephedra	Ephedra Root
Radix et Caulis Jixueteng	Ji Xue Teng	Millettia	Millettia Root and Vine; Chicken Blood Vine
Radix et Ramus Litseae Cubebae	Dou Chi Jiang	Litsea	Aromatic Litsea Root and Stem
Radix et Rhizoma Oryzae Glutinosae	Nuo Dao Gen Xu	Oryza	Sweet Rice Root and Rhizome
Radix et Rhizoma Polygoni Cuspidati	Hu Zhang	Polygonum	Giant Knotweed Rhizome
Radix et Rhizoma Rhei	Da Huang	Rheum	Rhubarb Root and Rhizome

Pharmaceutical	Pinyin	Botanical	Common
Radix et Rhizoma Veratri	*Li Lu*	*Veratrum*	*Veratrum Root*
Radix Euphorbiae Kansui	*Gan Sui*	*Euphorbia*	*Kansui Spurge Root*
Radix Euphorbiae seu Knoxiae	*Jing Da Ji*	*Euphorbia or Knoxia*	*Peking Spurge Root*
Radix Gentianae Longdancao	*Long Dan Cao*	*Gentiana*	*Chinese Gentian Root*
Radix Gentianae Qinjiao	*Qin Jiao*	*Gentiana*	*Large-Leaf Gentian Root*
Radix Ginseng	*Bai Shen*	*Panax*	*Rock Candy cured White Ginseng Root*
Radix Ginseng	*Ji Lin Shen*	*Panax*	*Jilin Wild Ginseng*
Radix Ginseng	*(Hong) Ren Shen*	*Panax*	*Ginseng Root steamed until red*
Radix Ginseng	*Shen Xu*	*Panax*	*Rock Candy cured White Ginseng Root Tail*
Radix Ginseng	*Sheng Shai Shen*	*Panax*	*Dried Ginseng Root*
Radix Ginseng	*Ye Shan Shen*	*Panax*	*Wild Ginseng*
Radix Glehniae Littoralis	*Bei Sha Shen*	*Glehnia*	*Beech Silver-top Root; Northern Sand Root*
*Radix Glycyrrhizae Praeparata**	*Zhi Gan Cao*	*Glycyrrhiza*	*Honey-fried Licorice Root*
Radix Glycyrrhizae Uralensis	*Gan Cao*	*Glycyrhiza*	*Licorice Root*
*Radix Gossypii Hirsuti**	*Mian Hua Gen*	*Gossypium*	*Cotton Root*
*Radix Ilicis Pubescentis**	*Mao Dong Qing*	*Ilex*	*Pubescent Holly Root*
Radix Isatidis seu Baphicacanthi	*Ban Lan Gen*	*Isatis*	*Isatis Root; Woad Root*
Radix Lateralis Aconiti Carmichaeli Praeparata	*(Hei)Fu Zi*	*Aconitum*	*Prepared Sichuan Aconite Root*
Radix Ledebouriella Divaricatae	*Fang Feng*	*Ledebouriella*	*Siler Root; Ledebouriella Root*
Radix Ligustici Chuan Xiong	*Chuan Xiong*	*Ligusticum*	*Sichuan Lovage Root*
Radix Linderae Strychnifoliae	*Wu Yao*	*Lindera*	*Spicebush Root*
Radix Lithospermi seu Arnebiae	*Zi Cao*	*Lithospermum*	*Groomwell Root*
Radix Morindae Officinalis	*Ba Ji Tian*	*Morinda*	*Morinda Root*
Radix Paeoniae Lactiflorae	*Bai Shao*	*Paeonia*	*White Peony Root*
Radix Paeoniae Rubra	*Chi Shao*	*Paeonia*	*Red Peony Root*
Radix Panacis Quinquefolii	*Xi Yang Shen*	*Panax*	*American Ginseng Root*
Radix Peucedani	*Qian Hu*	*Peucedanum*	*Hogfennel Root*
Radix Phytolaccae	*Shang Lu*	*Phytolacca*	*Poke Root*
Radix Platycodi Grandiflori	*(Ku) Jie Geng*	*Platycodon*	*Ballonflower Root; Bellflower Root; Bitter Jie Geng*
Radix Polygalae Tenuifoliae	*Yuan Zhi*	*Polygala*	*Chinese Senega Root; Seneca Snakeroot*

Pharmaceutical	Pinyin	Botanical	Common
Radix Polygoni Multiflori	He Shou Wu	Polygonum	Fleeceflower Root; Fo-Ti Root
Radix Pseudoginseng	San Qi	Panax	Pseudoginseng Root; Notoginseng Root
Radix Pseudostellariae Heterophyllae	Tai Zi Shen	Pseudostellaria	Prince Ginseng Root
Radix Puerariae	Ge Gen	Pueraria	Kudzu Root
Radix Pulsatillae Chinensis	Bai Tou Weng	Pulsatilla	Pulsatilla Root; Anemone Root
Radix Ranunculi Ternati*	Mao Zhao Cao	Ranunculus	Buttercup Root
Radix Rehmanniae Glutinosae	Sheng Di Huang	Rehmannia	Fresh Chinese Foxglove Root
Radix Rehmanniae Glutinosae Conquitae	Shu Di Huang	Rehmannia	Wine-cooked Chinese Foxglove Root
Radix Rhapontici seu Echinops	Lou Lu	Rhaponticum or Echinops	Rhaponticum Root; Echinops Root
Radix Rubiae Cordifoliae	Qian Cao Gen	Rubia	Madder Root
Radix Salviae Miltiorrhizae	Dan Shen	Salvia	Red Sage Root
Radix Sanguisorbae Officinalis	Di Yu	Sanguisorba	Burnet-bloodwort Root
Radix Saussureae Lappae	Mu Xiang	Saussurea	Costus Root; Aucklandia
Radix Scrophulariae Ningpoensis	Xuan Shen	Scrophularia	Figwort Root
Radix Scutellariae Baicalensis	Huang Qin	Scutellaria	Scute; Baical Skullcap Root
Radix Sophorae Flavenscentis	Ku Shen	Sophora	Bitter Ginseng Root
Radix Sophorae Tonkinensis	Shan Dou Gen	Sophora	Pigeon Pea Root
Radix Stellariae Dichotomae	Yin Chai Hu	Stellaria	Stellaria Root
Radix Stemonae	Bai Bu	Stemona	Stemona Root
Radix Stephaniae Tetrandrae	Han Fang Ji	Stephania	Stephania Root
Radix Tinosporae Capillipes*	Jin Guo Lan	Tinospora	Tinospora Root
Radix Trichosanthis Kirilowii	Tian Hua Fen	Trichosanthes	Snakegourd Root
Ramulus Cinnamomi Cassiae	Gui Zhi	Cinnamomum	Cinnamon Twig
Ramulus cum Uncis Uncariae	Gou Teng	Uncaria	Gambir vine Stems and Hooks
Ramulus Mori Albae	Sang Zhi	Morus	Mulberry Twig
Ramulus Nelumbinis Nuciferae	Lian Geng	Nelumbo	Lotus Stem
Ramulus Perillae*	Zi Su Geng	Perilla	Perilla Stem
Ramulus Sangjishang	Sang Ji Sheng	Loranthus or Viscum	Mulberry Mistletoe Stem
Ramus Lonicerae Japonicae	Jin Yin Teng	Lonicera	Honeysuckle Stem
Ramus Tinosporae Sinensis	Kuan Jin Teng	Tinospora	Tinospora Stem

Pharmaceutical	Pinyin	Botanical	Common
Realgar	Xiong Huang	Realgar	Realgar; Arsenic Disulfide
Receptaculum Nelumbinis Nuciferae	Lian Fang	Nelumbo	Mature Lotus Receptacle
Resina Asafoetidae*	E Wei	Ferula	Asafoetida Gum-resin; Devil's Dung
Resinae Myrrhae	Mo Yao	Commiphora	Myrrh Gum-resin
Rhizoma Acori Graminei	Shi Chang Pu	Acorus	Sweetflag Rhizome
Rhizoma Alismatis Orientalitis	Ze Xie	Alisma	Water Plantain Rhizome
Rhizoma Alpiniae Officinari	Gao Liang Jiang	Alpinia	Lesser Galangal Rhizome
Rhizoma Anemoni Altaicae*	Jiu Jie Chang Pu	Anemone	Altaica Rhizome
Rhizoma Arisaematis	(Sheng) Tian Nan Xing	Arisaema	Raw Jack-in-the-Pulpit Rhizome
Rhizoma Arisaematis Praeparatae	Zhi Nan Xing	Arisaema	Prepared Jack-in-the-Pulpit Rhizome
Rhizoma Atractylodis	Cang Zhu	Atractylodes	Atractylodes Rhizome
Rhizoma Atractylodis Macrocephalae	Bai Zhu	Atractylodes	White Atractylodes Rhizome
Rhizoma Belamcandae Chinensis	She Gan	Belamcanda	Belamcanda Rhizome; Blackberry Lily Rhizome
Rhizoma Bletillae Striatae	Bai Ji	Bletilla	Bletilla Rhizome
Rhizoma Cibotii Barometz	Gou Ji	Cibotium	Chain Fern Rhizome
Rhizoma Cimicifugae	Sheng Ma	Cimicifuga	Black Cohosh Rhizome; Bugbane Rhizome
Rhizoma Coptidis	Huang Lian	Coptis	Coptis; Golden Thread Rhizome
Rhizoma Corydalis Yanhusuo	Yan Hu Suo	Corydalis	Corydalis Rhizome
Rhizoma Curculiginis Orchioidis	Xian Mao	Curculigo	Golden Eye-grass Rhizome
Rhizoma Curcumae	E Zhu	Curcuma	Zedoary Tumeric Rhizome
Rhizoma Curcumae Longae	Jiang Huang	Curcuma	Tumeric Rhizome
Rhizoma Cyperi Rotundi	Xiang Fu	Cyperus	Cyperus Rhizome; Nut-grass Rhizome; Sedge Rhizome
Rhizoma Dioscoreae Hypoglaucae	Bei Xie	Dioscorea	Hypoglauca Yam Rhizome; Fish-poison Yam Rhizome
Rhizoma Dioscoreae Nipponicae*	Chuan Shan Long	Dioscorea	Japanese Dioscorea Rhizome
Rhizoma Drynariae	Gu Sui Bu	Drynaria	Drynaria Rhizome
Rhizoma Dryopteridis	Dong Bei Guan Zhong	Dryopteris	Dryopteris Rhizome
Rhizoma et Radix Ligustici	Gao Ben	Ligusticum	Straw Weed Rhizome and Root; Chinese Lovage Rhizome and Root
Rhizoma et Radix Notopterygii	Qiang Huo	Notopterygium	Notopterygium Rhizome and Root

Pharmaceutical

Pharmaceutical	Pinyin	Botanical	Common
*Rhizoma Fagopyri Cynosi**	*Jin Qiao Mai*	*Fagopyrum*	*Wild Buckwheat Rhizome*
Rhizoma Gastrodiae Elatae	*Tian Ma*	*Gastrodia*	*Gastrodia Rhizome*
Rhizoma Guanzhong	*Guan Zhong*	*Dryopteris*	*Shield-fern Rhizome*
Rhizoma Homalomenae Occultae	*Qian Nian Jian*	*Homalomena*	*Homalomena Rhizome*
Rhizoma Imperatae Cylindricae	*Bai Mao Gen*	*Imperata*	*Woolly Grass Rhizome; White Grass Rhizome*
*Rhizoma Paridis Polyphyllae**	*Zao Xiu*	*Paris*	*Paris Rhizome*
Rhizoma Phragmitis Communis	*Lu Gen*	*Phragmites*	*Reed Rhizome; Corrizo Rhizome*
Rhizoma Picrorhizae	*Hu Huang Lian*	*Picrorhiza*	*Picrorhiza Rhizome*
Rhizoma Pinelliae Ternatae	*(Fa) Ban Xia*	*Pinellia*	*Prepared Pinellia Rhizome*
Rhizoma Pinelliae Ternatae	*(Sheng) Ban Xia*	*Pinellia*	*Raw Pinellia Rhizome*
Rhizoma Polygonati	*Huang Jing*	*Polygonatum*	*Siberian Solomon Seal Rhizome*
Rhizoma Polygonati Odorati	*Yu Zhu*	*Polygonatum*	*Fragrant Solomon's Seal Rhizome; Polygonatum*
Rhizoma et Radix Cynanchi Baiqian	*Bai Qian*	*Cynanchum*	*Cynanchum Rhizome and Root*
*Rhizoma Smilacis China**	*Ba Qia*	*Smilax*	*Smilax Rhizome*
Rhizoma Smilacis Glabrae	*Tu Fu Ling*	*Smilax*	*Glabrous Greenbrier Rhizome*
Rhizoma Sparganii Stoloniferi	*San Leng*	*Sparganium*	*Bur-reed Rhizome*
Rhizoma Typhonii Gigantei	*Bai Fu Zi*	*Typhonium*	*Typhonium Rhizome*
Rhizoma Zingiberis Officinalis	*Gan Jiang*	*Zingiber*	*Dried Ginger Rhizome*
Rhizoma Zingiberis Officinalis Recens	*Sheng Jiang*	*Zingiber*	*Fresh Ginger Rhizome*
*Rhizoma Zingiberis**	*Pao Jiang*	*Zingiber*	*Quick-fried Ginger Rhizome*
Saccharum Granorum	*Yi Tang*	*Saccharum Granorum*	*Barley Malt Sugar/Syrup*
Sanguis Draconis	*Xue Jie*	*Dracaena*	*Dragon's Blood Resin*
Scapus et Inflorescentia Eriocaulonis Buergeriani	*Gu Jing Cao*	*Eriocaulon*	*Pipewort Scapus*
Sclerotium Omphaliae Lapidescens	*Lei Wan*	*Omphalia*	*Omphalia Fungus Fruiting Body*
Sclerotium Polypori Umbellati	*Zhu Ling*	*Polyporus*	*Polyporus Sclerotium*
Sclerotium Poriae Cocos	*Fu Ling*	*Poria*	*Hoelen; China Root; Tuckahoe; Indian Bread*
Sclerotium Poriae Cocos Pararadicis	*Fu Shen*	*Poria Cocos*	*Tuckahoe Spirit*
Sclerotium Poriae Cocos Rubrae	*Chi Fu Ling*	*Poria*	*Red Hoelen; Red Tuckahoe*
Scolopendra Subspinipes	*Wu Gong*	*Scolopendra*	*Centipede*

Pharmaceutical	Pinyin	Botanical	Common
Secretio Bufonis	Chan Su	Bufo	Dried Skin Secretion of Toad
Secretio Moschus	She Xiang	Moschus	Musk; Musk Deer Navel Gland Secretion
Semen Albutili seu Malvae	Dong Kui Zi	Malva or Abutilon	Musk Mallow Seed; Malva Seed
Semen Allii Tuberosi	Jiu Zi	Allium	Chinese Leek Seed
Semen Alpiniae Katsumadai	Cao Dou Kou	Alpinia	Wild Cardamon Seed; Katsumada's Galangal Seed
Semen Arecae Catechu	Bing Lang	Areca	Betel Nut
Semen Astragali Complanati	Sha Yuan Ji Li	Astragalus	Flattened Milk-vetch Seed
Semen Benincasae Hispidae	Dong Gua Ren	Benincasa	Wintermelon Seed; Wax Gourd Seed
Semen Biotae Orientalis	Bai Zi Ren	Biota	Arbor-Vitae Seed
Semen Broussonetiae Papyriferae*	Chu Shi Zi	Broussonetia	Broussonetia Seed
Semen Cannabis Sativae	Huo Ma Ren	Cannabis	Hemp Seed; Marihuana Seed
Semen Cassiae	Jue Ming Zi	Cassia	Cassia Seed
Semen Celosiae Argenteae	Qing Xiang Zi	Celosia	Celosia Seed
Semen Citri Reticulatae*	Ju He	Citrus	Tangerine Seed
Semen Coicis Lachryma-jobi	Shu Yi Ren	Coix	Dry-Fried Coix Seed
Semen Coicis Lachryma-jobi	Yi Yi Ren	Coix	Coix Seed; Job's Tears Seed
Semen Croton Tiglii	Ba Dou	Croton	Croton Seed
Semen Cucurbitae Moschatae	Nan Gua Zi	Cucurbita	Pumpkin Seed and Husk
Semen Cuscutae Chinensis	Tu Si Zi	Cuscuta	Dodder Seed
Semen Dolichoris Lablab	Bian Dou	Dolichos	Hyacinth Bean
Semen Euphorbiae Lathyridis*	Xu Sui Zi	Euphorbia	Caper Spurge Seed; Moleplant Seed
Semen Euryales Ferocis	Qian Shi	Euryale	Euryale Seed
Semen Ginkgo Bilobae	Bai Guo	Ginkgo	Ginkgo Nut
Semen Glycinis Germinatum	Dou Juan	Glycine	Young Soybean Sprout
Semen Hydnocarpi Anthelminticae	Da Feng Zi	Hydnocarpus	Chaulmoogra Seed
Semen Juglandis Regiae	Hu Tao Ren	Juglans	Walnut
Semen Leonuri Heterophylli	Chong Wei Zi	Leonurus	Motherwort Seed
Semen Lepidii seu Descurainiae	Ting Li Zi	Lepidium or Descurainia	Tansy Mustard Seed
Semen Litchi Chinensis	Li Zhi He	Litchi	Leechee Nut
Semen Momordicae Cochinchinensis	Mu Bie Zi	Momordica	Momordica Seed
Semen Myristicae Fragrantis	Rou Dou Kou	Myristica	Nutmeg Seed

Pharmaceutical

Pharmaceutical	Pinyin	Botanical	Common
Semen Nelumbinis Nuciferae	Lian Zi	Nelumbo	Lotus Seed
Semen Oroxyli Indici	Mu Hu Die	Oroxylum	Oroxylum Seed
Semen Oryzae Sativae*	Jing Mi	Oryza	Rice Grain
Semen Perillae Frutescentis	Zi Su Zi	Perilla	Perilla Seed
Semen Persicae	Tao Ren	Prunus	Peach Seed (Kernel)
Semen Pharbitidis	Qian Niu Zi	Pharbitis	Morning Glory Seed
Semen Phaseoli Calcarati	Chi Xiao Dou	Phaseolus	Aduki Bean
Semen Phaseoli Radiati	Lu Dou	Phaseolus	Mung Bean
Semen Plantaginis	Che Qian Zi	Plantago	Plantago Seed; Plantain Seed
Semen Pruni	Yu Li Ren	Prunus	Bush Cherry Seed
Semen Pruni Armeniacae	(Bei) Xing Ren	Prunus	(Northern) Apricot Seed
Semen Pruni Armeniacae	(Nan) Xing Ren	Prunus	(Southern) Apricot Seed
Semen Raphani Satavi	Lai Fu Zi	Raphanus	Radish Seed
Semen Sesami Indici	Hei Zhi Ma	Sesamum	Black Sesame Seed
Semen Sinapsis Albae	Bai Jie Zi	Brassica	White Mustard Seed
Semen Glycinis Praeparatum	Dan Dou Chi	Glycine	Prepared (Fermented) Soybean
Semen Sterculiae Scaphigerae	Pang Da Hai	Sterculia	Sterculia Seed
Semen Strychni	Ma Qian Zi	Strychnos	Nux-vomica Seed
Semen Torreyae Grandis	Fei Zi	Torreya	Torreya Seed
Semen Trichosanthis	Gua Lou Ren	Trichosanthes	Snakegourd Seed
Semen Trigonellae Foeni-graeci	Hu Lu Ba	Trigonella	Fenugreek Seed
Semen Tritici Aestivi Levis	Fu Xiao Mai	Triticum	Wheat Chaff/Grain
Semen Vaccariae Segetalis	Wang Bu Liu Xing	Vaccaria	Cow Soapwort Seed
Semen Zanthoxyli Bungeani	Chuan Jiao Mu	Zanthoxylum	Sichuan Pepper Seed
Semen Zanthoxyli Bungeani	(Chuan) Jiao Mu	Zanthoxylum	Sichuan Pepper Seed
Semen Ziziphi Spinosae	Suan Zao Ren	Ziziphus	Sour Jujube Seed; Zizyphus
Smithsonitum	Lu Gan Shi	Smithsonitum	Smithsonite; Calamine
Spica Prunellae Vulgaris	Xia Ku Cao	Prunella	Selfheal Spike; Heal all Spike
Spina Gleditsiae Sinensis	Zao Jiao Ci	Gleditsia	Honeylocust Spine; Soap Bean Spine
Spora Lygodii Japonici	Hai Jin Sha	Lygodium	Japanese Climbing Fern Spore
Squama Manitis Pentadactylae	Chuan Shan Jia	Manis	Anteater-Scales; Pangolin Scales
Stalactitum	E Guan Shi	Stalactitum	Stalactite Tubular Tip
Stamen Nelumbinis Nuciferae	Lian Xu	Nelumbo	Lotus Stamen

Pharmaceutical	Pinyin	Botanical	Common
Stigma Crocus Sativae	*Xi Hong Hua*	*Crocus*	*Stigma of the True Saffron Flower*
Strichopus Japonicus	*Hai Shen*	*Strichopus*	*Sea Cucumber; Sea Slug*
Stylus Zeae Mays	*Yu Mi Xu*	*Zea*	*Cornsilk*
Styrax Liquidis	*Su He Xiang*	*Liquidambar*	*Rose Maloes Resin*
Succinum	*Hu Po*	*Succinum*	*Amber; Fossilized Resin of Pine Tree*
Succus Bambusae	*Zhu Li*	*Bambusa*	*Dried Bamboo Sap*
Sulphur	*Liu Huang*	*Sulphur*	*Sulphur*
*Tabani Bivittati**	*Meng Chong*	*Tabanus*	*Gadfly*
Talcum	*Hua Shi*	*Talcum*	*Talc; Soapstone*
Terra Flava Usta	*Fu Long Gan*	*Terra Flava Usta*	*Ignited Wood Stove Earth*
*Testis et Penis Otariae**	*Hai Gou Shen*	*Phoca*	*Male Seal Sexual Organs*
*Testis et Penis Canis**	*Guang Gou Shen*	*Canis*	*Male Dog Sexual Organs*
*Testis et Penis Cervi**	*Hua Lu Shen*	*Cervus*	*Male Deer Sexual Organs*
*Testis et Penis Equii**	*Hei Lu Shen*	*Equus*	*Male Horse Sexual Organs*
Thallus Algae	*Kun Bu*	*Laminaria or Ecklonia*	*Kelp Thallus; Kombu Thallus*
Tuber Asparagi Cochinchinensis	*Tian Men Dong*	*Asparagus*	*Chinese Asparagus Tuber*
Tuber Curcumae	*Yu Jin*	*Curcuma*	*Tumeric Tuber*
Tuber Dioscoreae Bulbiferae	*Huang Yao Zi*	*Dioscorea*	*Dioscorea Tuber*
Tuber Ophiopogonis Japonici	*Mai Men Dong*	*Ophiopogon*	*Creeping Lily-turf Tuber*
Vesica Fellea Bovus	*Niu Dan*	*Bos*	*Cow Gallbladder*
Vesica Fellea Ursi	*Xiong Dan*	*Ursus*	*Bear Gallbladder*
Zaocys Dhumnades	*Wu Shao She*	*Zaocys*	*Black-striped Snake*

Herb Name Cross Reference Keyed to Common Names

Common	Pinyin	Botanical	Pharmaceutical
(Northern) Apricot Seed	(Bei) Xing Ren	Prunus	Semen Pruni Armeniacae
(Southern) Apricot Seed	(Nan) Xing Ren	Prunus	Semen Pruni Armeniacae
Abalone Shell	Shi Jue Ming	Haliotis	Concha Haliotidis
Acalypha	Tie Xian	Acalypha	Herba Acalypae Australis*
Acanthopanax Rootbark.	Wu Jia Pi	Acanthopanax	Cortex Acanthopanacis Gracilistyli Radicis
Achyranthes Root	Huai Niu Xi	Achyranthes	Radix Achyranthis Bidentatae
Achyranthes Root	Tu Niu Xi	Achyranthes	Radix Achyranthis Aspera
Aconite Root	Wu Tou	Aconitum	Radix Aconiti
Actinolite	Yang Qi Shi	Actinolitum	Actinolitum
Aduki Bean	Chi Xiao Dou	Phaseolus	Semen Phaseoli Calcarati
Agrimony	Xian He Cao	Agrimonia	Herba Agrimoniae Pilosae
Ajuga	Bai Mao Xia Ku Cao	Ajuga	Herba Ajugae Decumbentis*
Akebia Fruit	Ba Yue Zha	Akebia	Fructus Akebiae
Akebia Stem	Mu Tong	Akebia	Caulis Mutong
Algae	Hai Dai	Laminaria	Herba Laminaria Japonicae
Aloe Vera Leaf	Lu Hui	Aloe	Herba Aloes
Aloeswood Secretion or Sap	Chen Xiang	Aquilaria	Lignum Aquilariae
Altaica Rhizome	Jiu Jie Chang Pu	Anemone	Rhizoma Anemoni Altaicae*
Alum; Potassium Aluminum Sulfate	Ming Fan	Alumen	Alumen
Amber; Fossilized Resin of Pine Tree	Hu Po	Succinum	Succinum
American Ginseng Root	Xi Yang Shen	Panax	Radix Panacis Quinquefolii
Ampelopsis Root	Bai Lian	Ampelopsis	Radix Ampelopsis Japonicae*
Amur Cork-tree Bark	Huang Bai	Phellodendron	Cortex Phellodendri
Androsace	Dian Di Mei	Androsace	Herba Androsacae Umbellatae*
Anemarrhena Root	Zhi Mu	Anemarrhena	Radix Anemarrhenae Asphodeloidis
Angelica Root	Bai Zhi	Angelica	Radix Angelicae Dahuricae
Anteater-Scales; Pangolin Scales	Chuan Shan Jia	Manis	Squama Manitis Pentadactylae

Common	Pinyin	Botanical	Pharmaceutical
Antelope Horn	*Ling Yang Jiao*	*Saiga*	*Cornu Antelopis*
Antler Powder from the dregs of cooking Antler Glue	*Lu Jiao Shuang*	*Cervus*	*Cornu Cervi Degelatinatium*
Antler; Deerhorn; Ossified Horn of the Mature Male Deer	*Lu Jiao*	*Cervus*	*Cornu Cervi*
Arbor-Vitae Seed	*Bai Zi Ren*	*Biota*	*Semen Biotae Orientalis*
Arborvitae Leafy Twig	*Ce Bai Ye*	*Biota*	*Cacumen Biotae Orientalis*
Ardisia Root	*Zhu Sha Gen*	*Ardisia*	*Radix Ardisiae Crenatae**
Aristolochia Root	*Guang Fang Ji*	*Aristolochia or Cocculus*	*Radix Aristolochiae Fangchi*
Aromatic Litsea Root and Stem	*Dou Chi Jiang*	*Litsea*	*Radix et Ramus Litseae Cubebae*
Aromatic Madder	*Xiang Ru*	*Elsholtzia*	*Herba Elsholtziae seu Moslae*
Artemisia	*Liu Ji Nu*	*Artemisia*	*Herba Artemisiae Anomalae*
Artificially Induced Cow Gallstons	*Ren Gong Niu Huang*	*Bos*	*Calculus Artificialis*
Asafoetida Gum-resin; Devil's Dung	*E Wei*	*Ferula*	*Resina Asafoetidae**
Asarum; Chinese Wild Ginger	*Xi Xin*	*Asarum*	*Herba cum Radice Asari*
Asiabell Root	*Dang Shen*	*Codonopsis*	*Radix Codonopsitis Pilosulae*
Atractylodes Rhizome	*Cang Zhu*	*Atractylodes*	*Rhizoma Atractylodis*
Avicularis; Knotweed	*Bian Xu*	*Polygonum*	*Herba Polygoni Avicularis*
Ballonflower Root; Bellflower Root; Bitter Jie Geng	*(Ku) Jie Geng*	*Platycodon*	*Radix Platycodi Grandiflori*
Bamboo Shavings	*Zhu Ru*	*Bambusa*	*Caulis Bambusae in Taenils*
Barbat Scullcap	*Ban Zhi Lian*	*Scutellaria*	*Herba Scutellariae Barbatae*
Barley Malt Sugar/Syrup	*Yi Tang*	*Saccharum Granorum*	*Saccharum Granorum*
Barley Sprout; Malted Barley	*Mai Ya*	*Hordeum*	*Fructus Hordei Vulgaris Germinatus*
Bat Dung or Feces	*Ye Ming Sha*	*Vespertilio*	*Excrementum Vespertilionis Murini*
Bear Gallbladder	*Xiong Dan*	*Ursus*	*Vesica Fellea Ursi*
Beech Silver-top Root; Northern Sand Root	*Bei Sha Shen*	*Glehnia*	*Radix Glehniae Littoralis*
Begonia	*Zi Bei Tian Kuei*	*Begonia*	*Herba Begoniae Fimbristipulatae*
Belamcanda Rhizome; Blackberry Lily Rhizome	*She Gan*	*Belamcanda*	*Rhizoma Belamcandae Chinensis*
Betel Nut	*Bing Lang*	*Areca*	*Semen Arecae Catechu*
Betelnut Husk	*Da Fu Pi*	*Areca*	*Pericarpium Arecae Catechu*
Birthwort Fruit	*Ma Dou Ling*	*Aristolochia*	*Fructus Aristolochiae*
Birthwort Root	*Qing Mu Xiang*	*Aristolochia*	*Radix Aristolochiae*

Common	Pinyin	Botanical	Pharmaceutical
Bitter Ginseng Root	*Ku Shen*	*Sophora*	*Radix Sophorae Flavenscentis*
Bitter Orange Fruit	*Zhi Ke*	*Citrus or Poncirus*	*Fructus Citri Aurantii*
Black Cardamon Fruit	*Yi Zhi Ren*	*Alpinia*	*Fructus Alpiniae Oxyphyllae*
Black Cohosh Rhizome; Bugbane Rhizome	*Sheng Ma*	*Cimicifuga*	*Rhizoma Cimicifugae*
Black Pepper Fruit	*Hu Jiao*	*Piper*	*Fructus Piperis Nigri*
Black Sesame Seed	*Hei Zhi Ma*	*Sesamum*	*Semen Sesami Indici*
Black-striped Snake	*Wu Shao She*	*Zaocys*	*Zaocys Dhumnades*
Bland Bamboo Leaf and Stem	*Dan Zhu Ye*	*Lophatherum*	*Herba Lophatheri Gracilis*
Bletilla Rhizome	*Bai Ji*	*Bletilla*	*Rhizoma Bletillae Striatae*
Boneset; Thoroughwort; Feverwort	*Pei Lan*	*Eupatorium*	*Herba Eupatorii Fortunei*
Borax; Sodium Tetraborate	*Peng Sha*	*Borax*	*Borax*
Broom Cyperus Seed	*Di Fu Zi*	*Kochia*	*Fructus Kochiae Scopariae*
Broomrape Fleshy Stem	*Rou Cong Rong*	*Cistanche*	*Herba Cistanches Deserticolae*
Broussonetia Seed	*Chu Shi Zi*	*Broussonetia*	*Semen Broussonetiae Papyriferae**
Brucea Fruit	*Ya Dan Zi*	*Brucea*	*Fructus Bruceae Javanicae*
Buddleia Flower	*Mi Meng Hua*	*Buddleia*	*Flos Buddleiae Officinalis Immaturus*
Bugleweed	*Ze Lan*	*Lycopus*	*Herba Lycopi Lucidi*
Bur-reed Rhizome	*San Leng*	*Sparganium*	*Rhizoma Sparganii Stoloniferi*
Burdock Seed	*Niu Bang Zi*	*Arctium*	*Fructus Arctii Lappae*
Burnet-bloodwort Root	*Di Yu*	*Sanguisorba*	*Radix Sanguisorbae Officinalis*
Bush Cherry Seed	*Yu Li Ren*	*Prunus*	*Semen Pruni*
Buttercup Root	*Mao Zhao Cao*	*Ranunculus*	*Radix Ranunculi Ternati**
Calcined Dragon Bone; Calcined Fossilized Bone	*Duan Long Gu*	*Os Draconis*	*Os Draconis*
Calcined Oyster Shell	*Duan Mu Li*	*Ostrea*	*Concha Ostreae*
Calcite	*Han Shui Shi*	*Calcitum*	*Calcitum*
Calcium Hydroxide	*Chen Shi Huei*	*Calcaria*	*Calcaria**
Callicarpa Leaf	*Zi Zhu*	*Callicarpa*	*Folium Callicarpae*
Calomel; Mercurous Chloride	*Qing Fen*	*Calomelas*	*Calomelas*
Cantharides; Chinese Blistering Beetle	*Ban Mao*	*Mylabris*	*Mylabris*
Caper Spurge Seed; Moleplant Seed	*Xu Sui Zi*	*Euphorbia*	*Semen Euphorbiae Lathyridis**
Carpesium	*Tian Ming Jing*	*Carpesium*	*Herba Carpesii*

Common	Pinyin	Botanical	Pharmaceutical
Carpesium Fruit	*He Shi*	*Carpesium or Daucus*	*Fructus Carpesii seu Daucusi*
Cassia Seed	*Jue Ming Zi*	*Cassia*	*Semen Cassiae*
Cattail Leaves	*Pu Hui*	*Typha*	*Folium Typhae*
Celosia Seed	*Qing Xiang Zi*	*Celosia*	*Semen Celosiae Argenteae*
Centipeda Herb	*E Bu Shi Cao*	*Centipeda*	*Herba Centipedae Minimae**
Centipede	*Wu Gong*	*Scolopendra*	*Scolopendra Subspinipes*
Chain Fern Rhizome	*Gou Ji*	*Cibotium*	*Rhizoma Cibotii Barometz*
Changium Root	*Ming Dang Shen*	*Changium*	*Radix Changii**
Charred Cattail Pollen	*Pu Huang Tan*	*Typha*	*Pollen Typhae Carbonisatus*
Charred Hawthorn Fruit or Berry	*Shan Zha Tan*	*Crataegus*	*Fructus Crataegi Carbonisatus*
Charred Human Hair	*Xue Yu Tan*	*Homo Sapiens*	*Crinis Carbonisatus Hominis*
Charred Windmill Palm Petiole	*Zong Lu Pi Tan*	*Trachycarpus*	*Fibra Stipulae Trachycarpi Carbonisatus*
Chaulmoogra Seed	*Da Feng Zi*	*Hydnocarpus*	*Semen Hydnocarpi Anthelminticae*
Cherokee Rose Fruit / Rosehip	*Jin Ying Zi*	*Rosa*	*Fructus Rosae Laevigatae*
Chicken Gizard Lining	*Ji Nei Jin*	*Gallus*	*Endothelium Corneum Gigeriae Galli*
Chinese Asparagus Tuber	*Tian Men Dong*	*Asparagus*	*Tuber Asparagi Cochinchinensis*
Chinese Cardamon Fruit	*Cao Guo*	*Amomum*	*Fructus Amomi Tsao-Ko*
Chinese Caterpillar Fungus	*Dong Chong Xia Cao*	*Cordyceps*	*Cordyceps Sinensis*
Chinese Chive Bulb	*Xie Bai*	*Allium*	*Bulbus Allii*
Chinese Gentian Root	*Long Dan Cao*	*Gentiana*	*Radix Gentianae Longdancao*
Chinese Leek Seed	*Jiu Zi*	*Allium*	*Semen Allii Tuberosi*
Chinese Lobelia	*Ban Bian Lian*	*Lobelia*	*Herba Lobeliae Chinensis cum Radice*
Chinese Quince Fruit	*Mu Gua*	*Chaenomeles*	*Fructus Chaenomelis*
Chinese Senega Root; Seneca Snakeroot	*Yuan Zhi*	*Polygala*	*Radix Polygalae Tenuifoliae*
Chinese Soft-shell Turtle Shell	*Bie Jia*	*Amyda*	*Carapax Amydae Sinensis*
Chinese Sumac Bark	*Yan Fu Mu*	*Rhus*	*Cortex Rhois Chinensis**
Chinese Tulip Bulb	*Shan Ci Gu*	*Tulipa*	*Pseudobulbus Shancigu*
Chinese Wild Yam Root	*Shan Yao*	*Dioscorea*	*Radix Dioscoreae Oppositae*
Chlorite Schist; Lapis	*Meng Shi*	*Lapis Micae seu Chloriti*	*Lapis Micae seu Chloriti*
Chlorite Schist; Phlogopitum; Lapis	*Meng Shi*	*Lapis Micae seu Chloriti*	*Lapis Chloriti seu Micae*
Cicada Skin; Cicada Moulting	*Chan Tui*	*Cryptotympana*	*Periostracum Cicadae*

Common	Pinyin	Botanical	Pharmaceutical
Cinnabar; Red Mercury Sulfide	*Zhu Sha*	*Cinnabaris*	*Cinnabaris*
Cinnamon Bark	*Rou Gui*	*Cinnamomum*	*Cortex Cinnamomi Cassiae*
Cinnamon Twig	*Gui Zhi*	*Cinnamomum*	*Ramulus Cinnamomi Cassiae*
Clam Shell	*Hai Ge Ke*	*Cyclina*	*Concha Cyclinae Sinensis*
Clematis Root	*Wei Ling Xian*	*Clematis*	*Radix Clematidis*
Clove Flower-bud	*Ding Xiang*	*Eugenia*	*Flos Caryophylli*
Clubmoss	*Shen Jin Cao*	*Lycopodium*	*Herba Lycopodii Clavati**
Cnidium Seed	*She Chuang Zi*	*Cnidium*	*Fructus Cnidii Monnieri*
Cockle Shell: Ark Shell	*Wa Leng Zi*	*Arca*	*Concha Arcae*
Cockscomb Flower	*Ji Guan Hua*	*Celosia*	*Flos Celosiae Cristatae*
Coix Seed; Job's Tears Seed	*Yi Yi Ren*	*Coix*	*Semen Coicis Lachryma-jobi*
Coltsfoot Flower	*Kuan Dong Hua*	*Tussilago*	*Flos Tussilaginis Farfarae*
Commelina	*Ya Zhi Cao*	*Commelina*	*Herba Commelinae**
Copper Sulphate; Blue Vitriol	*Dan Fan*	*Chalcanthitum*	*Chalcanthitum**
Coptis; Golden Thread Rhizome	*Huang Lian*	*Coptis*	*Rhizoma Coptidis*
Coral-bean Bark	*Hai Tong Pi*	*Erythrina*	*Cortex Erythrinae*
Cornsilk	*Yu Mi Xu*	*Zea*	*Stylus Zeae Mays*
Corydalis Rhizome	*Yan Hu Suo*	*Corydalis*	*Rhizoma Corydalis Yanhusuo*
Costus Root; Aucklandia	*Mu Xiang*	*Saussurea*	*Radix Saussureae Lappae*
Cotton Root	*Mian Hua Gen*	*Gossypium*	*Radix Gossypii Hirsuti**
Cow Gallbladder	*Niu Dan*	*Bos*	*Vesica Fellea Bovus*
Cow Soapwort Seed	*Wang Bu Liu Xing*	*Vaccaria*	*Semen Vaccariae Segetalis*
Creeping Lily-turf Tuber	*Mai Men Dong*	*Ophiopogon*	*Tuber Ophiopogonis Japonici*
Croton Seed	*Ba Dou*	*Croton*	*Semen Croton Tiglii*
Crystalized Volatile Oil of the Camphor Tree	*Zhang Nao*	*Cinnamomum*	*Camphora*
Cubeba Fruit	*Bi Cheng Qie*	*Piper*	*Fructus Cubebae*
Cuttle-fish Bone	*Hai Piao Xiao*	*Sepia or Sepiella*	*Os Sepiae seu Sepiellae*
Cyathula Root	*Chuan Niu Xi*	*Cyathula*	*Radix Cyathulae Officinalis*
Cynanchum Rhizome and Root	*Bai Qian*	*Cynanchum*	*Rhizoma et Radix Cynanchi Baiqian*
Cynanchum Root	*Ge Shan Xiang*	*Cynanchum*	*Radix Cynanchi Auriculati*
Cynomorium Fleshy Stem	*Suo Yang*	*Cynomorium*	*Herba Cynomorii Songarici*
Cyperus Rhizome; Nut-grass Rhizome; Sedge Rhizome	*Xiang Fu*	*Cyperus*	*Rhizoma Cyperi Rotundi*

Common	Pinyin	Botanical	Pharmaceutical
Dalbergia Heartwood	*Jiang Xiang*	*Dalbergia*	*Lignum Dalbergiae Odoriferae*
Dandelion	*Pu Gong Ying*	*Taraxacum*	*Herba Taraxaci Mongolici cum Radice*
Daphne Flower	*Yuan Hua*	*Daphne*	*Flos Daphnes Genkwa*
Dead Stiff Body of Sick Silkworm Larvae	*Jiang Can*	*Bombyx*	*Bombyx Batryticatus*
Dendrobium Stem	*Shi Hu*	*Dendrobium*	*Herba Dendrobii*
Dichroa Leaf	*Shu Qi*	*Dichroa*	*Folium Dichroae Febrifugae*
Dichroa Root	*Chang Shan*	*Dichroa*	*Radix Dichroae Febrifugae*
Dioscorea Tuber	*Huang Yao Zi*	*Dioscorea*	*Tuber Dioscoreae Bulbiferae*
Dittany Root Bark	*Bai Xian Pi*	*Dictamnus*	*Cortex Dictamni Dasycarpi Radicis*
Dodder Seed	*Tu Si Zi*	*Cuscuta*	*Semen Cuscutae Chinensis*
Dog Bone	*Gou Gu*	*Canis*	*Os Canine*
Dogwood Fruit; Asiatic Cornelian Cherry Fruit	*Shan Zhu Yu*	*Cornus*	*Fructus Corni Officinalis*
Donkey Hide Gelatin; Ass Skin Glue	*E Jiao*	*Equus*	*Gelatinum Corii Asini*
Dragon Bone; Fossilized Bone	*Long Gu*	*Os Draconis*	*Os Draconis*
Dragon Tooth; Fossilized Tooth	*Long Chi*	*Dens Draconis*	*Dens Draconis*
Dragon's Blood Resin	*Xue Jie*	*Dracaena*	*Sanguis Draconis*
Dried Bamboo Sap	*Zhu Li*	*Bambusa*	*Succus Bambusae*
Dried Ginger Rhizome	*Gan Jiang*	*Zingiber*	*Rhizoma Zingiberis Officinalis*
Dried Paste of Concentrated Decoction of Black or White Cutch	*Er Cha*	*Acacia or Uncaria*	*Pasta Acacia seu Uncaria*
Dried Persimmon Fruit	*Shi Bing*	*Diospyros*	*Fructus Diospyri Kaki**
Dried Skeleton of Luffa Sponge	*Si Gua Lou*	*Luffa*	*Fasciculus Vascularis Luffae*
Dried Skin Secretion of Toad	*Chan Su*	*Bufo*	*Secretio Bufonis*
Dry-Fried Coix Seed	*Shu Yi Ren*	*Coix*	*Semen Coicis Lachryma-jobi*
Drynaria Rhizome	*Gu Sui Bu*	*Drynaria*	*Rhizoma Drynariae*
Dryopteris Rhizome	*Dong Bei Guan Zhong*	*Dryopteris*	*Rhizoma Dryopteridis*
Duckweed	*Fu Ping*	*Spirodela or Lemna*	*Herba Lemnae seu Spirodelae*
Earthworm	*Di Long*	*Pheretima*	*Lumbricus*
Eclipta	*Han Lian Cao*	*Eclipta*	*Herba Ecliptae Prostratae*
Eleagnus Leaf	*Hu Tui Ye*	*Eleagnus*	*Folium Eleagni Pungens*
Elecampane	*Jin Fei Cao*	*Inula*	*Herba Inulae*
Elecampane Flower	*Xuan Fu Hua*	*Inula*	*Flos Inulae*

Common	Pinyin	Botanical	Pharmaceutical
Ephedra Root	Ma Huang Gen	Ephedra	Radix Ephedrae
Ephedra Stem	Ma Huang	Ephedra	Herba Ephedrae
Epimedium	Yin Yang Huo	Epimedium	Herba Epimedii
Eucommia Bark	Du Zhong	Eucommia	Cortex Eucommiae Ulmoidis
Euryale Seed	Qian Shi	Euryale	Semen Euryales Ferocis
Evodia Fruit	Wu Zhu Yu	Evodia	Fructus Evodiae Rutaecarpae
Fennel Fruit	Xiao Hui Xiang	Foeniculum	Fructus Foeniculi Vulgaris
Fenugreek Seed	Hu Lu Ba	Trigonella	Semen Trigonellae Foeni-graeci
Figwort Root	Xuan Shen	Scrophularia	Radix Scrophulariae Ningpoensis
Finger Citron Flower	Fo Shou Hua	Citrus	Flos Citri Sarcodactylis
Finger Citron Fruit	Fo Shou	Citrus	Fructus Citri Sarcodactylis
Flattened Milk-vetch Seed	Sha Yuan Ji Li	Astragalus	Semen Astragali Complanati
Fleeceflower Root; Fo-Ti Root	He Shou Wu	Polygonum	Radix Polygoni Multiflori
Fleeceflower Stem; Fo-Ti Stem	Ye Jiao Teng	Polygonum	Caulis Polygoni Multiflori
Fluorite	Zi Shi Ying	Fluoritum	Fluoritum
Flying Squirrel Feces	Wu Ling Zhi	Trogopterus or Pteromys	Excrementum Trogopteri seu Pteromi
Forsythia Fruit; Golden Bells	Lian Qiao	Forsythia	Fructus Forsythiae Suspensae
Fragrant Solomon's Seal Rhizome; Polygonatum	Yu Zhu	Polygonatum	Rhizoma Polygonati Odorati
Frankincense Gum-resin	Ru Xiang	Boswellia	Gummi Olibanum
Fresh Chinese Foxglove Root	Sheng Di Huang	Rehmannia	Radix Rehmanniae Glutinosae
Dried Ginseng Root	Sheng Shai Shen	Panax	Radix Ginseng
Fresh Ginger Rhizome	Sheng Jiang	Zingiber	Rhizoma Zingiberis Officinalis Recens
Fresh Ginger Skin	Sheng Jiang Pi	Zingiber	Cortex Zingiberis Officinalis Recens
Fresh Water Turtle Shell	Gui Ban	Chinemys	Plastrum Testudinis
Gadfly	Meng Chong	Tabanus	Tabani Bivittati*
Gallnut of Chinese Sumac	Wu Bei Zi	Rhus/Melaphis	Galla Rhois Chineneis
Gambir vine Stems and Hooks	Gou Teng	Uncaria	Ramulus cum Uncis Uncariae
Gardenia Fruit	Zhi Zi	Gardenia	Fructus Gardeniae Jasminoidis
Garlic Bulb	Da Suan	Allium	Bulbus Allii Sativi
Gastrodia Rhizome	Tian Ma	Gastrodia	Rhizoma Gastrodiae Elatae
Gecko Lizard	Ge Jie	Gekko	Gekko

Common	Pinyin	Botanical	Pharmaceutical
Geranium; Heronbill; Cranebill	Lao Guan Cao	Erodium or Geranium	Herba Erodii seu Geranii*
Giant Knotweed Rhizome	Hu Zhang	Polygonum	Radix et Rhizoma Polygoni Cuspidati
Ginkgo Leaf	Yin Guo Ye	Ginkgo	Folium Ginkgo Bilobae
Ginkgo Nut	Bai Guo	Ginkgo	Semen Ginkgo Bilobae
Ginseng Leaf	Ren Shen Ye	Panax	Folium Ginseng
Ginseng Root Neck	Ren Shen Lu	Panax	Cervix Ginseng
Ginseng Root steamed until red	(Hong) Ren Shen	Panax	Radix Ginseng
Glabrous Greenbrier Rhizome	Tu Fu Ling	Smilax	Rhizoma Smilacis Glabrae
Glorybower Leaf	Chou Wu Tong	Clerodendron	Folium Clerodendri Trichotomi
Goat Horn	Shan Yang Jiao	Naemorhedis	Cornu Naemorhedis
Gold	Huang Jin	Aurum	Aurum*
Golden Eye-grass Rhizome	Xian Mao	Curculigo	Rhizoma Curculiginis Orchioidis
Grains-of-Paradise Flower	Sha Ren Hua	Amomum	Flos Amomi
Grains-of-Paradise Fruit or Seeds	Sha Ren	Amomum	Fructus seu Semen Amomi
Grains-of-Paradise Shell	Sha Ren Ke	Amomum	Pericarpium Amomi
Groomwell Root	Zi Cao	Lithospermum	Radix Lithospermi seu Arnebiae
Groundsel	Qian Li Guang	Senecio	Herba Senecionis Scandentis*
Gynura Leaf	Ju Ye San Qi	Gynura	Folium Gynurae*
Gypsum; Calcium Sulphate	Shi Gao	Gypsum	Gypsum Fibrosum
Halloysite; Red Kaolin	Chi Shi Zhi	Halloysitum Rubrum	Halloysitum Rubrum
Hawksbill Turtle Shell	Dai Mao	Eretmochelys	Carapax Eretmochelydis Imbricatae*
Hawthorn Ripe Fruit or Berry	Shan Zha Rou	Crataegus	Fructus Crataegi
Hawthorn Unripe Fruit or Berry	Shan Zha	Crataegus	Fructus Crataegi
Hematite; Iron Ore	Dai Zhe Shi	Haematitum	Haematitum
Hemp Seed; Marihuana Seed	Huo Ma Ren	Cannabis	Semen Cannabis Sativae
Hoelen; China Root; Tuckahoe; Indian Bread	Fu Ling	Poria	Sclerotium Poriae Cocos
Hogfennel Root	Qian Hu	Peucedanum	Radix Peucedani
Holly Leaf	Si Ji Qing	Ilex	Folium Ilicis Chinensis*
Homalomena Rhizome	Qian Nian Jian	Homalomena	Rhizoma Homalomenae Occultae
Honey	Feng Mi	Mel	Mel*

Common	Pinyin	Botanical	Pharmaceutical
Honey-fried Licorice Root	Zhi Gan Cao	Glycyrrhiza	Radix Glycyrrhizae Praeparata*
Honeylocust Fruit; Soap Bean Fruit	Zao Jiao	Gleditsia	Fructus Gleditsiae Sinensis
Honeylocust Spine; Soap Bean Spine	Zao Jiao Ci	Gleditsia	Spina Gleditsiae Sinensis
Honeysuckle Flower	Jin Yin Hua	Lonicera	Flos Lonicerae Japonicae
Honeysuckle Stem	Jin Yin Teng	Lonicera	Ramus Lonicerae Japonicae
Hornet Nest; Wasp Nest	Lu Feng Fang	Polistes	Nidus Vespae
Horsetail; Scouring Rush; Shavegrass	Mu Zei	Equisetum	Herba Equiseti Hiemalis
Houttuynia; Fish Smell Plant	Yu Xing Cao	Houttuynia	Herba cum Radice Houttuyniae Cordatae
Human Placenta	Zi He Che	Homo Sapiens	Placenta Hominis
Hyacinth Bean	Bian Dou	Dolichos	Semen Dolichoris Lablab
Hyacinth Bean Flower	Bian Dou Hua	Dolichos	Flos Dolichoris Lablab
Hydrangea Flower	Ba Xian Hua	Hydrangea	Flos Hydrangeae Macrophyllae*
Hypoglauca Yam Rhizome; Fish-poison Yam Rhizome	Bei Xie	Dioscorea	Rhizoma Dioscoreae Hypoglaucae
Ignited Wood Stove Earth	Fu Long Gan	Terra Flava Usta	Terra Flava Usta
Immature (Green) Tangerine Peel	Qing Pi	Citrus	Pericarpium Citri Reticulatae Viride
Immature Bitter Orange Fruit	Zhi Shi	Citrus or Poncirus	Fructus Immaturus Citri Aurantii
Indigo	Qing Dai	Indigo	Indigo Pulverata Levis
Iron Filing	Sheng Tie Luo	Frusta Ferri	Frusta Ferri
Isatis Leaf; Woad Leaf	Da Qing Ye	Isatis	Folium Isatidis Daqingye
Isatis Root; Woad Root	Ban Lan Gen	Isatis	Radix Isatidis seu Baphicacanthi
Ivy	Chang Chun Teng	Hedera	Herba Hederae Nepalensis*
Japanese Climbing Fern	Jin Sha Teng	Lygodium	Herba Lygodii Japonici
Japanese Climbing Fern Spore	Hai Jin Sha	Lygodium	Spora Lygodii Japonici
Japanese Dioscorea Rhizome	Chuan Shan Long	Dioscorea	Rhizoma Dioscoreae Nipponicae*
Japanese Elder Bark	Lu Ying	Sambucus	Cortex Sambuci*
Japanese Thistle	Da Ji	Cirsium	Herba seu Radix Cirsii Japonici
Jilin Wild Ginseng	Ji Lin Shen	Panax	Radix Ginseng
Jujube Fruit; Chinese Black Date	Da Zao	Ziziphus	Fructus Ziziphi Jujubae
Jujube Fruit; Chinese Red Date	Hong Zao	Ziziphus	Fructus Ziziphi Jujubae
Kadsura Stem	Hai Feng Teng	Piper	Caulis Piperis Futokadsurae

Common	Pinyin	Botanical	Pharmaceutical
Kansui Spurge Root	*Gan Sui*	*Euphorbia*	*Radix Euphorbiae Kansui*
Kariyat; Green Chiretta	*Chuan Xin Lian*	*Andrographis*	*Herba Andrographitis Paniculatae*
Kelp Thallus; Kombu Thallus	*Kun Bu*	*Laminaria or Ecklonia*	*Thallus Algae*
Knotty Pine Wood	*Song Jie*	*Pinus*	*Lignum Pini Nodi*
Korean Ash Bark	*Qin Pi*	*Fraxinus*	*Cortex Fraxini*
Kudzu Flower	*Ge Hua*	*Pueraria*	*Flos Puerariae*
Kudzu Root	*Ge Gen*	*Pueraria*	*Radix Puerariae*
Ladybell Root; Southern Sand Root	*Nan Sha Shen*	*Adenophora*	*Radix Adenophorae*
Laquer	*Gan Qi*	*Rhus*	*Lacca Sinica Exsiccatae*
Large-Leaf Gentian Root	*Qin Jiao*	*Gentiana*	*Radix Gentianae Qinjiao*
Leech	*Shui Zhi*	*Hirudo*	*Hirudo seu Whitmania*
Leechee Nut	*Li Zhi He*	*Litchi*	*Semen Litchi Chinensis*
Leopard Bone	*Bao Gu*	*Panthera*	*Os Leopardis*
Lesser Galangal Rhizome	*Gao Liang Jiang*	*Alpinia*	*Rhizoma Alpiniae Officinari*
Licorice Root	*Gan Cao*	*Glycyrhiza*	*Radix Glycyrrhizae Uralensis*
Lily Bulb	*Bai He*	*Lilium*	*Bulbus Lilii*
Limonite	*Yu Liang Shi*	*Limonite*	*Limonite*
Litharge; Galena	*Mi Tuo Seng*	*Lithargyrum*	*Lithargyrum*
Long Pepper Fruit	*Bi Ba*	*Piper*	*Fructus Piperis Longi*
Long-noded Pit Viper Snake	*Bai Hua She*	*Agkistrodon*	*Agkistrodon seu Bungarus*
Longan Fruit Flesh	*Long Yan Rou*	*Euphoria*	*Arillus Euphoriae Longanae*
Loquat Leaf	*Pi Pa Ye*	*Eriobotrya*	*Folium Eriobotryae Japonicae*
Loropetalum Bark	*Ji Mu*	*Loropetalum*	*Cortex Loropetali**
Lotus Leaf	*He Ye*	*Nelumbo*	*Folium Nelumbinis Nuciferae*
Lotus Plumule	*Lian Xin*	*Nelumbo*	*Plumula Nelumbinis Nuciferae*
Lotus Rhizome Node	*Ou Jie*	*Nelumbo*	*Nodus Nelumbinis Nuciferae Rhizomatis*
Lotus Seed	*Lian Zi*	*Nelumbo*	*Semen Nelumbinis Nuciferae*
Lotus Stamen	*Lian Xu*	*Nelumbo*	*Stamen Nelumbinis Nuciferae*
Lotus Stem	*Lian Geng*	*Nelumbo*	*Ramulus Nelumbinis Nuciferae*
Lucid Ganoderma; Reishi	*Ling Zhi*	*Ganoderma*	*Fructificatio Ganodermae Lucidi**
Luffa Skin	*Si Gua Pi*	*Luffa*	*Pericarpium Luffa Acutangulae*
Lysimachia	*Jin Qian Cao*	*Lysimachia*	*Herba Lysimachiae*
Macaque Gallstone	*Hou Zao*	*Macaca*	*Calculus Macacae Mulattae*
Madder Root	*Qian Cao Gen*	*Rubia*	*Radix Rubiae Cordifoliae*

Common	Pinyin	Botanical	Pharmaceutical
Magnetite; Magnetic Iron Ore; Loadstone	Ci Shi	Magnetitum	Magnetitum
Magnolia Bark	Hou Po	Magnolia	Cortex Magnoliae Officinalis
Magnolia Flower	Hou Po Hua	Magnolia	Flos Magnoliae Officinalis
Magnolia Flower	Xin Yi Hua	Magnolia	Flos Magnoliae
Mahonia Leaf	Shi Da Gong Lao	Mahonia	Folium Mahoniae*
Male Deer Sexual Organs	Hua Lu Shen	Cervus	Testis et Penis Cervi*
Male Dog Sexual Organs	Guang Gou Shen	Canis	Testis et Penis Canis*
Male Horse Sexual Organs	Hei Lu Shen	Equus	Testis et Penis Equii*
Male Seal Sexual Organs	Hai Gou Shen	Phoca	Testis et Penis Otariae*
Manchurian Lilac Bark	Bao Ma Zi	Syringa	Cortex Syringae*
Matrimony Vine Fruit; Wolfberry Fruit	Gou Qi Zi	Lycium	Fructus Lycii
Matrimony-vine Rootbark; Wolfberry Bark	Di Gu Pi	Lycium	Cortex Lycii Radicis
Mature Antler Glue; Mature Antler Gelatin	Lu Jiao Jiao	Cervus	Colla Cornu Cervi
Mature Lotus Receptacle	Lian Fang	Nelumbo	Receptaculum Nelumbinis Nuciferae
Medicated Leaven	Shen Qu	Massa Fermentata	Massa Fermentata
Melon Pedicle	Gua Di	Cucumis	Pedicellus Cucumeris
Mercury	Shui Yin	Hydrargyrum	Hydrargyrum
Millettia Root and Vine; Chicken Blood Vine	Ji Xue Teng	Millettia	Radix et Caulis Jixueteng
Mimosa Tree Bark; Silktree Bark	He Huan Pi	Albizzia	Cortex Albizziae Julibrissin
Mimosa Tree Flower; Silktree Flower	He Huan Hua	Albizzia	Flos Albizziae Julibrissin*
Mirabilite; Glauber's Salt	Mang Xiao	Mirabilitum	Mirabilitum
Momordica Fruit	Luo Han Guo	Momordica	Fructus Momordicae Grosvenori
Momordica Leaf	Luo Huo Guo Ye	Momordica	Folium Momordicae Grosvenori
Momordica Seed	Mu Bie Zi	Momordica	Semen Momordicae Cochinchinensis
Morinda Root	Ba Ji Tian	Morinda	Radix Morindae Officinalis
Morning Glory Seed	Qian Niu Zi	Pharbitis	Semen Pharbitidis
Mother-of-Pearl Shell	Zhen Zhu Mu	Pteria	Concha Margaritiferae
Motherwort	Yi Mu Cao	Leonurus	Herba Leonuri Heterophylli
Motherwort Seed	Chong Wei Zi	Leonurus	Semen Leonuri Heterophylli
Mugwort Leaf	Ai Ye	Artemisia	Folium Artemisiae Argyi
Mulberry Fruit Bud	Sang Shen	Morus	Fructus Mori Albae
Mulberry Leaf	Sang Ye	Morus	Folium Mori Albae

Common	Pinyin	Botanical	Pharmaceutical
Mulberry Mistletoe Stem	Sang Ji Sheng	Loranthus or Viscum	Ramulus Sangjishang
Mulberry Rootbark	Sang Bai Pi	Morus	Cortex Mori Albae Radicis
Mulberry Twig	Sang Zhi	Morus	Ramulus Mori Albae
Mung Bean	Lu Dou	Phaseolus	Semen Phaseoli Radiati
Musk Mallow Seed; Malva Seed	Dong Kui Zi	Malva or Abutilon	Semen Albutili seu Malvae
Musk; Musk Deer Navel Gland Secretion	She Xiang	Moschus	Secretio Moschus
Myrobalan Fruit	He Zi	Terminalia	Fructus Terminaliae Chebulae
Myrrh Gum-resin	Mo Yao	Commiphora	Resinae Myrrhae
Northern Schisandra Fruit	Wu Wei Zi	Schisandra	Fructus Schisandrae Chinensis
Notopterygium Rhizome and Root	Qiang Huo	Notopterygium	Rhizoma et Radix Notopterygii
Nutmeg Seed	Rou Dou Kou	Myristica	Semen Myristicae Fragrantis
Nux-vomica Seed	Ma Qian Zi	Strychnos	Semen Strychni
Oldenlandia	Bai Hua She She Cao	Oldenlandia	Herba Oldenlandiae Diffusae
Omphalia Fungus Fruiting Body	Lei Wan	Omphalia	Sclerotium Omphaliae Lapidescens
Ophicalcite	Hua Rui Shi	Ophicalcitum	Ophicalcitum
Opium Poppy Husk	Ying Su Ke	Papaver	Pericarpium Papaveris Somniferi
Oriental Wormwood	Yin Chen Hao	Artemisia	Herba Artemisiae Yinchenhao
Oroxylum Seed	Mu Hu Die	Oroxylum	Semen Oroxyli Indici
Ox or Water Buffalo Gallstone	Niu Huang	Bos or Bubalis	Calculus Bovis seu Calculus Bubali
Oyster Shell	Mu Li	Ostrea	Concha Ostreae
Paederia Stem	Ji Shi Teng	Paederia	Caulis Paederiae*
Pagoda Tree Flower Bud	Huai Hua Mi	Sophora	Flos Sophorae Japonicae Immaturus
Pagoda Tree Fruit	Huai Jiao	Sophora	Fructus Sophorae Japonicae
Paris Rhizome	Zao Xiu	Paris	Rhizoma Paridis Polyphyllae*
Partially-blossoming Chinese Tea Rose Flower	Yue Ji Hua	Rosa	Flos et Fructus Rosae Chinensis
Patchouli; Agastache	Huo Xiang	Agastache or Pogostemon	Herba Agastaches seu Pogostemi
Patrinia; Thiaspi	Bai Jiang Cao	Patrinia or Thiaspi	Herba cum Radice Patriniae
Peach Seed (Kernel)	Tao Ren	Prunus	Semen Persicae
Peanut Skin	Hua Sheng Yi	Arachis	Pericarpium Arachi*
Pear Peel	Li Pi	Pyrus	Pericarpium Pyri*
Pearl	Zhen Zhu	Pteria	Margarita

Common	Pinyin	Botanical	Pharmaceutical
Peking Spurge Root	*Jing Da Ji*	*Euphorbia or Knoxia*	*Radix Euphorbiae seu Knoxiae*
Peppermint; Spearmint; Field Mint	*Bo He*	*Mentha*	*Herba Menthae Haplocalycis*
Perilla Leaf	*Zi Su Ye*	*Perilla*	*Folium Perillae Frutescentis*
Perilla Seed	*Zi Su Zi*	*Perilla*	*Semen Perillae Frutescentis*
Perilla Stem	*Zi Su Geng*	*Perilla*	*Ramulus Perillae**
Persimmon Calyx	*Shi Di*	*Diospyros*	*Calyx Diospyri Kaki*
Picrorhiza Rhizome	*Hu Huang Lian*	*Picrorhiza*	*Rhizoma Picrorhizae*
Pigeon Pea Root	*Shan Dou Gen*	*Sophora*	*Radix Sophorae Tonkinensis*
Pill-bearing Spurge	*Ze Qi*	*Euphorbia*	*Herba Euphorbiae Helioscopiae*
Pink Flower Herb	*Qu Mai*	*Dianthus*	*Herba Dianthi*
Pipe-fish	*Hai Long*	*Solenognathus*	*Hailong*
Pipewort Scapus	*Gu Jing Cao*	*Eriocaulon*	*Scapus et Inflorescentia Eriocaulonis Buergeriani*
Plantago Seed; Plantain Seed	*Che Qian Zi*	*Plantago*	*Semen Plantaginis*
Plantago; Plantain	*Che Qian Cao*	*Plantago*	*Herba Plantaginis*
Poke Root	*Shang Lu*	*Phytolacca*	*Radix Phytolaccae*
Polygonum	*Guan Ye Liao*	*Polygonum*	*Herba Polygoni Perfoliati**
Polyporus Sclerotium	*Zhu Ling*	*Polyporus*	*Sclerotium Polypori Umbellati*
Pomegranate Husk or Rind	*Shi Liu Pi*	*Punica*	*Pericarpium Punicae Granati*
Pomegranate Root Bark	*Shi Liu Gen Pi*	*Punica*	*Cortex Punicae Granati Radicis*
Potentilla	*Fan Bai Cao*	*Potentilla*	*Herba Potentillae Discoloris**
Powdered Jack-in-the-Pulpit Rhizome mixed with Cow Bile	*Dan Nan Xing*	*Arisaema*	*Pulvis Arisaemae cum Felle Bovis*
Praying Mantis Egg Case	*Sang Piao Xiao*	*Paratenodera*	*Ootheca Mantidis*
Prepared Alum	*Ku Fan*	*Alumen Praeparatum*	*Alumen Praeparatum*
Prepared (Fermented) Soybean	*Dan Dou Chi*	*Glycine*	*Semen Glycinis Praeparatum*
Prepared Jack-in-the-Pulpit Rhizome	*Zhi Nan Xing*	*Arisaema*	*Rhizoma Arisaematis Praeparatae*
Prepared Pinellia Rhizome	*(Fa) Ban Xia*	*Pinellia*	*Rhizoma Pinelliae Ternatae*
Prepared Sichuan Aconite Root	*(Hei)Fu Zi*	*Aconitum*	*Radix Lateralis Aconiti Carmichaeli Praeparata*
Prince Ginseng Root	*Tai Zi Shen*	*Pseudostellaria*	*Radix Pseudostellariae Heterophyllae*
Privet Fruit; Waxtree Fruit	*Nu Zhen Zi*	*Ligustrum*	*Fructus Ligustri Lucidi*
Processed Resin of Borneol Camphor	*Bing Pian*	*Dryobalanops*	*Borneol*

Common	Pinyin	Botanical	Pharmaceutical
Processed Resin of Styrax Benzoin	An Xi Xiang	Styrax	Benzoinum
Pseudoginseng Flower; Notoginseng Flower	San Qi Hua	Panax	Flos Pseudoginseng
Pseudoginseng Root; Notoginseng Root	San Qi	Panax	Radix Pseudoginseng
Pteris	Feng Wei Cao	Pteris	Herba Pterii*
Pubescent Angelica Root	Du Huo	Angelica	Radix Angelicae Pubescentis
Pubescent Holly Root	Mao Dong Qing	Ilex	Radix Ilicis Pubescentis*
Puffball Fruiting Body	Ma Bo	Lasiosphaera	Fructificatio Lasiosphaerae seu Calvatiae
Pulsatilla Root; Anemone Root	Bai Tou Weng	Pulsatilla	Radix Pulsatillae Chinensis
Pumice	Fu Hai Shi	Pumice	Pumice
Pumpkin Seed and Husk	Nan Gua Zi	Cucurbita	Semen Cucurbitae Moschatae
Puncture Vine Fruit; Caltrop Fruit	Bai Ji Li	Tribulus	Fructus Tribuli Terrestris
Pure Mirabilite; Pure Sodium Sulphate; Pure Glauber's Salt	Xuan Ming Fen	Mirabilitum	Mirabilitum Purum
Purple Aster Root	Zi Wan	Aster	Radix Asteris Tatarici
Purslane	Ma Chi Xian	Portulaca	Herba Portulacae Oleraceae
Pyrite	Zi Ran Tong	Pyritum	Pyritum
Pyrola	Lu Xian Cao	Pyrola	Herba Pyrolae*
Pyrrosia Leaf	Shi Wei	Pyrrosia	Folium Pyrrosiae
Quick-fried Ginger Rhizome	Pao Jiang	Zingiber	Rhizoma Zingiberis*
Radish Seed	Lai Fu Zi	Raphanus	Semen Raphani Satavi
Ramie Root	Zhu Ma Gen	Boehmeria	Radix Boehmeriae Niveae*
Rangoon Creeper Fruit	Shi Jun Zi	Quisqualis	Fructus Quisqualis Indicae
Raspberry Fruit Bud	Fu Pen Zi	Rubus	Fructus Rubi Chingii
Raw Cattail Pollen	(Sheng) Pu Huang	Typha	Pollen Typhae
Raw Jack-in-the-Pulpit Rhizome	(Sheng) Tian Nan Xing	Arisaema	Rhizoma Arisaematis
Raw Pinellia Rhizome	(Sheng) Ban Xia	Pinellia	Rhizoma Pinelliae Ternatae
Realgar; Arsenic Disulfide	Xiong Huang	Realgar	Realgar
Red Dogbane Whole Herb or Leaf	Luo Bu Ma	Apocynum	Herba seu Folium Apocyni Veneti*
Red Hoelen; Red Tuckahoe	Chi Fu Ling	Poria	Sclerotium Poriae Cocos Rubrae
Red Lead Oxide	Qian Dan	Minium	Minium
Red Peony Root	Chi Shao	Paeonia	Radix Paeoniae Rubra
Red Sage Root	Dan Shen	Salvia	Radix Salviae Miltiorrhizae

Common	Pinyin	Botanical	Pharmaceutical
Red Tangerine Peel	Ju Hong	Citrus	Pars Rubra Epicarpii Citri Erythrocarpae
Reed Rhizome; Corrizo Rhizome	Lu Gen	Phragmites	Rhizoma Phragmitis Communis
Rhaponticum Root; Echinops Root	Lou Lu	Rhaponticum or Echinops	Radix Rhapontici seu Echinops
Rhinoceros Horn	Xi Jiao	Rhinoceros	Cornu Rhinoceri
Rhodea	Wan Nian Qing	Rhodea	Herba Rhodeae Japonicae*
Rhododendron Leaf	Man Shan Hong	Rhododendron	Folium Rhododendri*
Rhubarb Root and Rhizome	Da Huang	Rheum	Radix et Rhizoma Rhei
Rice Grain	Jing Mi	Oryza	Semen Oryzae Sativae*
Rice Paper Pith	Tong Cao	Tetrapanax	Medulla Tetrapanacis Papyriferi
Rice Sprout	Gu Ya	Oryza	Fructus Oryzae Sativae Germinatus
Rock Candy cured White Ginseng Root	Bai Shen	Panax	Radix Ginseng
Rock Candy cured White Ginseng Root Tail	Shen Xu	Panax	Radix Ginseng
Rorippa	Han Cai	Rorippa	Herba Rorippae*
Rose Maloes Resin	Su He Xiang	Liquidambar	Styrax Liquidis
Round Cardamon Fruit; Cluster Fruit	Bai Dou Kou	Amomum	Fructus Amomi Kravanh
Rush Pith	Deng Xin Cao	Juncus	Medulla Junci Effusi
Safflower	Hong Hua	Carthamus	Flos Carthami Tinctorii
Salvia	Ji Ning	Salvia	Herba Salviae Plebeia*
Sandalwood Heartwood	Tan Xiang	Santalum	Lignum Santali Albi
Sappan Heartwood	Su Mu	Caesalpinia	Lignum Sappan
Sargassum Seaweed	Hai Zao	Sargassum	Herba Sargassii
Sargentodoxa Stem	Hong Teng	Sargentodoxa	Caulis Sargentodoxae Cuneatae
Saururus	San Bai Cao	Saururus	Herba Saururi Chinensis*
Saxifrage	Hu Er Cao	Saxifrage	Herba Saxifragae Stoloniferae*
Schizonepeta Stem or Bud	Jing Jie	Schizonepeta	Herba Schizonepetae Tenuifoliae
Scorpion	Quan Xie	Buthus	Buthus Martensi
Scurfy Pea Fruit	Bu Gu Zhi	Psoralea	Fructus Psoraleae Corylifoliae
Scute; Baical Skullcap Root	Huang Qin	Scutellaria	Radix Scutellariae Baicalensis
Sea Cucumber; Sea Slug	Hai Shen	Strichopus	Strichopus Japonicus
Sea Horse	Hai Ma	Hippocampus	Hippocampus
Sedum	Jing Tian San Qi	Sedum	Herba Sedi*

Common	Pinyin	Botanical	Pharmaceutical
Selaginella	*Shi Shang Bai*	*Selaginella*	*Herba Selaginellae Doederleinii*
Selfheal Spike; Heal all Spike	*Xia Ku Cao*	*Prunella*	*Spica Prunellae Vulgaris*
Senna Leaf	*Fan Xie Ye*	*Cassia*	*Folium Sennae*
Shepherd's Purse	*Ji Cai*	*Capsella*	*Herba Capsellae**
Shield-fem Rhizome	*Guan Zhong*	*Dryopteris*	*Rhizoma Guanzhong*
Siberian Solomon Seal Rhizome	*Huang Jing*	*Polygonatum*	*Rhizoma Polygonati*
Sichuan Aconite	*Chuan Wu*	*Aconitum*	*Radix Aconite Carmichaeli*
Sichuan Chinaberry Fruit; Sichuan Pagoda Tree Fruit; Neem Fruit	*Chuan Lian Zi*	*Melia*	*Fructus Meliae Toosendan*
Sichuan Chinaberry Root Bark; Sichuan Pagoda Tree Root Bark; Neem Root Bark	*Ku Lian Gen Pi*	*Melia*	*Cortex Meliae Radicis*
Sichuan Chinaberry Tree Bark; Sichuan Pagoda Tree Bark; Neem Tree Bark	*Ku Lian Mu Pi*	*Melia*	*Cortex Meliae*
Sichuan Lovage Root	*Chuan Xiong*	*Ligusticum*	*Radix Ligustici Chuan Xiong*
Sichuan Pepper Fruit	*Chuan Jiao*	*Zanthoxylum*	*Pericarpum Zanthoxyli Bungeani*
Sichuan Pepper Seed	*Chuan Jiao Mu*	*Zanthoxylum*	*Semen Zanthoxyli Bungeani*
Sichuan Pepper Seed	*(Chuan) Jiao Mu*	*Zanthoxylum*	*Semen Zanthoxyli Bungeani*
Siler Root; Ledebouriella Root	*Fang Feng*	*Ledebouriella*	*Radix Ledebouriella Divaricatae*
Siliceous Secretions of Bamboo	*Tian Zhu Huang*	*Bambusa*	*Concretio Silicea Bambusae Textillis*
Silkworm Feces	*Can Sha*	*Bombyx*	*Excrementum Bombycis Mori*
Silver	*Xiao Shi*	*Niter*	*Niter**
Small Thistle; Field Thistle	*Xiao Ji*	*Cephalanoplos*	*Herba Cephalanoplos*
Smilax Rhizome	*Ba Qia*	*Smilax*	*Rhizoma Smilacis China**
Smithsonite; Calamine	*Lu Gan Shi*	*Smithsonitum*	*Smithsonitum*
Snake Skin Slough	*She Tui*	*Zaocys*	*Exuviae Serpentis*
Snakegourd Fruit	*Gua Lou*	*Trichosanthes*	*Fructus Trichosanthis*
Snakegourd Peel	*Gua Lou Pi*	*Trichosanthes*	*Pericarpium Trichosanthis*
Snakegourd Root	*Tian Hua Fen*	*Trichosanthes*	*Radix Trichosanthis Kirilowii*
Snakegourd Seed	*Gua Lou Ren*	*Trichosanthes*	*Semen Trichosanthis*
Sour Jujube Seed; Zizyphus	*Suan Zao Ren*	*Ziziphus*	*Semen Ziziphi Spinosae*
Southern Schisandra Fruit	*Nan Wu Wei Zi*	*Schisandra*	*Fructus Schisandrae Sphenantherae*
Spicebush Root	*Wu Yao*	*Lindera*	*Radix Linderae Strychnifoliae*
St. Paul's Wort	*Xi Xian Cao*	*Siegesbeckia*	*Herba Siegesbeckiae*

Common	Pinyin	Botanical	Pharmaceutical
Stalactite Tubular Tip	E Guan Shi	Stalactitum	Stalactitum
Star Anise Fruit	Ba Jiao Hui Xiang	Illicium	Fructus Illicii*
Star Jasmine Stem	Luo Shi Teng	Trachelospermum	Caulis Trachelospermi Jasminoidis
Stellaria Root	Yin Chai Hu	Stellaria	Radix Stellariae Dichotomae
Stemona Root	Bai Bu	Stemona	Radix Stemonae
Stephania Root	Han Fang Ji	Stephania	Radix Stephaniae Tetrandrae
Sterculia Seed	Pang Da Hai	Sterculia	Semen Sterculiae Scaphigerae
Stigma of the True Saffron Flower	Xi Hong Hua	Crocus	Stigma Crocus Sativae
Stink Bug	Jiu Xiang Chong	Aspongopus	Aspongopus*
Stinking Elm Fruit Paste	Wu Yi	Ulmus	Praepartio Fructus Ulmi Macrocarpi
Stonecrop	Chui Pen Cao	Sedum	Herba Sedii Sarmentosi*
Straw Weed Rhizome and Root; Chinese Lovage Rhizome and Root	Gao Ben	Ligusticum	Rhizoma et Radix Ligustici
Sulphur	Liu Huang	Sulphur	Sulphur
Swallowort Root	Bai Wei	Cynanchum	Radix Cynanchi Baiwei
Sweet Jie Geng	Gan Jie Geng	Adenophora	Radix Adenophorae Trachelioidis
Sweet Rice Root and Rhizome	Nuo Dao Gen Xu	Oryza	Radix et Rhizoma Oryzae Glutinosae
Sweet Wormwood; Southernwood	Qing Hao	Artemisia	Herba Artemisiae Annuae
Sweetflag Rhizome	Shi Chang Pu	Acorus	Rhizoma Acori Graminei
Sweetgum Fruit	Lu Lu Tong	Liquidambar	Fructus Liquidambaris Taiwanianae
Talc; Soapstone	Hua Shi	Talcum	Talcum
Tallow Tree Root Bark	Wu Jiu Gen Pi	Sapium	Cortex Sappii Sebiferi Radicis*
Tamarisk	Cheng Liu	Tamarix	Cacumen Tamaricis Chinensis*
Tangerine Peel	Chen Pi	Citrus	Pericarpium Citri Reticulatae
Tangerine Seed	Ju He	Citrus	Semen Citri Reticulatae*
Tangkuei Head	Dang Gui Tou	Angelica	Caput Radicis Angelicae Sinensis
Tangkuei Root	Dang Gui	Angelica	Radix Angelicae Sinensis
Tangkuei Tail	Dang Gui Wei	Angelica	Extremas Radicis Angelicae Sinensis
Tansy Mustard Seed	Ting Li Zi	Lepidium or Descurainia	Semen Lepidii seu Descurainiae
Teasel Root	Xu Duan	Dipsacus	Radix Dipsaci Asperi
Tendrilled Fritillary Bulb	Chuan Bei Mu	Fritillaria	Bulbus Fritillariae Cirrhosae

Common

Common	Pinyin	Botanical	Pharmaceutical
Thalictrum	Tang Song Cao	Thalictrum	Herba Thalictri Foliolosi*
Thimbleberry	Mao Mei	Rubus	Herba Rubi Parvifolii*
Thin Cinnamon Bark from Young Trees	Guan Gui	Cinnamomum	Cortex Tubiformis Cinnamomi Cassiae
Thorowax Root; Hare's Ear Root	Chai Hu	Bupleurum	Radix Bupleuri
Thunberg Fritillary Bulb	Zhe Bei Mu	Fritillaria	Bulbus Fritillariae Thunbergii
Tiger Bone	Hu Gu	Panthera	Os Tigris
Tinospora Root	Jin Guo Lan	Tinospora	Radix Tinosporae Capillipes*
Tinospora Stem	Kuan Jin Teng	Tinospora	Ramus Tinosporae Sinensis
Torreya Seed	Fei Zi	Torreya	Semen Torreyae Grandis
Tree of Heaven Bark	Chun Pi	Ailanthus	Cortex Ailanthi Altissimae
Tree Peony Rootbark	Mu Dan Pi	Paeonia	Cortex Moutan Radicis
Tremella Fungus Fruiting Body	Bai Mu Er	Tremella	Fructificatio Tremellae Fuciformis
Tuckahoe Skin	Fu Ling Pi	Poria	Cortex Poriae Cocos
Tuckahoe Spirit	Fu Shen	Poria Cocos	Sclerotium Poriae Cocos Pararadicis
Tumeric Rhizome	Jiang Huang	Curcuma	Rhizoma Curcumae Longae
Tumeric Tuber	Yu Jin	Curcuma	Tuber Curcumae
Typhonium Rhizome	Bai Fu Zi	Typhonium	Rhizoma Typhonii Gigantei
Ume Plum Fruit; Black Plum Fruit	Wu Mei	Prunus	Fructus Pruni Mume
Veratrum Root	Li Lu	Veratrum	Radix et Rhizoma Veratri
Vervain	Ma Bian Cao	Verbena	Herba Verbenae*
Viola	Zi Hua Di Ding	Viola	Herba cum Radice Violae Yedoensitis
Vitex Fruit	Man Jing Zi	Vitex	Fructus Viticis
Walnut	Hu Tao Ren	Juglans	Semen Juglandis Regiae
Water Plantain Rhizome	Ze Xie	Alisma	Rhizoma Alismatis Orientalitis
Waterbuffalo Horn	Shui Niu Jiao	Bubalus	Cornu Bubali
Watermelon Fruit and Peel or Rind	Xi Gua	Citrullus	Fructus Citrulli Vulgaris
Wheat Chaff/Grain	Fu Xiao Mai	Triticum	Semen Tritici Aestivi Levis
White Arsenic	Pi Shi	Arsenolith	Arseolitum
White Atractylodes Rhizome	Bai Zhu	Atractylodes	Rhizoma Atractylodis Macrocephalae
White Bulb of Green Onion or Scallion	Cong Bai	Allium	Bulbus Allii Fistulosi
White Chrysanthemum Flower	(Bai) Ju Hua	Chrysanthemum	Flos Chrysanthemi Morifolii
White Mustard Seed	Bai Jie Zi	Brassica	Semen Sinapsis Albae

Common	Pinyin	Botanical	Pharmaceutical
White Peony Root	Bai Shao	Paeonia	Radix Paeoniae Lactiflorae
Wild Aconite	Cao Wu	Aconitum	Radix Aconiti Kusnezoffii
Wild Buckwheat Rhizome	Jin Qiao Mai	Fagopyrum	Rhizoma Fagopyri Cynosi*
Wild Cardamon Seed; Katsumada's Galangal Seed	Cao Dou Kou	Alpinia	Semen Alpiniae Katsumadai
Wild Chrysanthemum Flower	Ye Ju Hua	Chrysanthemum	Flos Chrysanthemi Indici
Wild Ginseng	Ye Shan Shen	Panax	Radix Ginseng
Wine-cooked Chinese Foxglove Root	Shu Di Huang	Rehmannia	Radix Rehmanniae Glutinosae Conquitae
Wingless Cockroach	Tu Bie Chong	Eupolyphaga	Eupolyphaga seu Opisthoplatia
Wintercherry Calyx or Fruit	Suan Jiang	Physalis	Calyx seu Fructus Physalis*
Wintermelon Fruit Peel; Wax Gourd Fruit Peel	Dong Gua Pi	Benincasa	Epicarpium Benincasae Hispidae
Wintermelon Seed; Wax Gourd Seed	Dong Gua Ren	Benincasa	Semen Benincasae Hispidae
Woolly Grass Rhizome; White Grass Rhizome	Bai Mao Gen	Imperata	Rhizoma Imperatae Cylindricae
Wooly Grass Flower; White Grass Flower	Bai Mao Hua	Imperata	Flos Imperatae Cylindricae
Xanthium Fruit; Cocklebur Fruit	Cang Er Zi	Xanthium	Fructus Xanthii Sibirici
Yellow Chrysanthemum Flower	(Huang) Ju Hua	Chrysanthemum	Flos Chrysanthemi Morifolii
Yellow Milk-vetch Root	Huang Qi	Astragalus	Radix Astragali Membranaceus
Young Chinese Rose Flower	Mei Gui Hua	Rosa	Flos Rosae Rugosae
Young Deer Antler Velvet	Lu Rong	Cervus	Cornu Cervi Parvum
Young Soybean Sprout	Dou Juan	Glycine	Semen Glycinis Germinatum
Zedoary Tumeric Rhizome	E Zhu	Curcuma	Rhizoma Curcumae

Appendices

Appendix A

Supplies Needed for a Start-up Pharmacy

When ready to set up a Chinese herbal pharmacy few supplies are needed other than a well-selected inventory of herbs. A triple-beam scale is recommended for weighing medicinals; a mortar and pestle, preferably made of brass or marble for crushing heavier substances; a blender for grinding up softer herbs. Finally, zip log or small paper bags work well for packaging herbal formulas for patients. Labeling laws suggest notations of the patient's name, date of expiration and ingredients on the bag of medicinals.

Appendix B lists 175 primary herbs commonly used in the most basic formulas. When developing an inventory, it is helpful to decide on a budget and compare prices of herbs between suppliers. Varying quality between suppliers must be considered as well.

Appendix C lists herb companies that sell bulk herbs or granules. Most suppliers have catalogs and/or websites. Please note that many suppliers will only sell to licensed professionals.

Most Chinese pharmacies use wooden drawers to store the medicinals. However, insects can travel between drawers whereas one-gallon glass jars prevent this from happening. Containers should be appropriately labeled. Having color pictures or samples of all herbs are very helpful in properly identifying your shipments. Most suppliers are very good about identifying each medicinal within a shipment but mislabeling or no labeling does occur.

Herbs have a shelf life of about one year. Some last longer but potency may diminish with age. Inspect herbs frequently to check for molds or insects. Infestations occur more often in humid climates.

Appendix B

175 Herbs For A Start-up Pharmacy

This is a suggested list of herbs for practitioners who want to start a Chinese herbal pharmacy.

Ai Ye/ Artemisia

Ba Ji Tian/ Morinda

Bai Dou Kou/ Amomum

Bai Jie Zi/ Brassica

Bai Mao Gen/ Imperata

Bai Shao / Paeonia

Bai Tou Weng/ Pulsatilla

Bai Zhi/ Angelica

Bai Zhu/ Atractylodes

Bai Zi Ren/ Biota

Ban Lan Gen/ Isatis

Bei Sha Shen/ Glehnia

Bei Xie/ Dioscorea

Bi Ba/ Piper

Bian Dou/ Dolichos

Bing Lang/ Areca

Bo He/ Mentha

Cang Er Zi/ Xanthium

Ce Bai Ye/ Biota

Chai Hu/ Bupleurum

Che Qian Zi/ Plantago

Chen Pi/ Citrus

Chi Shao/ Paeonia

Chi Xiao Dou/ Phaseolus

Chuan Lian Zi/ Melia

Chuan Niu Xi/ Cyathula

Chuan Xiong/ Ligusticum

Da Fu Pi/ Areca

Da Huang/ Rheum

Da Qing Ye/ Isatis

Da Zao/ Ziziphus

Dan Dou Chi/ Glycine

Dan Shen/ Salvia

Dan Zhu Ye/ Lophatherum

Dang Gui/ Angelica

Dang Shen/ Codonopsis

Di Fu Zi/ Kochia

Di Gu Pi/ Lycium

Di Yu/ Sanguisorba

Dong Gua Ren/ Benincasa

Du Huo/ Angelica

Du Zhong/ Eucommia

E Jiao/ Equus

E Zhu/ Curcuma

(Fa) Ban Xia/ Pinellia
Fan Xie Ye/ Cassia
Fang Feng/ Ledebouriella
Fo Shou/ Citrus
Fu Ling/ Poria
Fu Pen Zi/ Rubus
Gan Cao/ Glycyrrhiza
Gan Jiang/ Zingiber
Gao Ben/ Ligusticum
Gao Liang Jiang/ Alpinia
Ge Gen/ Pueraria
Gou Qi Zi/ Lycium
Gou Teng/ Uncaria
Gua Lou Pi/ Trichosanthes
Gua Lou Ren/ Trichosanthes
Gui Zhi/ Cinnamomum
Hai Zao/ Sargassum
Han Fang Ji/ Stephania
He Shou Wu/ Polygonum
Hong Hua/ Carthamus
Hou Po/ Magnolia
Hu Huang Lian/ Picrorhiza
Hua Shi/ Talcum
Huai Niu Xi/ Achyranthes
Huang Bai/ Phellodendron
Huang Jing/ Polygonatum
Huang Lian/ Coptis
Huang Qi/ Astragalus
Huang Qin/ Scutellaria
Huo Ma Ren/ Cannabis
Huo Xiang/ Agastache
Ji Nei Jin/ Gallus
Ji Xue Teng/ Millettia
Jiang Huang/ Curcuma
Jie G eng/ Platycodon
Jin Qian Cao/ Lysimachia
Jin Yin Hua/ Lonicera
Jing Jie/ Schizonepeta
Ju Hua/ Chrysanthemum
Jue Ming Zi/ Cassia
Ku Shen/ Sophora
Kuan Dong Hua/ Tussilago
Kun Bu/ Laminaria
Lai Fu Zi/ Raphanus
Lian Qiao/ Forsythia
Lian Zi/ Nelumbo
Ling Zhi/ Ganoderma
Long Dan Cao/ Gentiana
Long Gu/ Os Draconis
Long Yan Rou/ Euphoria
Lu Gen/ Phragmites
Ma Huang/ Ephedra
Mai Men Dong/ Ophiopogon
Mai Ya/ Hordeum
Man Jing Zi/ Vitex
Mang Xiao/ Mirabilitum
Mu Dan Pi/ Paeonia
Mu Gua/ Chaenomeles
Mu Li/ Ostrea
Mu Tong/ Akebia

Mu Xiang/ Saussurea

Nan Sha Shen/ Adenophora

Niu Bang Zi/ Arctium

Pi Pa Ye/ Eriobotrya

Pu Gong Ying/ Taraxacum

Qian Cao Gen/ Rubia

Qian Hu/ Peucedanum

Qian Shi/ Euryale

Qiang Huo/ Notopterygium

Qin Jiao/ Gentiana

Qing Hao/ Artemisia

Qing Pi/ Citrus

Qu Mai/ Dianthus

Rou Cong Rong/ Cistanche

Rou Gui/ Cinnamonum

Sang Bai Pi/ Morus

Sang Ji Sheng/ Loranthus

Sang Ye/ Morus

Sha Ren/ Amomum

Shan Yao/ Dioscorea

Shan Zha/ Crataegus

Shan Zhu Yu/ Cornus

Shen Qu/ Massa Fermentata

Sheng Di Huang/ Rehmannia

Sheng Ma/ Cimicifuga

Shi Chang Pu/ Acorus

Shi Gao/ Gypsum

Shi Hu/ Dendrobium

Shi Wei/ Pyrrosia

Shu Di Huang/ Rehmannia

Suan Zao Ren/ Ziziphus

Tai Zi Shen/ Pseudostellaria

Tao Ren/ Prunus

Tian Hua Fen/ Trichosanthes

Tian Ma/ Gastrodia

Tian Nan Xing/ Arisaema

Tu Si Zi/ Cuscuta

Wei Ling Xian/ Clematis

Wu Jia Pi/ Acanthopanax

Wu Ling Zi/ Trogopterus

Wu Wei Zi/ Schisandra

Wu Yao/ Lindera

Wu Zhu Yu/ Evodia

Xi Xin/ Asarum

Xia Ku Cao/ Prunella

Xiang Fu/ Cyperus

Xiao Hui Xiang/ Foeniculum

Xin Yi Hua/ Magnolia

Xing Ren/ Prunus

Xu Duan/ Dipsacus

Xuan Shen/ Scrophularia

Yan Hu Suo/ Corydalis

Yi Mu Cao/ Leonurus

Yi Yi Ren/ Coix

Yi Zhi Ren/ Alpinia

Yin Chen Hao/ Artemisia

Yu Jin/ Curcuma

Yu Li Ren/ Prunus

Yu Zhu/ Polygonatum

Yuan Zhi/ Polygala

Ze Xie/ Alisma

Zhe Bei Mu/ Fritillaria

Zhi Ke/ Citrus

Zhi Mu/ Anemarrhena

Zhi Shi/ Citrus

Zhi Zi/ Gardenia

Zhu Ling/ Polyporus

Zhu Ru/ Bambusa

Zi Su Ye/ Perilla

Zi Su Zi/ Perilla

Zi Wan/ Aster

Appendix C

Suppliers of Bulk Chinese Medicinals

Brion Herbs Corporation
9250 Jeronimo Road
Irvine, CA 92718
Tel: 800-333-Herb, 714-587-1238
Fax: 800-557-1260

Chi Thanh Trading Co.
May Hing Import & Export
959 Grace Ave.
Oakland, CA 94608
Tel: 510-428-2783
Fax: 510-428-9347

Crane Enterprises (this company only sells herbs to licensed acupuncturists)
745 Falmouth Rd.
Mashpee, MA 02649
Tel: 800-227-4118, 508-539-1700
Fax: 508-339-2369
Website: www.craneherb.com

Golden Flower Chinese Herbs
P.O. Box 781
Placitas, NM 87043
Tel: 800-729-8509, 505-837-2040
Fax: 505-837-2052
Email: GFCH@aol.com
Website: www.gfcherbs.com

Internatural
Dept. CHH
P.O. Box 489
Twin Lakes, WI 53181 USA
Tel: 800-643-4221 (Order Line)
Tel: 262-889-8581 (Office Line)
Fax: 262-889-8591
Email: internatural@lotuspress.com
Website: www.internatural.com

Kwok Shing Import & Export
1818 Harrison St.
San Francisco, CA 94103
Tel: 800-326-1668
Fax: 415-861-1668

Lotus Herbs
1124 Hacienda Blvd.
La Puente, CA 91744
Tel: 800-478-4325, 626-916-1070
Fax: 800-856-3558, 626-917-7763
www.LotusHerbs.com

Lotus Light Enterprises
Dept. CHH
P.O. Box 1008
Silver Lake, WI 53170 USA
Tel: 800-548-3824 (Order Line)
Tel: 262-889-8501 (Office Line)
Fax: 262-889-8591
Email: lotuslightl@lotuspress.com
Website: www.lotuslight.com

Mayway Corporation
1338 Mandela Parkway
Oakland, CA 94607
Tel: 800-262-9929, 510-208-3113
Fax: 800-909-2828, 510-208-3069/3070
Email: sales@mayway.com
www.mayway.com

North South China Herbs, Inc.
1556 Stockton St.
San Francisco, CA 94133
Tel: 415-421-4907
Fax: 415-421-5576

Nu Herbs Company
3820 Penniman Ave.
Oakland, CA 94619
Tel: 800-233-4307, 510-534-4372
Fax: 800-550-1928, 510-534-4384
Website: www.NuHerbs.com

Qualiherbs
13839 Bentley Place
Cerritos, CA 90703
Tel: 800-533-5907, 562-802-0035
Fax: 562-802-0625
Email: qualiherb@worldnet.att.net
Website: www.herb.com.tw

Spring Wind Herb Company
2325 Fourth St, Ste 6
Berkeley, CA 94710
Tel: 800-588-4883, 510-849-1820
Fax: 510-849-4886
Website: www.springwind.com

Thorne Sales & Distributing (this company only sells herbs to licensed acupuncturists)
10 Westmont Road
Candler, NC 28715
Tel: 828-670-5464
Fax: 828-670-8610
Email: naturec@msn.com
Website: www.thornesales.com

Glass Jar Supplier:

E.D. Luce Prescription Packaging
7709 Somerset Blvd.
Paramount, CA 90723
Tel: 800-869-0571
Fax: 562-997-0117

Appendix D

Instructions for Cooking Loose Herbs

Please use this form as a sample to create your own instruction sheet for your clinic.

Please use a cooking pot that is made out of glass, pottery, enamel or stainless steel. Avoid aluminum or cast iron pots, as they will interfere with the medicinal functions of the herbs. Do not add honey, sugar, or other sweetener, or anything else to the tea. If you find the taste of the tea unpleasant, you may put a drop of lemon juice on your tongue or eat a few raisons to get rid of the after-taste. While cooking the herbs keep the lid on or slightly tilted to prevent water evaporation.

Empty one bag of herbs into your cooking pot and add ________ cups of water. Soak the herbs for about 10 minutes. Bring herbs to a boil, then lower stove to a medium/low flame and simmer for _______ minutes. Strain the liquid tea into a large container.

For the second boiling add _______ cups of fresh water to the already wet herbs. Again bring to a boil and simmer for _______ minutes. Strain the liquid tea into the container above.

Combine both decoctions. Throw the herbs away. The tea must be stored in the fridge to avoid spoilage. The herbal decoction will spoil like any food in the fridge after 8 - 10 days.

Drink _______ cup(s) _________ times a day before/after each meal. You may warm up each cup, but do not microwave the medicinal herb tea.

SPECIAL INSTRUCTIONS: FOLLOW ONLY IF CHECKED

Please call this office when you contract a cold or flu as the current herbs may not be appropriate for you during that disease process.

_____ Cook _____ slices of fresh ginger with each bag.

_____ Add herb(s) from small bag _______ minutes before the first cooking is finished.

_____ Cook herb(s) in small bag for _______ minutes before adding the remaining herbs.

Please note that Chinese herbs are very strong, so sometimes effects can be felt immediately. However, in chronic cases, you may need to take herbs for several months. The prescription should be re-evaluated at least every two weeks. Should you experience any unpleasant side effects such as irritability, nausea, diarrhea, headaches, or gas, or have further questions, please don't hesitate to call my office.

Bibliography

1. Bensky D, Barolet R. *Chinese Herbal Medicine: Formulas & Strategies*. Seattle, WA 1990. Eastland Press.
2. Bensky D, Gamble A. *Chinese Herbal Medicine: Materia Medica*. Seattle, WA 1993. Eastland Press.
3. Chengdu Institute of TCM. *The Chinese Herbal Medicine*. Shanghai, PRC. Shanghai Science and Technology Press.
4. Chen SY, Li F. *A Clinical Guide to Chinese Herbs and Formu lae*. New York, NY 1993. Churchill Livingstone.
5. Chen ZL, Chen M. *A Comprehensive Guide to Chinese Herbal Medicine*. Long Beach, CA 1992. Oriental Healing Arts Institute.
6. Chin WY; Keng H. *An Illustrated Dictionary of Chinese Medici nal Herbs*. Sebastopol, CA 1992. CRCS Publications.
7. Flaws B. *Fire in the Valley: The TCM Diagnosis & Treatment of Vaginal Diseases*. Boulder, CO 1991. Blue Poppy Press
8. Gansu Institute of New Medicine and Pharmacology. *Chinese Herbal Medicine 2nd edition*. Beijing, PRC 1982. The People's Medical Press.
9. Hempen CH, Engelhardt U. *Chinesische Diätetik*. München, Germany 1997. Urban & Schwarzenberg.
10. Hsu HY. *Commonly Used Chinese Herb Formulas with Illustra tions*. Long Beach, CA 1980. Oriental Healing Arts Institute.
11. Huang BS. *Syndromes of Traditional Chinese Medicine*. Harbin, PRC 1993. Heilongjiang Education Press.
12. Jiangsu Institute of New Medicine. *Encyclopedia of Chinese Herbal Medicine, 2nd edition.* Shanghai, PRC. Shanghai Science and Technology Press.
13. Junying G et al. *Herbal Formulas: Practical Traditional Chinese Medicine and Pharmacology*. Beijing, China 1991. New World Press.
14. Junying G, Wenquan H, Tianchi R, Xuifeng M. *Medicinal Herbs: Practical Traditional Chinese Medicine and Pharma cology*. Beijing, China 1991. New World Press.
15. Kim BD. *Chinese Herbology Vol 1, 2 and 3*. Santa Monica, CA 1984, 1985. Emperor's College of TCM.
16. Maciocia G. *The Foundations of Chinese Medicine*. New York, NY 1989. Churchill Livingston
17. Naeser M. *Outline Guide to Chinese herbal Patent Medicines in Pill Form*. Boston, MA 1990. Boston Chinese Medicine.
18. Ni M. *Chinese Herbology Made Easy*. Los Angeles, CA. Union of Tao and Man.
19. Reid D. *Chinese Herbal Medicine*. Boston, MA. 1987. Shambalah Publications
20. Rutiz J, Karsten Y, Kim BD. Herb Index. Santa Monica, CA 1985. Emperor's College of TCM.

21. Stoeger E; Friedl F. *Arzneibuch der Chinesischen Medizin.* Deutscher Apotheker Verlag Stuttgart 1992
22. Tierra M. *Planetary Herbology.* Twin Lakes, WI 1988. Lotus Press.
23. Tierra M. *The Way of Herbs.* New York, NY 1990. Pocket Books.
24. Veith I. *Huang Ti Nei Ching Su Wen, The Yellow Emperor's Classic of Internal Medicine.* Berkley, 1949. University of California Press.
25. Wiseman N. *English-Chinese, Chinese-English Dictionary of Chinese Medicine.* PRC 1995.
26. Yen, KY. *The Illustrated Chinese Materia Medica.* Taipei, Republic of China 1992. SMC Publishing.
27. Yeung H. *Handbook of Chinese Herbs and Formulas, Vol 1 & 2.* Los Angeles, CA 1983. Institute of Chinese Medicine.
28. Zeng N. *Class Notes.* Santa Fe, NM 1989-91. International Institute of Chinese Medicine
29. Zhang ZB. *Traditional Chinese Internal Medicine, 8th edition.* Shanghai, PRC 1985. Shanghai Science and Technology Press.
30. Zhongjing Z. *Treatise on Febrile Disease Caused by Cold.* Beijing, China 1986. New World Press.
31. Zhu CH. *Chinese Prepared Medicines.* Brookline, MA 1989. Paradigm Publications.

Pinyin Index

A

B

* Indicates the most frequently used herbs that are cited throughout the book.
Note: Herbs that are cited on more than 10 pages but are less common than those marked with an * are broken out into disharmony subentries.

C

Pinyin Index

D

E

F

H

J

M

N

Y

Z

English Index

A

B

C

D

E

English Index

G

H

I

J

K

Q

R

S

T

U

V

W

X

Y

Z

Disharmonies and Syndromes Index

A

B

C

D

E

F

G

H

I

J

K

L

O

P

Q

S

BOOKS OF RELATED INTEREST

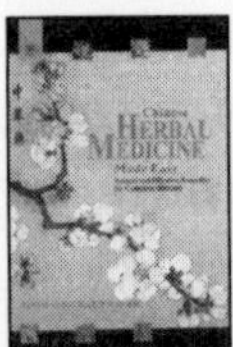

CHINESE HERBAL MEDICINE MADE EASY
Natural and Effective Remedies for Common Illnesses
Thomas Richard Joiner
ISBN: 81-7822-102-0

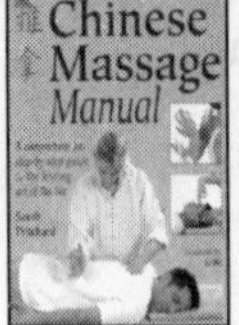

CHINESE MASSAGE MANUAL
A Comprehensive, Step-by-Step Guide to the Healing Art of Tui Na
Sarah Pritchard
ISBN: 81-7822-122-5

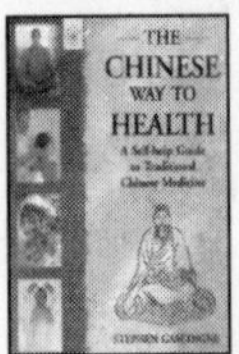

THE CHINESE WAY TO HEALTH
A Self-help Guide to Traditional Chinese Medicine
Dr. Stephen Gascoigne
ISBN: 81-7822-160-8

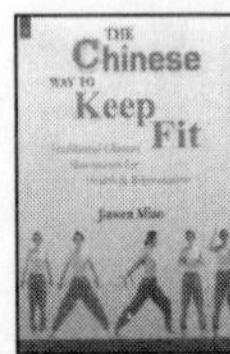

THE CHINESE WAY TO KEEP FIT
Information and Exercises
Jiawen Miao
ISBN: 81-7822-124-1

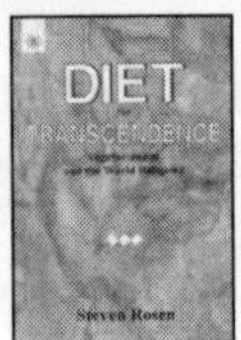

DIET FOR TRANSCENDENCE
Vegetarianism and the World Religions
Steven Rosen
ISBN: 81-7822-201-9

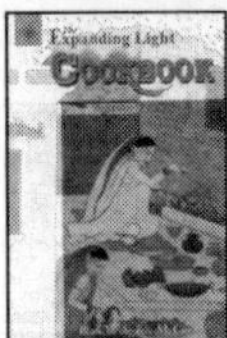

THE EXPANDING LIGHT COOKBOOK
Vegetarian Favorites
Blanche Agassy McCord
ISBN: 81-7822-052-0

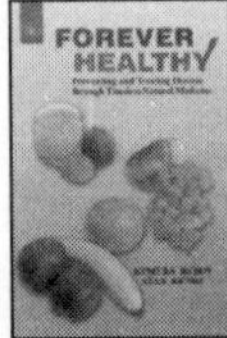

FOREVER HEALTHY
Preventing and Treating Disease through Timeless Natural Medicine
Kumuda Reddy & Stan Kendz
ISBN: 81-7822-171-3

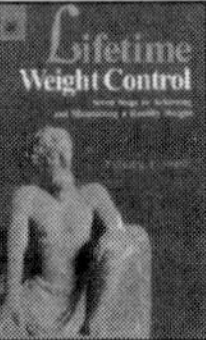

LIFETIME WEIGHT CONTROL
Seven Steps to Achieving and Maintaining a Healthy Weight
Patrick Fanning
ISBN: 81-7822-022-9

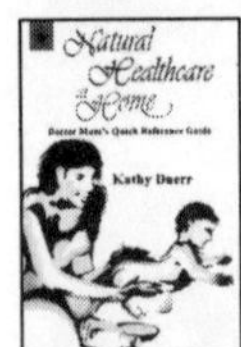

NATURAL HEALTHCARE AT HOME
Doctor Mum's Quick Reference Guide
Kathy Duerr
ISBN: 81-7822-017-2

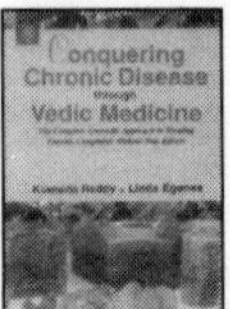

CONQUERING CHRONIC DISEASE THROUGH VEDIC MEDICINE
Kumuda Reddy, Linda Egenes
ISBN: 81-7822-169-1

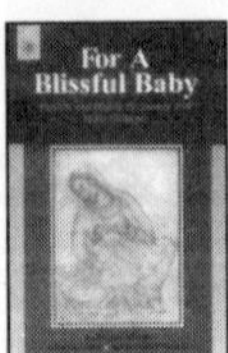

FOR A BLISSFUL BABY
Healthy and Happy Pregnancy with Vedic Medicine
Kumuda Reddy, Linda Egenes & Margaret Mullins
ISBN: 81-7822-170-5

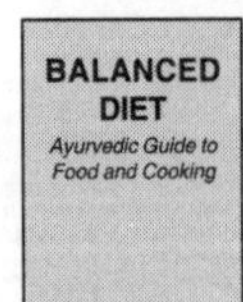

BALANCED DIET
Ayurvedic Guide to Food and Cooking
Joyce Bueker
ISBN: 81-7822-110-1